Clinical Handbook of Myocarditis

Clinical Handbook of Myocarditis

Edited by **Jeff Wilson**

FOSTER ACADEMICS

New Jersey

Published by Foster Academics,
61 Van Reypen Street,
Jersey City, NJ 07306, USA
www.fosteracademics.com

Clinical Handbook of Myocarditis
Edited by Jeff Wilson

International Standard Book Number: 978-1-63242-083-1 (Hardback)

Printed in China.

Contents

Preface

This handbook presents an important account of Myocarditis. Myocarditis is basically described as the inflammation of the heart muscle, which can turn out to be severe and potentially fatal in certain cases. This is an elaborative book consisting of a collection of analyses from top-notch international veterans on several aspects of myocarditis. It presents a clinical outlook on the disease and discusses elucidative reviews regarding its causes, diagnosis, treatment, and classification and also encompasses reviews of myocarditis in HIV-positive patients. The book also highlights the pathogenesis of myocarditis, elucidating mechanisms and pathways activated during viral infection and host immune reaction during the disease along with novel findings in the pathogenesis which may result in novel directions for clinical diagnosis, including utilization of novel biomarkers, and latest treatments of myocarditis.

The information shared in this book is based on empirical researches made by veterans in this field of study. The elaborative information provided in this book will help the readers further their scope of knowledge leading to advancements in this field.

Finally, I would like to thank my fellow researchers who gave constructive feedback and my family members who supported me at every step of my research.

Editor

Part 1

Myocarditis from Clinical Perspective

1

Myocarditis in Childhood: An Update on Etiology, Diagnosis and Management

Vedide Tavli and Baris Guven
Izmir Dr Behcet Uz Children's Hospital, Department of Pediatric Cardiology
Izmir

1. Introduction

Myocarditis is the term used to describe acute or chronic inflammation of the myocardium. For two decades, there has been increasing confrontations concerning the diagnosis, management and clinical outcome of the myocarditis. The cause of myocarditis frequently remains unknown. However, infections, systemic diseases, toxins and drugs have been reported being associated with inflammation of the myocardium (Kearney et al., 2001 & Mahrholdt H et al, 2006). The majority of cases are supposed to be due to infectious agents and it was recognized that any infectious agents could initiate myocarditis (Brodison & Swann, 2001). In North America and Europe, viral infection is the most common causes of myocarditis (Magnani & Dec, 2006). The true overall incidence of myocarditis remain obscure due to inconsistency of its definition and clinical manifestation in the paediatric population. Post-mortem study from Sweden reported incidence of myocarditis to be 1.06 % in 12.747 consecutive autopsies (Gravanis & Sternby, 1991). Since the clinical presentation of myocarditis is so variable, high index of suspicion is essential. Patients are asymptomatic and diagnosis is incidental in the majority of cases. The spectrum of disease ranges from nonspecific findings (chest pain, fever, myalgia, atrial or ventricular tachycardia) to acute heart failure and sudden death. Myocarditis as a cause of sudden death has been reported in up to 12% of young adults (Doolan et al., 2004). However, population based study from Finland (Kyto et al, 2007) documented that the incidence of fatal myocarditis (1.59 per 100000) was highest in infants under one year of age and incidence was lowest in young adults (5-24 years, 0.12-0.17/100000). Recently, Weber et al have also suggested that myocarditis is an infrequent, corresponding to approximately 2% of paediatric deaths (Weber et al., 2008).

Previous researches (Felker et al, 1999 & Lipshultz et al, 2003) strongly suggested that acute myocarditis may proceed to dilated cardiomyopathy. Diagnostic evaluation of a series of 1.278 patients (mean age: 50 years, range 15-87 years) with cardiomyopathy revealed that 9.8% of cases was diagnosed with myocarditis (Felker et al, 1999). In a paediatric study assessing the incidence of cardiomyopathy, viral myocarditis was found to be responsible for 27% of cases with dilated cardiomyopathy (Lipshultz et al, 2003). Moreover, in a prospective cohort study (Towbin et al, 2006), it has been shown that most common known cause of dilated cardiomyopathy is myocarditis (46%). Several mechanisms were postulated for progression of myocarditis to dilated cardiomyopathy, including direct viral injury,

autoimmune response of body through the effects of lymphocytes, natural killer cells, cytokines and apoptotic cell death (Kawai, 1999).
Diagnosis of acute myocarditis can be difficult owing to the lack of accepted and standardized criteria in addition to the nonspecific pattern of clinical presentation. The other issue hampered agreement on the most proper diagnostic criteria and documentation of cases, is broad diversity of aetiologies associated with myocarditis (Dec et al, 1985). At present, diagnosis has been made by use of pathological classification, commonly referred to as Dallas criteria (Aretz et al, 1987). The identification of inflammatory infiltrate with or without myocardial cell necrosis on conventionally stained myocardial tissue biopsy specimens is essential for histological diagnosis. On the basis of these criteria, myocarditis is described as active or borderline myocarditis in accordance with the presence or absence, respectively, of myocardial necrosis. The inflammatory infiltrate should be further identified as lymphocytic, eosinophilic or granulomatous (Figure 1). Sampling error, low sensitivity and specificity, discrepancy in expert interpretation remain limitations to the use of endomyocardial biopsy for diagnosis of acute myocarditis (Hauck et al, 1989 & Shanes et al, 1987). Inflammation in acute myocarditis may be focal, therefore it is challenging to biopsy the inflamed area of myocardium (Robinson et al, 2005). Additionally, it is invasive and potentially dangerous procedure, particularly in the paediatric patient (Checchia & Kulik, 2006). According to the some researchers (Parillo, 2001), this histopathological criteria could not be considered the gold standard for diagnosing acute myocarditis. Molecular pathological analyses, such as polymerase chain reaction (PCR) and in-situ hybridization allows rapid detection and documentation of the viral genetic material in the myocardium (Angelini et al, 2002 & Bock et al, 2010). In 2008, it was reported that immunohistological signs of myocarditis has been associated with poor outcome in myocarditis (Kindermann et al, 2008).

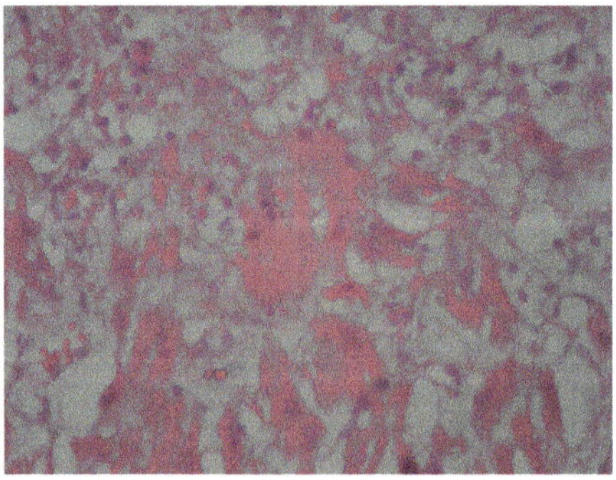

Fig. 1. The pathological diagnosis of viral myocarditis necessitates the manifestation of a inflammatory infiltrate associated with myocyte necrosis. The infiltrate consists of predominantly mononuclear cells (Stained by hematoxylin and eosin, magnification X 400; Text and image courtesy of Ragip Ortac, Gulden Diniz, Malik Ergin)

Therapy of myocarditis in children with inotropes and afterload reduction is usually sufficient. Although the long-term sequels are rare, dilated cardiomyopathy and sudden cardiac death may develop in clinical course. Extracorporeal membrane oxygenation and mechanical ventilations are other options for severe cases (Vashist & Singh, 2009). Newer therapeutic strategies such as intravenous immunoglobulin and immunosuppressive agents have been investigated with the improvements in understanding pathogenesis of the myocarditis (Drucker et al, 1994 & Camargo et al 2009). It is the aim of this review to give a brief and complete discussion of pathogenesis, diagnosis and management of myocarditis.

2. Etiology

The vast majority of myocarditis in the developed countries result from viral infections (Table 1). The causes other than infections are autoimmune-systemic diseases, toxins and hypersensitivity to drugs (Brodison & Swann, 2001). Enteroviruses (particularly Coxsackie) and adenovirus were recognized as the major cause of viral myocarditis (Baboonian& Treasure, 1997; Pauschinger et al, 1999). During the last decade, parvovirus B19 (PVB19) and human herpesvirus 6 (HHV6) have been described as new pathogens (Kuhl et al, 2003). Moreover, investigators from Germany found that PVB19 and HHV6 are the most common causes of biopsy-confirmed viral myocarditis (Kuhl et al, 2005 & Mahrholdt et al, 2006). An investigation analysing the potential role of PVB19 in the clinical setting of acute myocarditis revealed that PVB19 was the most common agent. Kuhl et al had also noticed that Dallas criteria was frequently negative in patients with positive PVB19 PCR and macrophages were augmented in virus positive cases (Kuhl et al, 2003). These findings support the postulation of Bowles et al that different viruses have various pathogenic mechanisms such as lymphocyte-dependent vs. macrophage-dependent (Bowles et al, 2005). Nevertheless, PVB19 DNA has also been revealed in the myocardium of healthy donors (Donosa et al, 2005), in hearts of adults with dilated cardiomyopathy (Lotze et al, 2004), and in hearts of the patients with lupus and amyloidosis (Kuethe et al, 2007), despite the number of subjects studies was small. From these results, the question arises whether PVB19 certainly cause the underlying heart disease or whether it is just spectator attending in the heart as a result of former infection which is usual in young adults or children. A study by Kuethe et al was conducted to investigate this question. They suggested that PVB19 displays lifelong persistence, identification of PVB19 DNA was not correlated with clinical symptoms and serological analysis should be standardized procedure for future studies considering prevalence of PVB19 (Kuethe et al, 2009).

Polymerase chain reaction (PCR) analyses of myocardium in children and adult patients have showed the existence of adenoviral genome in cases with myocarditis and dilated cardiomyopathy with a larger frequency than enterovirus (Pauschinger et al, 1999 & Bowles et al, 2003). Geographical variation in viral etiology is also remarkable that hepatitis C virus has been more commonly documented in Japanese patients and parvovirus B19 is more frequently detected by PCR in German population (Magnani & Dec, 2006). Matsumori et al found that hepatitis C virus infection is often found in cases with dilated cardiomyopathy and that hepatitis C virus have an crucial role in the pathogenesis of cardiomyopathy (Matsumori et al, 1995). It was also suggested that antiviral therapeutics against hepatitis C virus could be indicated in these cases. Other viruses linked with myocarditis include Epstein-Barr virus, cytomegalovirus, herpes simplex virus, influenza A-B and HIV (Magnani & Dec, 2006). Multiple infections with different viruses have also been detected in cases (approximately one quarter of all cases) with systolic left ventricular dysfunction (Kuhl et al, 2005). Influenza A and B may also involve a combined myocarditis risk, particularly in patients with pre-existing cardiovascular diseases (Friman et al, 1995). From the study (Bowles et al, 2003) conducted in 624 patients with myocarditis (116 neonates, 191 infants), it was concluded that most common amplified viral genomes in myocardial tissues included are adenovirus, cytomegalovirus, parvovirus and influenza A (ordered in decreasing frequency). It has been known that HIV may cause myocarditis and dilated cardiomyopathy (Breuckman et al, 2005). Direct viral injury, antiretroviral agents, coinfections and inhibition of contractility through HIV glycoprotein type I 120 play a role in the pathogenesis of myocarditis and dilated cardiomyopathy (Chen et al, 2002). The introduction of highly active antiretroviral therapy (HAART) has significantly reduced the incidence of HIV related- myocarditis. On the other hand, in developing countries where the supply of HAART is limited, researchers have observed increase in prevalence of HIV associated cardiomyopathy (Pugliese et al, 2000).

Viral			
Coxsackie virus	Respiratory syncytial virus		
Adenovirus	Vaccinia (smallpox vaccine)		
Human herpes virus	HIV		
Parvovirus B19	Influenza A and B		
Hepatitis C virus	Cytomegalovirus		
Epstein-Barr virus			
Bacterial			
Borrelia Burgdorferi	Streptoccus pneumoniae		
Mycobacterial	Treponema pallidum		
Mycoplasma pneumonia	Neisseria Meningitides		
Corynobacterium diphtheria	Rickettsia sp.		
Hemophilus influenza	Vibrio cholerae		
Parasitic-Fungal-Protozoal			
Ascaris sp.	Schistosomiasis		
Echinococcus granulosus	Larva migrans		
Aspergillus sp.	Candida		
Taenia Solium	Coccidioides		
Cryptococcus	Histoplasma		
Toxoplasma gondium	Tryponosoma cruzi		
Immunologic			
Rheumatic fever	Polymyositis, rheumatic arthritis		
Chagas disease	Sarcoidosis		
Systemic lupus erythamatosus	Thyrotoxicosis		
Diabetes Mellitus	Wegener's Granulomatosis		
Ulcerative colitis	Scleroderma		
Hypersensitivity-Drugs			
Amitriptyline	Amphotericin B	Arsenic	Scorpion envenomation
Anthracyclines	Electric shock	Penicilline	
Digoxin	Phenytoin	Copper	
Dobutamine	Colchicine	Isoniazide	
Cephalosporins	Iron	Lead	

Table 1. Main etiologies observed in myocarditis.

During the pandemic of influenza A (H1N1), myocarditis was documented in four children (80 children with H1N1 influenza) within a 30-day period (Bratincsak et al, 2010). In their retrospective review, three children had fulminant myocarditis, 1 with fatal outcome and 2 required extracorporeal membrane oxygenation support. From these findings, they assumed that new H1N1 influenza A virus is more frequently associated with a severe form of myocarditis that formerly encountered influenza strains. A study from Spain have also emphasized the importance of myocarditis as a risk factor for mortality.

Numerous bacterial infections may cause myocarditis, involvement of myocardium may have insidious course (electrocardiography changes) or may present with significant signs and symptoms. Fulminant septicaemia may result in myocarditis with fatal course. Most common causes of myocarditis associated with bacteraemia included are meningococcus, streptococcus and Listeria (Brodison&Swann, 1998). Borrelia burgdorferi causes Lyme carditis with acute or chronic course. Recently, a study o 207 children with early disseminated Lyme disease conducted by Costello et al found that 33 children (16%) had mild to fulminant myocarditis, 14 of whom had advanced atrioventricular block (none required permanent pacemaker). Lyme disease may rarely present with cardiomyopathy (Costello et al, 2009).

Various drugs implicated in the development of myocarditis including; anthracyclins, cyclophosphamide, cisplatin, 5-fluorourasil, Lithium, aminophylline, catecholamines, antibiotics (penicillines,), phenytoine and trastuzumab (Ellis&Disalvo, 2007). Myocyte injury may occur by direct toxic effect on heart or by provoking hypersensitivity reactions. Hypersensitivity reaction may be indicated fever, sinus tachycardia, peripheral eosinophilia and a rash that follows days to weeks after administration formerly well-accepted agent. Actually, it is not the drugs that heralds the reaction, but its metabolites (haptens) in the cases of hypersensitivity myocarditis. The pathological findings are indistinguishable and are independent of the drug involved. The inflammatory infiltrate predominantly consists of eosinophils, and can be located in focal areas, or diffusely within the myocardium with slight or no sign of necrosis, or substitute fibrosis. If the grade of myocardial inflammation or necrosis is severe, arrhythmias or hemodynamic collapse may likely occur. Eosinophilic necrotising myocarditis is an extreme form of hypersensitivity myocarditis that promptly cause cardiovascular collapse. Eosinophilic myocarditis has been documented following administration dobutamine and vaccines (Tetanus, small pox).

Systemic diseases that are related with active myocarditis include connective tissue diseases such as systemic lupus erythematosus, mixed connective tissue disease, systemic sclerosis, Churg-Strauss syndrome; celiac disease and Whipple's disease. Protozoal, helmintic and parasitic infections may also present with eosinophilic myocarditis. Myocardial abnormalities in SLE is multifactorial with coronary vasculitis, valvulopathy, hypertension, immune injury and drugs are the major contributors. Myocardial abnormalities are common in autopsy patients. However, clinically apparent myocarditis occurs in < 10 % of cases suggesting that the subclinical form is more frequent (Magnani&Dec, 2006).

Further understanding the etiology of myocarditis will illicit more direct therapeutic approaches such as vaccine and antiviral agents. Although some antiviral agents as ribavirin, oseltamivir and acyclovir have had moderate effect on influenza, RSV pneumonitis and CMV disease, currently there is no specific therapy approved for Enteroviruses, parvovirus B 19 and adenovirus. But, other options may be worth considering. A historical example of a promising therapy for viral myocarditis and prevention of dilated cardiomyopathy is that of decline in the incidence of endocardial fibroelastosis in children after initiation of mumps virus vaccine. It has been known that endocardial fibroelastosis is associated with congestive heart failure and death. Evidence from myocardial samples of patients with EFE supported the hypothesis that it is sequela of viral myocarditis, in particular of that due to mumps virus. Based on the chronology of the fading of the disease, Ni et al. suggested that it is likely that vaccination was responsible for the remarkable decrease in documented case of EFE. So it is logical to think that vaccination against parvovirus B19, echovirus and adenovirus could diminish cases of myocarditis and dilated cardiomyopathy.

3. Pathogenesis

Special attention to understanding the mechanism and pathogenesis of myocarditis have been increased since Gore and Saphir showed in 1947 that diphteric and rheumatic carditis separately comprised only 10% of a series of 1402 patients of myocarditis (Gore & Saphir, 1947). In 1970's, several investigators demonstrated the persistence of neutralizing antibodies to coxsackie B (CVB) in cases with cardiomyopathy than healthy subjects (Kawai, 1971, Kawai et al., 1978, Toshima et al., 1979). This finding supported the hypothesis of a viral cause underlying the pathogenesis of cardiomyopathy. Evidence from murine models helped understanding pathogenesis of myocarditis (Liu&Mason, 2001). Myocarditis in susceptible mice is characterized by 3 separate disease processes, direct viral or other infectious agent access to myocardium tissue rapidly evolves into the second phase (Figure 2). In second phase, also called autoimmune phase of disease, immunological activation is the main feature. During the last phase, signs of myocarditis usually disappear and the damaged myocytes are substituted by diffuse fibrosis. Misdiagnosis and inappropriate therapy are especially possible at the time of transitional period among the 3 phases. In the case of reinfection and autoimmune recurrence, confusion can be compounded.

3.1 Viremia

Currently, there are two models of coxsackie B virus 3 induced myocarditis. The first one provokes acute viral myocarditis with a significant damage to myocytes and sudden death of animals within a week of infection (Fuse et al., 2005). In the second model, some degree of mice seemed to advance acute viral myocarditis following an infection with a cardiotropic strain of CVB3 (Fairwather&Rose, 2007). There also models with CMV, HIV and adenovirus (O'Donoughe et al., 1990, Salone et al., 2003, Beischel et al., 2004). During the time of active viremia, cardiotropic RNA virus (Coxsackie B) is taken into cells by receptor mediated endocytosis and are directly translated interior to the cells to produce protein (Huber, 1993). The virus enters the cell by endothelial receptors, particularly coxsackie-adenovirus receptor (CAR). Additionally, coxsackie B1, B3 and B5 uses decay accelerating factor (Shafren et al., 1995); adenoviruses uses αv integrin as coreceptors for viral entry (Wickham et al., 1994). It has been shown that CAR is highly expressed in the heart and brain, peaking in the perinatal period with subsequently declining with age and it is identified on the entire surface of the myocardium (Kashimura et al., 2004). Therefore, one can explain the susceptibility of neonates and infants to coxsackie B 3 myocarditis on the basis of expression level and the location of CAR. Titers of viral antigens in the myocardium is highest on the fourth day of inoculation of virus (Tomioka et al., 1986). No neutralizing antibodies to the virus were present until day 4. The antibody titers elevate promptly on day 8 and 10 reach the highest level on day 14 (Kawai, 1999). The emergence of a rising antibody titers is closely linked to elimination of the virus from the myocardium.

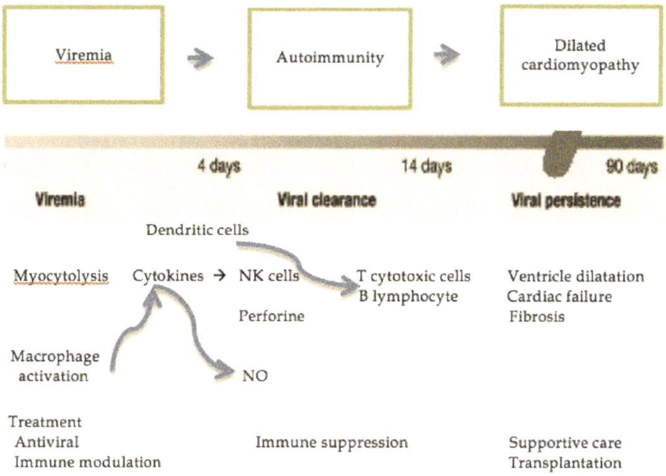

Fig. 2. Schematic drawings of pathophysiological processes of viral myocarditis. NO: Nitric oxide, NK: Natural killer cells.

3.2 Autoimmunity

First phase terminates with the stimulation of the host immune response that weakens viral proliferation but may also augment viral entry. Under ideal circumstances, immune system should normalize to a resting state once viral proliferation is limited. However, if host immune system stimulation persists unrestricted even with the elimination of the virus, autoimmune disease may develop, activating the second phase. This phase is distinguished by inflammatory cellular infiltration with natural killer cells and macrophages, then consequent expression of proinflammatory cytokines, especially interleukin-1, interleukin-2, TNF and interferon γ (Kawai, 1999, Matsumori et al., 1994). It has been shown that TNF triggers endothelial cells, recruits further inflammatory cells, more enhances cytokine production and has direct negative inotropic effects (Feldman&McNamara, 2000). Cytokines can also induce macrophages to express inducible nitric oxide synthase (NOS) in heart cells (Zaragoza et al., 1998). The role of NO in myocarditis is complicated. NO can reduce viral replication, and peroxynitrate production has strong antiviral effects (Zaragoza et al., 1997). Mice deficient in NOS were found to have greater viral titers and more widespread myocyte injury (Padalko et al., 2004). Alternatively, myosin induced autoimmune myocarditis animal model showed us that NOS expression in myocytes and macrophages is related with more severe inflammation, where NOS inhibitors can have potential to reduce myocarditis severity (Zaragoza et al., 1998, Mikami et al., 1997). Furthermore, improvement in myocarditis of the mouse model has been demonstrated by blocking IL-1b or TNF-a at the onset of the disease (Fairweather et al., 2004). Cihakova et al. also showed that the severity of CVB3 induced myocarditis as well as myosin-induced myocarditis is associated with the levels of IL-1b and IL-18 in the myocardium (Cihakova et al., 2008). T cells are activated in viral myocarditis by classical cell-mediated immunity. Viral peptide fragments are processed in the Golgi apparatus of the myocyte and presented to the cell. These prepared T-cells are capable of identifying the viral antigen and destroy the infected myocyte by

means of cytokine and perforine secretion (Ayach et al., 2003). But, persistent excited stimulation of the T cells is eventually harmful to the host, due to both direct T-cell mediated and cytokine-mediated cell damage diminish the number of contractile elements.
Continuous T-cell activation is induced through antigens intrinsic to the myocardium that share molecular mimicry with viral peptides. The virus may also prompt a TH2 reaction, stimulating more CD8 killer cells in the process. It can be explained partially by the presence of evidence that CD4/CD8 or p56lck knockout animals have a much better survival following coxsackie infection (Liu et al., 1995). Recently, it has been shown that CD4+ Th cell subset, referred as Th17 cells, are involved in several inflammatory diseases, including experimental autoimmune myocarditis and collagen induced arthritis (Aggarwal et al., 2003, Chen et al., 2006). In addition to the proinflammatory effects, evidence from previous works suggested that Th17 cells may facilitate the production of autoantibodies in the development of acute viral myocarditis (Yuan et al., 2009). In experimental study published last year (Yuan et al., 2010), they showed that IL-17 produced by Th17 may take part in the regulation of the equilibrium between antiviral immunity and autoimmunity in CAVB3-induce acute viral myocarditis and IL-17 will be a new therapeutic goal for viral myocarditis in future (Milenkovic et al., 2010).
Although the activation of CD4 cells also leads to B-cell clonal expansion and antibody production, antibodies might not be the critical initiating factor that directs the advancing of the myocarditis. The severity of myocarditis was also found to be dependent on the responding T-cell subset in T-cell knockout mice (Opavsky et al., 1999). But, it has been shown that antibodies are a significant modifier of the disease phenotype. In a study conducted in 1982, it was found that among 30% of cases with suspected myocarditis, as well as in 18/19 patients with proven viral infection due to coxsackie, influenza A or mumps virus (Maisch et al., 1982). They also showed that antimyolemmal antibodies was correlated with the degree of in vitro induced cytolysis of rat myocytes.
Adenoviral myocarditis differs from coxsackie virus in the setting of pathogenesis (Hayder&Müllbacher, 1996). The amount of CD2, CD3 and CD45ROt lymphocytes detected in the adenovirus-infected cases was decreased compared with those patients who had myocarditis with other pathogens (Pauschinger et al., 1999). It was also demonstrated that 71% of PCR-positive adenoviral did not have inflammation histologically (Martin et al., 1994). One of the strategies of adenovirus for modulating immune response is that interaction of adenoviral encoded proteins with host immune components. These proteins may protect cells from tumor necrosis factor mediated lysis, as well as downregulation of major histocompatibility complex class I antigen expression. On the other side, adenoviral E1a encoded proteins are able to encourage the induction of apoptosis and inhibition of interleukin-6 (IL-6) expression (Davison et al., 2003). Besides this, it restricts IL-6 signal transduction pathways. These functions of E1A may be relevant to the occurrence of dilated cardiomyopathy. HIV has been identified within myocytes and is related with interference of myocyte integrity and replacement of endocardial fibrosis. Therefore, it was suggested that HIV myocarditis may share similar pathogenic mechanism of those of coxsackie (d'Amati et al., 2001).
It should be underlined that the natural killer (NK) cells is also important in the pathogenesis of myocardial inflammation. These finding corroborate those observed in a prior animal study, in which animals depleted of their NK cells previous to infection with coxsackievirus develop a more severe myocarditis (Godeny et al., 1987). The NK cells particularly reduce the nonenveloped virus infection by destroying the infected cells.

3.3 Dilated cardiomyopathy

Several remodelling mechanisms leading to dilated cardiomyopathy may be particular to myocarditis. The association of myocarditis to dilated cardiomyopathy has been moderately elucidated by molecular techniques. Badorff and Knowlton, demonstrated that dystrophin is cellular target for coxsackie B3 viral protease (Badorrff&Knowlton, 1999). It may provide one of the molecular mechanisms clarifying the significant ventricular dilatation that may develop immediately following viral infection. Furthermore, it was found that dystrophin deficiency augments host vulnerability to coxsackie virus infection (Xiong et al., 2002). This conclusion may result from the findings that more efficient liberation of the virus from the infected myocytes and is related with an increase in virus-mediated cytopathic effects. Proteases from other viruses (adenovirus and HIV) may also cleave cytoskeletal proteins (Chen et al., 1999, Shoeman et al., 1993).

Identification of viral RNA at early, intermediate and late stages of myocarditis has been demonstrated in animal models. That persistent myocyte viral gene expression may be a cause of progressive dilated cardiomyopathy. Some findings propose that the persisting viral RNA seems to be capable of replication. In 172 patients with biopsy-confirmed viral infection, persistent viral genome of enterovirus, parvovirus B19, and HHV-6 was found to be associated with on-going impairment in ejection fraction (Kuhl et al., 2005); But, in the lack of measurable virus titers, it appears likely that the replication can be done in a limited or transformed manner (Klingel et al., 1992). All the more so, such replication might produce novel antigenic non-infectious or defective interfering viral elements, sufficient to cause evolving myocardial injury (Kawai, 1999). Cytokines possibly will participate in the development of dilated cardiomyopathy (Ono et al., 1998). During the second phase, they stimulate the matrix metalloproteinases, such as elastase, colleganases and gelatinase. Moreover, various reports suggest that several different viruses perform as a trigger for apoptosis. In addition to an immune-mediated mechanism activated by viral infection and persistent viral RNA in the myocardium, apoptosis may provide the third mechanism to elucidate the development of dilated cardiomyopathy.

3.4 Host factors

It is not fully understood which factors may define susceptibility to viral myocarditis and the development of cardiomyopathy. There are still remaining issues to be answered as why is it that who are in proximity to each other may be infected with the identical virus, but all do not develop myocardial injury? Why do certain infected cases continue to develop mild versus severe myocarditis or cardiomyopathy. But, up to date, the presence of genetic and environmental factors have been documented that influence particularly to viral myocarditis. Risk factors associated with severe myocarditis include age, viral variant, exercise, mouse strain and sex (Woodruff, 1980). Biochemical alterations such as selenium deficiency, vitamin E deficiency (Beck et al., 2003) and mercury exposure (Illback et al., 1996) have been documented to increase the viral virulence. Host genetic configuration not only influences the pathogenic mechanism of disease but also affects the severity of myocarditis. HLA-DQ locus and CD45 polymorphisms were to found to be essential determinants for early viral infection (Tchilian et al., 2006). Several investigations documented the significant association between dilated cardiomyopathy and MHC class II antigens, primarily HLA DR4 (Carlquist et al., 1991, Limas&Limas, 1989). In the study published in the Annals of Human Genetics, it is documented that HLA-DQA1* 0501 and DQB1*0303 are related to genetic susceptibility to idiopathic dilated cardiomyopathy (IDC), while DQA1* 0201, DQB1*

0502 and DQB1* 0504 present protection from IDC (Liu et al., 2005). However, associations of MHC class II alleles with dilated cardiomyopathy are possibly affected by ethnicity, sex, age and geographical variations. Besides the MHC haplotype, non- MHC genes should be considered (Neu et al., 1987). Two non-MHC loci on murine chromosomes 1 and 6, referred as Eam1 and Eam2, respectively, might influence autoimmune myocarditis (Guler et al., 2005). These loci intersect with loci implicated in other autoimmune diseases, such as lupus and diabetes, might give a clue that various autoimmune disease could be controlled by related genetic mechanisms. Initial antiviral response by the host has been recognized to be mediated at least in part by Toll-like receptors. TLR3 was found to play a significant role in the host innate immune response to infection with several cardiotropic viruses. Recent data suggests that variations in TLR3 alter the innate immune response and might change host susceptibility to increased cardiovascular pathology (Gorbea et al., 2010).

4. Clinical features

As stated previously, clinical picture of myocarditis is extremely variable, ranging from asymptomatic ECG abnormalities to heart failure (Dec et al., 1985, Bowles et al., 2003). The term "*Acute* fulminant myocarditis" is used for cases with severe congestive heart failure or cardiogenic shock (Amabile et al., 2006). Age of child influences clinical presentation of myocarditis (Dec et al., 1985). Viral prodrome of flu-like illness, respiratory symptoms or gastroenteritis may precede symptoms of heart failure. Neonates and infants present with poor feeding, irritability or listlessness, diaphoresis, apnea and episodic pallor. Usual symptoms of congestive heart failure, as well as mild cyanosis and pallor are observed on physical examination. It should be emphasized that neonates and affected younger infants may have intrauterine myocarditis with chronic course (Bowles et al., 2003). For very young infants acquiring myocarditis in the peripartal period, the prognosis is very poor, with more than 90% of children dying. Previous studies have implicated the myocarditis as the cause of sudden death (Friedman et al., 1998, Bowles et al., 2003). In the retrospective study of Krous et al., they evaluated the infants who died of sudden death infant syndrome in a safe sleep environment, accidental suffocation or myocarditis were assessed, and they have noticed the manifestation of scattered inflammatory cells and necrotic myocyte were noticed (Krous et al., 2009). From this observation, they suggested that few scattered inflammation and necrotic myocyte were normal finding in the developing heart exposed to new environmental pathogens. However, degree of cardiac infiltration was found to be greater in infants who died of myocarditis. In German study published in 2004, researchers found that viral myocardial affection is the cause of death in cases with SIDS (Dettmeyer et al., 2004). Besides, it was proposed by authors that PVB19 seems to play a more significant role than presumed so far.

Recent history of viral disease 10 to 14 days preceding presentation typically occurs in older children and adolescents (Friedman et al., 1998). Nonspecific gastrointestinal and respiratory complaints are more common than chest pain (Vashist&Singh, 2009). Jugular venous distension and pulmonary rales may be seen, and the resting tachycardia may be obvious, unlike in neonates. Since symptoms of myocarditis vary considerably in children, diagnosis can be challenging. Durani and colleagues, documented that most patients present with complaints of shortness of breath having tachypnea at presentation (Durani et al., 2009). Vomiting (48%) and poor feeding (40%) are also commonly seen in myocarditis. The authors also observed that the diagnosis of myocarditis was missed on the first presentation to a physician in 83% of cases. In a retrospective review, of 31 children with probable and definite myocarditis, 57% were initially diagnosed as suffering pneumonia or asthma (Freedman et al., 2007). One point that deserves attention in these studies is the absence of other signs of congestive heart failure in the majority of cases with myocarditis. Only 50% of children had hepatomegaly and 34% had abnormal chest radiography. The electrocardiographic changes include sinus tachycardia with low voltage QRS complexes, inverted T waves typically occur in the clinical setting of myocarditis (Durani et al., 2009). Wide Q waves and ST segment changes as a pattern of myocardial infarction also may be observed. Supraventricular tachycardia, ventricular tachycardia or atrial fibrillation, as well as atrioventricular block may occur (Friedman et al., 1994). Of note, the sensitivity of electrocardiography in myocarditis is only 47% (Morgera et al., 1992). However, Freedman and colleagues found that sensitivity of electrocardiography as a screening test was 93% (Freedman et al., 2007). Additional interesting finding that is worth to mentioning that the presence of axis deviation (%37) in children with myocarditis. Although ventricular tachycardia is a rare initial manifestation of myocarditis, it may often develops in long-term follow up and may occasionally result in sudden death (Drory et al., 1991).

Myocarditis imitating an acute coronary syndrome has also been defined. Viral genomes were demonstrated in 71% of adult cases with normal coronary anatomy, clinically mimicking myocardial infarction. Parvovirus B19 was most common agent identified in this study (Kuhl et al., 2003). ECG criteria (wide Q waves in I, avL, V5 and V6, ST segment change > 2 mm, ventricular arrhythmias) was described for the diagnosis of myocardial infarction in children (Towbin et al., 1992). However, similar ECG findings can occur in myocarditis (Durani et al., 2009). Most common ECG findings in adult patients with myocarditis include ST segment elevation(55%), T wave inversion (27%), ST segment depression (27%) and pathological Q waves (%18) (Dec et al., 1992, Angelini et al., 2000). Myocardial infarction and myocarditis in neonates overlap and mimic each other (deVetten et al., 2011). Despite angiographically normal coronary anatomy, global or segmental wall motion abnormalities are commonly obvious (Angelini et al., 2000). Physicians should always bear in mind the possibility of acute myocarditis in younger cases who present with acute coronary syndromes when coronary risk factors are lacking, global rather than segmental left ventricular dysfunction is evident on echocardiography or ECG abnormalities encompass beyond a single coronary artery zone (Magnani&Dec, 2006).

5. Diagnosis

Although the misdiagnosis of the myocarditis is common, several diagnostic methods can aid physicians in making diagnosis of the myocarditis.

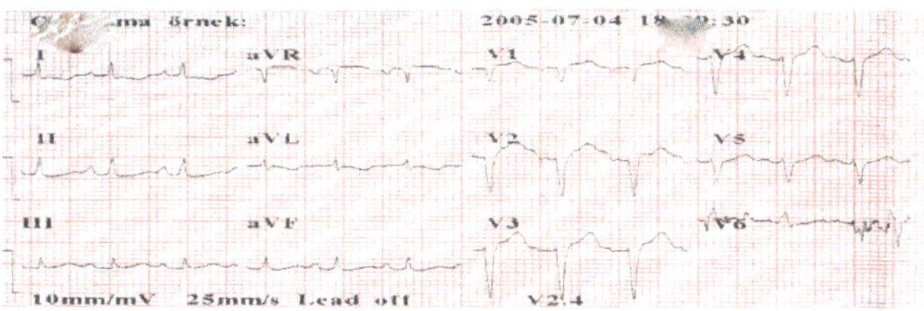

Fig. 3. 12 lead ECG in children with myocarditis. Negative T wave in DI, aVL, ST-T changes were noted in precordial leads.

5.1 Electrocardiography and chest radiography

Chest radiography and electrocardiography (ECG) can be used as first line diagnostic modality (Figure 3). Most common ECG changes are sinus tachycardia, axis deviation, ventricular hypertrophy and ST-T wave changes (Freedman et al., 2007). Moreover, evidence from previous studies suggests that the presence of northwest axis deviation, new left bundle branch block and abnormal QRS complexes is correlated with higher rates of transplantation or death (Magnani et al., 2006, Morgera et al.,1992, Nakashima et al., 1998, Greenwood et al. 1976). A recent adult study have shown that QRS prolongation is an independent predictor for transplantation or death in patients with suspected myocarditis (Ukena et al., 2011). In the majority of cases of myocarditis (up to 90%), abnormal chest radiography was documented (Durani et al., 2009, Freedman et al., 2007). Most common chest radiography finding is cardiomegaly, followed by pulmonary edema and pulmonary infiltrate (Figure 4).

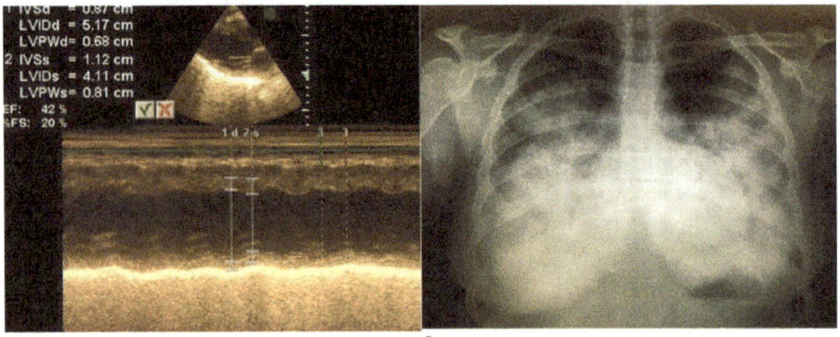

a b

Fig. 4. M-mode echocardiography (a) and chest x-ray (b) of an adolescent girl with presumed viral myocarditis. M-mode echocardiography demonstrating systolic dysfunction with flattened interventricular septum. In chest radiography, there was prominent diffuse vascular congestion that is compatible with pulmonary edema. 13 year old girl admitted our hospital with dyspnea and tachycardia. She had a history of preceding viral upper respiratory infection. The patient intubated and connected to mechanical ventilation on day one of emergency room admission. She died within 72 hours after initial presentation.

5.2 Laboratory finding

General markers for inflammation such as erythrocyte sedimentation rate and C-reactive protein in serum are commonly elevated. However, their usage in diagnosis of myocarditis is limited. Freedman et al. demonstrated that the most sensitive marker for myocarditis was an increased aspartate transaminase (AST). AST elevation was found in 85% of probable and definite cases of myocarditis (Freedman et al., 2007). On the other hand, C-reactive protein and erythrocyte sedimentation rate have been elevated in cases of myocarditis with a range of 27 to 56%. Cardiac troponin t (cTnT) has also been investigated as a diagnostic marker for acute myocarditis since 1990's. cTnT, a contractile protein unique to cardiac muscle, is vastly concentrated in the myocytes and will be released into the blood within hours after heart muscle injury. Following myocardial cell necrosis an increased concentration of cTnT is noticable in blood for more than a week. Cardiac troponin T measurements are especially useful in clinical settings in which traditional enzyme determinations fail to diagnose myocardial cell damage effectively. Likewise, cTnT is not reliably corresponded to increases in blood of cardiac enzymes or myoglobin in all cases of Wolff-Parkinson-White syndrome undergoing radiofrequency ablation. Cardiac troponin I, subunit of thin filament of contractile element of the myocardium, has high specificity (89%) and low sensitivity (34%) in adult patients with acute myocarditis, whereas cTnT has been documented to have a specificity of 83% and sensitivity of 71% in children. Moreover, higher levels of cTnT have been demonstrated to be a prognostic marker for poor outcome in adults presenting with acute myocarditis. Elevated levels of interleukin-10 (IL-10) and TNF appears to be predictor of fulminant myocarditis. Besides this, increase of serum Fas and Fas ligand levels, as well as immunohistological signs of inflammation (CD3 and/or CD68) on initial presentation are associated with fatal outcome in patients with acute myocarditis.

5.3 Echocardiography

Echocardiographic features of myocarditis are nonspecific. Patterns of echocardiography in myocarditis could mimic hypertrophic, dilated or right ventricular cardiomyopathy and as well as ischemic heart disease (Checcia&Kulik, 2006). Echocardiography can be used for assessing wall thickness, cardiac chamber size together with systolic and diastolic functions. Right ventricular dysfunction is relatively unusual. However, right ventricular dysfunction was found to be predictor of adverse outcome in patients with active myocarditis (Mendes et al., 1994). Left ventricular diastolic dysfunction with a restrictive pattern is also observed in most cases of myocarditis. Left ventricular wall thickening was found to be highest on days 1-3 after onset of acute myocarditis. It has also been noted that left ventricular thickening was more marked in the fulminant myocarditis (Felker et al., 2006). On the contrary to adult patients, echocardiographic findings of pediatric patients revealed that relatively thicker posterior wall was correlated with better prognosis and recovery (Carvalho et al., 1996). Segmental wall motion abnormalities are relatively frequent, but global hypokinesis is prevalent. Pericardial effusion commonly occurs. The presence of thrombi in ventricle has also been documented in up to 25% of cases (Daly et al., 1983).

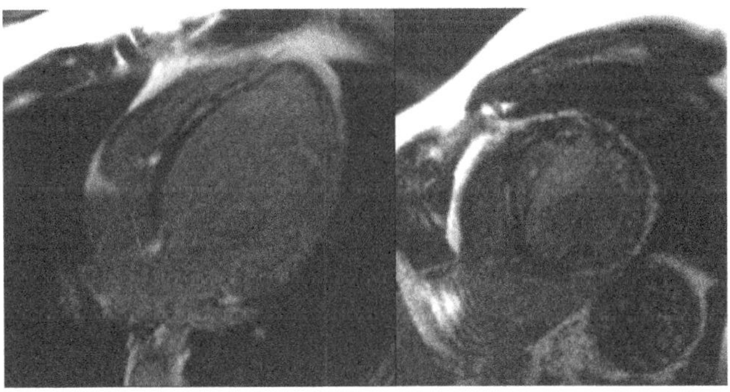

Fig. 5. Cardiac magnetic resonance imaging of acute myocarditis in a adolescent. In four chamber and short axis view, subepicardial late enhancement are noted. Text and image courtesy of Alper Yuksel, Yigit Goktay.

5.4 Magnetic resonance imaging

Current practice has focused on the use of cardiac magnetic resonance imaging (CMR) for the diagnosis of acute myocarditis (Gutberlet et al., 2008, Friedrich et al., 1998). CMR with a unique potential for tissue characterization, particularly with the utilization of T1 and T2 weighted images, can assess 3 markers of tissue injury, which is, hyperemia and capillary leakage, necrosis and fibrosis and intracellular and interstitial edema (Friedrich et al., 2009). CMR visualizes the entire myocardium, recognizing borders of inflammation from later modeling. Thus, it can be used to monitor lesions and be used to show the execution of endomyocardial biopsy, as well as it may be useful in the quantification of the magnitude of damage (Danti et al., 2009, Mahroldt et al., 2004). Goitein et al. demonstrated that cardiac MRI have a larger impact than echocardiography in verifying the existence of myocarditis and evaluating the extent of disease (Goitein et al., 2009). It has been shown that echocardiography is useful in revealing wall motion abnormalities, whereas cardiac MRI could actually identify the often subtle patchy myocardial inflammation (Friedrich et al., 1998). Gadolinium is used as a contrast agent due to ability to penetrate cells whose membranes ruptured and allows contrast agent to diffuse into the cells (Weinmann et al., 1984). Myocardial blood flow and edema, that is likely to be increased in tissues which are inflamed, could augment signal enhancement in MRI. But, cardiac MRI features can be missed on the first pass perfusion (Skouri et al., 2006). Delayed enhancement MRI permits visualization of necrotic and fibrotic myocardium (Friedrich et al., 2009). The observations obtained from the studies using contrast media-enhanced cardiac MRI indicate that pattern of myocarditic lesions occur predominantly in the lateral free wall and get localized to the subepicardial or intramyocardial regions (Mahroldt et al., 2004, Friedrich et al., 1998). The finding of lateral free wall involvement (subepicardial region) partially explain why some young patients with acute myocarditis can present with only ST elevation on ECG (Figure 5). Postmortem studies also showed that lateral wall was the preferred location in myocarditis (Theleman et al., 2001, Shirani et al., 1993). Subendocardial region involvement pattern which is typical for myocardial infarction was never seen in patients with acute myocarditis (Mahroldt et al., 2004). Mahroldt et al. also demonstrated that in the right ventricle half of septum, that is common location of EMB, had relatively low density of inflammatory cells. Apart from lateral free wall pattern, Marhold et al showed that HHV6 myocarditis had pattern that was located in midwall area of the interventricular septum. Pericardial effusion has also been reported in 32 to 57% of cases with myocarditis (Friedrich et al., 2009). Its presence, although not specific for myocarditis, is a supportive evidence for active inflammation.

Recently, International Consensus Group on Cardiovascular Magnetic Resonance suggested the diagnostic criteria, known as "Lake Louis Consensus Criteria" (Friedrich et al., 2009). Cardiac MRI should be made in the setting of clinically suspected myocarditis according to these criteria. It was also stated that maximum diagnostic accuracy can be accomplished with the presence of any two or more of the following criteria: Regional or global myocarditis signal increases in T2 weighted images, increased global myocardial early gadolinium enhancement ratio between myocardium and skeletal muscle (T1 weighted images) or presence of at least one focal lesion with nonischemic regional distribution (late gadolinium enhancement).

In a retrospective study published in 2009, researchers found that myocarditis in children is characterized mainly by subepicardial and transmural enhancement. Global hypokinesia, left ventricular dilatation, ejection fraction less than 30% and transmural myocardial involvement were discovered to be associated with poor outcome (Vashist et al., 2009).

5.5 Biopsy

Despite its limitations, EMB is the gold standard for diagnosis of myocarditis. Together with simultaneous PCR and immunohistology, rapid detection of the viral genome is possible (Checcia&Kulik, 2006). The Dallas criteria have regulated the definition of myocarditis (Aretz et al., 1987). Active myocarditis is considered if light microscopy shows infiltrating lymphocytes and cytolysis. One of the potential advantage of this procedure it may aid physician in determining the management of myocarditis. Children with viral myocarditis may benefit from therapy with immune suppression while patients with cardiomyopathy may not (Liu et al., 2001). Several issues have to be considered before making a decision about biopsy. As stated earlier, some complications such as pneumothorax, dysrhythmia, perforation and death, may occur during the procedure, and it can be hazardous for particularly pediatric patients (Pophal et al., 1999). Limited sensitivity of EMB that is related with sampling error should also be evaluated (Hauck et al., 1989). Substantial controversy exist with respect to diagnostic criteria for examining tissue specimens. Poor interobserver variability may limit the utility of Dallas criteria (Shanes et al., 1987). A scientific statement from the American Heart Association, The American College of Cardiology and European Society of Cardiology published in 2007, has evaluated the role of EMB in myocarditis (Cooper et al., 2007). Various clinical scenarios have been described. Of these only two have received class I recommendation for EMB (Table). In a retrospective review analyzing the morbidity and mortality of EMB in children, highest risk was found in children with suspected myocarditis on inotropic support (Pophal et al., 1999). Authors also found that risk of biopsy in small children (< 10 kg) or sick infants was extreme. Compared with established risk of EMB in adults, there is an increased risk in children. Thus, careful risk-benefit analysis should be therefore undertaken for each patient.

6. Treatment

In spite of the significant progress in understanding the mechanisms of myocarditis pathogenesis in last two decades, advances in treatment strategies are still limited and the supportive care is the principal therapy. Most patients with acute myocarditis presenting with dilated cardiomyopathy respond favorably to standard anticongestive therapy including afterload reduction, diuretics, angiotensin converting enzyme inhibitors and the introduction of β blockers such as carvedilol or metoprolol succinate once the acute phase is controlled. Various experimental studies with β adrenoreceptor inhibitors or agonists showed different effects in acute myocarditis. Treatment with propranolol in mice infected with encephalomyocarditis virus (EMCV) reduced the severity of myocarditis and mortality (Wang et al., 2005). On the other hand, carvedilol, non selective β blocker, improved the survival and decreased the virus replication of mice infected with EMCV through the enhancement of IL-12 and IFN-γ production, whereas metoprolol had no effect on this murine model (Nishio et al., 2003). Despite the lack of extensive studies in pediatric patients, administration of carvedilol has been found to be associated with improvement of left ventricle function and clinical symptoms and normalization of antioxidant enzyme activity (Bajcetic et al., 2008). Similar to effects of β blockers, ACE inhibitors and angiotensin receptor blockers have been documented to lessen viral myocardial injury in murine models (Yamamoto et al., 2003). It is also proposed that early introduction of beta-blockers and ACE inhibitors might prevent the remodelling that advances to dilated cardiomyopathy (Ellis&DiSalvo, 2007). Phosphodiesterase inhibitors such as milrinone, if well tolerated, can be really helpful. A recent multi-institutional analysis revealed that milrinone was used most often for vasoactive support in children (Klugman et al., 2009). Anticoagulants should be considered if ejection fraction is severely decreased or in the setting of atrial arrhythmia (Gunthard et al., 2009). Digoxin should be used in low dose and with caution in patients with viral myocarditis since high dose digoxin was proven to increase mortality in animals with EMVC induced myocarditis as well as elevate intracardiac production of cytokines (Matsumori et al., 1999). Ventilation and oxygenation could be best achieved with continuous positive airway pressure (CPAP) or other non-invasive methods. CPAP, unloads inspiratory muscles and leads to decreased left ventricular afterload without compromising cardiac index via increasing intrathoracic pressure. Medications used for intubation can cause hypotension and acute cardiovascular collapse, thus CPAP also avoids this and is an outstanding adjunctive therapy for cardiac failure and myocarditis (Bradley et al., 1992, Naughton et al., 1995).

Extracorporeal membrane oxygenation support and ventricular assist device might be particularly useful for patients with fulminant myocarditis. Extracorporeal membrane oxygenation may also be considered in those who are in the recovery phase from acute myocarditis (Sezai et al., 2007). For patients with cardiogenic shock because of the acute myocarditis who worsen despite ideal medical therapy, extracorporeal membrane oxygenation and ventricular assist device may help as a bridge to transplant (Moloney et al., 2005). The full mobilization, survival rates up to 90% for fulminant myocarditis and decreased anticoagulation make these pulsatile ventricular assist device systems as the alternative choice of therapy for children (Patopov et al., 2007). Cardiac transplantation is reserved only for patients who are intractable with medical management and mechanical circulatory support. Almost half of the annual cardiac transplantation cases are performed for idiopathic dilated cardiomyopathy, at least 10% of which represent as myocarditis (Ellis&DiSalvo, 2007).

6.1 Immune therapy

It is well known that the long term morbidity and mortality following viral myocarditis seem to be dependent on cellular and humoral immunity abnormalities. Therefore, many investigations have been conducted to search the use of immunosuppressants and immune-modulator agents for treatment of acute myocarditis and dilated cardiomyopathy. However, debate still persists on whether immune therapy for acute myocarditis is useful or not. Initial adult studies investigating the effect of prednisone with or without azathioprine and cyclosporine demonstrated a slight improvement in left ventricular function. But, this improvement was temporary (Mason et al., 1995, Parillo et al., 1989). In a study conducted by Parillo et al., patients were grouped as reactive or nonreactive on the basis of histopathology, immunoglobulin deposition on EMB, an increased erythrocyte sedimentation rate or a positive gallium scan. At three months, reactive patients who were treated with prednisone (60 mg daily) had a statistically significant increase in ejection fraction compared with controls. After six months, improvement seen earlier was no longer present. In 1995, the Myocarditis Treatment Trial failed to show neither an improvement in left ventricle ejection fraction at 28 weeks nor an improvement in survival up to 4.3 years (Mason et al., 1995). Although a few uncontrolled studies showed benefit with several immune suppressive agents, meta analysis of adult studies did not confirm a significant favourable effect of immunosuppression (Garg et al., 1998, Maisch et al., 1998). There were also investigations to evaluate the results of immune suppressive regime in children with acute myocarditis (Chan et al., 1991, Camargo et al., 1995). However, studies in children are inadequate and yet, no randomized controlled trials are present. In a study (Camargo et al., 1995) conducted among 68 children with severe dilated cardiomyopathy, patients were classified into either conventional treatment or given one of three immune suppressive agents, prednisolone, prednisolone plus azathioprine and prednisolone with cyclosporine. Children taking immunosuppression treatment with a second agent, demonstrated enhanced hemodynamic parameters, as well as histological improvement in inflammation. A meta analysis (Hia et al., 2004) assessing the impact of immunosuppression on the outcome of acute myocarditis in children was published in 2004. Better outcome was observed among children who received immunosuppressive therapy. On the other hand, the findings were not statistically significant. Randomized large controlled studies are needed to conclude that immunosuppressive therapy is beneficial for outcome of children with acute myocarditis. On the contrary, one trial published in 1997, demonstrated that survival was improved with the treatment of cyclosporine and corticosteroids in patients with giant cell myocarditis (Cooper et al., 1997). A different approach has also been investigated, in which Wojnicz et al. used HLA expression on endomyocardial specimens to classify inflammatory cohort (Wojnicz et al., 2001). Of 202 patients with dilated cardiomyopathy, 84 patients with increased HLA expression were randomized to receive either placebo or immunosuppression for 3 months. After 2 years, significant improvement in ejection fraction and end diastolic diameter were noted only among the immunosuppressive group.

It was suggested that intravenous immunoglobulin (IVIG) may be an useful therapy for acute myocarditis due to its both antiviral and immunomodulating effects. Previously, it has been shown that IVIG may be used in several autoimmune disorders, including idiopathic thrombocytopenic purpura, systemic vasculitis and Kawasaki disease (Rosen et al., 1993, Wolf et al., 1996). Up to date, there are no randomized controlled studies evaluating the use of IVIG to treat the children with acute myocarditis. A systemic review conducted by Robinson et al., evaluated the use of intravenous immunoglobulin therapy in acute myocarditis in both adults and children (Robinson et al., 2005). They determined that intravenous immunoglobulin might be useful in the presence of ongoing or active infection which may be causing obstinate cardiac failure. In a study conducted in children with presumed viral myocarditis, high dose IVIG treatment was found to be associated with improved recovery of left ventricular function and with a tendency of better survival (Drucker et al., 1994). In adults, the results of a randomized clinical trail suggested that for patients with recent onset dilated cardiomyopathy, IVIG did not enhance an improvement in ejection fraction (McNamara et al., 2001). However, in this cohort, ejection fraction was increased considerably during follow-up and short term prognosis remained favourable. Despite the presence of several case reports indicating that adults treated with intravenous immunoglobulin reveal better cardiac function, Cochrane review of IVIG administration in myocarditis and dilated cardiomyopathy demonstrated no benefit in adults (McNamara et al., 1997, Tedeschi et al., 2002). On the other hand, little is known about the exact mechanisms responsible for potential benefits of IVIG in the therapy of patients with acute myocarditis. Several studies both in the clinical setting and experimental models propose that immunoglobulin may reduce inflammatory cytokines that have direct negative inotropic effects and decrease the oxidative stress (Kishimoto et al., 2003).

Numerous cases with myocarditis recover spontaneously. It is hard to know if the noted improvement is a consequence of therapy with IVIG or immunosuppression versus natural course of the disease. Therefore, studies assessing immunomodulation and immune suppressive agents were problematic to decode into an applicable, routine treatment for children and adults with acute myocarditis. One should also consider that initiating agents for acute myocarditis and following clinical course may change from time to time and by geographic site. Although such a controversy remains to be settled, IVIG may be used only in selected pediatric patients with acute myocarditis.

6.2 Antiviral treatment & vaccines

While viral infection is the most frequent cause of myocarditis, it might be possible to think that vaccines and antiviral agents might be helpful in the treatment of myocarditis. It is obvious that studies using polymerase chain reaction identified viral genomes in patients with acute myocarditis (Bowles et al., 2003). Bu, there are a few studies which demonstrated that requirement for transplantation and mortality was not dependent on the presence of viral genome (Kindermann et al., 2008, Kuhl et al., 2005). So, many investigators suggested that the presence of viral antigens or nucleotides in the myocardium alone is not satisfactory to prove that the virus is the cause of myocarditis (Matsumori et al., 2007). Since the diagnosis of viral myocarditis is frequently challenging and the diagnostic approaches have not been established or standardised, the number of clinical trials for virus proven myocarditis is limited. For that reason, in order to investigate therapeutic and preventative methods for myocarditis, various animal models have been developed. Several promising new agents including peroxisome proliferator activated gamma receptor activator, rapamycine, pycogenol, SUNC8079 and mycophenol mofetil have been studied in murine models of myocarditis during the last decade (Komiyoshi et al., 2005, Ellis&DiSalvo, 2007, Matsumori, 2007). It has been demonstrated that these agents decrease the severity of myocarditis and improve cardiac function, blocks activation of NF-κ, blocks mRNA expression of key cytokines (IL-1, IL-6 and TNF) and stabilizes mast cell (Matsumori, 2007). Synergistic effect of IFN- α and ribavirin has been demonstrated against both EMCV and coxsackie virus infection (Okada et al., 1992, Matsumori, 2007). IFN- β has reported to be effective in studies including small number of patients with left ventricular dysfunction whose biopsy specimens were positive for adenovirus or enterovirus (Kuhl et al., 2003).
Although various strategies for the prevention of acute myocarditis have been studied in murine models, up to now, there have been no vaccination trial in humans. Vaccination against mumps, rubella, poliomyelitis, measles and influenza has made myocarditis consequent to these infections quite rare and increases the arguments on whether vaccination against other cardiotropic viruses might prevent myocarditis in the future. A classical example in this regard was supported by the study of EFE described previously (Ni et al., 1997). The mumps virus vaccine has entirely eliminated this form of dilated cardiomyopathy. It is unlikely that antiviral vaccines to battle this disease will be improved in the near future due to low incidence of the disease.

6.3 Physical activity

Recommendations concerning physical activity affirm that all patients with presumed or definite myocarditis discontinue competitive sports and undergo a prudent convalescence period around six months after the onset of clinical manifestations. Athletes may return to sports activity if LV function, dimensions and wall motions return to normal, markers of inflammation in blood have resolved, 12-lead ECG has normalized and clinically relevant arrhythmias are absent on Holter ECG or graded exercise testing (Maron et al., 2005).

7. Outcome

Prognosis of myocarditis is as changed as its clinical presentations. Although the fewer data are available on the natural history of myocarditis in children, it is proposed that the outcomes in pediatric patients presenting with acute heart failure secondary to acute myocarditis tends to be more positive than the prognosis with dilated cardiomyopathy (Drucker et al., 1994, Lee et al., 1999). In a retrospective analysis of 36 children with histologically proven lymphocytic myocarditis (Lee et al., 1999), excellent outcomes have been demonstrated in children with myocarditis, especially those surviving 72 hours after presentation. Gagliardi and colleagues, classified 114 children into three groups as acute myocarditis, borderline myocarditis and non-inflammatory cardiomyopathy according to histological analysis (Gagliardi et al., 2004). Best survival rate (97%) was found in acute myocarditis group. They suggested that this high long term survival rate of this cohort may be due to effect of short term immunosuppressive therapy. On the other hand, in a multi-center study including children and adults, difference in outcomes between age groups was noted (Bowles et al., 2003). Survival rate for neonates and infants (33 and 45%, respectively) were significantly lower than the other groups. Survival rate was noted to be greatest in adolescent age group. A retrospective study involving 28 children with acute myocarditis, analysed the predictors of outcome. It was observed that ejection fraction < 30%, shortening fraction < 15%, left ventricle dilatation and moderate to severe mitral regurgitation at admission were associated with poor outcome (Kuhn et al., 2004). However, it was understood from the findings of adult trials that syncope, right ventricle dysfunction, elevated pulmonary artery pressure and advanced New York Heart Association functional class were predictors of increased probability of death or requirement for transplantation (Mendes et al, 1994, McCarthy et al., 2000, Magnani&Dec, 2006, Kindermann et al., 2008). Histological classification and severity of symptoms may also give a clue about prognosis. Giant cell myocarditis has a chance of 89% of death or transplantation. Surprisingly, acute fulminant myocarditis may have a better prognosis (Ellis & DiSalvo, 2007).

In general, transplantation is needed in 1-8% of patients with acute myocarditis (Ellis & DiSalvo, 2007). In spite of severe disease at presentation, there is a probability of improvement. Patients should not be listed promptly unless recovery is believed extremely unlikely despite judicious management.

8. Conclusion

Myocarditis in children is challenging given a variety of clinical manifestations that may share common pediatric illnesses such as respiratory infections and gastrointestinal disorders. A high index suspicion is so vital in the diagnosis. With the introduction of new additional diagnostic modalities including cardiac magnetic resonance imaging and biomarkers, cases will be identified easily in the future that would have been formerly missed. Myocarditis causes dilated cardiomyopathy in a significant portion of children. Prognosis for cases with acute viral myocarditis is much better than cases with established cases of dilated cardiomyopathy. Therefore, prompt diagnosis and early effective supportive care are crucial. Even if, much improvement has been achieved in pathogenesis, diagnosis and treatment of myocarditis, many questions remain to be answered and indicate the necessity for additional investigations.

9. References

Aggarwal, S., Ghilardi, N., Xie, M. H., de Sauvage, F. J., and Gurney, A. L. (2003). Interleukin-23 promotes a distinct CD4 T cell activation state characterized by the production of interleukin-17. J. Biol. Chem. 278, 1910–1914.

Amabile N, Fraisse A, Bouvenot J, et al: Outcome of acute fulminant myocarditis in children. Heart (British Cardiac Society) 2006;92:1269-1273.

Angelini A, Calzolari V, Calabrese F, Boffa GM, Maddalena F, Chioin R, Thiene G. Myocarditis mimicking acute myocardial infarction: role of endomyocardial biopsy in the differential diagnosis. Heart. 2000;84:245–250.

Angelini A, Crosato M, Boffa GM, Calabrese F, Calzolari V, Chioin R, Daliento L, Thiene G. Active vs. borderline myocarditis: clinicopathological correlates and prognostic implications. Heart 2002;87:210–215.

Aretz HT, Billingham ME, Edwards WD, Parker MM, Factor SM, Fallon JT & Fenoglio JJ. Myocarditis: a histopathologic definition and classification. Am J Cardiovasc Pathol. 1987;1:3–14.

Ayach B, Fuse K, Martino T, Liu P. Dissecting mechanisms of innate and acquired immunity in myocarditis. Curr Opin Cardiol. 2003 May;18(3):175-81.

Baboonian C, Treasure T. Meta-analysis of the association of enteroviruses with human heart disease. Heart. 1997;78:539–543.

Badorff C, Knowlton K. Role of CVB protease 2A in dystrophin destruction. Nat Med. 1999;5:320 -326.

Bajcetic M, Kokic Nikolic A, Djukic M, Kosutic J, Mitrovic J, Mijalkovic D, Jovanovic I, Simeunovic S, Spasic MB, Samardzic R. Effects of carvedilol on left ventricular function and oxidative stress in infants and children with idiopathic dilated cardiomyopathy: a 12-month, two-center, open-label study. Clin Ther. 2008 Apr;30(4):702-14.

Balaji S, Wiles HB, Sens MA, et al. Immunosuppressive treatment for myocarditis and borderline myocarditis in children with ventricular ectopic rhythm. Br Heart J 1994; 72: 354–359.

Beck MA, Levander OA, Handy J: Selenium deficiency and viral infection. J Nutr 2003;133(5 Suppl 1):1463S-1467S.

Beischel J, Larson DF, Yu Q, Yang B, Sepúlveda RT, Kelley T, Watson RR. Dilated cardiomyopathy in retrovirally infected mice: a novel model for silent viral DCM? Cardiovasc Toxicol. 2004;4(4):317-25.

Bock CT, Klingel K, Kandolf R. (2010) Human parvovirus B19-associated myocarditis. N Engl J Med 362:1248–1249.

Bowles NE, Ni J, Kearney DL, Pauschinger M, Schultheiss HP, McCarthy R, Hare J, Bricker JT, Bowles KR & Towbin JA. Detection of viruses in myocardial tissues by polymerase chain reaction: evidence of adenovirus as a common cause of myocarditis in children and adults. J Am Coll Cardiol. 2003;42:466–472.

Bowles NE, Bowles KR, Towbin JA. Viral genomic detection and outcome in myocarditis. Heart Fail Clin 2005; 1:407–417.

Bradley TD, Holloway RM, McLaughlin PR, et al. Cardiac output response to continuous positive airway pressure in congestive heart failure. Am Rev Respir Dis 1992; 145: 377–382.

Bratincsak A, El-Said HG, Bradley JS, Shayan K, Grossfeld PD, Cannavino CR. Fulminant Myocarditis Associated With Pandemic H1N1 Influenza A Virus in Children. J Am Coll Cardiol 2010; 55:928–929.

Breuckmann F, Neumann T, Kondratieva J, et al: Dilated cardiomyopathy in two adult human immunodeficiency positive(HIV+) patients possibly related to highly active antiretroviral therapy (HAART). Eur J Med Res 2005;10:395-399

Brodison A, Swann JW. Myocarditis: a review. The Journal of infection. 1998 Sep;37(2):99-103.

Camargo PR, Snitcowsky R, da Luz PL, et al: Favorable effects of immunosuppressive therapy in children with dilated cardiomyopathy and active myocarditis. Pediatr Cardiol 1995;16:61-68.

Camargo PR, Okay TS, Yamamoto L, et al. Myocarditis in children and detection of viruses in myocardial tissue: implications for immunosuppressive therapy. Int J Cardiol 2009.

Carlquist, J. F., Menlove, R. L., Murray, M. B., O'Connell, J. B., and Anderson, J. L. (1991). HLA class II (DR and DQ) antigen associations in idiopathic dilated cardiomyopathy. Validation study and meta-analysis of published HLA association studies. Circulation 83,515–522.

Chan KY, Iwahara M, Benson LN, et al: Immunosuppressive therapy in the management of acute myocarditis in children: a clinical trial. J Am Coll Cardiol 1991;17:458-460.

Checchia PA, Kulik TJ. Acute viral myocarditis: diagnosis. Pediatr Critical Care Med 2006; 7: S8–S11.

Chen F, Shannon K, Ding S, et al: HIV type 1 glycoprotein 120 inhibits cardiac myocyte contraction. AIDS Res Hum Retrovir 2002;18:777-784.

Chen, P.H., Ornelles, D.A. & Shenk, T. The adenovirus L3 23-kilodalton proteinasecleaves the amino-terminal head domain from cytokeratin 18 and disrupts the cytokeratinnetwork of HeLa cells. J. Virol. 67, 3507–3514 (1993).

Chen, Y., Langrish, C. L., McKenzie, B., Joyce-Shaikh, B., Stumhofer, J. S., McClanahan, T., Blumenschein, W., Churakovsa, T., Low, J., Presta, L., Hunter, C. A., Kastelein, R. A., et al. (2006). Anti-IL-23 therapy inhibits multiple inflammatory pathways and ameliorates autoimmune encephalomyelitis. J. Clin. Invest. 116, 1317–1326.

Cihakova, D., Barin, J. G., Afanasyeva, M., Kimura, M., Fairweather, D., Berg, M., Talor, M. V., Baldeviano, G. C., Frisancho, S., Gabrielson, K., Bedja, D., and Rose, N. R. (2008). Interleukin-13 protects against experimental Autoimmune myocarditis by regulating macrophage differentiation. Am. J. Pathol. 172, 1195–1208.

Cooper LT Jr, Berry GJ, Shabetai R. Idiopathic giant-cell myocarditis— natural history and treatment. Multicenter Giant Cell Myocarditis Study Group Investigators. N Engl J Med. 1997;336:1860 –1866.

Cooper LT, Baughman KL, Feldman AM, et al: The role of endomyocardial biopsy in the management of cardiovascular disease: a scientific statement from the American Heart Association, the American College of Cardiology, and the European Society of Cardiology. Circulation 2007;116:2216-2233.

Costello JM, Alexander ME, Greco KM, et al: Lyme carditis inchildren: presentation, predictive factors, and clinical course. Pediatrics 2009;123:e835-e841.

d'Amati G, di Gioia CR, Gallo P. Pathological findings of HIV associated cardiovascular disease. Ann N Y Acad Sci. 2001;946:23– 45.

Daly K, Monaghan M, Richardson P, et al: Significant incidence of mural thrombi in acute myocarditis—indications for early anticoagulation (abstract). J Am Coll Cardiol 1983;1:584.

Danti M, Sbarbati S, Alsadi N, et al. Cardiac magnetic resonance imaging: diagnostic value and utility in the follow-up of patients with acute myocarditis mimicking myocardial infarction. Radiol Med 2009; 114:229–238.

Davison AJ, Benko M, Harrach B. Genetic content and evolution of adenoviruses. *J Gen Virol* 2003;84:2895â€"2908.

de Vetten L, Bergman KA, Elzenga NJ, van Melle JP, Timmer A, Bartelds B. Neonatal myocardial infarction or myocarditis? Pediatr Cardiol. 2011 Apr;32(4):492-7. Epub 2011 Jan 8.

Dec GW, Palacios IF, Fallon JT, Aretz HT, Mills J, Lee DC, Johnson RA. Active myocarditis in the spectrum of acute dilated cardiomyopathies: clinical features, histologic correlates, and clinical outcome. New England Journal of Medicine. 1985;312:885–890.

Dec GW, Waldman H, Southern J, Fallon JT, Hutter AM, Palacios I. Viral myocarditis mimicking acute myocardial infarction. J Am Coll Cardiol. 1992;20:85- 89.

Dettmeyer R, Baasner A, Schlamann N, Padosch SA, Haag R, Kandolf R, Madea B. Role of virus-induced myocardial infections in sudden infant death syndrome:a prospective postmortem study. Ped Research 2004;55:947–52.

Donoso Mantke O, Meyer R, Prosch S, et al. High prevalence of cardiotropic viruses in myocardial tissue from explanted hearts of heart transplant recipients and heart donors: a 3-year retrospective study from a German patients' pool. J Heart Lung Transplant 2005; 24:1632–8.

Doolan A, Langlois N, Semsarian C. Causes of sudden cardiac death in young Australians. *Med J Aust. 2004*;180:110 -112.

Drory Y, Turetz Y, Hiss Y, Lev B, Fishman EZ, Pines A, Kramer MR. Sudden unexpected death in persons less than 40 years of age. Am J Cardiol. 1991;68:1388 -1392.

Drucker NA, Colan SD, Lewis AB, et al. Gamma-globulin treatment of acute myocarditis in the pediatric population. Circulation 1994; 89:252–257.

Durani Y, Egan M, Baffa J, et al. Pediatric myocarditis: presenting clinical characteristics. Am J Emerg Med 2009; 27:942–947.

Ellis CR, Di Salvo T. Myocarditis: basic and clinical aspects. Cardiol Rev 2007; 15: 170–177.

Fairweather, D., Afanasyeva, M., and Rose, N. R. (2004). Cellular immunity: A role for cytokines. In "Handbook of Systemic Autoimmune Diseases: The Heart in Systemic Autoimmune Diseases" (A. Doria, and and P. Pauletto, Eds.), pp. 3–7. Elselvier, Amsterdam.

Fairweather, D., and Rose, N. R. (2007). Coxsackievirus-induced myocarditis in mice: A model of autoimmune disease for studying immunotoxicity. Methods 41, 118–122.

Feldman AM, McNamara D. Myocarditis. N Engl J Med. 2000;343:1388–1398.

Felker GM, Hu W, Hare JM, Hruban RH, Baughman KL, Kasper EK. The spectrum of dilated cardiomyopathy: the Johns Hopkins experience with 1,278 patients. Medicine (Baltimore). 1999;78:270 -283

Felker GM, Boehmer JP, Hruban RH, et al: Echocardiographic findings in fulminant and acute myocarditis. J Am Coll Cardiol2000;36:227-232.

Freedman SB, Haladyn JK, Floh A, et al. Pediatric myocarditis: emergency department clinical findings and diagnostic evaluation. Pediatrics 2007;120:1278–1285.

Friedman RA, Kearney DL, Moak JP, et al. Persistence of ventricular arrhythmia after resolution of occult myocarditis in children and young adults. *J Am Coll Cardiol* 1994;24:780-783.

Friedman RA, Schowengerdt KO, Towbin JA. Myocarditis. In: Bricker JT, Garson A Jr, Fisher DJ, et al., eds. *The Science and Practice of Pediatric Cardiology*. 2nd ed. Baltimore: Williams & Wilkins, 1998: 1777-1794.

Friedrich MG, Strohm O, Schulz-Menger J, et al: Contrast media enhanced magnetic resonance imaging visualizes myocardial changes in the course of viral myocarditis. Circulation 1998;97:1802-1809.

Friedrich MG, Sechtem U, Schulz-Menger J, et al: Cardiovascular magnetic resonance in myocarditis: A JACC White Paper. J Am Coll Cardiol 2009;53:1475-1487.

Friman G, Wesslen L, Fohlman Jet al. The epidemiology of infectious myocarditis, lymphocytic myocarditis and dilated cardiomyopathy. Eur Heart J 1995; 16 (Suppl. O): 36-41.

Fuse, K., Chan, G., Liu, Y., Gudgeon, P., Husain, M., Chen, M., Yeh, W. C., Akira, S., and Gagliardi MG, Bevilacqua M, Bassano C, et al. Long term follow up of children with myocarditis treated by immunosuppression and of children with dilated cardiomyopathy. Heart 2004; 90: 1167–1171.

Garg A, Shiau J, Guyatt G. The ineffectiveness of immunosuppressive therapy in lymphocytic myocarditis: an overview. Ann Intern Med 1998; 129: 317–322.

Godeny EK, Gauntt CJ. Murine natural killer cells limit coxsackievirus B3 replication. *J Immunol* 1987;139:913-918.

Goitein O, Matetzky S, Beinart R, et al. Acute myocarditis: noninvasive evaluation with cardiac MRI and transthoracic echocardiography. AJR Am J Roentgenol 2009; 192:254–258.

Gorbea C, Makar KA, Pauschinger M, Pratt G, Bersola JL, Varela J, David RM, Banks L, Huang CH, Li H, Schultheiss HP, Towbin JA, Vallejo JG, Bowles NE. A role for Toll-like receptor 3 variants in host susceptibility to enteroviral myocarditis and dilated cardiomyopathy.J Biol Chem. 2010 Jul 23;285(30):23208-23. Epub 2010 May 14.

Gore I, Saphir O. Myocarditis: a classification of 1402 cases. Am Heart J. 1947;34:827–830.

Gravanis, MB. ; Sternby, NH. (1991) Incidence of myocarditis. A 10-year autopsy study from Malmö, Sweden. *Archives of Pathology & Laboratory Medicine*, Vol.115 No. 5, (April 1991), pp. 390-392, ISSN 1543-2165.

Greenwood RD, Nadas AS, Fyler DC: The clinical course of primary myocardial disease in infants and children. Am Heart J 1976;92:549-560.

Guler, M. L., Ligons, D. L., Wang, Y., Bianco, M., Broman, K. W., and Rose, N. R. (2005). Two autoimmune diabetes loci influencing T cell apoptosis control susceptibility toexperimental autoimmune myocarditis. J. Immunol. 174, 2167–2173.

Gunthard J, Stocker F, Bolz D, et al. Dilated cardiomyopathy and thrombo-embolism. Eur J Pediatr 1997; 156: 3–6.

Gutberlet M, Spors B, Thoma T, et al: Suspected chronic myocarditis at cardiac MR: diagnostic accuracy and association with immunohistologically detected inflammation and viral persistence.Radiology 2008;246:401-409.

Hampton TG, Crumpacker CS, Abelmann WH, Amende I, Morgan JP. 2005. Propranolol ameliorates and epinephrine exacerbates progression of acute and chronic viral myocarditis. Am J PhysiolHeart Circ Physiol 289:H1577–H1583.

Hauck AJ, Kearney DL, Edwards WD. Evaluation of postmortem endomyocardial biopsy specimens from 38 patients with lymphocytic myocarditis: implications for role of sampling error. Mayo Clin Proc. 1989;64:1235–1245.

Hayder H, Müllbacher A. Molecular basis of immune evasion strategies by adenoviruses. Immunol Cell Biol. 1996 Dec;74(6):504-12.

Hia CP, Yip WC, Tai BC, et al. Immunosuppressive therapy inacute myocarditis: an 18 year systematic review. Arch Dis Child 2004; 89: 580–584.

Huber SA. Animal models: immunological aspects. In: Banatvla JE, ed. Viral Infections in the Heart. London, UK: Edward Arnold; 1993: 82–109.

Ilback NG, Wesslen L, Fohlman J, et al: Effects of methyl mercury on cytokines, inflammation and virus clearance in acommon infection (coxsackie B3 myocarditis). Toxicol Lett 1996;89:19-28.

Kamiyoshi Y, Takahashi M, Yokoseki O, et al. Mycophenolate mofetil prevents the development of experimental autoimmune myocarditis. J Mol Cell Cardiol. 2005;39:467- 477.

Kashimura T, Kodama M, Hotta Y, et al: Spatiotemporal changes of coxsackievirus and adenovirus receptor in rat hearts during postnatal development and in cultured cardiomyocytes of neonatal rat. Virchows Arch 2004;444:283-292.

Kawai C, Matsumori A, Kitaura Y, Takatsu T. Viruses and the heart: viral myocarditis and cardiomyopathy. Prog Cardiol. 1978;7:141–162.

Kawai C. From myocarditis to cardiomyopathy: mechanisms of inflammation and cell death: learning from the past for the future. Circulation.1999;99:1091–1100.

Kawai C. Idiopathic cardiomyopathy: a study on the infectious-immune theory as a cause of the disease. Jpn Circ J. 1971;35:765–770.

Kearney MT, Cotton JM, Richardson PJ & Shah AM. Viral myocarditis and dilated cardiomyopathy: mechanisms, manifestations, and management. Postgrad Med J 2001; 77:4–10.

Kindermann I, Kindermann M, Kandolf R, Klingel K, Bultmann B, Muller T, Lindinger A, Böhm M. Predictors of outcome in patients with suspected myocarditis. Circulation 2008;118:639–648.

Kishimoto C, Shioji K, Kinoshita M, Iwase T, Tamaki S, Fujii M, Murashige A, Maruhashi H, Takeda S, Nonogi H, Hashimoto T. Treatment of acute inflammatory cardiomyopathy with intravenous immunoglobulin ameliorates left ventricular function associated with suppression of inflammatory cytokines and decreased oxidative stress. Int J Cardiol. 2003 Oct;91(2-3):173-8.

Klingel K, Hohenadl C, Canu A, Albrecht M, Seemann M, Mall G, Kandolf R. Ongoing enterovirus-induced myocarditis is associated with persistent heart muscle infection: quantitative analysis of virus replication, tissue damage, and inflammation. Proc Natl Acad Sci U S A. 1992;89:314 -318.

Klugman D, Berger JT, Sable CA, He J, Khandelwal SG, Slonim AD. Pediatric patients hospitalized with myocarditis: a multi-institutional analysis. Pediatr Cardiol. 2010 Feb;31(2):222-8.

Krous HF, Ferandos C, Masoumi H, et al. Myocardial inflammation, cellular death, and viral detection in sudden infant death caused by SIDS, suffocation, or myocarditis. Pediatr Res 2009; 66:17–21.

Kuethe F, Lindner J, Matschke K, Wenzel JJ, Norja P, Ploetze K, Schaal S, Kamvissi V,Bornstein SR, Schwanebeck U & Modrow S. Prevalence of parvovirus B19 and human bocavirus DNA in the heart of patients with no evidence of dilated cardiomyopathy or myocarditis. Clin Infect Dis. 2009 Dec 1;49(11):1660-6.

Kuethe F, Sigusch HH, Hilbig K, et al. Detection of viral genome in the myocardium: lack of prognostic and functional relevance in patients with acute dilated cardiomyopathy. Am Heart J 2007; 153:850–8.

Kuhl U, Pauschinger M, Schwimmbeck PL, et al. Interferon-beta treatment eliminates cardiotropic viruses and improves left ventricular function in patients with myocardial persistence of viral genomes and left ventricular dysfunction. Circulation. 2003;107:2793–2798

Kuhl U, Pauschinger M, Bock T, et al. Parvovirus B19 infection mimicking acute myocardial infarction. Circulation 2003; 108:945–950.

Kuhl U, Pauschinger M, Seeberg B, et al. Viral persistence in the myocardium is associated with progressive cardiac dysfunction. Circulation 2005;112:1965—70.

Kuhn B, Shapiro ED, Walls TA, et al. Predictors of outcome of myocarditis. Pediatr Cardiol 2004; 25: 379–384.

Kyto V, Saraste A, Voipio-Pulkki LM, et al. Incidence of fatal myocarditis: a population-based study in Finland. Am J Epidemiol 2007;165:570–4.

Lee KJ, McCrindle BW, Bohn DJ, et al. Clinical outcomes of acute myocarditis in childhood. Heart 1999; 82: 226–233.

Limas, C. J., and Limas, C. (1989). HLA antigens in idiopathic dilated cardiomyopathy. Br.Heart. J. 62, 379–383.

Lipshultz SE, Sleeper LA, Towbin JA, et al. The incidence of pediatric cardiomyopathy in two regions of the United States. N Engl J Med 2003;348:1647-55.

Liu P, Penninger J, Aitken K, Sole M, Mak T. The role of transgenic knockout models in defining the pathogenesis of viral heart disease. Eur Heart J. 1995 Dec;16 Suppl O:25-7.

Liu PP, Mason JW. Advances in the understanding of myocarditis. Circulation. 2001;104:1076 -1082.

Liu W, Li WM, Sun NL. HLA-DQA1, -DQB1 polymorphism and genetic susceptibility to idiopathic dilated cardiomyopathy in Hans of northern China. Ann Hum Genet. 2005 Jul;69(Pt 4):382-8.

Liu, P. P. (2005). Myeloid differentiation factor-88 plays a crucial role in the pathogenesis of coxsackievirus B3-induced myocarditis and influences type I interferon production. Circulation 112, 2276–2285.

Lotze U, Egerer R, Tresselt C, et al. Frequent detection of parvovirus B19 genome in the myocardium of adult patients with idiopathic dilated cardiomyopathy. Med Microbiol Immunol 2004; 193:75–82.

Magnani JW, Danik HJ, Dec Jr GW, et al: Survival in biopsy proven myocarditis: a long-term retrospective analysis of the histopathologic, clinical, and hemodynamic predictors. Am Heart J 2006;151:463-470.

Magnani JW, Dec GW: Myocarditis: current trends in diagnosis and treatment. Circulation 2006;113:876-890.

Mahrholdt H, Goedecke C, Wagner A, et al: Cardiovascular magnetic resonance assessment of human myocarditis: a comparison to histology and molecular pathology. Circulation 2004;109: 1250-1258.

Mahrholdt H, Wagner A, Deluigi CC, Kispert E, Hager S, Meinhardt G, Vogelsberg H, Fritz P, Dippon J, Bock CT, Klingel K, Kandolf R & Sechtem U. Presentation, patterns of myocardial damage, and clinical course of viral myocarditis. Circulation 2006;114:1581–1590.

Maisch B, Trostel-Soeder R, Strechemesser E, et al. Diagnostic relevance of humoral and cell-mediated immune reactions in patients with acute viral myocarditis. *Clin Exp Immunol* 1982;48:533-545

Maisch B, Herzum M, Hufnagel G, et al. Immunosuppressive treatment for myocarditis and dilated cardiomyopathy. Eur Heart J 1995; 16 Suppl O: 153–161.

Maron BJ, Ackerman MJ, Nishimura RA, et al: Task Force 4: HCM and other cardiomyopathies, mitral valve prolapse, myocarditis, and Marfan syndrome. J Am Coll Cardiol 2005;45:1340-1345.

Martin AB, Webber S, Fricker FJ, Jaffe R, Demmler G, Kearney D, Zhang YH, Bodurtha J, Gelb B, Ni J, et al. Acute myocarditis. Rapid diagnosis by PCR in children. Circulation. 1994 Jul;90(1):330-9.

Mason JW, O'Connell JB, Herskowitz A, et al. A clinical trial of immunosuppressive therapy for myocarditis. The myocarditis treatment trial investigators. N Engl J Med 1995; 333: 269–275.

Matsumori A, Igata H, Ono K, et al: High doses of digitalis increase the myocardial production of proinflammatory cytokines and worsen myocardial injury in viral myocarditis: a possible mechanism of digitalis toxicity. Jpn Circ J 1999;63:934-940.

Matsumori A, Matoba Y, Sasayama S. Dilated cardiomyopathy associated with hepatitis C virus infection. Circulation. 1995;92:2519 -2525.

Matsumori A, Yamada T, Suzuki H, Matoba Y, Sasayama S. Increased circulating cytokines in patients with myocarditis and cardiomyopathy. Br Heart J. 1994;72:561–566.

Matsumori A. Treatment options in myocarditis: what we know from experimental data and how it translates to clinical trials.Herz. 2007 Sep;32(6):452-6.

McCarthy III RE, Boehmer JP, Hruban RH, et al: Long-term outcome of fulminant myocarditis as compared with acute (nonfulminant) myocarditis. N Engl J Med 2000;342:690-695.

McNamara DM, Rosenblum WD, Janosko KM, et al. Intravenous immune globulin in the therapy of myocarditis and acute cardiomyopathy. Circulation 1997; 95: 2476–2478.

McNamara DM, Holubkov R, Starling RC, et al: Controlled trial of intravenous immune globulin in recent-onset dilated cardiomyopathy. Circulation 2001;103:2254-2259.

Mendes LA, Dec GW, Picard MH, et al. Right ventricular dysfunction: an independent predictor of adverse outcome in patients with myocarditis. Am Heart J 1994; 128: 301–307.

Mikami S, Kawashima S, Kanazawa K, Hirata K, Hotta H, Kayashi Y, Itoh H, Yokoyama M. Low-dose N omega-nitro-L-arginine methyl ester treatment improves survival rate and decreases myocardial injury in a murine model of viral myocarditis induced by Coxsackievirus B3. Circ Res. 1997;81:504 -511.

Milenkovic M, Arsenović-Ranin N, Stojić-Vukanić Z, Bufan B, Vučićević D, Jančić I. Quercetin ameliorates experimental autoimmune myocarditis in rats. J Pharm Pharm Sci. 2010;13(3):311-9.

Moloney ED, Egan JJ, Kelly P, et al. Transplantation for myocarditis: a controversy revisited. J Heart Lung Transplant. 2005;24:1103–1110.

Moncada S, Liew FY, Lowenstein CJ. The role of inducible nitric oxide synthase in the host response to coxsackievirus myocarditis. Proc Natl Acad Sci U S A. 1998;95:2469 - 2474.

Morgera T, Di Lenarda A, Dreas L, et al: Electrocardiography ofmyocarditis revisited: clinical and prognostic significance of electrocardiographic changes. Am Heart J 1992;124:455-467.

Nakashima H, Katayama T, Ishizaki M, et al: Q wave and non-Q wave myocarditis with special reference to clinical significance. Jpn Heart J 1998;39:763-774.

Naughton MT, Rahman MA, Hara K, et al. Effect of continuous positive airway pressure on intrathoracic and left ventricular transmural pressures in patients with congestive heart failure. Circulation 1995; 91: 1725–1731.

Neu, N., Rose, N. R., Beisel, K. W., Herskowitz, A., Gurri-Glass, G., and Craig, S. W. (1987). Cardiac myosin induces myocarditis in genetically predisposed mice. J. Immunol. 139, 3630–3636.

Ni J, Bowles NE, Kim YH, et al. Viral infection of the myocardium in endocardial fibroelastosis. Molecular evidence for the role of mumps virus as an etiologic agent. Circulation 1997;95:133–9.

Nishio R, Shioi T, Sasayama S, Matsumori A. 2003. Carvedilol increases the production of interleukin-12 and interferon-gamma and improves the survival of mice infected with the encephalomyocarditis virus. J Am Coll Cardiol 41:340–345.

O'Donoghue HL, Lawson CM, Reed WD. Autoantibodies to cardiac myosin in mouse cytomegalovirus myocarditis. Immunology. 1990 Sep;71(1):20-8.

Okada I, Matsumori A, Matoba Y, et al. Combination treatment with ribavirin and interferon for coxsackievirus B3 replication. J Lab Clin Med 1992;120:569–73.

Ono K, Matsumori A, Shioi T, et al. Cytokine gene expression after myocardial infarction in rat hearts: possible implication in left ventricular remodeling. Circulation. 1998;98:149 -156.

Opavsky MA, Penninger J, Aitken K, Wen WH, Dawood F, Mak T, Liu P. Susceptibility to myocarditis is dependent on the response of T lymphocytes to coxsackieviral infection. Circ Res. 1999;85:551–558.

Padalko E, Ohnishi T, Matsushita K, Sun H, Fox-Talbot K, Bao C, Baldwin WM, Lowenstein CJ. Peroxynitrite inhibition of coxsackievirus infection by prevention of viral RNA entry. Proc Natl Acad Sci U S A. 2004;101:11731–11736.

Parrillo JE, Cunnion RE, Epstein SE, et al. A prospective, randomized, controlled trial of prednisone for dilated cardiomyopathy. N Engl J Med 1989; 321: 1061–1068.

Parrillo JE. Inflammatory cardiomyopathy (myocarditis): which patients should be treated with anti-inflammatory therapy? Circulation. 2001; 104:4–6.

Pauschinger M, Bowles NE, Fuentes-Garcia FJ, et al. Detection of adenoviral genome in the myocardium of adult patients with idiopathic left ventricular dysfunction. Circulation. 1999;99:1348–1354.

Pophal SG, Sigfusson G, Booth KL, et al. Complications of endomyocardial biopsy in children. J Am Coll Cardiol 1999; 34: 2105–2110.

Potapov EV, Stiller B, Hetzer R. Ventricular assist devices in children: current achievements and future perspectives. Pediatr Transplant 2007; 11: 241–255.

Pugliese A, Isnardi D, Saini A, et al: Impact of highly active antiretroviral therapy in HIV positive patients with cardiac involvement. J Infect 2000;40:282-284.

Robinson J, Hartling L, Vandermeer B, et al. Intravenous immunoglobulin for presumed viral myocarditis in children and adults. Cochrane Database Syst Rev 2005:CD004370.

Robinson JL, Hartling L, Crumley E, et al. A systematic review of intravenous gamma globulin for therapy of acute myocarditis. BMC Cardiovasc Disord 2005; 5: 12.

Rosen FS. Putative mechanisms of the effect of intravenous gama- globulin. Clin Immunol Immunopathol 1993;67:S41–3.

Salone B, Martina Y, Piersanti S, et al: Integrin alpha3beta1 is an alternative cellular receptor for adenovirus serotype 5. J Virol 2003;77:13448-13454.

Sezai A, Hata M, Niino T, et al. Mechanical circulatory support for fulminant myocarditis. Surg Today 2008; 38: 773–777.

Shafren DR, Bates RC, Agrez MV, et al: Coxsackieviruses B1, B3, and B5 use decay accelerating factor as a receptor for cell attachment. J Virol 1995;69:3873-3877.

Shanes JG, Ghali J, Billingham ME, Ferrans VJ, Fenoglio JJ, Edwards WD, Tsai CC, Saffitz JE, Isner J, Forner S. Interobserver variability in the pathologic interpretation of endomyocardial biopsy results. Circulation. 1987;75:401– 405.

Shirani J, Freant LJ, Roberts WC. Gross and semiquantitative histologic findings in mononuclear cell myocarditis causing sudden death, and implications for endomyocardial biopsy. Am J Cardiol. 1993;72:952–957.

Shoeman, R.L. et al. Cleavage of human and mouse cytoskeletal and sarcomeric proteins by human immunodeficiency virus type 1 protease. Actin, desmin, myosin, and tropomyosin. Am. J. Pathol. 142, 221–230 (1993).

Skouri HN, Dec GW, Friedrich MG, Cooper LT. Noninvasive imaging in myocarditis. J Am Coll Cardiol 2006; 48:2085–2093.

Tchilian, E. Z., Gil, J., Navarro, M. L., Fernandez-Cruz, E., Chapel, H., Misbah, S., Ferry, B.,Renz, H., Schwinzer, R., and Beverley, P. C. (2006). Unusual case presentations associated with the CD45 C77G polymorphism. Clin. Exp. Immunol. 146, 448-454.

Tedeschi A, Airaghi L, Giannini S, et al. High-dose intravenous immunoglobulin in the treatment of acute myocarditis. A case report and review of the literature. J Intern Med 2002; 251:169–173.

Theleman KP, Kuiper JJ, Roberts WC. Acute myocarditis sudden death without heart failure. Am J Cardiol. 2001;88:1078–1083.

Tomioka N, Kishimoto C, Matsumori A, Kawai C. Effects of prednisolone on acute viral myocarditis in mice. J Am Coll Cardiol. 1986;7:868–872.

Toshima H, Ohkita Y, Shingu M. Clinical features of acute coxsackie B viral myocarditis. Jpn Circ J. 1979 May;43(5):441-4.

Towbin JA, Bricker JT, Garson A Jr. Electrocardiographic criteria for diagnosis of acute myocardial infarction in childhood. *Am J Cardiol* 1992;69:1545-1548.

Ukena C, Mahfoud F, Kindermann I, Kandolf R, Kindermann M, Böhm M. Prognostic electrocardiographic parameters in patients with suspected myocarditis. Eur J Heart Fail. 2011 Apr;13(4):398-405. Epub 2011 Jan 14.

Vashist S, Singh GK. Acute myocarditis in children: current concepts and management. Curr Treat Options Cardiovasc Med 2009; 11:383–391.

Vashist S, Woodard PK, Grady M, Singh G. MRI characteristics of acute myocarditis in pediatric patients: patterns and predictors of outcomes [abstract]. St Louis Washington University School of Medicine; 2009.

Wang JF, Meissner A, Malek S, Chen Y, Ke Q, Zhang J, Chu V, Hampton TG, Crumpacker CS, Abelmann WH, Amende I, Morgan JP. Propranolol ameliorates and epinephrine exacerbates progression of acute and chronic viral myocarditis. Am J Physiol Heart Circ Physiol. 2005 Oct;289(4):H1577-83. Epub 2005 May 27.

Weinmann HJ, Brasch RC, Press WR, Wesbey GE. Characteristics of gadolinium-DTPA complex: a potential NMR contrast agent. Am J Roentgenol. 1984;142:619–624.

Wickham TJ, Filardo EJ, Cheresh DA, et al: Integrin alpha v beta 5 selectively promotes adenovirus mediated cell membrane permeabilization. J Cell Biol 1994;127:257-264.

Wojnicz R, Nowalany-Kozielska E, Wojciechowska C, Glanowska G, Wilczewski P, Niklewski T, Zembala M, Polonski L, Wodniecki J,Rozek MM. Randomized, placebo-controlled study for immunosuppressive treatment of inflammatory dilated cardiomyopathy: two-year follow-up results. Circulation. 2001;104: 39–45.

Wolf HM, Eibl MM. Immunomodulatory effect of immunoglobulins Clin Exp Rheum 1996;14(Suppl 15):S17–25.

Woodruff JF. Viral myocarditis: A review. *Am J Pathol* 1980;101:427-484.

Xiong D, Lee GH, Badorff C, Dorner A, Lee S, Wolf P, Knowlton KU. Dystrophin deficiency markedly increases enterovirus-induced cardiomyopathy: a genetic predisposition to viral heart disease. Nat Med. 2002 Aug;8(8):872-7. Epub 2002 Jul 15.

Yamamoto K, Shioi T, Uchiyama K, et al. Attenuation of virus-induced myocardial injury by inhibition of the angiotensin II type 1 receptor signal and decreased nuclear factor-kappa B activation in knockout mice. J Am Coll Cardiol. 2003;42:2000 - 2006

Yuan J, Yu M, Lin QW, Cao AL, Yu X, Dong JH, Wang JP, Zhang JH, Wang M, Guo HP, Liao YH. Neutralization of IL-17 inhibits the production of anti-ANT autoantibodies in CVB3-induced acute viral myocarditis. Int Immunopharmacol. 2010 Mar;10(3):272-6. Epub 2009 Nov 20.

Yuan J, Yu M, Lin QW, Cao AL, Yu X, Dong JH, Wang JP, Zhang JH, Wang M, Guo HP, Cheng X, Liao YH. Th17 cells contribute to viral replication in coxsackievirus B3-induced acute viral myocarditis. J Immunol. 2010 Oct 1;185(7):4004-10. Epub 2010 Aug 27.

Zaragoza C, Ocampo C, Saura M, Leppo M, Wei XQ, Quick R, Moncada S, Liew FY, Lowenstein CJ The role of inducible nitric oxide synthase in the host response to Coxsackievirus myocarditis. . Proc Natl Acad Sci U S A. 1998 Mar 3;95(5):2469-74.

Zaragoza C, Ocampo CJ, Saura M, McMillan A, Lowenstein CJ. Nitric oxide inhibition of Coxsackie replication in vivo. J Clin Invest. 1997; 100:1760 –1767.

2

Clinical Presentation

Rafid Fayadh Al-Aqeedi
Hamad Medical Corporation, Cardiology and Cardiovascular Surgery Department
Qatar

1. Introduction

Myocarditis is a clinical syndrome characterized by inflammation of myocardium. It can be produced by a myriad of etiologies including infectious, autoimmune, myocardial toxins, hypersensitivity reactions and physical agents. Virtually any infectious agent can produce myocardial inflammation and injury. Human myocarditis is most frequently caused by viral infection. Ongoing viral infection, myocardial destruction, and adverse remodeling can lead to persistent ventricular dysfunction and dilated cardiomyopathy. The modern molecular techniques have facilitated new insights into inflammatory autoimmune processes that affect the myocardium and ultimately result in acute or chronic dilated cardiomyopathy.

The clinical manifestations are highly variable, ranging from asymptomatic electrocardiographic or echocardiographic abnormalities to acute myocardial infarction-like syndrome, overt congestive heart failure, fulminant condition with new atrial or ventricular arrhythmias or profound cardiogenic shock and death. Myocarditis is occasionally the unrecognized culprit in cases of sudden cardiac death. Autopsy series have reported much higher rates of myocarditis than expected with overt clinical manifestation from different etiological agents. The prospective postmortem data have implicated myocarditis in sudden cardiac death of young adults at rates of 8.6 percent to 12 percent (Doolan et al., 2004; Fabre & Sheppard, 2005). Furthermore, it has been identified as a cause of dilated cardiomyopathy in 9 percent of cases in a large prospective series (Felker et al., 1999).

The clinical history in patients presented with myocarditis remains essential to envelop a wide variety of etiologies in the clinical scenarios, many of which are infectious (Brodison & Swann, 1998). In the past 10 years, however, viruses, including adenovirus, parvovirus B19, hepatitis C, and herpes virus 6, have emerged as significant pathogens (Mahrholdt et al., 2006). The geographical distribution can be of relevance for some forms of myocarditis. In selected countries, Chagas disease, Lyme myocarditis, acute rheumatic fever and disorders associated with advanced human immune deficiency virus infection are significant causes. Other important infrequent clinicopathologic variants in the etiological spectrum are systemic disorders like giant cell myocarditis, cardiac sarcoidosis and eosinophilic myocarditis. Additionally, drugs, vaccinations, toxins, physical agents like radiation, heat stroke and hypothermia can be the key point for some rare clinical diagnoses. The physical examination in patients with myocarditis might be normal, but more severe cases frequently evident for significant physical findings. Although histological findings remains the gold standard for establishing the diagnosis of myocarditis, low risk patients are often given a presumptive diagnosis if imaging studies and a compatible clinical scenario suggest new onset cardiomyopathy. The clinical manifestations of suspected patients with myocarditis will be discussed in details.

2. Clinicopathological classification

Over the past two decades, a great deal of confusion may be traced to the changing diagnostic criteria, multifaceted classifications, and varying patterns of infectious disease. The details of classifications will be discussed in other chapter in this book.

The morphologic criteria for the diagnosis of myocarditis by means of endomyocardial biopsy interpretation was proposed by the Dallas criteria authors in 1986 who defined myocarditis as a process characterized by the presence of an inflammatory cell infiltration of the myocardium with necrosis and/or degeneration of myocytes that is not typical of the myocardial damage of ischemic heart disease. The inflammatory cells are typically lymphocytic but may also include eosinophilic, neutrophilic, giant cells, granulomatous, or mixed cellularity infiltration. The amount of inflammation and its distribution may be mild, moderate, or severe and focal, confluent, or diffuse, respectively. A retrospective study of 112 consecutive patients with biopsy-confirmed myocarditis demonstrated, 55 percent lymphocytic; 22 percent borderline (inflammatory cellular infiltrate with no evidence of myocyte necrosis); 10 percent granulomatous; 6 percent giant cell and 6 percent eosinophilic form of myocarditis (Magnani et al., 2006). The viral etiology of myocarditis is thought to be the primary causative agents in most cases. However, a direct causative relationship still less well established in many clinical occasions. The majority of these cases are classified as lymphocytic myocarditis.

The Dallas criteria considered to be the first attempt to develop standardized histopathological description of biopsy samples from patients presented with myocarditis (Aretz et al., 1987). However, the histopathology alone can be inadequate to identify the presence of active myocarditis. Some clinicians feel that the definition is too narrow owing to the limitation by variable interpretation, lack of clinical prognostic values, and low sensitivity (Baughman, 2006). A combination of histopathologic characteristics and clinical criteria has been proposed in 1991 (Lieberman et al., 1991) as an alternative scheme to be utilized in the diagnosis of myocarditis. Histologic evidence of myocarditis was demonstrated in 35 of 348 patients submitted to endomyocardial biopsy over 5 years. Analysis of the histologic findings and clinical course of these patients resulted in a clinicopathologic classification of myocarditis in which four clinical subgroups are identified.

2.1 Fulminant myocarditis

The fulminant myocarditis is less frequent form of presentation. Patients presents with acute heart failure and cardiogenic shock up to two weeks after a distinct viral prodrome. They have severe cardiovascular compromise and may require mechanical circulatory support. Multiple foci of active myocarditis are typical. The histopathologic finding does not match the clinical phenotypic severity. The ventricular dysfunction often normalizes if patients survive the acute illness or results in death (McCarthy et al., 2000). In one series, 14 of 147 patients (10.2 percent) with clinical myocarditis presented in a fulminant fashion, with the triad of hemodynamic compromise, rapid onset of symptoms (usually within 2 weeks), and fever (McCarthy et al., 2000). On follow up, 93 percent of the original cohorts were alive and transplant free 11 years following initial biopsy, compared with only 45 percent in those with more classic forms of acute myocarditis.

2.2 Acute myocarditis

Classically, patients with acute myocarditis presents with a less distinct onset of illness with nonspecific symptoms related to the heart. Viral prodrome occurs between 20 and 80 percent of the cases, can be readily missed by the patient, and thus cannot be relied upon for diagnosis. They present with an established ventricular dysfunction and may respond to immunosuppressive therapy or their condition may progress to dilated cardiomyopathy. In a series of 245 patients with clinically suspected myocarditis, the most common symptoms include fatigue (82 percent); dyspnea on exertion (81 percent); arrhythmias (55 percent, both supraventricular and ventricular); palpitations (49 percent); and chest pain at rest (26 percent), (Kuhl et al., 2005). The presentation can mimic acute coronary syndromes in view of troponin release, ST segment elevation on electrocardiogram, and segmental wall motion abnormalities on echocardiogram.

2.3 Chronic active myocarditis

This group of patients with chronic active myocarditis represents the majority of older adult with myocarditis. They are also presents with a less distinct onset of illness and often insidious with symptoms compatible with moderate ventricular dysfunction such as fatigue and dyspnea. Affected patients may initially respond to immunosuppressive therapy but often have clinical and histologic relapses and develop ventricular dysfunction associated with chronic inflammatory changes, and mild to moderate fibrosis on histological study including giant cells.

2.4 Chronic persistent myocarditis

This group of patients with chronic persistent myocarditis, whom also presents with a less distinct onset of illness, is characterized by a persistent histological infiltrate, often with foci of myocyte necrosis but without ventricular dysfunction, despite other cardiovascular symptoms such as chest pain or palpitation.

The previously depicted four forms are still used to describe the clinical presentation and progression of myocarditis, particularly in the absence of ongoing histological evaluation. These categories may also provide some prognostic information and may suggest which patients can or cannot benefit from immunosuppressive therapy.

A new diagnostic criteria derived from limited data was proposed in 2009. The Lake Louise Consensus Criteria utilizes the cardiac magnetic resonance imaging (CMR) for the diagnosis of myocarditis (Friedrich et al., 2009). The CMR enhances the ability to detect myocardial inflammation through noninvasive means, as well as to improve diagnostic accuracy. In these criteria, four major domains are considered when making the diagnosis including, clinical presentation compatible with myocarditis, evidence of new or recent onset myocardial damage, increased T2 signal or delayed enhancement on CMR (compatible with myocardial edema and inflammation), and endomyocardial biopsy evidence of myocardial inflammation. The use of CMR appears suitable to identify patients with significant ongoing inflammation, which may be especially important for patients with recurrent or persisting symptoms and in patients with new onset heart failure. The awareness came out that the recommendations proposed by these criteria are based on limited data and that not all centers will be able to apply all components of the suggested protocol.

3. Clinical manifestation

Myocarditis is synonymous with inflammatory cardiomyopathy which has a wide range of clinical presentation, from subtle to devastating clinical scenario that contributes to the difficulties in diagnosis and classification of this disorder. There are few population-based, epidemiologic studies which have defined the presenting symptoms of acute myocarditis; this is due to the absence of a safe and sensitive noninvasive test that can confirm the diagnosis. Worldwide, the true frequency of disease in its less severe forms, whether clinical or subclinical, across various age segments of the population are more difficult to appreciate. Table 1 summarized the most significant clinical manifestations and physical findings in patients presented with myocarditis. Typically myocarditis has a bimodal age distribution in the general population, with the acute presentation more commonly seen in young children and teenagers. In contrast, the presenting symptoms are more subtle and insidious, often with dilated cardiomyopathy and heart failure in the older adult population. Most studies of acute myocarditis reported a slight preponderance in male patients (Caforio et al., 2007). The male-to-female ratio is 1.5 to 1, which may be related to a protective effect of natural hormone variations on immune responses in women (Schwartz et al., 2004). The variable clinical manifestation of myocarditis in part reflects the variability in histological disease severity. Myocardial inflammation may be focal or diffuse, involving any or all cardiac chambers. Severe, diffuse myocarditis can result in a clinical manifestation of acute dilated cardiomyopathy.

Many patients with myocarditis present with a nonspecific illness characterized by fatigue, mild dyspnea, and myalgias. Most cases of viral myocarditis are subclinical; therefore, the patient infrequently seeks medical attention during acute illness. These subclinical cases may have transient electrocardiographic abnormalities. The reported antecedent infectious viral syndrome is highly variable, ranging from 10 percent to 80 percent of patients with viral myocarditis (Baboonian & Treasure, 1997; Feldman & McNamara, 2000; Imazio et al., 2008; Mason et al., 1995). The appearance of cardiac specific symptoms occurs primarily in the subacute virus clearing phase; therefore, patients commonly present two weeks after the acute viremia.

A few patients present acutely with fulminant congestive heart failure secondary to widespread myocardial involvement. Animal models have lead to a much greater understanding of the fulminant clinical course of myocarditis in which a rapid progression, severe ventricular dysfunction and cardiovascular collapse occurs (Ellis & Di Salvo, 2007). Fulminant myocarditis, manifested by severe hemodynamic compromise requiring high dose vasopressor support or mechanical circulatory support, was identified in 15 of 147 patients (10.2 percent) in a large prospective study (McCarthy et al., 2000). Fulminant cases were additionally characterized by a distinct viral prodrome, fever, and abrupt onset (generally <3 days) of advanced heart failure symptoms. These patients typically have severe global left ventricular dysfunction and minimally increased left ventricular end-diastolic dimensions. Of note, either borderline or active lymphocytic myocarditis can produce this dramatic clinical presentation. The histological features of chronic myocarditis are usually produced a more subtle clinical course. Adults may present with heart failure years after initial index event of myocarditis.

Clinical manifestations

1. Subclinical presentation (most cases of viral myocarditis)
2. Nonspecific symptoms (e.g fatigue, arthralgias and myalgias)
3. Clinical presentation, including :
   - Shortness of breath, orthopnea or paroxysmal nocturnal dyspnea
   - Pedal edema
   - Chest pain (concomitant pericarditis)
   - Palpitation (arrhythmias)
   - Presyncope or syncope (atrioventricular block)
   - Sudden cardiac death (dysrhythmic death)
   - Fever
   - Flu-like syndrome (e.g pharyngitis or tonsillitis)
   - Thromboembolic symptoms (systemic or pulmonary)

Physical findings

1. Normal or unremarkable findings
2. Relevant physical signs, including :
   - Tachypnea
   - Cyanosis
   - Elevated jugular venous pressure
   - Tachycardia
   - Signs of cardiovascular collapse and shock
   - Diffuse apex beat and laterally displaced (cardiomegaly)
   - Diminished intensity of first heart sound
   - Third and fourth heart sound summation gallops
   - Murmurs of mitral or tricuspid valves regurgitation
   - Pericardial friction rub and effusion (concomitant myopericarditis)
   - Bibasilar crackles
   - Hepatomegaly
   - Ascites
   - Peripheral edema

Table 1. The most significant clinical manifestations and physical findings in patient with myocarditis

The medical history may embrace a number of hints that merits an emphasis. Previous history of rheumatic heart disease or symptoms defined by Jones criteria e.g. fever or arthralgia can be a clue for the clinical diagnosis acute rheumatic fever. History of tick bite may correlate with suspected Lyme disease. Patients treated for neoplastic disorders with chemotherapeutic agents like doxorubicin may draw attention to anthracyclines-induced myocarditis. History of travel to Central or South America can be a clue for the diagnosis of Chagas disease. Additionally, giant-cell myocarditis should be considered in patients with acute dilated cardiomyopathy associated with thymoma, autoimmune disorders, ventricular tachycardia, or high-grade heart block. Furthermore, an unusual cause of myocarditis, such as cardiac sarcoidosis, should be suspected in patients who present with chronic heart

failure, dilated cardiomyopathy and new ventricular arrhythmias, or second-degree or third degree heart block or who do not have a response to standard care (Yazaki et al., 1998).
In the European Study of the Epidemiology and Treatment of Inflammatory Heart Disease, a 3055 patients with suspected acute or chronic myocarditis were screened, of them 72 percent had dyspnea, 32 percent had chest pain, and 18 percent had arrhythmias (Hufnagel et al., 2000). The most important clinical manifestations in patients with myocarditis are as followed:

3.1 Shortness of breath

Dyspnea on exertion and fatigue are common. A history of shortness of breath at rest, orthopnea, pedal edema or paroxysmal nocturnal dyspnea is suggestive of congestive heart failure. Dyspnea is due to left ventricular dysfunction causes elevated left ventricular diastolic pressure and low cardiac output.

3.2 Chest pain

Chest pain is usually associated with concomitant pericarditis. Chest discomfort is reported in one third of patients. The pain is most commonly described as a pleuritic, sharp, stabbing precordial pain. It may be substernal and squeezing and, therefore, difficult to distinguish from that typical of ischemic pain. However, myocarditis can be masquerading as an acute coronary syndrome both clinically and on the electrocardiogram, particularly in younger patients (Angelini et al., 2000). In one series of 34 patients with known normal coronary anatomy presenting with symptoms and electrocardiographic changes consistent with an acute coronary syndrome, 11 (32 percent) of the patients were found to have myocarditis on biopsy (Dec et al., 1992). Sarda et al., using myocardial indium111-labeled antimyosin antibody and rest thallium imaging, identified 35 of 45 patients (78 percent) who presented with acute chest pain, ischemic electrocardiographic abnormalities, and elevated cardiac biomarkers as having diffuse or focal myocarditis. However biopsy verification of actual myocarditis was not undertaken in this series. Complete recovery of left ventricular function occurred at six months in 81 percent of these patients (Sarda et al., 2001). Some presentations of myocarditis, especially those related to parvovirus B19, present like an acute lateral wall myocardial infarction. The ischemia associated with myocarditis may be due to localized inflammation or occasionally, due to coronary artery spasm (McCully et al,. 2005). It is essential for clinicians to consider acute myocarditis in younger patients who present with acute coronary syndromes when coronary risk factors are absent, electrocardiographic abnormalities extend beyond a single coronary artery territory or global rather than segmental left ventricular dysfunction is evident on echocardiography.

3.3 Palpitation, presyncope or syncope

Palpitation is a common presentation in patient with myocarditis. Presyncope or syncope in a patient with a presentation consistent with myocarditis may be a signal for high-grade atrioventricular block and risk for sudden death. Small focal inflammation in electrically sensitive areas may be the etiology of patients whose initial presentation is sudden death.

3.4 Fever

Fever with or without sweats and chills occur in 20 percent of patients presenting with myocarditis. A history of fever or flu-like syndrome in form of pharyngitis, tonsillitis, or upper respiratory tract infection before admission occurs in 50 percent of patients (Imazio et al., 2008).

3.5 Other symptoms

Apart from the nonspecific symptoms recognized like malaise, myalgias and arthralgias, other extracardiac symptoms may identify infectious, toxic agents or autoimmune diseases affecting the heart and resulting in a myocarditis. A viral prodrome of fever, myalgias, and muscle tenderness may precede viral myocarditis, while a delayed hypersensitivity reaction may be first apparent from a cutaneous rash. Rash, fever, peripheral eosinophilia, or a temporal relation with recently initiated medications or the use of multiple medications suggest a possibility of hypersensitivity myocarditis.

The clinical diagnosis of myocarditis is challenging due to its varying presentation, nonspecific symptoms and physical findings. Accordingly, a high level of clinical suspicion is warranted and a presumptive diagnosis usually made based on patient demographics and the clinical course.

4. Physical examination

The physical examination of patient presented with myocarditis is frequently normal. Mild cases of patients with myocarditis may appear to have a simple viral syndrome. More acutely ill patients with acute myocarditis have the classic signs of circulatory impairment due to congestive heart failure. Patients may shows signs of fluid overload including elevated jugular venous pressure, bibasilar crackles, hepatomegaly, ascites and peripheral edema. More severe cases may show cardiovascular collapse and signs of shock. In addition to the signs of fluid overload, the physical examination may reveal direct evidence of cardiovascular signs in symptomatic patients. Tachypnea and tachycardia are common. Tachycardia is often out of proportion to fever. Cyanosis may occur as well. The apex beat may be diffuse and laterally displaced suggesting cardiomegaly. Heart auscultation may reveal diminished intensity of first heart sound. The third and occasionally fourth heart sound summation gallops may be noted with impaired ventricular function, particularly when biventricular acute myocardial involvement results in systemic and pulmonary congestion. If the right or left ventricular dilatation is severe, auscultation may reveal murmurs of mitral or tricuspid valves regurgitation. Table 1 summarized the most significant clinical manifestations and physical findings in patients presented with myocarditis.

A pericardial friction rub and effusion may become evident in some patients with diffuse inflammation as a result of myopericarditis. Pericardial tamponade was reported in very rare occasions. Pleural friction rub may develop as the inflammatory process involves surrounding structures. In cases where a dilated cardiomyopathy has developed, signs of peripheral or pulmonary thromboembolism may be encountered. Certain physical findings may imply a specific cause of myocarditis. Enlarged lymph nodes might suggest systemic sarcoidosis. A pruritic, maculopapular rash may suggest a hypersensitivity reaction, often to a drug or toxin. Acute rheumatic fever can present with the modified Jones criteria.

5. Electrocardiogram findings

Generally, the Electrocardiogram (ECG) is a sensitive means in myocarditis. However, its diagnostic value is limited by the low specificity and a wide diversity of changes which

observed during the course of disease. The ECG must be timely repeated, since minor abnormalities detected initially may become subsequently more apparent.
The ECG findings associated with myocarditis may include first, second or third degree atrioventricular block, intraventricular conduction delay (widened QRS complex), bundle branch or fascicle block, reduced R wave height, abnormal Q waves, ST-T segment changes or low voltage. In one report, either ST-segment elevation or T-wave inversion is present as the most sensitive ECG criterion in <50% of patients, even during the first weeks of the disease (Morgera et al., 1992). A gradual increase in the width of the QRS complex may be a sign of exacerbation of myocarditis. Frequent premature beats, supraventricular tachycardia and atrial fibrillation may arise as well. Arrhythmias such as sinus arrest, ventricular tachycardia, ventricular fibrillation or asystole may occur and threaten the life of patients with myocarditis. Hence, continuous ECG monitoring is crucial to detect potentially fatal arrhythmias.

6. Clinical manifestation of complications

Despite the fact that a substantial number of myocarditis are never coming to medical attention, a less frequent form of myocarditis is fulminant and leads rapidly to cardiovascular collapse and shock that required mechanical ventilation support. In contradiction, if these patients survive the first 3-4 weeks of illness they have almost complete recovery and far fewer long term complications compared with those patients with more indolent courses (Chau et al., 2006; Khabbaz et al., 2007). Generally, there are a number of well recognized complications that may encounter in the variety of clinical scenarios of patients with myocarditis.

6.1 Congestive heart failure

In many patients who develop heart failure, fatigue and decreased exercise capacity are the initial manifestations. However, diffuse, severe myocarditis, if rapid in evolution, can result in acute myocardial failure and cardiogenic shock. Signs of right ventricular failure include increased jugular venous pressure, hepatomegaly, and peripheral edema may supervene. The decline in right ventricular function "protects" the left side of the circulation so that signs of left ventricular failure may not be seen. If, however, there is predominant left ventricular involvement, the patient may present with the symptoms of pulmonary congestion including dyspnea, orthopnea, pulmonary crackles, and, in severe cases, acute pulmonary edema. Patients with persistent viral genome expression show limited recovery of left ventricular function, decreased stroke volume index and more stiffness of the ventricle with the resultant long-term morbidity of heart failure and a mortality of nearly 25 percent (Fuse et al., 2000).

6.2 Arrhythmias

A number of arrhythmias may be seen during the clinical course of myocarditis. Sinus tachycardia is more frequent than serious atrial or ventricular arrhythmias, while palpitations secondary to premature atrial or, more often, ventricular premature complexes are common. Ventricular arrhythmias and variable heart blocks are uncommon, but well recognized clinical presentations (Hosenpud et al., 1986; Marboe & Fenoglio et al., 1988). Persistent complex ventricular arrhythmias after apparent resolution of myocarditis were reported in children and young adults as well (Friedman et al., 1994).

Several series have examined the frequency of myocarditis among patients evaluated for life threatening ventricular arrhythmias that occurred in the absence of structural heart disease (Strain et al., 1983; Sugrue et al., 1984; Vignola et al., 1984). These patients tended to be young (younger than 50 years) and to have normal or near-normal left ventricular systolic function. The frequency of syncope or cardiac arrest as reported has ranged from 8 percent to 61 percent (Strain et al., 1983; Sugrue et al., 1984). Biopsy evidence of myocarditis among patients without structural heart disease has ranged from 8 percent to 50 percent. On the other hand, patients with ventricular arrhythmias due to lymphocytic or granulomatous myocarditis stay at higher risk. Sustained ventricular tachycardia or new heart block in the setting of rapidly progressive congestive heart failure suggests giant cell myocarditis. Granulomatous myocarditis has been associated more frequently with life threatening ventricular arrhythmias, syncope, and high-grade atrioventricular block requiring temporary or permanent ventricular pacing than has lymphocytic myocarditis (Davidoff et al., 1991; Fleming & Bailey, 1981; Sekiguchi et al., 1996). Furthermore, granulomatous myocarditis might be suspected in patients who present with apparently chronic dilated cardiomyopathy yet with new ventricular arrhythmias or heart block or who do not have a response to optimal care (Yazaki et al., 1998).

6.3 Sudden cardiac death

The risk of sudden dysrhythmic death in patients with myocarditis is increasingly appreciated in the current morbidity and mortality data. The discovery of myocarditis in 1 to 9 percent of routine postmortem examinations suggests that myocarditis is a major cause of sudden, unexpected death (Feldman & McNamara, 2000).

Although heart failure and cardiomyopathy are more common clinical presentations, patients with myocarditis may present with syncope or unexpected sudden cardiac death, presumably due to ventricular tachycardia or fibrillation (Drory et al., 1991; Eckart et al., 2004; Maron et al., 2003; Theleman et al., 2001). Myocarditis is a significant cause of sudden, unexpected death in adults younger than age 40 years and elite young athletes. In these presumably healthy individuals, autopsy findings have revealed myocarditis in up to 20 percent of cases (Wesslen et al., 1996). In an autopsy series of patients under age 40 who presented with sudden death in the absence of known heart disease, myocarditis was responsible for 22 percent of cases under age 30 and 11 percent in older subjects (Drory et al., 1991). In another autopsy study of sudden death occurring in 1866competitive athletes, myocarditis was present in 6 percent of the cardiovascular deaths (Maron et al., 2009). In one more series of autopsies in military recruits, myocarditis accounted for 20 percent of deaths due to identifiable structural cardiac abnormalities (Eckart et al., 2004).

6.4 Dilated cardiomyopathy

A substantial subset of symptomatic cases of postviral or lymphocytic myocarditis present with a syndrome of heart failure and dilated cardiomyopathy. A clinical and pathologic syndrome that is similar to dilated cardiomyopathy (DCM) may develop after resolution of viral myocarditis in animal models and biopsy proven myocarditis in human subjects (Gilbert & Mason, 1987). This has led to speculation that DCM may develop in some individuals as a result of subclinical viral myocarditis. Theoretically, an episode of myocarditis could initiate a variety of autoimmune reactions that injure the myocardium and ultimately result in the development of DCM. These abnormalities in immune regulation and the variety of antimyocardial antibodies present in DCM are consistent with this hypothesis. Enteroviral RNA sequences may be found in heart biopsy samples in DCM but with a very variable frequency (0–30 percent), (Bowles et al., 1986; Giacca et al., 1994). Furthermore, analysis of human viruses other than enteroviruses suggests that adenoviruses, herpes, and cytomegalovirus can also cause myocarditis and potentially DCM, particularly in children and young subjects (Martin et al., 1994; Pauschinger et al., 1999).

In most acute cases of lymphocytic myocarditis, left ventricular function improves over one to six months with standard heart failure care. However a substantial minority will develop a persistent inflammation that leads to chronic cardiomyopathy. In the patients who develop chronic cardiomyopathy, the risk of heart transplantation and death is high. In a large review of 1230 cases of initially unexplained cardiomyopathy, 9 percent were thought to be due to myocarditis (Felker et al., 2000). A similar prevalence of 10 percent was noted in the Myocarditis Treatment Trial in which endomyocardial biopsy was performed in over 2200 patients with unexplained heart failure of less than two years duration (Mason et al., 1995).

6.5 Thromboembolism

Thromboembolism, arterial and venous, is more evident in patients with left ventricular dysfunction, and appears to be quite frequent complication in certain forms of myocarditis and cardiomyopathies. Additionally, the risk of thromboembolism from either tissue or thrombus from the biopsy site is higher in left ventricular biopsy. Right-sided thromboembolism can be due to thrombus from the venous access sheath especially with the internal jugular approach. The possibility of some small added diagnostic yield by taking biopsy samples of the left ventricle in addition to the right is outweighed by the small attendant risk of systemic embolism.

Thromboembolism is frequent in advanced Chagas disease, and its occurrence is probably underestimated (Bestetti, 2000; Samuel et al., 1983). At autopsy, 73 percent of patients have left or right ventricular mural thrombi, with evidence of pulmonary or systemic embolization in 60 percent (Arteaga-Fernandez et al., 1989). The apical aneurysm typical of Chagas disease is particularly prone to the formation of thrombi and is associated with a high incidence of thromboembolic events (Fernandes et al., 1987). Furthermore, there is a high incidence of thromboembolism in population with peripartum cardiomyopathy. Thrombi are the result of the hypercoagulable state of pregnancy and of stasis and turbulent flow in the dilated heart. Thrombi often form in patients with lower left ventricular ejection fraction (<35 percent), (Amos et al., 2006; Sliwa et al., 2006). Higher mortality rates have been reported to be due to thromboembolism as well (Ford et al., 2000).

6.6 Recurrent myocarditis

The clinical course of myocarditis in the majority of patients is self-limited and there is complete resolution of myocardial inflammation without further relapse or sequelae. However, the disease has been observed to recur in a similar scenario to initial presentation, which then may resolve spontaneously or be associated with heart failure, arrhythmias, or death. Chronic myocarditis may be considered to be one of the mechanisms of the process of recurrence. Recurrence was reported to in 10 to 25 percent of patients after apparent resolution of the initial illness (Daly et al., 1984; Dec et al., 1985). Recurrence of myocarditis

is well recognized in patients with acute rheumatic fever. It is also demonstrated in subsequent pregnancies after peripartum cardiomyopathy and recurrence should be suspected if ventricular function subsequently deteriorates (Dec et al., 1985). Women should be counseled to avoid pregnancy after a diagnosis of peripartum cardiomyopathy. Recurrence was also described in giant cell myocarditis in transplanted heart which responded to intensive immunosuppression. History of third time recurrences of active myocarditis proven by endomyocardial biopsy associated with complete atrioventricular block was described as well and viral studies showed no evidence of recent infection (Kanazawa et al., 2004). Another report present recurrent viral myocarditis and vaccine-associated myocarditis in a single patient with complete reversal of the cardiomyopathy and return to normal cardiac function (Makaryus et al., 2006). Moreover, some cases were observed to have recurrent myocarditis after tapering of immunosuppressive therapy and previous biopsy specimens showing healed myocarditis.
One report indicated that pericarditis on initial presentation may be associated with a higher rate of recurrence of myocarditis (Fowler et al., 1973). However, in reality, there are no reliable predictors that identify patients likely to have recurrence.

7. Manifestations of specific forms of myocarditis

Specific clinical forms of myocarditis of variable etiologies will be described below. Table 2 summarized some key clinical hints among specific forms of myocarditis that help with the clinical diagnosis

7.1 Viral myocarditis

Amongst the multiple infectious etiologies which have been implicated as the cause of clinically significant acute myocarditis, viral myocarditis being the most common and the enterovirus coxsackie B being the most significant. Numerous seroepidemiologic and molecular studies were linked coxsackievirus B to outbreaks of myocarditis occurred before the 1990s. The spectrum of viruses that were detected in endomyocardial biopsy samples shifted from coxsackievirus B to adenovirus in the late 1990s. In the last decade a number of reports implicate new viruses in the etiology of myocarditis and dilated cardiomyopathy. The parvovirus B19 was identified in patients with myocarditis in Germany (Kühl et al., 2005; Mahrholdt et al., 2006) and hepatitis C virus was reported in Japan (Matsumori 2005, 2006) as well.
Early studies suggested that cardiac involvement occurred in 3.5 to 5 percent of patients during outbreaks of coxsackievirus infection (Gerzen et al., 1972; Grist & Bell, 1969). Most cases of enteroviral myocarditis or pericarditis occur in children and young adults in whom more than two-thirds are male. In the majority of patients, active myocarditis remains unsuspected because the subclinical and self-limited pattern of presentation or the presence of myocarditis may infer only by the finding of transient electrocardiographic ST-T-wave abnormalities. In addition, subtle cardiac symptoms and signs may be overshadowed by the systemic manifestations of the underlying infection or disease process. Clinically, the patients give a history of a preceding upper respiratory febrile illness or a flu-like syndrome, and viral nasopharyngitis or tonsillitis may be evident. In the United States Myocarditis Treatment Trial, 89 percent of subjects reported a syndrome consistent with a viral prodrome (Mason et al., 1995). The patient may also have fever, myalgias, and muscle tenderness that is followed by chest pain, dyspnea or arrhythmias, and occasionally heart

failure. A pericardial friction rub is documented in half of cases, and the electrocardiogram shows ST segment elevations or ST- and T-wave abnormalities. Most adults recover completely and only a minority of cases progress to chronic dilated cardiomyopathy.

Clinical clues	Clinical diagnosis	Comments
Preceding upper respiratory febrile or flu-like illness (viral nasopharyngitis or tonsillitis)	Viral myocarditis	Often self-limited
Patients present with chronic heart failure, dilated cardiomyopathy and new arrhythmias or heart block with no response to standard care	Sarcoid myocarditis	Enlarged lymph nodes suggest systemic sarcoidosis
Cutaneous rash (pruritic, maculopapular), fever, peripheral eosinophilia or a temporal relation with recently initiated medications or the use of multiple medications	Hypersensitive/ eosinophilic myocarditis	
Patients treated anti-neoplastic chemotherapeutic agents	Anthracyclines-induced myocarditis	
History of travel to Central or South America, Systemic or pulmonary thromboembolism	Chagas disease	The apical aneurysm is typical in advanced disease
History of residence or travel through the endemic area; previous tick bites; prior or current erythema migrans lesions and coexistence of neurologic dysfunction	Lyme disease	Varying degrees of atrioventricular conduction block is common
Previous history of rheumatic heart disease or symptoms defined by Jones criteria e.g. erythema marginatum, polyarthralgia, chorea, subcutaneous nodules fever or arthralgia	Acute rheumatic fever	
Heart failure developing in the last month of pregnancy or within 5 months following delivery	Peripartum cardiomyopathy	Higher incidence of thromboembolism (hypercoagulable state of pregnancy). More often when left ventricular ejection fraction <35 %
Sustained ventricular tachycardia in rapidly progressive heart failure associated with thymoma, autoimmune disorders, or high-grade heart block	Giant-cell myocarditis	Syncope or sudden death develop due to ventricular arrhythmias or heart block

Table 2. Some key clinical hints among specific forms of myocarditis that help with the clinical diagnosis.

In addition to the coxsackievirus B, other members of the genus Enterovirus (coxsackievirus A, echovirus, and poliovirus) and many other viruses have also been associated less frequently with myocarditis; these viruses include influenza virus, Epstein-Barr virus, cytomegalovirus, human herpesvirus (Kindermann et al., 2008) and varicella-zoster virus. Myocarditis and pericarditis were reported in association with influenza virus infection during the 1918–1919 pandemic. Unusually, myocarditis has also been described as a complication of mumps in a severe but usually self-limited form. Molecular diagnostic assays have implicated mumps virus in some cases of endocardial fibroelastosis following myocarditis as well. In more recent study of 172 patients with a biopsy sample showing myocarditis, the most common viruses were parvovirus B19, 36.6 percent; enterovirus, 32.6 percent; co-infection with HHV-6 and parvovirus B19, 12.6 percent human herpesvirus 6 (HHV-6), 10.5 percent; adenovirus, 8.1 percent (Kuhl et al., 2005).

The novel influenza virus A (H1N1) pandemic began in Mexico in 2009 and rapidly spread worldwide. The cardiac complications of H1N1 infection were uncommonly reported. Sudden death as a result of myocarditis was a rare recognized complication in otherwise immunocompetent individuals, despite the absence of significant respiratory tract infection. A report from Japan described 10 patients presented with fulminant myocarditis which was confirmed by endomyocardial biopsy in 6 patients, 8 of the cases were rescued (Ukimura et al., 2009). Also, a documented influenza myocarditis was reported due to 2009 pandemic H1N1 virus occurred in a previously healthy adult (Haessler et al., 2010). Another reported fatal case of acute myocarditis in an immunocompetent young woman, the autopsy revealed a predominantly lymphocytic myocarditis (Gdynia et al., 2011). On the other hand, cases diagnosed with fulminant myocarditis were described in pediatric population with fatal outcomes within a 30-day of presentation (Bratincsák et al., 2010).

Though viral myocarditis is most often self-limited and without sequelae, fulminant condition with arrhythmias, heart failure occurs. Arrhythmias are common and are occasionally difficult to manage. Patients with fulminant myocarditis may require mechanical cardiopulmonary support or cardiac transplantation, but the majority survived and many demonstrate substantial recovery of ventricular function. Patients with myocarditis and pulmonary hypertension are at a particularly high risk of death. Deaths attributed to heart failure, tachyarrhythmias, and heart block has been reported and it seems prudent to monitor the electrocardiogram of patients with arrhythmias, especially during the acute illness. In some patients, myocarditis simulates acute myocardial infarction, with chest pain, electrocardiographic changes, and elevated serum levels of myocardial enzymes. Additionally, viral myocarditis are assumed to be the major causes of chronic dilated cardiomyopathy, some cases of myocarditis may recur as well, however the number of cases with acute myocarditis that progresses to chronic dilated cardiomyopathy remains anonymous.

7.2 Human immunodeficiency virus (HIV) myocarditis

The human immunodeficiency virus type I (HIV-1) infection that causes the acquired immunodeficiency syndrome (AIDS) has became a worldwide pandemic. It has been identified for more than 3 decades, during which time a number of factors may altered the nature of cardiac manifestation. Notably, the survival in adult with HIV infection and AIDS is prolonged as a result of earlier detection and the use of highly active antiretroviral therapy (HAART), (Hoover et al., 1993; Palella et al., 1998). On the other hand, disorders such as hypertension, hyperglycemia, hyperlipidemia, lipodystrophy and coronary artery disease appeared to add further comorbidity to HIV infection (Fisher & Lipshultz, 2001; Friis-Møller et al., 2007; Tershakovec et al., 2004).

Human immunodeficiency virus is the most common cardiac pathologic finding at autopsy in HIV infected patients with prevalence as high as 70 percent (Anderson et al., 1988; Baroldi et al., 1988, Lewis, 1989). Myocarditis identified at autopsy or on endomyocardial biopsy in HIV-infected patients is most often nonspecific and manifested as focal, inflammatory lymphocytic infiltrates without myocyte necrosis. However, it is uncertain whether the myocarditis so frequently observed at autopsy is clinically relevant.

Myocarditis should be considered in any HIV-infected patient with dyspnea or cardiomegaly. It is most often present with signs and symptoms of congestive heart failure or asymptomatic left ventricular (LV) dysfunction established by echocardiography. Of note, the clinical features of concomitant noncardiac disorders may mask cardiac involvement and steer to inaccurate approach, since myocardial manifestations due of HIV infection may respond at least transiently to standard therapy. A prospective long-term clinical and echocardiographic follow-up study of asymptomatic HIV-positive patients showed a mean annual incidence of progression to dilated cardiomyopathy of 15.9 cases per 1,000 patients. The exact pathogenesis of myocarditis in the AIDS is unclear. Possible direct action of HIV on the myocardial tissue or an autoimmune process induced by HIV, possibly in association with other cardiotropic viruses. It is difficult to assess the clinical significance of viral infection of the myocardium in HIV infected patients. A histologic diagnosis of myocarditis was reported in 83 percent of patients with dilated cardiomyopathy. This significant proportion had focal, nonspecific lymphocytic myocarditis (Barbaro et al., 1998).

Dilated cardiomyopathy can be subclinical or may present with overt clinical findings. Cardiac involvement is often subclinical as echocardiographic studies have demonstrated LV dysfunction in 41 percent of asymptomatic HIV-positive individuals (Corallo et al., 1988). However, in the primary care setting, AIDS cardiac complications are unusual. One autopsy series demonstrated no cardiac disease in 115 consecutive autopsies of patients who died of AIDS-related complications (Lewis, 1989). In one series of 416 HIV-positive patients from Rwanda without a previous history of cardiovascular disease and not receiving HAART reported an echocardiographically evident dilated cardiomyopathy in 17.7 percent (Twagirumukiza et al., 2007). The overt clinical involvement is seen in 10 percent of HIV patients, and the most common clinically significant finding is a dilated cardiomyopathy associated with typical findings of congestive heart failure, namely edema and shortness of breath.

Apart from the clinical manifestation which may be seen as a direct consequence of HIV infection, a more likely, as a consequence of possible etiologies related to non-HIV cardiotrophic viral infection, postviral autoimmune mechanism, drug toxicity or neoplastic infiltration by Kaposi sarcoma or lymphoma.

Since the introduction of HAART regimens there has been a marked reduction in the incidence of myocarditis and opportunistic infections, which has led to a nearly 30 percent reduction in HIV-associated cardiomyopathy (Barbaro, 2005). Opportunistic infections include bacteria, fungi, protozoa, and viruses are the most frequent cause of morbidity and mortality in AIDS which is identified in 10 to 15 percent of cases (Hofman et al., 1993). However, symptomatic disease appears to be rare. Toxoplasma gondii is the most frequently documented infectious cause of myocarditis associated with AIDS. Myocardial toxoplasmosis described in 1 to 16 percent autopsy series of patients dying of AIDS (Anderson et al., 1988; Baroldi et al., 1988; Matturri et al., 1990). Cytomegalovirus is another common opportunistic infection in patients with late stage AIDS that can cause myocarditis in selected patients (Barbaro et al., 1998; Niedt & Schinella, 1985). Other virus identified within the myocardium of HIV-infected or AIDS patients, either at antemortem endomyocardial biopsy or from autopsy material, have included Epstein-Barr and coxsackie B virus in adults (Barbaro et al., 1998; Dittrich et al., 1988) These viruses may be present as either primary infection or as coinfection and can occur with or without associated myocarditis and with or without associated LV dysfunction. Other infections like, myocardial tuberculosis appears to be rare (Miller-Catchpole et al., 1989). Fungal myocarditis is another unusual complication of disseminated infection that is identified most often at autopsy. Various fungal organisms identified in the myocardium at autopsy with associated myocarditis. Cardiac cryptococcus has been diagnosed in association with congestive heart failure and resolved after therapy (Kinney et al., 1989; Lafont et al., 1987; Lewis et al., 1985).

Other possible etiologies of LV dysfunction are drug toxicity from either abuse of illicit substances or iatrogenic disease from agents used in the therapy for AIDS. Alcohol, cocaine, or heroin may contribute to LV dysfunction in many cases (Brown et al., 1991; Peng et al., 1989; Soodini & Morgan, 2001). Therapeutic agents implicated as potential cardiac toxins include zidovudine (d'Amati et al., 1992; Herskowitz et al., 1992), interleukin-2 (Samlowski et al., 1989) and interferon alfa-2 (Deyton et al., 1989; Zimmerman et al., 1994). Neoplastic infiltration of the heart by Kaposi sarcoma is frequently seen at autopsy and usually associated with widespread disease in the terminal phases of AIDS (Silver et al., 1984). Non-Hodgkin lymphoma is also observed in this setting and also associated with widespread disease (Holladay et al., 1992).

7.3 Bacterial myocarditis

Nowadays, myocarditis of infectious etiology caused by non-viral agents is less frequent worldwide. Bacterial involvement of the heart is uncommon, but when it does occur, it is usually as a complication of endocarditis. Various bacteria include (*Corynebacterium diphtheriae, Streptococcus pyogenes, Staphylococcus aureus, Haemophilus pneumoniae, Salmonella* spp., *Neisseria gonorrhoeae, Leptospira, Borrelia burgdorferi, Treponema pallidum, Brucella, Mycobacterium tuberculosis*, Actinomyces, *Chlamydia* spp., *Coxiella brunetti, Mycoplasma pneumoniae* and *Rickettsia* spp). Bacteria like streptococcal and staphylococcal species and *Bartonella, Brucella, Leptospira,* and *Salmonella* species can spread to the myocardium as a consequence of severe cases of endocarditis. Some forms of bacterial myocarditis will be discussed below.

7.3.1 Diphtheritic myocarditis

Worldwide, the most common bacterial cause of myocarditis is diphtheria. As early as 1806, a relationship between infection (diphtheria) and chronic heart disease was postulated, but it was not until the 1970s, with the advent of endomyocardial biopsy, that the diagnosis of myocarditis could be established during life.

The risk of developing cardiac toxicity is proportional to the severity of local infection. *Corynebacterium diphtheriae* produce toxins that inhibit protein synthesis that can cause myocarditis and leads to a dilated, flabby, hypocontractile heart. The manifestations of diphtheritic myocarditis include various dysrhythmias, conduction disturbances, and dilated cardiomyopathy. Cardiomegaly and severe congestive heart failure typically appear after the first week of illness. However, clinically evident cardiac manifestation like dyspnea, decreased heart sounds, gallop rhythm or cardiac dilatation is much less common, occurring in 10 to 25 percent of all patients with diphtheria (Morgan et al., 1963).

Myocarditis occurred in 22 percent of 656 hospitalized patients with diphtheria in the Kyrgyz Republic in 1995; 7 percent of patients with myocarditis and 2 percent of patients without myocarditis died (Kadirova et al., 2000). Myocarditis as evidenced by electrocardiographic changes such as ST-T wave changes, QTc prolongation, and/or first-degree heart block can be detected in as many as two-thirds of cases, often occurring when local respiratory symptoms are improving (Boyer & Weinstein, 1963; Lumio et al., 1948). The conduction system is frequently involved. The complete heart block result from diphtheritic myocarditis was almost always fatal before temporary cardiac pacemakers were developed. Diphtheritic myocarditis considered the most serious complication and remains the major cause of mortality (Kneen et al., 2004). The death rate is highest during the first week of illness particularly among patients with bull-neck diphtheria and among patients with myocarditis who develop ventricular tachycardia, atrial fibrillation, or complete heart block.

7.3.2 Lyme myocarditis

Lyme disease is an inflammatory disease caused by infection with the spirochete *Borrelia burgdorferi*. In United States, carditis occurs in approximately 5 percent, while, it is less frequent in Europe, affecting approximately 0.3 to 4.0 percent of untreated adults (Cox et al., 1991). This difference may be related to infection by different organisms.

A careful history should address risk factors or possible evidence of *B. burgdorferi* infection particularly in the presence of atrioventricular conduction abnormalities (McAlister et al., 1989). These include history of residence or travel through an endemic area; previous tick bites; prior or current erythema migrans lesions and coexistence of objective or subjective neurologic dysfunction compatible with neurologic Lyme disease. Cardiac Lyme disease occurs during the early disseminated phase of the disease, usually within weeks to a few months after infection (Fish, 2008). In a patient with suspected Lyme disease after a tick bite, the possibility of coinfection with Ehrlichia (ehrilichiosis) and Babesia (babesiosis) should be considered as both can also cause myocarditis.

There is a male predominance of approximately 3:1 in cardiac Lyme disease (Vlay, 1993). Patients with cardiac involvement may be asymptomatic and clinically inapparent. However, some patients develop symptomatic myocarditis with cardiac muscle dysfunction and/or associated pericarditis (Vlay et al., 1991) (Lorcerie et al., 1987). Symptoms mainly include palpitations, shortness of breath, chest pain, presyncope or syncope. In a review of 84 patients with Lyme carditis, the United States Centers for Disease Control and Prevention reported palpitations in 69 percent, conduction abnormalities in 19 percent, myocarditis in 10 percent and left ventricular failure 5 percent (Ciesielski et al., 1989). Endomyocardial biopsy samples resemble idiopathic lymphocytic myocarditis, and rarely the spirochetal organisms are identified (Cox et al., 1991; McAlister et al., 1989; Stanek et al., 1990).

Atrioventricular conduction block of varying degrees are the most common manifestation of Lyme carditis. In some patients, heart block is the first and only manifestation of Lyme disease (Kimball et al., 1989). Patients may present with first degree heart block but can progress to second degree or complete heart block over a short period of time (Peeters et al., 1990). One review of 52 patients with Lyme carditis found that 87 percent had atrioventricular block, which was usually symptomatic (McAlister et al., 1989). Wenckebach periodicity occurred in 40 percent and complete atrioventricular block in 50 percent; other findings include bundle branch and fascicular blocks, which are rare. In another report, 38 percent of patients with Lyme carditis required a temporary pacemaker (Goldings & Jericho, 1986). Patients with a PR interval greater than 300 milliseconds carry a highest risk for progression to complete heart block, which may develop rapidly (Steere et al., 1980). Complete heart block caused by Lyme disease typically resolves within one week, and more minor conduction disturbances within six weeks (Fish, 2008; McAlister et al., 1989). More reports showed heart block usually persists for 3 to 42 days and often resolves spontaneously (Costello et al., 2009; Cox et al., 1991; Steere et al., 1980; van der Linde et al., 1989). In Europe, scattered case reports have suggested that *B. burgdorferi* may, in isolated cases, be a cause of chronic cardiomyopathy (Bartůnek et al., 2006; Palecek et al., 2010). This has not been shown in the United States. A small Dutch series evaluated 42 patients with dilated cardiomyopathy (Vlay et al., 1991). Nine were seropositive for anti-B. burgdorferi; six recovered fully, two had a partial response, and one showed no improvement.

7.3.3 Salmonella myocarditis

Typhoid fever is a life-threatening illness rarely complicated by myocarditis. Salmonella myocarditis may produce variable clinical manifestations from latent to severe clinical forms, such as acute congestive heart failure or sudden cardiac death (Al-Aqeedi et al., 2009; Burt et al., 1990). Postmortem studies suggest that myocarditis is a major cause of sudden unexpected death in young adults and may account for 20 percent of cases (Feldman & McNamara, 2000).

7.3.4 Yersinia myocarditis

Myocarditis sometimes occurs as a complication of Yersinia. Clinical evidence of Campylobacter-associated myocarditis described in association with *Campylobacter* spp. enteritis (Kotilainen et al., 2006). Mild, self-limited myocarditis accompanies 10 percent of cases of Yersinia induced arthritis and can occur independently. Typical manifestations include cardiac murmurs and transient electrocardiographic abnormalities, such as prolongation of the PR interval and nonspecific ST-segment and T wave changes. The syndrome of Yersinia-induced arthritis and carditis can be confused with acute rheumatic fever.

7.3.5 Legionella myocarditis

Myocardial involvement is a rare manifestation of Legionella infection, though, the most common extrapulmonary site of Legionnaires' disease is the heart. Numerous reports have described myocarditis, pericarditis, postcardiotomy syndrome, and prosthetic valve endocarditis (Antonarakis et al., 2006; Lowry & Tompkins, 1993; Tompkins et al., 1988). Most cases have been hospital acquired. Legionella carditis in the adult population is invariably seen in association of pneumonia, however, isolated Legionella myocardial involvement without associated pneumonia have been reported (Burke et al., 2009).

7.3.6 Mycoplasma myocarditis

Cardiac abnormalities rarely reported in conjunction with *Mycoplasma pneumoniae* infection including myocarditis and pericarditis (Martin & Bates, 1991; Paz & Potasman, 2002).

Myocarditis has been described in rare autopsy reports as well. Cardiac manifestations include rhythm disturbances, congestive heart failure, chest pain, and conduction abnormalities on the electrocardiogram.

7.3.7 Q fever myocarditis

Myocarditis, though uncommon, may be a particularly severe manifestation of Q fever. A study of 1070 patients with acute Q fever from southern France, 1 percent had pericarditis, and 1 percent had myocarditis. In other series of 1276 patients with Q fever over a 15-year period, only eight developed myocarditis but two were among only 12 total patients with Q fever who died (Fournier et al., 2001). Q fever may also cause endocarditis which usually occurs in patients with previous valvular damage or immunocompromise particularly a bicuspid aortic valve or a prosthetic valve.

7.3.8 Chlamydial myocarditis

Chlamydial infection also has been reported in association with clinical manifestations of myocarditis (Mavrogeni et al., 2008).

7.3.9 Relapsing fever myocarditis

Relapsing fever is an arthropod-borne infection characterized by recurrent episodes of fever, caused by spirochetes of the genus Borrelia. The first episode of illness tends to be the most severe. Myocarditis appears to be common in both louse-borne and tick-borne relapsing fever. Clinical and electrocardiographic evidence of myocarditis and myocardial dysfunction includes a prolonged QTc interval, commonly a galloping third heart sound, elevated central venous pressure, arterial hypotension, and rare pulmonary congestion. Heart involvement has been prominent in fatal cases (Wengrower et al., 1984).

7.4 Acute rheumatic fever

Acute rheumatic fever (ARF) is a nonsuppurative complication of group A streptococcus pharyngitis that occurs two to four weeks following infection and arises as an autoimmune response to extracellular or somatic bacterial antigens that share similar epitopes in human tissue. Rheumatic fever remains one of the most important cardiovascular diseases that cause significant cardiac morbidity and mortality in developing countries (Hutchison, 1998). In developed countries, ARF is generally preceded by pharyngitis but not skin infection (Guidelines for the diagnosis of rheumatic fever, JAMA 1992). However, data from endemic regions with ARF and rheumatic heart disease suggest a less clear association (McDonald et al., 2004, 2006; Noel et al., 2005).

Acute rheumatic fever occurs most frequently in children from 5 to 15 years of age. The incidence of rheumatic heart disease in patients with a history of ARF is variable; in general, valvular damage manifesting as a murmur later in life is likely to occur in about 50 percent of patients with evidence of carditis at initial presentation (Albert et al., 1995; Meira et al., 2005). The myocardial lesions consist of nonspecific lymphocytic myocarditis and Aschoff nodules. The latter are pathognomonic of ARF. Myocarditis is often indicated by cardiomegaly and/or congestive heart failure (CHF) particularly in the absence of a significant pericardial effusion. The presence of valvulitis is established clinically by auscultatory findings. Although CHF in rheumatic fever patients traditionally has been ascribed to severe myocardial inflammation, endomycardial biopsy in patients with rheumatic carditis does not show significant evidence of myocyte damage (Narula et al., 1993). In addition, echocardiographic left ventricular ejection fraction and indices of myocardial contractility remain normal in patients with rheumatic carditis even in the presence of CHF (Essop et al., 1993). Further, CHF occurs only in the presence of hemodynamically significant valvular lesions.

The diagnosis of ARF is established largely on clinical grounds. The clinical manifestations initially described by Jones (Jones, 1944). Subsequently revised and lastly the established guidelines for the diagnosis of rheumatic fever reviewed by the American Heart Association Working Group in 2002 (Ferrieri, 2002). The five major manifestations include migratory arthritis, carditis and valvulitis, central nervous system involvement (eg, Sydenham chorea), erythema marginatum and subcutaneous nodules. Whereas, the four minor manifestations include, arthralgia, fever, elevated acute phase reactants (erythrocyte sedimentation rate, C-reactive protein) and prolonged PR interval. The probability of ARF is high in the setting of group A streptococcal infection followed by two major manifestations or one major and two minor manifestations. Strict adherence to the Jones criteria in areas of high prevalence may result in under detection of the disease. This was illustrated in a report of 555 cases of confirmed ARF among Australian aboriginals in whom monoarthritis and low-grade fever were important manifestations (Carapetis & Currie, 2001).

7.5 Chagas myocarditis

Chagas disease is a protozoan infection due to *Trypanosoma cruzi*; transmitted by an insect vector, produces an extensive myocarditis that typically becomes evident years after the initial infection. It is a major public health problem in endemic areas and in immigrants from rural Central or South America. Chagas myocarditis is by far the most common form of cardiomyopathy in Latin American countries (Schofield & Dias, 1991). Chagas disease consists of acute and chronic phases. During the chronic phase, many patients present the indeterminate form. The latter describes patients who have positive serology, but no symptoms, physical signs, or laboratory evidence of organ involvement (Dias, 1989).

7.5.1 Acute phase

The first signs of acute Chagas' disease develop at least 1 week after contact with the infected vector. Local skin indurated erythema and swelling produces the typical portal of entry lesions at the skin known as chagomas accompanied by local lymphadenopathy. The conjunctiva portal of entry may result in a unilateral painless periorbital edema and swelling of the palpebrae (Romana's sign). Infection can also occur through blood transfusion, congenital transmission, and, much less often, organ transplantation, laboratory accident, breast feeding, and oral contamination (Benchimol Barbosa, 2006). Although heart transplantation for Chagas cardiomyopathy has been successfully performed, reactivation of *Trypanosoma cruzi* is common. These initial local signs may be followed by malaise, fever sweating, myalgias anorexia, and a morbilliform rash may also appear. Generalized lymphadenopathy and hepatosplenomegaly may develop. Cardiac failure occur secondary to myocarditis; cardiac involvement is present in over 90 percent of those in whom the diagnosis is made (Pinto et al., 2004). The frequency and severity of myocarditis are inversely proportional to age (Dias & Kloetzel, 1968). The acute symptoms resolve spontaneously in virtually all patients, who then enter the asymptomatic or indeterminate phase of chronic T. cruzi infection. The electrocardiogram normalized in over 90 percent of patients after one year.

The indeterminate form usually lasts 10 to 30 years and only approximately 30 percent of the patients develop overt cardiac disease. Most patients remain asymptomatic throughout life. The natural history of this phase of disease is characterized by subtle degree of cardiac involvement and gradual appearance of clinical or electrocardiographic markers of cardiac involvement, which signals the onset of the chronic phase. In one review, progression from indeterminate to the full-blown clinical form in the chronic phase occurred at approximately 2 percent per year (Dias, 1989). In another report, 38.3 percent of patients with positive serology but without symptoms developed chagasic cardiomyopathy over a 10-year period (Coura et al., 1985). About 50 percent of patients remain with the indeterminate form indefinitely (Marin-Neto et al., 2003).

7.5.2 Chronic phase

The chronic form is characterized by dilatation of several cardiac chambers, fibrosis and thinning of the ventricular wall, aneurysm formation (especially at the left ventricular apex), and mural thrombi.

Chronic progressive heart failure is the rule and is associated with poor survival. Mortality associated with the chronic phase almost exclusively due to cardiovascular involvement. The cause of death is sudden cardiac death in 55 to 65 percent, progressive heart failure in 25 to 30 percent, and stroke in 10 to 15 percent (Rassi et al., 2001). Symptoms and physical signs at this stage of the disease arise from three basic syndromes that often coexist in the same patient, heart failure, cardiac dysrhythmia, and thromboembolism (systemic and pulmonary). Heart failure in Chagas heart disease is usually biventricular and commonly presented with fatigue. However, right-sided failure manifested with increased jugular venous pressure, peripheral edema, ascites, and hepatomegaly is characteristically more pronounced than those of left-sided failure manifested with dyspnea and pulmonary rales. Both systolic and diastolic dysfunction can occur (Sousa et al., 1988). Cardiac examination typically reveals the findings of murmurs of mitral and tricuspid regurgitation, wide splitting of the second heart sound due to right bundle branch block and prominent diffuse apical thrust.

Cardiac arrhythmias may cause palpitation, lightheadedness, dizziness, or syncope. Autonomic dysfunction results in marked abnormalities in the heart rate changes. Chest pain is common symptom and usually atypical in Chagas heart disease. It may mimic angina due to abnormal coronary vasomotion postulated as underlying mechanism (Marin-Neto et al., 1992). Sudden cardiac death accounts for 55 to 65 percent of deaths in CD; the real frequency of this complication is probably underestimated, particularly in rural areas (Rassi et al., 2001). Sudden cardiac arrest can occur even in previously asymptomatic patients (Rassi Júnior et al., 1995). However, most patients have severe underlying heart disease, including ventricular aneurysms at multiple sites (posterior-lateral, inferior basal, or apical), which is a characteristic finding in Chagas heart disease (Rassi Júnior et al., 1995). Sudden death is usually precipitated by exercise, and can be caused by VT or fibrillation, asystole, or complete AV block (Mendoza et al., 1986). The electrocardiogram is abnormal in most patients with cardiac involvement and typically shows right bundle branch block, left anterior hemiblock and diffuse ST-T changes, which may progress to complete atrioventricular block.Ventricular arrhythmia may also be seen in form of premature beats that may be multiform and runs of nonsustained ventricular tachycardia. The severity of ventricular arrhythmias tends to correlate with the degree of LV dysfunction. Other changes like, abnormal Q waves, various degrees of atrioventricular block, QT interval prolongation and variation in the QT interval (QT dispersion) are frequent findings (Salles et al., 2003).Virtually all types of atrial and ventricular arrhythmias occur frequently, atrial fibrillation and low QRS voltage may be observed in advanced disease.

A potentially serious complication of chronic Chagas heart disease is thromboembolism. In a review of 1345 autopsies, cardiac thrombus or thromboemboli reported in 44 percent; both right and left cardiac chambers equally affected (Samuel et al., 1983). Although thromboembolic phenomena were more common in the systemic circulation, pulmonary embolism accounted for 14 percent of deaths. Cardioembolism appears to be an important cause of acute ischemic stroke. One series of 94 patients with Chagas disease in Brazil reported higher rate of cardioembolism (56 versus 9 percent) as compared to control group (Carod-Artal et al., 2005). Stroke was also reported significantly more frequent in patients who had Chagas disease related cardiomyopathy compared with patients who had other cardiomyopathies (15.0 versus 6.3 percent), (Oliveira-Filho et al., 2005). Echocardiography or contrast ventriculography may reveal a left ventricular apical aneurysm, regional wall motion abnormalities,or diffuse cardiomyopathy. The cause of death is either intractable CHF or an arrhythmia, with a minority of patients dying from embolic phenomena.

7.6 Fungal myocarditis

The incidence of invasive fungal disease has dramatically increased over the past few decades corresponding to the rising number of immunocompromised patients. Cardiac fungal infection, especially myocarditis, may be difficult to recognize clinically and may in itself produce a fatal outcome. Myocardial involvement frequently occurs in disseminated fungal infection in which multiple organs often affected. Conditions that appear predisposing to fungal infection are human immunodeficiency virus infection, medication like, corticosteroids, antineoplastic agents or broad-spectrum antibiotics, alone or in combination with invasive medical procedures (Nosanchuk, 2002). Candida was the most frequently observed organism, while Aspergillus was the second most frequent fungus to involve the heart. Rarely Cryptococcus identified as a cause of myocarditis as well.

7.7 Eosinophilic and hypersensitivity myocarditis

The association between eosinophilia (eosinophil count >500/mm3) and heart disease was first identified by Loeffler (Loeffler, 1936). A specific eosinophilic form of myocarditis identified following drug-induced hypersensitivity reactions and systemic hypereosinophilic syndromes (Taliercio et al., 1985).

Eosinophilic myocarditis is characterized by a predominantly mature eosinophils infiltration of the myocardium and other organ systems. It occurs in association with systemic diseases such as hypereosinophilic syndrome, Churg-Strauss syndrome and Löffler's endomyocardial fibrosis. Also it may occur in association with cancer, parasitic, helminthic or protozoal infections such as Chagas disease, toxoplasmosis, schistosomiasis, trichinosis, hyatid cysts and visceral larval migrans (Corradi et al., 2004; Corssmit et al., 1999; Spodick, 1997). Eosinophilic myocarditis has been reported after vaccination for several diseases, including smallpox (Arness et al., 2004; Barton et al., 2008). Acute eosinophilic necrotizing myocarditis is a rare aggressive form of eosinophilic myocarditis and may represent an extreme form of hypersensitivity myocarditis which characterized by acute onset and rapidly results in cardiovascular deterioration and circulatory collapse carried high mortality rates (Cooper & Zehr, 2005). The clinical manifestations of eosinophilic myocarditis may include right and left congestive heart failure, endocardial and valvular fibrosis leading to regurgitation, and formation of endocardial thrombi. Clinical awareness warranted when presentation may mimics acute myocardial infarction, with ischemic chest pain and ST-segment elevation on electrocardiography (Galiuto et al., 1997).

Hypersensitivity myocarditis is a form of eosinophilic myocarditis due to autoimmune reaction affecting the heart muscle, often induced by drug. It is often first discovered at postmortem examination. In one series, the prevalence of clinically undetected hypersensitivity myocarditis in explanted hearts ranged from 2.4 to 7 percent (Wu et al., 2002).

Numerous drugs have been implicated in hypersensitivity myocarditis including, antibiotics (Burke et al., 1991) like penicillins, cephalosporins and sulfonamides; antipsychotics (Killian et al., 1999) like clozapine and tricyclic antidepressants (Ansari et al., 2003; Burke et al., 1991; Kounis et al., 1989); others like methyldopa, hydrochlorothiazide, furosemide, tetracycline, azithromycin, aminophylline, phenytoin and benzodiazepines (Ben m'rad et al., 2009; Pursnani et al., 2009; Taliercio et al., 1985). Hypersensitivity myocarditis not constantly develop early in the course of medication. Patients taking the antipsychotic agent clozapine have been reported to develop myocarditis more than two years after the drug was started (Haas et al., 2007). Prolonged continuous infusion of dobutamine has also been associated with hypersensitivity myocarditis which has been reported in 2.4 to 23 percent (Spear, 1995; Takkenberg et al., 2004). Cocaine also rarely produce a hypersensitivity myocarditis, unlike the hypereosinophilic syndrome, peripheral eosinophilia is typically absent (Isner & Chokshi, 1991).

Clinically, the presentation often heralded by fever, peripheral eosinophilia and a drug rash that occurs days to weeks after administration of a previously well-tolerated agent. Electrocardiographic abnormalities show nonspecific ST segment changes or infarct patterns (Fenoglio et al., 1981). Myocardial involvement varies but usually does not result in fulminant heart failure or hemodynamic collapse. However, some patients present with sudden death or rapidly progressive heart failure (Burke et al., 1991; Galiuto et al., 1997).

Eosinophilic myocarditis can be a manifestation of eosinophilia-myalgia syndrome, which is a multisystem disease caused by ingestion of contaminants in L-tryptophan containing products (Belongia et al., 1990), characterized by peripheral eosinophilia and generalized disabling myalgias (Martin et al., 1990). Eosinophils, lymphocytes, macrophages, and fibroblasts accumulate in the affected tissues, but their role in pathogenesis is unclear. The disease is frequently evolves into a chronic course but can be fatal in up to 5% of patients.

7.8 Giant cell myocarditis

Idiopathic giant cell myocarditis is a rare inflammatory disease that often affects previously healthy young adults and frequently fatal type of myocarditis (Cooper et al., 2008). The pathogenesis of this disorder is not known. It is identified by the presence of multinucleated giant cells associated with eosinophils and myocyte destruction in the absence of granulomas on endomyocardial biopsy. It is thought to be primarily autoimmune in nature because of the reported comorbidity with a variety of autoimmune disorders (Cooper et al., 1997), thymoma, (Kilgallen et al., 1998) and drug hypersensitivity (Daniels et al., 2000).

Idiopathic giant cell myocarditis is usually a fulminant form of myocarditis and characterised by a history of rapid progression of severe heart failure associated with refractory sustained ventricular arrhythmias. Giant-cell myocarditis is sometimes distinguished from the much more common postviral myocarditis by the presence of ventricular tachycardia, heart block, and a downhill clinical course, despite optimal clinical care. In the series of 63 patients with giant cell myocarditis enrolled in the multicenter Giant Cell Myocarditis Treatment Trial, 75 percent identified with heart failure symptoms as the primary presentation, 14 percent with ventricular arrhythmia and heart block in 5 percent (Cooper et al., 1997). Most patients will require cardiac transplantation, the median survival from the onset of symptoms of less than 6 months and has an 89 percent rate of death or transplantation. This represents a significantly worse outcome compared to lymphocytic or viral myocarditis. Despite a 25 percent incidence of post-transplantation recurrence of giant cell myocarditis detected by biopsy, the 5-year survival after transplantation is about 71 percent which is comparable to survival after transplantation for cardiomyopathy.

7.9 Systemic lupus erythematosus myocarditis

Acute myocarditis is an uncommon manifestation of systemic lupus erythematosus (SLE), with a prevalence of 8 to 25 percent in different studies (Apte et al., 2008; Mandell, 1987). Myocarditis frequently asymptomatic but less often may accompany other manifestations of acute SLE. In particular pericarditis, commonly occur in about two-thirds of patients, and generally follows a benign course, however tamponade or constriction may occur infrequently.

Myocarditis generally parallels the activity of the disease and, although common histologically, rarely results in clinical heart failure unless associated with hypertension. African American ethnicity is associated with a higher risk of myocarditis compared with Hispanic and Caucasian ethnicity (Apte et al., 2008). Myocarditis should be suspected if there is resting tachycardia disproportionate to body temperature, ST and T wave electrocardiographic abnormalities and unexplained cardiomegaly. The cardiomegaly may be associated with symptoms and signs of heart failure, conduction abnormalities or arrhythmias (Moder et al., 1999). Patients with SLE are at increased risk for myocardial ischemia due to accelerated atherosclerosis or coronary arteritis. Endocardial involvement with fibrinous endocarditis (Libman & Sachs, 1924) is another serious manifestation can lead to valvular insufficiencies or embolic events. Likewise patients with the antiphospholipid syndrome have a higher incidence of valvular disease, a variety of thrombotic disorders, myocardial infarction, pulmonary hypertension, and cardiomyopathy. Myocardial biopsy reveal mononuclear cells infiltration distinguish active myocarditis from fibrosis and other causes of cardiomyopathy (Schattner & Liang, 2003) or rarely cardiotoxicity induced by hydroxychloroquine (Keating et al., 2005). Inflammation may lead to fibrosis that may be manifested clinically as dilated cardiomyopathy.

7.10 Sarcoid myocarditis

It is a granulomatous form of myocarditis. The clinical evidence of myocardial involvement is present in approximately 5 percent of patients with sarcoidosis. However, an autopsy series have reported higher rates of about 25 percent of subclinical cardiac involvement (Chapelon-Abric et al., 2004; Kim et al., 2009; Thomsen & Eriksson et al., 1999). The clinical manifestations of cardiac sarcoidosis are largely nonspecific and may precede, follow, or occur concurrently with involvement of other organs. Sarcoid heart disease should be considered in the evaluation of an otherwise healthy young or middle aged person with cardiac symptoms or in a patient with known sarcoidosis who develops arrhythmias, conduction disease, or heart failure. Patients who present with apparently chronic dilated cardiomyopathy yet with new ventricular arrhythmias or second-degree or third degree heart block or who do not have a response to optimal care are more likely to have cardiac sarcoidosis (Yazaki et al., 1998). Cardiac symptoms were reported in 101 patients, when cardiac sarcoidosis was diagnosed in 84 percent compared to 4 percent in asymptomatic patients (Smedema et al., 2005). Endomyocardial biopsy shows characteristic noncaseating granulomas. However, the diagnosis can also be inferred if there is a tissue diagnosis of sarcoidosis from an extracardiac source in the presence of a cardiomyopathy of unknown origin.

The electrocardiographic abnormalities found in nearly 70 percent of patients with sarcoidosis (Chapelon-Abric et al., 2004). Cardiac involvement with sarcoidosis may produce clinical symptoms and electrocardiographic findings simulating myocardial infarction. Conduction abnormalities in form of first-degree heart block due to disease of the atrioventricular node or bundle of His, and various types of intraventricular conduction defects, are common among patients with cardiac sarcoidosis (Chapelon-Abric et al., 2004). These lesions may initially be silent, but can progress to complete heart block and cause syncope (Yoshida et al., 1997). Sustained or nonsustained ventricular tachycardia and ventricular premature beats are the second most common presentation of cardiac sarcoidosis; electrocardiography reveals ventricular arrhythmias in as many as 22 percent of patients with sarcoidosis (Sekiguchi et al., 1980). Supraventricular arrhythmias are infrequent. Sudden death due to ventricular tachyarrhythmias or conduction block accounts for 25 to 65 percent of deaths due to cardiac sarcoidosis, however, sudden death can occur in the absence of a previous cardiac event (Reuhl et al., 1997; Soejima & Yada, 2009; Yazaki et al., 2001). Both systolic and diastolic heart failure can occur. Left ventricular aneurysms develop in patients with extensive involvement of the myocardium. Mitral incompetence may occur with cardiac sarcoidosis due to associated systolic dysfunction and left ventricular dilation or due to papillary muscle involvement by sarcoid granulomas (Sato et al., 2008). Tricuspid regurgitation with atrioventricular block secondary to infiltration of tricuspid valves and conduction system by sarcoid granulomas has been reported as well (Goyal & Aragam, 2006). A left atrial granulomatous mass resembling myxoma has been reported too (Abrishami et al., 2004).

7.11 Peripartum cardiomyopathy

The syndrome is a rare disorder of pregnancy. It was recognized in 1937, as a distinct clinical entity (Gouley et al., 1937). Currently, the etiology of peripartum cardiomyopathy (PPCM) remains unclear. However, there is compelling data from animal and human studies suggesting that PPCM is actually a type of myocarditis arising from an infectious, autoimmune, or idiopathic etiology. The relationship between pregnancy and viral myocarditis was first published in 1968 (Farber & Glasgow, 1970). Endomyocardial biopsies in women with PPCM have demonstrated myocarditis in many patients. The highest incidence of myocarditis reported in PPCM was 76 percent (Midei et al., 1990), however much lower incidence was reported (8.8 percent), which found to be comparable to an age and sex matched control population undergoing transplantation for idiopathic dilated cardiomyopathy (9.1 percent), (Rizeq et al., 1994). Viral genomes of parvovirus B19, human herpes virus 6, Epstein-Barr virus, and human cytomegalovirus revealed in endomyocardial biopsy specimens from patients with PPCM (Bultmann et al., 2005). Other reported data linked with Chlamydial infection (Cenac et al., 2003).

Women present with heart failure during the peripartum period and become manifested in the last month of pregnancy or within 5 months of the delivery without apparent etiology for the heart failure can be found. The clinical scenario is challenging because many normal women in the last month of a normal pregnancy experience dyspnea, fatigue and pedal edema, symptoms can mimic early congestive cardiac failure. Physical examination can be significant for signs of right and left heart failure. Symptoms and signs that should raise the suspicion of heart failure include paroxysmal nocturnal dyspnea, chest pain, nocturnal cough, new regurgitant murmurs, pulmonary crackles, elevated jugular venous pressure and hepatomegaly. The electrocardiogram usually demonstrates a normal sinus or sinus tachycardia rhythm, but frequent ectopy and other atrial arrhythmias may also be present. Left ventricular hypertrophy, inverted T waves, Q waves, and nonspecific ST-T changes have also been reported (Brown & Bertolet, 1998). Recurrence in a subsequent pregnancy has been reported. However, significant improvement occurs in up to 50 percent of affected women; others are left with a progressive dilated cardiomyopathy.

8. Conclusion

The clinical signs and symptoms of myocarditis are highly variable. A thorough medical history with emphasis on possible causes is essential. A scrupulous awareness to ample clinical scenarios is essential for clinicians, particularly when the cases are lacking apparent etiologies or the presentations being similar to acute myocardial infarction, asymptomatic left ventricular systolic dysfunction, unexplained ventricular tachyarrhythmias or cardiogenic shock. Clinician need to be attentive when evidence of myocardial damage not attributable to epicardial coronary artery disease, primary valvular disease or noninflammatory causes. Usually, most cases of myocarditis are self limited and a spontaneous improvement occurs in a substantial number of patients with lymphocytic disease but is rarely, if ever, observed with granulomatous myocarditis. While routine diagnostic endomyocardial biopsy is not required in most cases of suspected acute myocarditis, the need for biopsy will depend upon the time course and severity of the clinical presentation.

Better understanding of the clinicopathologic aberration that characterize the diverse clinical scenarios and more comprehensive understanding of the natural history of the various subtypes of myocarditis should assist clinicians for better approach and subsequently plan more effective therapy in the future.

9. Acknowledgment

The authors would like to acknowledge Sahera Khalil Al-Nnadaf (H.D.) who actively contributed in preparation and assembly of this chapter.

10. References

Abrishami, B., O'Connel, C., Sharma, O. (2004). Cardiac sarcoidosis with presentation of large left atrial mass. *Curr Opin Pulm Med*, Vol.10, p. 397.

Akhras, F., Dubrey, S., Gazzard, B. (1994). Emerging patterns of heart disease in HIV infected homosexual subjects with and without opportunistic infections; a prospective colour flow Doppler echocardiographic study. *Eur Heart J*, Vol.15, pp. 68-75.

Al-aqeedi, RF., Kamha, A., Al-aani, FK. (2009). Salmonella myocarditis in a young adult patient presenting with acute pulmonary edema, rhabdomyolysis, and multi-organ failure *Journal of Cardiology*, Vol.54, pp. 475-479.

Albert, DA., Harel, L., Karrison, T. (1995). The treatment of rheumatic carditis: a review and meta-analysis. *Medicine (Baltimore)*, Vol.74, p. 1.

Arness, MK., Eckart, RE., Love, SS. (2004). Myopericarditis following smallpox vaccination. *Am J Epidemiol*, Vol.160, pp. 642-651.

Amos, AM., Jaber, WA., Russell, SD. (2006). Improved outcomes in peripartum cardiomyopathy with contemporary. *Am Heart J*, Vol.152, pp. 509-513.

Anderson, DW., Virmani, R., Reilly, JM. (1988). Prevalent myocarditis at necropsy in the acquired immunodeficiency syndrome. *J Am Coll Cardiol*, Vol.11, pp. 792-799.

Angelini, A., Calzolari, V., Calabrese, F. (2000). Myocarditis mimicking acute myocardial infarction: role of endomyocardial biopsy in the differential diagnosis. *Heart*, Vol.84, p. 245.

Ansari, A., Maron, BJ., Berntson, DG. (2003). Drug-induced toxic myocarditis. *Tex Heart Inst J*, Vol.30, pp. 76 -79.

Antonarakis, ES., Wung, PK., Durand, DJ. (2006). An atypical complication of atypical pneumonia. *Am J Med*, Vol.119, p. 824.

Apte, M., McGwin, G, Jr., Vilá, LM. (2008). Associated factors and impact of myocarditis in patients with SLE from LUMINA, a multiethnic US cohort (LV). *Rheumatology (Oxford)*, Vol.47, p. 362.

Aretz, HT., Billingham, ME., Edwards, WD. (1987). Myocarditis: a histopathologic definition and classification. *Am J Cardiovasc Pathol*, Vol.1, pp. 3-14.

Arteaga-Fernandez, E., Barretto, AC., Ianni, BM. (1989). Cardiac thrombosis and embolism in patients having died of chronic Chagas cardiopathy. *Arq Bras Cardiol*, Vol.52, pp. 189-192.

Baboonian, C. & Treasure, T. (1997). Meta-analysis of the association of enteroviruses with human heart disease. *Heart*, Vol.78, pp. 539 -543.

Barbaro, G., Di Lorenzo, G., Grisorio, B. (1998). Cardiac involvement in the acquired immunodeficiency syndrome: a multicenter clinical-pathological study. Gruppo Italiano per lo Studio Cardiologico dei pazienti affetti da AIDS Investigators. *AIDS Res Hum Retroviruses*, Vol.14, p. 1071.

Barbaro, G., Di Lorenzo, G., Grisorio, B. (1998). Gruppo Italiano per lo Studio Cardiologico dei Pazienti Affetti da AIDS. Incidence of dilated cardiomyopathy and detection of HIV in myocardial cells of HIV-positive patients. *N Engl J Med*, Vol.339, pp. 1093-1099.

Barbaro, G. (2005). Reviewing the cardiovascular complications of HIV infection after the introduction of highly active antiretroviral therapy. *Curr Drug Targets Cardiovasc Haematol Disord*, Vol.5, p. 337.

Baroldi, G., Corallo, S., Moroni, M. (1988). Focal lymphocytic myocarditis in acquired immunodeficiency syndrome (AIDS): a correlative morphologic and clinical study in 26 consecutive fatal cases. *J Am Coll Cardiol*, Vol.12, pp. 463-469.

Barton, M., Finkelstein, Y., Opavsky, M. (2008). Eosinophilic myocarditis temporally with conjugate meningococcal C and hepatitis B vaccines in children. *Pediatr Infect Dis J*, Vol.27, pp. 831-835.

Bartůnek, P., Gorican, K., Mrázek, V. (2006). Lyme borreliosis infection as a cause of dilated cardiomyopathy. *Prague Med Rep*, Vol.107(2), pp. 213-226.

Baughman, KL. (2006). Diagnosis of myocarditis: death of Dallas criteria. *Circulation*, Vol.113, pp. 593-595.

Belongia, EA., Hedberg, CW., Gleich, GJ. (1990). An investigation of the cause of the eosinophilia-myalgia syndrome associated with tryptophan use. *N Engl J Med*, Vol.323, p. 357.

Benchimol Barbosa, PR. (2006). The oral transmission of Chagas' disease: an acute form of infection responsible for regional outbreaks. *Int J Cardiol*, Vol.112, p. 132.

Ben m'rad, M., Leclerc-Mercier, S., Blanche, P. (2009). Drug-induced hypersensitivity syndrome: clinical and biologic disease patterns in 24 patients. *Medicine (Baltimore)*, Vol.88, p. 131.

Bestetti, R. (2000). Stroke in a hospital-derived cohort of patients with chronic Chagas' disease. *Acta Cardiol*, Vol.55, pp. 33-38.

Bowles, NE., Richardson, PJ., Olsen, ECJ. (1986). Detection of Coxsackie-B virus specific RNA sequences in myocardial biopsy samples from patients with myocarditis and dilated cardiomyopathy. *Lancet*, Vol.1, pp. 1120–1128.

Boyer, NH. & Weinstein, L. (1948). Diphtheritic myocarditis. *N Engl J Med*, Vol.239, p. 913.

Bratincsák, A., El-Said, HG., Bradley, JS. (2010). Fulminant myocarditis associated with pandemic H1N1 influenza A virus in children. *J Am Coll Cardiol*, Vol.9, pp. 928-929.

Brodison, A. & Swann, JW. (1998). Myocarditis: a Review. *J Infection*, Vol.37, pp. 99–103.

Brown, CS. & Bertolet, BD. (1998). Peripartum cardiomyopathy: a comprehensive review. *Am J Obstet Gynecol*, Vol.178, pp. 409-414.

Brown, J., King, A., Francis, CK. (1991). Cardiovascular effects of alcohol, cocaine, and acquired immune deficiency. *Cardiovasc Clin*, Vol.21, pp. 341-376.

Bultmann, BD., Klingel, K., Nabauer, M. (2005). High prevalence of viral genomes and inflammation in peripartum cardiomyopathy. *Am J Obstet Gynecol*, Vol.193, pp. 363–365.

Burke, AP., Saenger, J., Mullick, F. (1991). Hypersensitivity myocarditis. *Arch Pathol Lab Med*, Vol.115, pp. 764-769.

Burke, PT., Shah, R., Thabolingam, R. (2009). Suspected Legionella-induced perimyocarditis in an adult in the absence of pneumonia: a rare clinical entity. *Tex Heart Inst J*, Vol.36(6), pp. 601-613.

Burt, CR., Proudfoot, JC., Roberts, M. (1990). Fatal myocarditis secondary to Salmonella septicemia in a young adult. *J Emerg Med*, Vol.8, pp. 295 – 297.

Caforio, A., Calabrese, F., Angelini, A. (2007). A prospective study of biopsy-proven myocarditis: prognostic relevance of clinical and aetiopathogenetic features at diagnosis. *Eur Heart J*, Vol.28, pp. 1326-1333.

Carapetis, JR. & Currie, BJ. (2001). Rheumatic fever in a high incidence population: the importance of monoarthritis and low grade fever. *Arch Dis Child*, Vol.85, p. 223.

Carod-Artal, FJ., Vargas, AP., Horan, TA. (2005). Chagasic cardiomyopathy is independently associated with ischemic stroke in Chagas disease. *Stroke*, Vol.36, p. 965.

Cenac, A., Djibo A., Chaigneau, C. (2003). Are anti-Chlamydia pneumoniae antibodies prognosis indicators for peripartum cardiomyopathy? *J Cardiovasc Risk*, Vol.10, pp. 195–199.

Chapelon-Abric, C., de Zuttere, D., Duhaut, P. (2004). Cardiac sarcoidosis: a retrospective study of 41 cases. *Medicine (Baltimore)*, Vol.83, p. 315.

Chau, EM., Chow, WH., Chiu, C. (2006). Treatment and outcome in biopsy proven fulminant myocarditis in adults. *Int J Cardiol*, (June 2006) Vol.110 (3), pp. 405-406.

Ciesielski, CA., Markowitz, LE., Horsley, R. (1989). Lyme disease surveillance in the United States, 1983-1986. *Rev Infect Dis*, 11 Suppl, Vol.6, pp. S1435.

Cooper, LT., Jr, Berry, GJ., Shabetai, R. (1997). Idiopathic giant-cell myocarditis--natural history and treatment. Multicenter Giant Cell Myocarditis Study Group Investigators. *N Engl J Med*, Vol.336, pp. 1860–1866.

Cooper, LT. & Zehr, KJ. (2005). Biventricular assist device placement and immunosuppression as therapy for necrotizing eosinophilic myocarditis. *Nat Clin Pract Cardiovasc Med*, Vol.2, pp. 544-548.

Cooper, LT., Jr, Hare, JM., Tazelaar, HD. (2008). Usefulness of immunosuppression for giant cell myocarditis. *Am J Cardiol*, Vol.102, pp. 1535.

Corallo, S., Mutinelli, MR., Moroni, M. (1988). Echocardiography detects myocardial damage in AIDS: prospective study in 102 patients. *Eur Heart J*, Vol.9, pp. 887-892.

Corradi, D., Vaglio, A., Maestri, R. (2004). Eosinophilic myocarditis in a patient with idiopathic hypereosinophilic syndrome: insights into mechanisms of myocardial cell death. *Hum Pathol*, Vol.35, pp. 1160-1163.

Corssmit, EP., Trip, MD., Durrer, JD. (1999). Löffler's endomyocarditis in the idiopathic hypereosinophilic syndrome. *Cardiology*, Vol.91, p. 272-276.

Costello, JM., Alexander, ME., Greco, KM. (2009). Lyme carditis in children: presentation, predictive factors, and clinical course. *Pediatrics*, Vol.123, pp. e835.

Coura, JR., de Abreu, LL., Pereira, JB. (1985). Morbidity in Chagas' disease. IV. Longitudinal study of 10 years in Pains and Iguatama, Minas Gerais, Brazil. *Mem Inst Oswaldo Cruz*, Vol.80, p. 73.

Cox, J. & Krajden, M. (1991). Cardiovascular manifestations of Lyme disease. *Am Heart J*, Vol.122, pp. 1449-1455.

d'Amati, G., Kwan, W., Lewis, W. (1992). Dilated cardiomyopathy in a zidovudine-treated AIDS patient. *Cardiovasc Pathol*, Vol.1, pp. 317-320.

Daly, K., Richardson, PJ., Olsen, EG. (1984). Acute myocarditis. Role of histological and virological examination in the diagnosis and assessment of immunosuppressive treatment. *Br Heart J*, Vol.51, pp. 30-35.

Daniels, P., Tazelaar, H., Edwards, W. (2000). Giant cell myocarditis as a manifestation of drug hypersensitivity. *Cardiovasc Pathol*, Vol.9, pp. 287-291.

Davidoff, R., Palacios, I., Southern, J. (1991). Giant cell versus lymphocytic myocarditis. A comparison of their clinical features and long-term outcomes. *Circulation*, Vol.83, pp. 953-961.

Dec, GW Jr., Palacios, IF., Fallon, JT. (1985). Active myocarditis in the spectrum of acute dilated cardiomyopathies. Clinical features, histologic correlates, and clinical outcome. *N Engl J Med*, Vol.312, pp. 885-890.

Dec, GW Jr., Waldman, H., Southern, J. (1992). Viral myocarditis mimicking acute myocardial infarction. *J Am Coll Cardiol*, Vol.20, p. 85.

Deyton, LR., Walker, RE., Kovacs, JA. (1989). Reversible cardiac dysfunction associated with interferon alfa therapy in AIDS patients with Kaposi's sarcoma. *N Engl J Med*, Vol.321, pp. 1246-1249.

Dias, JC. & Kloetzel, K. (1968). The prognostic value of the electrocardiographic features of chronic Chagas' disease. *Rev Inst Med Trop Sao Paulo*, Vol.10, p. 158.

Dias, JC. (1989). The indeterminate form of human chronic Chagas' disease A clinical epidemiological review. *Rev Soc Bras Med Trop*, Vol.22, p. 147.

Dittrich, H., Chow, L., Denaro, F. (1988). Human immunodeficiency virus, coxsackievirus, and cardiomyopathy. *Ann Intern Med*, Vol.108, p. 308.

Doolan, A., Langlois, N., Semsarian, C. (2004). Causes of sudden cardiac death in young Australians. *Med J Aust*, Vol.180, pp. 110 -112.

Drory, Y., Turetz, Y., Hiss, Y. (1991). Sudden unexpected death in persons less than 40 years of age. *Am J Cardiol*, Vol.68, pp. 1388-1392.

Eckart, RE., Scoville, SL., Campbell, CL. (2004). Sudden death in young adults: a 25-year review of autopsies in military recruits. *Ann Intern Med*, Vol.141, p. 829.

Ellis, CR. & Di Salvo, T. (2007). Myocarditis: basic and clinical aspects. *Cardiol Rev*, Jul-Aug. Vol.15(4), pp. 170-177.

Essop, MR., Wisenbaugh, T., Sareli, P. (1993). Evidence against a myocardial factor as the cause of left ventricular dilation in active rheumatic carditis. *J Am Coll Cardiol*, Vol.22, pp. 826-829.

Fabre, A. & Sheppard, MN. (2005). Sudden adult death syndrome and other non ischaemic causes of sudden cardiac death: a UK experience. *Heart*, Vol.92(3), pp. 316-320.

Farber, PA., Glasgow, LA., (1970). Viral myocarditis during pregnancy: encephalomyocarditis virus infection in mice. *Am Heart J*, Vol.80, pp. 96–102.

Feldman, AM. & McNamara, D. (2000). Myocarditis. *N Engl J Med*, Vol.343, pp. 1388–1398.

Felker, GM., Hu, W., Hare, JM. (1999). The spectrum of dilated cardiomyopathy: the Johns Hopkins experience with 1,278 patients. *Medicine (Baltimore)*, Vol.78, pp. 270 -283.

Felker, GM., Thompson, RE., Hare, JM. (2000). Underlying causes and long-term survival in patients with initially unexplained cardiomyopathy. *N Engl J Med*, Vol.342, p. 1077.

Fenoglio, JJ, Jr., McAllister, HA, Jr., Mullick, FG. (1981). Drug related myocarditis. I. Hypersensitivity myocarditis. *Hum Pathol*, Vol.12, p. 900.

Fernandes, SO., de Oliveira, MS., Teixeira, Vd. (1987). Endocardial thrombosis and type of left vortical lesion in chronic Chagasic patients. *Arq Bras Cardiol*, Vol.48, pp. 17-19.

Ferrieri, P. Jones Criteria Working Group. (2002). Proceedings of the Jones Criteria workshop. *Circulation*, Vol.106, p. 2521.

Fish, AE., Pride, YB., Pinto, DS. (2008). Lyme carditis. *Infect Dis Clin North Am*, Vol.22, p. 275.

Fisher, SD. & Lipshultz, SE. (2001). Epidemiology of cardiovascular involvement in HIV disease and AIDS. *Ann N Y Acad Sci*, Vol.946, p. 13.

Fleming, HA. & Bailey, SM. (1981). Sarcoid heart disease. *J R Coll Physicians Lond*, Vol.15, pp. 245-253.

Ford, RF., Barton, JR., O'brien, JM. (2000). Demographics, management, and outcome of peripartum cardiomyopathy in a community hospital. *Am J Obstet Gynecol*, Vol.182, pp. 1036-8.

Fournier, PE., Etienne, J., Harle, JR. (2001). Myocarditis, a rare but severe manifestation of Q fever: report of 8 cases and review of the literature. *Clin Infect Dis*, Vol.32, pp. 1440.

Fowler, NO. & Manitsas, GT. (1973). Infectious pericarditis. *Prog Cardiovasc Dis*, Vol.16, pp. 323-336.

Friedman, RA., Kearney, DL., Moak, JP. (1994). Persistence of ventricular arrhythmia after resolution of occult myocarditis in children and young adults. *J Am Coll Cardiol*, Vol.24, pp. 780-783.

Friedrich, MG., Sechtem, U., Schulz-Menger, J. (2009). Cardiovascular magnetic resonance in myocarditis: A JACC White Paper. *J Am Coll Cardiol*, Vol.53, pp. 1475-1487.

Friis-Møller, N. & Reiss, P. (2007). DAD Study Group. Class of antiretroviral drugs and the risk of myocardial infarction. *N Engl J Med*, Vol.356, p. 1723.

Fuse, K., Kodama, M., Okura, Y. (2000). Predictors of disease course in patients with acute myocarditis. *Circulation*, Dec 5, Vol.102(23), pp. 2829-2835.

Galiuto, L., Enriquez-Sarano, M., Reeder, GS. (1997). Eosinophilic myocarditis manifesting as myocardial infarction: early diagnosis and successful treatment. *Mayo Clin Proc*, Vol.72, pp. 603-610.

Gdynia, G., Schnitzler, P., Brunner, E. (2011). Sudden death of an immunocompetent young adult caused by novel (swine origin) influenza A/H1N1-associated myocarditis. *Virchows Arch*, Mar, Vol.458(3), pp. 371-376.

Gerzen, P., Granath, A., Holmgren, B. (1972). Acute myocarditis. A follow-up study. *Br Heart J*, Vol.34, p. 575.

Giacca, M., Severini, GM., Mestroni, L. (1994). Low frequency of detection by nested polymerase chain reaction of enterovirus ribonucleic acid in endomyocardial tissue of patients with idiopathic dilated cardiomyopathy. *J Am Coll Cardiol*, Vol.24, pp. 1033–1040.

Gilbert, EM. & Mason, JW. (1987). Immunosuppressive therapy of myocarditis. In: Engelmeier RS, JB O'Connell, eds. *Drug Therapy in Dilated Cardiomyopathy and Myocarditis*. New York: Marcel Dekker, pp. 233–263.

Goldings, EA. & Jericho, J. (1986). Lyme disease. *Clin Rheum Dis*, Vol.12, p. 343.

Gouley, BA., McMillan, TM., bellet, S. (1937). Idiopathic myocardial degeneration associated with pregnancy and especially the puerperium. *Am J Med Sci*, Vol.19, pp. 185–199.

Goyal, SB. & Aragam, JR. (2006). Cardiac sarcoidosis with primary involvement of the tricuspid valve. *Cardiol Rev*, Vol.14, p. e12.

Grist, NR. & Bell, EJ. (1969). Coxsackie viruses and the heart. *Am Heart J*, Vol.77, p. 295.

Guidelines for the diagnosis of rheumatic fever. Jones Criteria, 1992 update. (1992). Special Writing Group of the Committee on Rheumatic Fever, Endocarditis, and Kawasaki Disease of the Council on Cardiovascular Disease in the Young of the American Heart Association. *JAMA*, Vol.268, p. 2069.

Haas, SJ., Hill, R., Krum, H. (2007). Clozapine-associated myocarditis: a review of 116 cases of suspected myocarditis associated with the use of clozapine in Australia during 1993-2003. *Drug Saf*, Vol.30, p. 47.

Haessler, S., Paez A., Rothberg M. (2010). 2009 Pandemic H1N1-associated Myocarditis in a Previously Healthy Adult. *Clin Microbiol Infect*, Jul 15. Vol.17(4), pp. 572-574.

Heidenreich, PA., Eisenberg, MJ., Kee, LL. (1995). Pericardial effusion in AIDS. Incidence and survival. *Circulation*, Vol.92, pp. 3229-3234.

Herskowitz, A., Willoughby, SB., Baughman, KL. (1992). Cardiomyopathy associated with antiretroviral therapy in patients with HIV infection: a report of six cases. *Ann Intern Med*, Vol.116, pp. 311-313.

Hofman, P., Drici, MD., Gibelin, P. (1993). Prevalence of toxoplasma myocarditis in patients with the acquired immunodeficiency syndrome. *Br Heart J* Vol.70, p. 376.

Holladay, AO., Siegel, RJ., Schwartz, DA. (1992). Cardiac malignant lymphoma in acquired immune deficiency syndrome. *Cancer*, Vol.70, pp. 2203-2207.

Hoover, DR., Saah, AJ., Bacellar, H. (1993). Clinical manifestations of AIDS in the era of pneumocystis prophylaxis. Multicenter AIDS Cohort Study. *N Engl J Med*, Vol.329, pp. 1922-1926.

Hosenpud, JD., McAnulty, JH., Niles, NR. (1986). Unexpected myocardial disease in patients with life threatening arrhythmias. *Br Heart J*, Vol.56, pp. 55-61.

Hufnagel, G., Pankuweit, S., Richter, A. (2000). The European Study of Epidemiology and Treatment of Cardiac Inflammatory Diseases (ESETCID): first epidemiological results. *Herz*, Vol.25, pp. 279-285.

Hutchison, SJ. (1998). Acute rheumatic fever. *J Infect*, Vol.36, pp. 249-253.

Imazio, M., Cecchi, E., Demichelis, B. (2008). Myopericarditis versus viral or idiopathic acute pericarditis. *Heart*, Vol.94, pp. 498-501.

Isner, JM. & Chokshi, SK. (1991). Cardiovascular complications of cocaine. *Curr Probl Cardiol*, Vol.16, pp. 89-123.

Jones, TD. (1944). The diagnosis of rheumatic fever. *JAMA*, Vol.126, p. 481.

Kadirova, R., Kartoglu, HU., Strebel, PM. (2000). Clinical characteristics and management of 676 hospitalized diphtheria cases, Kyrgyz Republic,. *J Infect Dis*, 181 Suppl 1, pp. S110-115.

Kanazawa, H., Hata, N., Yamamoto, E. (2004). Recurrent myocarditis of unknown etiology. *J Nippon Med Sch*, Aug. Vol.71(4), pp. 292-296.

Keating, RJ., Bhatia, S., Amin, S. (2005). Hydroxychloroquine-induced cardiotoxicity in a 39-year-old woman with systemic lupus erythematosus and systolic dysfunction. *J Am Soc Echocardiogr*, Vol.18, p. 981.

Khabbaz, Z., Grinda, JM., Fabiani, JN. (2007). Extracorporeal life support: an effective and noninvasive way to treat acute necrotizing eosinophilic myocarditis. *J Thorac Cardiovasc Surg*, Apr, Vol.133(4), pp. 1122-3, author reply pp. 1123-1124.

Kilgallen, CM., Jackson, E., Bankoff, M. (1998). A case of giant cell myocarditis and malignant thymoma: a postmortem diagnosis by needle biopsy. *Clin Cardiol*, Vol.21, pp. 48-51.

Killian, JG., Kerr, K., Lawrence, C. (1999). Myocarditis and cardiomyopathy associated with clozapine. *Lancet*, Vol.354, pp. 1841–1845.

Kim, JS., Judson, MA., Donnino, R. (2009). Cardiac sarcoidosis. *Am Heart J*, Vol.157, p. 9.

Kimball, SA., Janson, PA., LaRaia, PJ. (1989). Complete heart block as the sole presentation of Lyme disease. *Arch Intern Med*, Vol.149, p. 1897.

Kindermann, I., Kindermann, M., Kandolf, R. (2008). Predictors of outcome in patients with suspected myocarditis. *Circulation*, Vol.118, pp. 639-648. [Erratum, *Circulation*, (2008). Vol.118(12), p. e493.]

Kinney, EL., Monsuez, JJ., Kitzis, M. (1989). Treatment of AIDS-associated heart disease. *Angiology*, Vol.40, pp. 970-976.

Kneen, R., Nguyen, MD., Solomon, T. (2004). Clinical features and predictors of diphtheritic cardiomyopathy in Vietnamese children. *Clin Infect Dis*, Vol.39, pp. 1591.

Kotilainen, P., Lehtopolku, M., Hakanen, AJ. (2006). Myopericarditis in a patient with Campylobacter enteritis: a case report and literature review. *Scand J Infect Dis*, Vol.38(6-7), pp. 549-552.

Kounis, NG., Zavras, GM., Soufras, GD. (1989). Hypersensitivity myocarditis. *Ann Allergy*, Vol.62, pp. 71-74.

Kühl, U., Pauschinger, M., Noutsias, M. (2005). High prevalence of viral genomes and multiple viral infections in the myocardium of adults with "idiopathic" left ventricular dysfunction. *Circulation*, Vol.111, pp. 887-893.

Kuhl, U., Pauschinger, M., Seeberg, B. (2005). Viral persistence in the myocardium is associated with progressive cardiac dysfunction. *Circulation*, Sep 27, Vol.112(13), pp. 1965-1970.

Lafont, A., Wolff, M., Marche, C. (1987). Overwhelming myocarditis due to Cryptococcus neoformans in an AIDS patient. *Lancet*, Vol.2, pp. 1145-1146.

Lewis, W. (1989). AIDS: cardiac findings from 115 autopsies. *Prog Cardiovasc Dis*. 32, pp. 207-215.

Lewis, W., Lipsick, J., Cammarosano, C. (1985). Cryptococcal myocarditis in acquired immune deficiency syndrome. *Am J Cardiol*, Vol.55, p. 1240.

Libman, E. & Sacks, B. (1924). A hitherto undescribed form of valvular and mural endocarditis. *Arch Intern Med*, Vol.33, pp. 701–737.

Lieberman, EB., Hutchins, GM., Herskowitz, A. (1991). Clinicopathologic description of myocarditis. *J Am Coll Cardiol*, Vol.18, pp. 1617-1626.

Loeffler, W. (1936). Endocarditis parietalis fibroplastica mit. Bluteosinophilie.*Schweiz Med Wochenschr*, Vol.17, pp. 817-820.

Lorcerie, B., Boutron, MC., Portier, H. (1987). Pericardial manifestations of Lyme disease. Ann *Med Interne (Paris)*, Vol.138, p. 601.

Lowry, PW. & Tompkins, LS. (1993). Nosocomial legionellosis: a review of pulmonary and extrapulmonary syndromes. *Am J Infect Control*, Vol.21, p. 21.

Lumio, JT., Groundstroem, KW., Melnick, OB. Electrocardiographic abnormalities in patients with diphtheria: a prospective study. *Am J Med*, Vol.116, p. 78.

Magnani, JW., Suk-Danik, HJ., Dec, GW. (2006). Survival in biopsy proven myocarditis: a long-term retrospective analysis of the histopathologic, clinical, and hemodynamic predictors. *Am Heart J*, Vol.151(2), pp. 463-470.

Mahrholdt, H., Wagner, A., Deluigi, CC. (2006). Presentation, Patterns of Myocardial Damage, and Clinical Course of Viral Myocarditis. *Circulation*, Vol.114, pp. 1581-1590.

Makaryus, AN., Revere, DJ., Steinberg, B. (2006). Recurrent reversible dilated cardiomyopathy secondary to viral and streptococcal pneumonia vaccine-associated myocarditis. *Cardiol Rev*, Jul-Aug, Vol.14(4), pp. e1-4.

Mandell, BF. (1987). Cardiovascular involvement in systemic lupus erythematosus. *Semin Arthritis Rheum*, Vol.17, p. 126.

Marboe, CC. & Fenoglio, JJ Jr. (1988). Pathology and natural history of human myocarditis. *Pathol Immunopathol Res*, Vol.7, pp. 226-239.

Marin-Neto, JA., Marzullo, P., Marcassa, C. (1992). Myocardial perfusion abnormalities in chronic Chagas' disease as detected by thallium-201 scintigraphy. *Am J Cardiol*, Vol.69, p. 780.

Marin-Neto, JA., Simões, MV., Maciel, BC. (2003). *Specific diseases: cardiomyopathies and pericardial diseases. Other cardiomyopathies. In: Evidence-Based Cardiology,* 2nd ed, Yusuf, S., Cairns, JA., Camm, AJ. (Eds), BMJ Books, London, p.718.

Maron, BJ., Carney, KP., Lever, HM. (2003). Relationship of race to sudden cardiac death in competitive athletes with hypertrophic cardiomyopathy. *J Am Coll Cardiol*, Vol.41, p. 974.

Maron, BJ., Doerer, JJ., Haas, TS. (2009). Sudden deaths in young competitive athletes: analysis of 1866 deaths in the United States, 1980-2006. *Circulation*, Vol.119, pp. 1085-1092.

Martin, AB., Webber, S., Fricker, FJ. (1994). Acute myocarditis: rapid diagnosis by PCR in children. *Circulation*, Vol.90, pp. 330–339.

Martin, RE. & Bates, JH. (2004). Atypical pneumonia. *Infect Dis Clin North Am*, Vol.5, p. 585.

Martin, RW., Duffy, J., Engel, AG. (1990). The clinical spectrum of the eosinophilia-myalgia syndrome associated with L-tryptophan ingestion. Clinical features in 20 patients and aspects of pathophysiology. *Ann Intern Med*, Jul 15, Vol.113(2), pp. 124-134.

Mason, JW., O'Connell, JB., Herskowitz, A. (1995). A clinical trial of immunosuppressive therapy for myocarditis. The Myocarditis Treatment Trial Investigators. *N Engl J Med*, Vol.333, pp. 269–275.

Matsumori, A. (2005). Hepatitis C virus infection and cardiomyopathies. *Circ Res*, Vol.96, pp. 144-147.

Matsumori, A., Shimada, T., Chapman, NM. (2006). Myocarditis and heart failure associated with hepatitis C virus infection. *J Card Fail*, Vol.12, pp. 293-298.

Matturri, L., Quattrone, P., Varesi, C. (1990). Cardiac toxoplasmosis in pathology of acquired immunodeficiency syndrome. *Panminerva Med*, Vol.32, pp. 194-196.

Mavrogeni, S., Manoussakis, M., Spargias, K. (2008). Myocardial involvement in a patient with chlamydia trachomatis infection. *J Card Fail*, Vol.14(4), pp. 351-353.

McAlister, HF., Klementowicz, PT., Andrews, C. (1989). Lyme carditis: an important cause of reversible heart block. *Ann Intern Med*, Vol.110, pp. 339-345.

McCarthy, RE., Boehmer, JP., Hruban, RH. (2000). Long-term outcome of fulminant myocarditis as compared with acute (non-fulminant) myocarditis. *N Engl J Med*, Vol.342, pp. 690–695.

McCully, RB., Cooper, LT., Schreiter, S. (2005). Coronary artery spasm in lymphocytic myocarditis: a rare cause of acute myocardial infarction. *Heart*, Vol.91, p. 202.

McDonald, M., Currie, BJ., Carapetis, JR. (2004). Acute rheumatic fever: a chink in the chain that links the heart to the throat? *Lancet Infect Dis*, Vol.4, p. 240.

McDonald, MI., Towers, RJ., Andrews, RM. (2006). Low rates of streptococcal pharyngitis and high rates of pyoderma in Australian aboriginal communities where acute rheumatic fever is hyperendemic. *Clin Infect Dis*, Vol.43, p. 683.

Meira, ZM., Goulart, EM., Colosimo, EA. (2005). Long term follow up of rheumatic fever and predictors of severe rheumatic valvar disease in Brazilian children and adolescents. *Heart*, Vol.91, p. 1019.

Mendoza, I., Camardo, J., Moleiro, F. (1986). Sustained ventricular tachycardia in chronic chagasic myocarditis: electrophysiologic and pharmacologic characteristics. *Am J Cardiol*, Vol.57, p. 423.

Midei, MG., DeMent, SH., Feldman, AM. (1990). Peripartum myocarditis and cardiomyopathy. *Circulation*, Vol.81, pp. 922–928.

Miller-Catchpole, R., Variakojis, D., Anastasi, J. (1989). The Chicago AIDS autopsy study: opportunistic infections, neoplasms, and findings from selected organ systems with a comparison to national data. Chicago Associated Pathologists. *Mod Pathol*, Vol.2, pp. 277-294.

Moder, KG., Miller, TD., Tazelaar, HD. (1999). Cardiac involvement in systemic lupus erythematosus. *Mayo Clin Proc*, Vol.74, p. 275.

Morgan, BC. (1963). Cardiac complications of diphtheria. *Pediatrics*, Vol.32, p. 549.

Morgera, T., Di Lenarda, A., Dreas, L. (1992). Electrocardiography of myocarditis revisited: clinical and prognostic significance of electrocardiographic changes. *Am Heart J*, Vol.124, pp. 455- 467.

Narula, J., Chopra, P., Talwar, KK. (1993). Does endomyocardial biopsy aid in the diagnosis of active rheumatic carditis? *Circulation*, Vol.88, pp. 2198-2205.

Niedt, GW. & Schinella, RA. (1985). Acquired immunodeficiency syndrome. Clinicopathologic study of 56 autopsies. *Arch Pathol Lab Med*, Vol.109, p. 727.

Noel, TP., Zabriskie, J., Macpherson, CN. (2005). Beta-haemolytic streptococci in school children 5-15 years of age with an emphasis on rheumatic fever, in the tri-island state of Grenada. *West Indian Med J*, Vol.54, p. 22.

Nosanchuk, JD. (2002). Fungal myocarditis. *Front Biosci*, Jun 1, Vol.7, pp. 1423-1438.

Oliveira-Filho, J., Viana, LC., Vieira-de-Melo, RM. (2005). Chagas disease is an independent risk factor for stroke: baseline characteristics of a Chagas Disease cohort. *Stroke*, Vol.36, p. 2015.

Palecek, T., Kuchynka, P., Hulinska, D. (2010). Presence of Borrelia burgdorferi in endomyocardial biopsies in patients with new-onset unexplained dilated cardiomyopathy. *Med Microbiol Immunol*, May, Vol.199(2), pp. 139-143.

Palella, FJ Jr., Delaney, KM., Moorman, AC. (1998). Declining morbidity and mortality among patients with advanced human immunodeficiency virus infection. HIV Outpatient Study Investigators. *N Engl J Med*, Vol.338, pp. 853-860.

Pauschinger, M., Doerner, A., Kuehl, U. (1999). Enteroviral RNA replication in the myocardium of patients with left ventricular dysfunction and clinically suspected myocarditis. *Circulation*, Vol.99, pp. 889–895.

Paz, A. & Potasman, I. (2002). Mycoplasma-associated carditis. Case reports and review. *Cardiology*, Vol.97(2), pp. 83-88.

Peeters, AJ., Dijkmans, BAC., Sedney, MI. (1990). Lyme borreliosis: A hidden cause of heart block in pacemaker treated males. *IV International Conference on Lyme Borreliosis*, Stockholm, Sweden.

Peng, SK., French, WJ., Pelikan, PC. (1989). Direct cocaine cardiotoxicity demonstrated by endomyocardial biopsy. *Arch Pathol Lab Med*, Vol.113, pp. 842-845.

Pinto, AY., Valente, SA., Valente Vda, C. (2004). Emerging acute Chagas disease in Amazonian Brazil: case reports with serious cardiac involvement. *Braz J Infect Dis*, Vol.8, p. 454.

Pursnani, A., Yee, H., Slater, W. (2009). Hypersensitivity myocarditis associated with azithromycin exposure. *Ann Intern Med*, Vol.150, p. 225.

Rassi, A Jr., Rassi, SG., Rassi, A. (2001). Sudden death in Chagas' disease. *Arq Bras Cardiol*, Vol.76, p. 75.

Rassi Júnior, A., Gabriel Rassi, A., Gabriel Rassi, S. (1995). Ventricular arrhythmia in Chagas disease. Diagnostic, prognostic, and therapeutic features. *Arq Bras Cardiol*, Vol.65, p. 377.

Reuhl, J., Schneider, M., Sievert, H. (1997). Myocardial sarcoidosis as a rare cause of sudden cardiac death. *Forensic Sci Int*, Vol.89, p. 145.

Rizeq, MN., Rickenbacher, PR., Fowler, MB. (1994). Incidence of myocarditis in peripartumcardiomyopathy. *Am J Cardiol*, Vol.74, pp. 474–477.

Salles, G., Xavier, S., Sousa, A. (2003). Prognostic value of QT interval parameters for mortality risk stratification in Chagas' disease: results of a long-term follow-up study. *Circulation*, Vol.108, p. 305.

Samlowski, WE., Ward, JH., Craven, CM. (1989). Severe myocarditis following high-dose interleukin-2 administration. *Arch Pathol Lab Med*, Vol.113, pp. 838-841.

Samuel, J., Oliveira, M., Correa De Araujo, RR. (1983). Cardiac thrombosis and thromboembolism in chronic Chagas' heart disease. *Am J Cardiol*, Vol.52, pp. 147-151.

Sarda, L., Colin, P., Boccara, F. (2001). Myocarditis in patients with clinical presentation of myocardial infarction and normal coronary angiograms. *J Am Coll Cardiol*, Vol.37, p. 786.

Sato, Y., Matsumoto, N., Kunimasa, T. (2008). Multiple involvements of cardiac sarcoidosis in both left and right ventricles and papillary muscles detected by delayed-enhanced magnetic resonance imaging. *Int J Cardiol*, Vol.130, p. 288.

Schattner, A. & Liang, MH. (2003). The cardiovascular burden of lupus: a complex challenge. *Arch Intern Med*, Vol.163, p. 1507.

Schofield, CJ. & Dias, JC. (1991). A cost-benefit analysis of Chagas disease control. *Mem Inst Oswaldo Cruz*, Vol.86, p. 285.

Schwartz, J., Sartini, D., Huber, S. (2004). Myocarditis susceptibility in female mice depends upon ovarian cycle phase at infection. *Virology*, Vol.330, pp. 16-23.

Sekiguchi, M., Numao, Y., Imai, M. (1980). Clinical and histopathological profile of sarcoidosis of the heart and acute idiopathic myocarditis. Concepts through a study employing endomyocardial biopsy. I. Sarcoidosis. *Jpn Circ J*, Vol.44, p. 249.

Sekiguchi, M., Yazaki, Y., Isobe, M. (1996). Cardiac sarcoidosis: diagnostic, prognostic, and therapeutic considerations. *Cardiovasc Drugs Ther*, Vol.10, pp. 495-510.

Silver, MA., Macher, AM., Reichert, CM. (1984). Cardiac involvement by Kaposi's sarcoma in acquired immune deficiency syndrome (AIDS). *Am J Cardiol*, Vol.53, pp. 983-985.

Sliwa, K., Fett, J., Elkayam, U. (2006). Peripartum cardiomyopathy. *Lancet*, Vol.368, pp. 687-693.

Smedema, JP., Snoep, G., van Kroonenburgh, MP. (2005). Cardiac involvement in patients with pulmonary sarcoidosis assessed at two university medical centers in the Netherlands. *Chest*, Vol.128, p. 30.

Soejima, K. & Yada, H. (2009). The work-up and management of patients with apparent or subclinical cardiac sarcoidosis: with emphasis on the associated heart rhythm abnormalities. *J Cardiovasc Electrophysiol*, Vol.20, p. 578.

Soodini, G. & Morgan, JP. (2001). Can cocaine abuse exacerbate the cardiac toxicity of human immunodeficiency virus? *Clin Cardiol*, Vol.24, pp. 177-181.

Sousa, AC., Marin-Neto, JA., Maciel, BC. (1988). Systolic and diastolic dysfunction in the indeterminate, digestive and chronic cardiac forms of Chagas' disease. *Arq Bras Cardiol*, Vol.50, p. 293.

Spear, GS. (1995). Eosinophilic explant carditis with eosinophilia: ? hypersensitivity to dobutamine infusion. *J Heart Lung Transplant*, Vol.14, pp. 755-760.

Spodick, DH. (1995). Eosinophilic myocarditis. *Mayo Clin Proc*, Vol.72, p. 996.

Stanek, G., Klein, J., Bittner, R. (1990). Isolation of Borrelia burgdorferi from the myocardium of a patient with longstanding cardiomyopathy. *N Engl J Med*, Vol.322, pp. 249-252.

Steere, AC., Batsford, WP., Weinberg, M. (1980). Lyme carditis: cardiac abnormalities of Lyme disease. *Ann Intern Med*, Vol.93, p. 8.

Strain, JE., Grose, RM., Factor, SM. (1983). Results of endomyocardial biopsy in patients with spontaneous ventricular tachycardia but without apparent structural heart disease. *Circulation*, Vol.68, pp. 1171-1181.

Sugrue, DD., Holmes, DR Jr., Gersh, BJ. (1984). Cardiac histologic findings in patients with life-threatening ventricular arrhythmias of unknown origin. *J Am Coll Cardiol*, Vol.4, pp. 952-957.

Takkenberg, JJ., Czer, LS., Fishbein, MC. (2004). Eosinophilic myocarditis in patients awaiting heart transplantation. *Crit Care Med*, Vol.32, p. 714.

Taliercio, CP., Olney, BA., Lie, JT. (1985). Myocarditis related to drug hypersensitivity. *Mayo Clin Proc*, Vol.60, pp. 463-468.

Tershakovec, AM., Frank, I., Rader, D. (2004). HIV-related lipodystrophy and related factors. Atherosclerosis, Vol.174, p. 1.

Theleman, KP., Kuiper, JJ., Roberts, WC. (2001). Acute myocarditis (predominately lymphocytic) causing sudden death without heart failure. *Am J Cardiol*, Vol.88, p. 1078.

Thomsen, TK. & Eriksson, T. (1999). Myocardial sarcoidosis in forensic medicine. *Am J Forensic Med Pathol*, Vol.20, p. 52.

Tompkins, LS., Roessler, BJ., Redd, SC. (1988). Legionella prosthetic-valve endocarditis. *N Engl J Med*, Vol.318, p. 530.

Twagirumukiza, M., Nkeramihigo, E., Seminega, B. (2007). Prevalence of dilated cardiomyopathy in HIV-infected African patients not receiving HAART: a multicenter, observational, prospective, cohort study in Rwanda. *Curr HIV Res*, Vol.5, p. 129.

Ukimura, A., Izumi, T., Matsumori, A. (2010). Clinical Research Committee on Myocarditis Associated with 2009 Influenza A (H1N1) Pandemic in Japan organized by Japanese Circulation Society. Collaborators (16) . A national survey on myocarditis associated with the 2009 influenza A (H1N1) pandemic in Japan. *Circ J*, Oct, Vol.74(10), pp. 2193-9.

van der Linde, MR., Crijns, HJ., Lie, KI. (1989). Transient complete AV block in Lyme disease. Electrophysiologic observations. *Chest*, Vol.96, pp. 219.

Vasan, RS., Shrivastava, S., Vijayakumar, M. (1996). Echocardiographic evaluation of patients with acute rheumatic fever and rheumatic carditis. *Circulation*, Vol.94, pp. 73-82.

Vignola, PA., Aonuma, K., Swaye, PS. (1984). Lymphocytic myocarditis presenting as unexplained ventricular arrhythmias: diagnosis with endomyocardial biopsy and response to immunosuppression. *J Am Coll Cardiol*, Vol.4, pp. 812-819.

Vlay, SC. (1993). *Cardiac manifestations in Lyme disease*, Coyle, P (Ed), Mosby-Yearbook, St Louis.

Vlay, SC., Dervan, JP., Elias, J. (1991). Ventricular tachycardia associated with Lyme carditis. *Am Heart J*, Vol.121, p. 1558.

Wengrower, D., Knobler, H., Gillis, S. (1984). Myocarditis in tick-borne relapsing fever. *J Infect Dis*, Vol.149, p. 1033.

Wesslen, L., Pahlson, C., Lindquist, O. (1996). An increase in sudden unexpected cardiac deaths among young Swedish orienteers during 1979-1992. *Eur Heart J*, Vol.17, pp. 902-910

Wu, L., Cooper, LT., Kephart, G. (2002). The Eosinophil in Cardiac Disease. In: Cooper L, ed. *Myocarditis: From Bench to Bedside*, Humana Press, Totowa, NJ, p. 437.

Yazaki, Y., Isobe, M., Hiramitsu, S. (1998). Comparison of clinical features and prognosis of cardiac sarcoidosis and idiopathic dilated cardiomyopathy. *Am J Cardiol*, Vol.82, pp. 537-40.

Yazaki, Y., Isobe, M., Hiroe, M. (2001). Prognostic determinants of long-term survival in Japanese patients with cardiac sarcoidosis treated with prednisone. *Am J Cardiol*, Vol.88, p. 1006.

Yoshida, Y., Morimoto, S., Hiramitsu, S. (1997). Incidence of cardiac sarcoidosis in Japanese patients with high-degree atrioventricular block. *Am Heart J*, Vol.134, p. 382.

Zimmerman, S., Adkins, D., Graham, M. (1994). Irreversible, severe congestive cardiomyopathy occurring in association with interferon alpha therapy. *Cancer Biother*, Vol.9, pp. 291-299.

3

Viral Myocarditis: Physiopathology and Diagnosis

Andréoletti Laurent
Head of the clinical and molecular Virology Unit, University medical centre and EA research team at the Medicine Faculty of Reims
France

1. Introduction

In Europe and the USA, viral aetiologies largely prevail over other causes of myocarditis as previously indicated by recent data demonstrating the molecular detection of cardiotropic viruses in human cardiac biopsy samples (Kühl et al., 2005a). Clinical presentations of the myocarditis range from non-specific systemic symptoms (fever, myalgias, palpitations, or exertional dyspnea) to fulminant hemodynamic collapse (5 to 10 cases per million inhabitants and per year) and sudden cardiac death (Feldman & McNamara, 2000; Magnani & Dec, 2006).

Acute myocarditis remains a complex and challenging diagnosis in cardiology (Magnani & Dec, 2006). This cardiomyopathy is defined histologically by the Dallas criteria as an"inflammation of the myocardium" associated with necrosis and an absence of ischaemia (Aretz et al., 1987; Cooper, 2009; Dennert et al., 2008; Felmann & McNamara, 2000). The use of the Dallas criteria in the diagnosis of myocarditis is associated with poor sensitivity and specificity, mainly because of the sampling error related to the often focal distribution of the specific histological lesions in cardiac tissue and because of the variability in pathological interpretation (Baughman, 2006; Mahrholdt et al., 2004). Moreover, the Dallas classification does not consider local quantification and differentiation of inflammatory cells and does not take into account viral infection and autoimmune regulation in cardiac tissues (Dennert et al., 2008). To improve the histological diagnosis, additional virological and immunological evaluations of cardiac tissues are required using immunohistochemical and PCR techniques, which allow identification and quantification of inflammatory cells and viral infection markers (Dennert et al., 2008). The diagnostic gold standard is endomyocardial biopsy with the histological Dallas criteria in association with new immunohistochemical and viral PCR analyses of cardiac tissues (Cooper et al., 2007). This new diagnostic approach can lead to better identification of the aetiological cause of the myocarditis and can improve the clinical management of viral myocarditis. This chapter chronicles the advances in understanding the physiopathology of viral acute and chronic myocarditis and in the development of new molecular techniques for an accurate and valuable virological diagnosis.

2. Human viral cardiac infection: proofs of concept and clinical relevance

Common human pathogenic DNA or RNA viruses can be responsible for acute or chronic endomyocardial tissue infection (Andréoletti et al., 1995; 2009; Kühl et al., 2005a). The detection of components (DNA or RNA genomes or viral proteins) of these viral agents by molecular techniques such as polymerase chain reaction (PCR) and/or immunohistochemical techniques demonstrating the viral protein expression in the cytoplasm of myocytes, was associated with an inflammation of the myocardium (acute myocarditis), arrhythmias, loss of contractility (Andréoletti et al., 2009; Cooper, 2009; Dennert et al., 2008). Moreover in serial of human cases, the presence of viral persistence was evidenced in the myocardium and associated with a left ventricular systolic dysfunction in relation to a reduction in the contractile function of the myocytes (Andréoletti et al., 2000; Badorff et al., 2001). Additional proofs of concept were that: (I) a longitudinal clinical investigation showed that the type of virus, the clinical presentation and the type of histological damage appeared to be related to the clinical course of the cardiac disease; (II) longitudinal clinical studies indicated that the immune clearance of the virus during or after the acute phase was correlated with an improvement of the left ventricular ejection fraction [LVEF] (Kühl et al. 2005b); (III) acute and chronic myocarditis as well as dilated cardiomyopathy (DCM) were reproduced in immunocompetent animal models following experimental viral infections (Andréoletti et al., 1997; Huber, 1993; Matsumori & Kawai, 1982). Altogether these clinical and experimental data supported the pathophysiological role of several human viruses in the genesis and the evolution of myocarditis and the DCM. Although up to 90% of people will be infected by at least one or more of these viruses in their life without getting their heart injured with associated clinical signs, only a few number will develop clinical symptoms. Therefore, it is highly suspected that a certain genetic background either related to immune alterations or to an improved susceptibility to viral cardiac infection (viral receptor or co-receptors polymorphisms) may be a prerequisite to develop clinical symptoms of myocarditis and/or progression to DCM following virus heart tissue infection. In addition, it has been shown that dystrophin mutations may make easier the development and progression of myocarditis and cardiac failure during coxsackievirus B3 infection, whereas dystrophin and/or sarcoglycan disruption by viral proteases account for myocardial injury (Andréoletti et al., 2007; Badorff et al., 2001; Lee et al., 2000). Human genetic studies of patients with myocarditis are rare and only 2 reports show an association between myocarditis and genetic factors such as HLA-DQ locus and CD45 polymorphism (Yajima & Knowlton, 2009). Future clinical investigations should therefore focus on the understanding of the underlying genetic susceptibility and related immune responses that explain why some patients are susceptible to develop clinical symptoms of acute myocarditis following viral infection, whereas other subjects clinically recover or progress to an 'idiopathic' DCM after the initial phase of the viral cardiac infection.

3. The pathophysiological mechanisms of viral myocarditis

The current understanding of the immunopathologcial phases of myocarditis derives largely from enterovirus-induced myocarditis in murine models (Andréoletti et al, 1997; Cooper et al., 2007; Liu & Mason, 2001; Yajima & Knowlton, 2009). During the enterovirus (virus Coxsackie B) natural course of infection, the data obtained from experimental murine models allowed the identification of three distinct pathophysiological phases defined as acute, sub-acute and chronic myocarditis (Cooper, 2003; Feldman & McNamara, 2000; Yajima & Knowlton, 2009) (Figure 1).

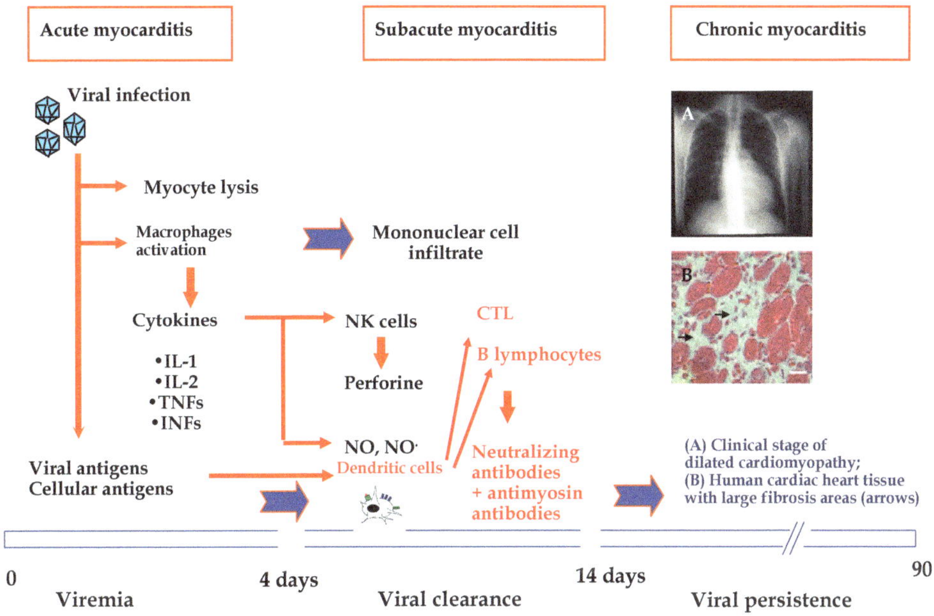

Fig. 1. Immunopathological phases of viral myocarditis.

3.1 Acute myocarditis during the initial Virus invasion

During the period of active viremia, cardiotropic RNA or DNA viruses interact with specific vascular endothelial cell receptors before to be translated in the endomyocardial target cells to produce viral proteins (Huber, 1993; Li et al., 2000) (Table 1). Mechanisms of viral entry into the host cell remains crucial and are of major interest because each of them is putative target for novel therapeutics. Before to interact specifically with the virus, expression of levels of the virus receptors for CVB3, PVB19, HVV6 (CAR/DAF, P-Antigen/ Alpha5-beta1 integrin and CD46, respectively) on endovascular endothelial cells of coronary vessels modulate the diffusion of these viral agents into the vessels and their subsequent translation into the endomyocardial target cells (Khül et al., 2005a; Yajima & Knowlton, 2009). Some inflammatory mechanisms as a primary persistent infection by HHV6 or PVB19 may modulate cell membrane receptors and /or immune suppression and preventing virus clearance; altogether these mechanisms could facilitate an endomyocardial super infection by a second viral agent as described in 27 % of virus positive DCM patients (Khül et al., 2005a) (Table 1).

Common cardiotropic Viruses	Detection Methods	Cardiovascular tissular Localization	Cellular Receptor / Coreceptor Involved	References
Adenovirus	EM	Cardiomyocytes, fibroblasts, endothelial cells	CAR / Integrins ($\alpha v\beta 3$ and $\alpha v\beta 5$)	Shi et al., 2009; Wickham et al., 1993
Enterovirus/ Coxsackievirus B	IHC, ISH	Cardiomyocytes	CAR / DAF	Shi et al., 2009; Coyne & Bergelson, 2006
Parvovirus B19	ISH, LCM + PCR	Endothelial cells, cardiomyocytes	Gb4Cer / Integrin ($\alpha 5\beta 1$); Ku80 autoantigen	Bultmann et al., 2003; Bönsch et al., 2010
Human Herpes Virus 6	In vitro Infection	Endothelial cells	CD46	Caruso et al., 2002; Santoro et al., 1999
Cytomegalovirus	ISH	Cardiomyocytes	Integrins ($\alpha 2\beta 1$, $\alpha 6\beta 1$, and $\alpha v\beta 3$)	Feire et al., 2004; Kyto et al., 2005
Epstein-Barr Virus	ISH	Lymphocytes B	CD21	Chimenti et al., 2004; Takano et al., 2008
Influenza Virus	ISH	Macrophages, Lymphocytes	ND	Cioc et al., 2002

EM indicated electron microscopy; IHC, immunohistochemistry ; ISH, in situ hybridrization; LCM + PCR, polymerase chain reaction using tissue samples isolated with laser capture microdissection; CAR, coxsackie and adenovirus receptor; DAF, decay accelerating factor ; CD, cluster of differentiation and ND, not determined

Table. 1. Cardiovascular tissular localization of common cardiotropic viruses and local suspected cellular receptors involved in the process of infection.

At the beginning of human viral infection, the first line of immune defense consists in the innate immune response (NKT cells, monocytes and macrophages). Cell-mediated immunity also plays an important role in viral clearing. Cytotoxic (CD8+) cells recognize degraded viral protein fragments that are presented by major histocompatibility-complex class I antigens on the myocyte surface (Seko et al., 1990) (Figure 1). The Toll-like receptors located at the surface or inside of dendritic cells (more particularly the Toll-like-receptors 4, 7, and 8 in the case of virus Coxsackie B infection) could recognize certain viral proteins or genomic and then activate intracellular signals (NF-kB pathways) responsible for a fast synthesis and secretion of pro-inflammatory cytokines as interferons and chemokines and also nitric oxide (Ayach et al., 2003; Kawai, 1999; Matsumori et al., 1994) (Figure 1). The pro-inflammatory cytokines then attract and activate many immune system cell lines to the site of the viral infection and they are directly responsible for cardiac myocytes lysis and also for lost of cardiomyocyte contractility and apoptosis cell-dead (Feldman & McNamara, 2000; Ventéo et al., 2010) (Figure 1).

3.2 Sub-acute myocarditis with an activation of the immune system and the development of autoimmunity

The activation of the immune system at the time of the viral invasion reaches to the initiation of specific cellular immunity response and to the immune shift towards a specific immune response. The viral particles are captured by antigen processing cells (APC) and degraded within the Golgi apparatus before being presented at the cell surface by the major histocompatibility complex class I (MHC class I) to the CD8+ lymphocytes. These primed T cells capable to detect the viral antigen will destroy the infected cardiac cells through cytokines or perforines secretion (Kawai, 1999, Matsumori et al., 1994). In addition, some myocardic cellular antigens of the host present can share epitopic similarities (molecular mimicry) with viral antigens therefore inducing an autoimmune trait that can sustain the inflammatory response and therefore the chronic inflammation phases (Figure 1). This sub-acute phase is known to be linked to autoimmune responses as many patients produce auto-antibodies and auto-reactive T cells against heart proteins (Domenico & Gaetano, 2006; Feldman & McNamara, 2000) and the amplification of this phenomenon can lead to the destruction of cardiomyocytes. The mechanisms linking enteroviral infection with sub-acute myocarditis, relapses and post inflammatory heart failure could be mainly mediated by dendritic cells (DCs) that are specialized in antigen processing and presentation and most important in priming of T cells within lymph nodes. The EV-induced autoimmune myocarditis may require activation of these cells via CD40 with Toll like receptors (TLRs 3, 4, 7) or RNA helicases (RIG-I, MAD-5) co-stimulation (Kramer et al., 2008). Moreover in human infections, it is clear that human enteroviruses (HEVs) can escape from immunological system by decreasing the specific functions of immunity cell system (Oldstone, 2006). Recently it has been demonstrated that Enteroviruses could infect and consequently modify the maturation process and some specialized functions of DCs (Kramer et al., 2007). Therefore, Enteroviruses or some of its components could activate or decrease some DCs functions acting as modulators of innate response system or autoimmunity (Kramer et al., 2007).

3.3 Chronic myocarditis with a potential evolution to the dilated cardiomyopathy clinical stage

After the active virus replication resulting in acute and sub acute myocarditis phases, the pathological signs of myocarditis generally disappeared and the destroyed myocytes are replaced by diffuse fibrosis (Dec et al., 1985) (Figure 1). At this stage, a progressive heart bi-ventricular dilatation with a cardiac failure can be observed and has been related to cardiac persistent or chronic viral replication mechanisms (Andréoletti et al., 2000; Badorff et al., 1999) (Figure 1). This persistent or chronic viral infection could be related with various cardiac cell dysfunctions as impairment of Ca+ efflux in cardiomyocytes and of loss of cell contractility, apoptosis balance deregulation, cleavage of dystrophine, modulation of cellular signalling pathways or alteration of the extracellular matrix (Andréoletti et al., 2009; Dennert & McNamara, 2009; Kawai, 2009; Khül et al., 2008a).

4. The Virological mechanisms of cardiac infection

4.1 Acute viral myocarditis

Viruses generally infect human beings by fecal-oral (enteroviruses, *parvovirus* B19, *Herpesviruses*) or respiratory routes (enteroviruses, *influenza viruses A & B, parainfluenza viruses I II III*) and they usually perform a first phase of multiplication into the airway epithelial cells of the higher respiratory tract or tonsils; this can be followed by a potential rapid invasion of the lower respiratory tract as observed during influenza virus infection. After this initial and local replication phase, the viruses can diffuse by lymphatic way to the general circulation (viremic phase) allowing them to reach the cardiac tissues. In the heart, the virus infects and replicate actively into the cardiac myocytes but also into the cardiac fibroblasts that can play the role of reservoir cells for a persistent infection (Andréoletti et al., 2009). During this active phase of replication, the development of the classical clinical signs of myocarditis is usually observed (Andréoletti et al., 2007; Magnani & Dec, 2006).

4.2 The chronic persistent viral Infection in heart tissues

4.2.1 The enterovirus model

After the acute myocarditis phase, persistence can be observed as described during human cardiac enterovirus (EV) infection. In some previous published studies, detection of viral genome has been demonstrated in patients with myocarditis and in patients with DCM, but it is unusual that replication competent virus can be isolated from the myocardium in patients with myocarditis (Andréoletti et al., 2009; Chapman & Kim, 2008a; Copper, 2009). The concept that EV endomyocardial persistent infections are the etiological cause of a subset of idiopathic DCM cases is supported by the detection of enterovirus genomic sequences and enteroviral capsid protein VP1 in up to 35 % of explanted heart tissues from end-stage DCM patients (Andreoletti et al. 2009; Li et al., 2000). In a previous published study, we observed that enteroviruses can persist with or without active viral replication in cardiac tissue of patients with end-stage dilated cardiomyopathy (Andréoletti et al., 2000). Enterovirus genome was detected in 25 of 70 patients with IDCM and, of these patients positive for genomic RNA, only 3 exhibited antigenomic RNA and VP1 antigen that demonstrated active viral replication, whereas 22 had latent infection characterized by the absence of antigenomic RNA associated with or not with VP1 antigen expression. No viral component was detected in control subjects (Andréoletti et al., 2000). These findings demonstrated that a small percentage of patients with end-stage chronic cardiac diseases had active enterovirus replication in their myocardium. Moreover, we demonstrated that enteroviral capsid protein VP1 was present in myocardial tissues from some patients with dilated cardiomyopathy and suggested that the pattern of VP1 detection may correlate with disease stage and severity. These data suggested that viral protein synthesis might be involved in persistent enterovirus infection in the pathogenesis of DCM (Li et al., 2000). It was observed that the ratio of positive- to negative-strand enteroviral RNA was greater with active virus replication than with persistent virus infection where a viral capsid protein synthesis activity was also evidenced in heart cardiac tissues (Andréoletti et al., 2000; Li et al., 2000, Chapman & Kim, 2008a). This slow viral replication could be explained by the existence of 5'NC genomic deleted viral forms that could be related to the development of slow replicating viral forms in heart tissues (Chapman et al., 2008b). As persistent expression of CVB proteins and 2Aprotease (2Apro) alone are sufficient for induction of cardiomyopathy in the mouse and as detection of HEV TD genomes in adult human heart disease is likely due to persistent HEV TD genomes, there is now a new hypothetical mechanism to link of acute viral myocarditis with postviral DCM (Chapman et al. 2008b).

4.2.2 The Parvovirus B19 model

Concerning the Parvovirus B19 virus, a persistent infection was detected in intra-cardiac endothelial cells of small arterioles and veins of patients with chronic cardiomyopathies by in situ hybridization and PCR techniques. This persistent PVB19 infection associated with a low viral replication may be associated with endothelial dysfunction, impairment of myocardial microcirculation, penetration of inflammatory cells and secondary myocyte necrosis. (Duechting et al., 2008). The molecular mechanisms responsible for the reactivation of latent parvovirus B19 infection, the influence of immune activation triggering parvovirus B19 replication and chronic myocarditis, and immune-independent viral pathogenesis remains to be assessed (Bock et al., 2010).

4.3 The chronic latent viral cardiac infections

In cases of *herpesviruses* (HSV1, HSV-2 , HCMV, HHV-6) cardiac infection a latent phase can occur subsequently to the acute phase of infection as demonstrated in a mice model (Grodums & Zbitnew, 1976). During this HSV experimental latent infection, HSV-DNA can be identified as agents of a persistent heart infection in cardiomyocytes, fibroblasts or Schwann cells, which has be seen in unmyelitinated axons in murine heart tissues. In human subjects, CMVH was detected in cardiomyocytes and in cardiac fibroblasts of patients with histological proven myocarditis (Schönian et al., 1995). Moreover, it was not possible to detect viral mRNA coding for structural proteins known as late proteins but only mRNA coding for viral enzymatic proteins (early proteins) related to the regulation of viral replication or associated with the HCMV DNA replication (Lenzo et al., 2002) Whatever, the cellular sites as well as the mechanisms of latency and reactivation of the *herpesviruses* (EBV, HCMV and HHV6) in human heart tissues remain to be assessed (Andréoletti et al., 2009; Cooper, 2009; Dennert et al., 2008).

5. Viral causes for human acute or chronic myocarditis

Human Enteroviruses, (*picornaviridae*), specifically Coxsackie group B serotypes, Parvovirus B19, HHV6 of the B type and the adenovirus are the most frequently etiological viral agents implicated in the acute myocarditis of the child or the young adult (<35 year-old) (Andréoletti et al., 2009; Bowles et al., 2003; Feldman & McNamara, 2000; Kühl et al., 2005b; Magnani & Dec, 2006) (Table 2). Moreover HHV-1, Adenovirus, myxoviruses and also paramyxoviruses including respiratory syncytial virus (RSV), *influenza* and *parainfluenza* strains can also induce an acute infection of cardiac tissue as previously demonstrated in reported acute myocarditis cases developed in immunocompetent patients (Bowles et al., 2003; Dennert et al., 2008). Other viruses as EBV or CMV are also associated with this pathology after heart transplantation. HIV or HCV can be also etiological agents of myocarditis (Matsumori et al., 2006; Sudano et al., 2006) (Table 2).
Recent data showed that it was possible to detect viruses in 71% of the cases of acute myocarditis using molecular techniques for the virological analysis of cardiac biopsy samples (Table 2) (Kühl et al., 2003). Co-infections were found in more than 12% of the cases, generally associating HHV6 and Parvovirus B19. HHV6 seems to be an important cofactor of myocarditis due to Parvovirus B19. HHV6 may enhance the pathogenicity of Parvovirus B19 through alterations of the extracellular matrix and modulation of the expression levels of the PVB19) receptor (P-antigen) on endothelial cells facilitating infections of the coronary vascular endothelium (Table 2) (Kühl et al., 2005a).
Concerning chronic myocarditis, there is no clinical data from transverse or longitudinal studies indicating the incidence of various viral causes of cardiac infection. However, viral persistence in the myocardium was associated with ventricular dysfunction whereas viral genome clearance was related to the hemodynamic improvement (Kühl et al. 2005a, 2005b). As in the cases of acute myocarditis, recent studies showed the interest to test a broad panel of cardiotropic viruses at the DCM stage. Thus, in a case series of 245 patients with clinically suggested DCM, one or more viruses were detected in 67% of the cases (Table 2) (Kühl et al.,

Human cardiotropic Viruses	Acute myocarditis	Dilated Cardiomyopathy	References
Human enteroviruses	14 - 33 %	8 - 35%	Li et al. 2000; Andréoletti et al. 2000, Kühl et al. 2005a, 2005b
Parvovirus B19 (PrvB19)	<1 - 37%	51%	Kühl et al. 2005a, 2005b
Human Herpes Virus 6 (HHV6)	11%	6-22%	Kühl et al. 2005a, 2005b, Mahrhodt et al.2004
Adenovirus	8.1 - 23%	2 - 12%	Kühl et al. 2005a, 2005b, Bowles et al. 2003
Multiple infections (60% of cases = PrvB19+HHV6)	12%	27%	Kühl et al. 2005a, 2005b
Rare viral causes in immunocompetent patients* (non restrictive list)			
Cytomegalovirus (CMVH)	3%	0.8%	Kühl et al. 2005a, 2005b
Epstein Barr Virus (EBV)	<1%	2%	Kühl et al. 2005a, 2005b
Herpes Simplex Virus (HSV)	<1%	-	Kühl et al. 2005a, 2005b
Influenza viruses	<1 - 2%	-	Kühl et al. 2005a, 2005b
Hepatitis C	-	-	-
HIV	-	-	-

*(-) Not determined; * Prevalence determined in cases of solid organ transplantation.*

Table. 1. Prevalence of viruses detected by molecular biology-based techniques in cardiac tissue samples taken from patients with acute myocarditis or dilated cardiomyopathy.

2005a). Moreover in these patients, the absence of associated myocardial inflammation suggests that viral persistence can be responsible for a modulation of the immune response, which would be decreased from the beginning of the chronic phase of myocarditis (Kawai, 1999; Yajima & Knowlton, 2009).

6. Diagnosis of viral causes of myocarditis

Many common human viruses can be the etiological cause of acute or chronic myocarditis in children or young adult patients (Andréoletti et al., 2009). Because of the large number and serotypes of human viruses potentially responsible for cardiac infection the clinical interest of viral serological assay remains of a limited interest in clinical practice (Mhafoud et al., 2011). A recent European study demonstrated that virus serology has no relevance for the diagnosis of myocardial infection in young adults; this study indicated that comparatively to the molecular analysis of endomyocardial biopsy tissues, the positive predictive value was 25% and that the negative predictive value was 49% (Mhafoud et al., 2011).Therefore the etiological diagnosis of viral myocarditis is based on the detection of the viruses or viral components (proteins or genomes) in peripheral blood samples at the time of viremia phase (clinically characterized by fever), but also at the entry and the excretion sites (throat, urine and stool samples), and in heart tissue samples that corresponds to the organ site of viral replication. Therefore, endomyocardial biopsy remains the gold standard for unequivocally establishing the histopathological and virological diagnosis of unexplained cardiomyopathies as acute or chronic myocarditis (Li et al., 2000; Mahrholdt et al., 2004). Its clinical impact on prognosis and treatment largely depends on establishing a rapid and standardized set of diagnostic methods including histopathological and virological analyses of endomyocardial tissue taken by endomyocardial biopsy (Aretz et al., 1987; Mahrholdt et al., 2004).

6.1 Endomyocardial biopsy (EMB)

As recommended by the Heart Failure Society of America and the Heart Failure Association of the European Society of Cardiology, the implementation of a right or left ventricular EMB is indicated in the case of acute symptoms of heart failure refractory to standard management, a substantial worsening of ejection fraction despite optimized pharmacological therapy, the development of hemodynamically significant arrhythmias, an heart failure with concurrent rash, fever, or peripheral eosinophilia, an history of collagen vascular disease such as systemic lupus, erythematosus, scleroderma, or polyarteritis nodosum, and a new-onset cardiomyopathy in the presence of known amyloidosis, sarcoidosis, or hemochromatosis when no obvious cause, in particular ischemic, could be established (Mahrholdt et al., 2004). EMB remains the gold standard for unequivocally establishing the diagnosis of unexplained cardiomyopathy Li et al., 2000). However, its sensitivity and its specificity are limited by the often-focal distribution of the specific histological lesions (Baughman, 2006).

Cardiac biopsy samples should be obtained in more than one area of the right ventricular septum and the number of samples should range from 5 to 10 of a volume from 1 to 2 mm^3. Five of these samples should be fixed in neutralized 10% formalin or 10% PFA; five should be flash-frozen or placed immediately conserved at -80°C to perform further classical or molecular virological techniques (Mahrholdt et al., 2004). Interestingly, it has been recently demonstrated that there were no differences in the number of positive left ventricular-EMB, right ventricular-EMB, or left ventricular- and right ventricular-EMB findings when related to the site of cardiovascular magnetic resonance- based late gadolinium enhancement. Preferential biopsy in regions showing late gadolinium enhancement on cardiovascular magnetic resonance does not increase the number of positive diagnoses of myocarditis. (Yilmaz et al., 2010).

6.2 Histopathological evaluation of cardiac biopsy samples

Histological evaluation of cardiac biopsies from patients with clinically suspected myocarditis is routinely done according to the Dallas criteria (Cooper, 2009). Since myocarditis is a focal disease, 4 to 5 biopsy samples obtained in more than one area of the right ventricular septum should be analysed for light microscopic examination and immunohistochemical assays (Mahrholdt et al., 2004). For routine light microscopy examination, EMB tissue is embedded in paraffin and serial sections are obtained and stained with hematoxylin, eosin. Masson trichrome or Sirius red can be useful for a better evaluation of the fibrosis (Cooper, 2009). Additional slides have to be performed for subsequent immunohistochemical assays (Aretz et al., 1987; Mahrholdt et al., 2004).

To improve the histological diagnosis, additional immunological evaluation of cardiac tissues is required with immunohistochemical techniques allowing quantification, identification, and differentiation of inflammatory cells (Aretz et al., 1987). Criteria for immunohistological diagnosis in the EMB of inflammatory cardiomyopathy is specified quantitatively as >14 infiltrating leukocytes/mm^2, preferably T-lymphocytes or activated T-cells. If foci of T-lymphocytes are present, active myocarditis can be diagnosed due to the nature of the infiltrate even when the critical level of 14 leukocytes/mm^2 is not reached (Aretz et al., 1987). Subsequent biopsies will allow reliable follow-up of the myocarditis with a semi-quantitative evaluation of myocardial inflammation, necrosis and healing. If the levels of inflammation appear unchanged from the most recent previous cardiac biopsies, the term ongoing (or persistent) myocarditis will be used (Cooper, 2009).

Finally in cases of clinically suspected viral myocarditis or unexplained cardiomyopathy, Dallas criteria have to be associated with classical immunohistological assays for the identification of inflammatory cells and also for the detection of viral capsid or early or late antigens in EMBs (Andréoletti et al., 2009).

6.3 Classical virological analyses of samples taken from patients with myocarditis

The etiological diagnosis of viral myocarditis, specifically during the acute phase corresponding to the acute viral infection, is based on the detection of the viruses or viral components (proteins or genomes) in heart biopsy tissue samples and additionally to detection of viral genomes in peripheral biological samples as whole blood (viremia) , throat (classical entry site of viruses) and urine and stool samples. The direct virological techniques are now based on molecular biology (PCR, RT-PCR) and immunohistochemical assays for EMBs. By comparison, the contribution of viral serological assays to the clinical diagnosis of acute or chronic myocarditis is relatively poor and the serological assays are of interest only for a late and retrospective diagnosis of viral myocarditis (Dennert et al., 2009). However, Hepatitis C and B and HIV serologies should be systematic in a patients suffering from acute or chronic myocarditis (Aretz et al., 1987).

Using classical molecular techniques, the genome of enteroviruses, adenoviruses, human hepatitis viruses or *herpesviruses* can be detected in 40 to 70 % of the cardiac tissues of patients suffering from an histological-proven acute myocarditis (Table 1) (Badorff et al., 1999; Gravanis & Sternby, 1991). These molecular techniques must be performed on a pool of several EMBs taken, from different heart tissue areas that should be extracted together in order to optimize the efficiency of viral nucleic acid recovery rates (Mahrholdt et al., 2004). Some specialized laboratories use real-time PCR assays that allow a quantitative approach to estimate viral loads of the majority of cardiotropic viruses. However, no published data exist on the clinical value of real-time PCR viral loads and the determination of clinical thresholds that could be capable to differentiate a viral cardiac replicative infection from a persistent or latent viral endomyocardial infection. Only one published study reported a mean value of 500 copies of PVB19 genome per one microgram of extracted DNA as the clinical threshold related to a significant endomyocardial inflammation (Bock et al., 2010) Only the strategy of associated classical RT-PCR and PCR assays or PCR-microarrays for the detection of all the most common cardiotropic viruses can provide an accurate diagnosis of viral myocarditis. However, sampling error in this focal cardiac disease and the frequent late timing of EMB can also hamper the clinical application of these molecular assays after disease onset. Finally, a positive RT-PCR or PCR result can provide an etiological diagnosis and have to be evaluated into the clinical context, whereas negative PCR results do not exclude a viral-related cardiac disease. Moreover, the only use of the molecular techniques cannot distinguish an active from a persistent viral cardiac infection. Therefore during the clinical course of myocarditis, the immunohistochemical detection of *enterovirus, adenovirus or parvovirus B19* capsid proteins or *herpesviruses* late proteins is necessary in order to differentiate a viral cardiac infection with replication activities from a persistent or latent cardiac infection (Matsumori et al, 2006; Sudano et al., 2006). In the present time, the combination of molecular and immunohistochemical assays on cardiac tissue samples provides a reliable diagnostic strategy for a complete diagnosis of a potential viral-induced acute or latent/persistent cardiac infections. The direct detection of viral genomes in association with the immunohistochemical detection of *viral* capsid or late proteins in cardiac tissues is crucial to characterize the phase of the viral infection (acute or persistent/chronic) and therefore to specifically adapt the therapeutic strategies (Andréoletti et al., 2009; Badorff et al., 1999; Gravanis & Sternby, 1991; Sudano et al., 2006).

6.4 Use of new techniques for the virological analyses of heart samples taken from patients with myocarditis or dilated cardiomyopathy

In the present time, classical real time PCR techniques allow a reliable qualitative detection of viral genomes in cardiac tissues of patients in cases of medical diagnosis of hypokinetic cardiomyopathies (Cooper, 2009) or in series of post mortem or explanted heart tissues (Andréoletti et al., 2000, Dennert et al., 2008; Cooper, 2009). The two critical points remain the number of endomyocardial biopsies (5 to 10) their anatomic origin as well the extraction phase that determine the quality of and the sensitivity of detection of the DNA or RNA viral genomic sequences (Cooper, 2009). The standardization of the extraction phase is now possible by the use of semi-automated or totally automated use of standardized procedure using certified available systems (Renois et al.,2010). A pool of several EMBs taken, from different heart tissue areas have to be extracted together in order to optimize the efficiency of viral nucleic acid recovery rates (Copper, 2009; Dennert et al., 2008). Combination of such automated extraction procedures with monoplex or multiplex classical real time RT PCR techniques can allow an international standardization of the molecular qualitative or quantitative detection of DNA or RNA cardiotropic viruses in human endomyocardial biopsies.

It is now possible to use new multiplex amplification assays followed by a microarray hybridization system allowing a simultaneous of 9 to 12 cardiotropic viruses (herpesviruses or human enteroviruses) in a single analysis. We experienced this system in our laboratory and we observed that multiplex PCR-microarray assay provided a consistently robust qualitative detection of at least 9 viruses in on reaction tube (HSV1, HSV2, CMVH, VZV, HHV6, HHV7, HHV8, enteroviruses species A & B) (unpublished data). We showed that there was a 100% concordance for positive virus detection results and that the theoretical limits of detection were as low as 10 genome copies for CVB3 Nancy per microgram of total RNA. Because the system used intergrated a internal extraction and ampliciation control, it should be assumed that negative results indicate the absence of targeted viruses (Figure 2). The use of such systems could help to standardize the diagnostic detection of cardiotropic viruses in endomyocardial tissues and can be routinely used for a rapid viral detection and screening; however this system is only qualitative and cannot provide semi-quantitative or quantitative viral load values for each detected virus. Therefore in cases of a positive viral detection in cardiac tissues we currently use a second quantitative approach using standardized classical real time viral quantitative detection assays. The obtained results are standardized in viral genome copies per one ug of extracted DNA (Andréoletti et al., 2009, Bock et al., 2010) (Figure 2).

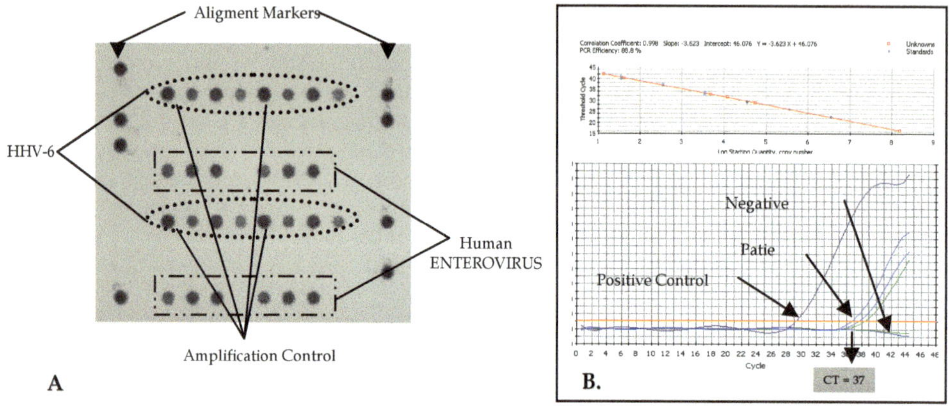

Fig. 2. Detection of a dual Human Enterovirus and HHV6 cardiac infection using a PCR-DNA microarray system in an adult patient with an idiopathic dilated cardiomyopathy. **A.** *PCR-DNA microarray system (CLART® Entherpex,Genomica, Madrid, Spain) allowing the detection and typing of 8 Human Herpes viruses and of the Human Enterovirus (HEVs) group. The study patient is co-infected by HHV-6 and Human Enterovirus (Poliovirus, Echovirus or Coxsackievirus).* **B.** *Quantitative detection of HEVs in biopsy heart tissues from the same idiopathic DCM patient using classical real time PCR assay and confirming the HEV cardiac infection Amplification curves obtained for positive and negative controls and one HEV positive DCM patient X. Positive control corresponded to the CVB3 Nancy strain; Negative control corresponded to healthy heart tissue; CT, cycle threshold.*

A new strategy for the molecular detection of cardiac viral infections couples broad-range PCR amplification to electrospray ionization/ mass spectrometry analysis (PCR/ESI-MS). Previous versions of this method were known commercially as the Ibis T5000 and the current commercial hardware platform that conducts the MS analysis is now known as the Abbott PLEX-ID (Ecker et al., 2008). This technique uses primers designed to genomic regions highly conserved regions across viral domains of life. The method was initially developed for the identification of viruses, including previously unknown or unculturable viral agents in samples where multiple microbes may be present, primarily for biodefense applications (Ecker et al., 2008). It is now being developed for diagnosis of human cardiac infections by our team (Figure 3). Preliminary data obtain from 52 heart biopsy samples taken from 24 patients with idiopathic DCM showed a Kappa test correlation of 0.7 +/- 0.22 between PleX-ID detection system and 8 monoplex Q rt-PCR assays. Among the 24 study patients, our findings indicated that EV (12.5%), PVB19 (12.5%) and dual EV-PVB19 (25%) infections were identified as major potential etiological causes of idiopathic DCM (personal data; not shown). Moreover this new system allowed a rapid semi-quantitative detection of EV associated with a genotyping identification of the EV strains (CVB3 or CVB5; personal data not shown) (Figure 3) .Finally this system allows a rapid and valuable quantitative detection and genotyping identification of common viruses in heart tissues and can be used in clinical practice for an accurate diagnostic of viral cardiac infection.

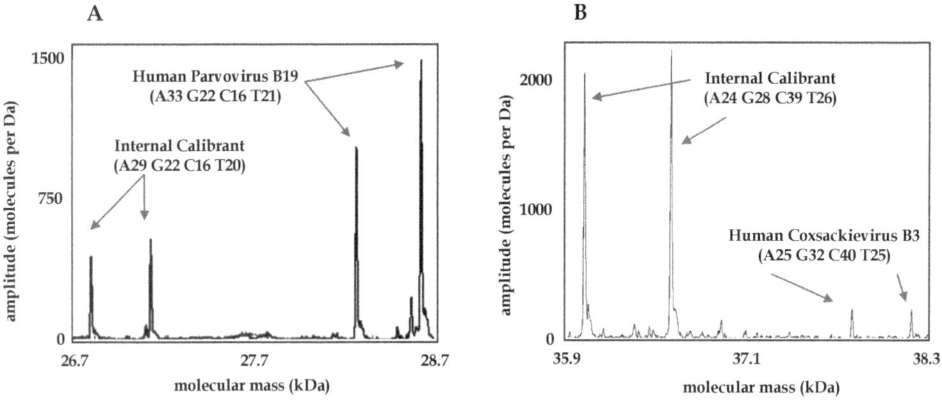

Fig. 3. Detection of parvovirus B19 (panel A) or coxsackievirus B3 (Panel B) in cardiac tissues of two patients (A and B) with idiopathic dilated cardiomyopathy using broad-range PCR amplification followed by ionisation and mass spectrometry analysis (personnal data 2011).

7. Conclusions and therapeutic perspectives

To improve histological diagnosis of viral myocarditis, additional virological evaluation of cardiac tissues is required with immunohistochemical and polymerase chain reaction (PCR) techniques allowing identification and quantification of viral infection markers. The diagnostic gold standard is endomyocardial biopsy (EMB) with the histological Dallas criteria, in association with new immunohistochemical and PCR analyses of cardiac tissues. These new viral diagnostic approaches can lead to better identification of the aetiology of myocarditis and can improve the clinical or therapeutic monitoring of viral causes of human myocarditis. Therapeutic strategies adapted specifically to the phase of the disease are currently under evaluation and may improve prognosis and clinical outcomes significantly. It might be more efficient to use positive immunomodulators (interleukins, interferon alpha, interferon gamma) alone or in combination with specific antiviral components such as ribavirin in the initial phase of the disease when viral replication activity can be detected in the cardiomyocytes (Külh et al., 2003). By contrast, immunosuppressive drugs would be more appropriate in the chronic phase of myocarditis, when no or low viral replication activities are detectable in cardiac tissues by immunohistochemistry assays.

Further specific strategies could consist to specifically block the entry of the virus in target cardiac cells, by preventing interaction of viruses with their cellular receptor and their consequent signalling amplification systems, such as the tyrosine kinase p56lck, phosphatase CD45 and downstream ERK1/2 (Dennert et al., 2008). Preventing direct viral damage using antiviral therapy is another possible approach by use of specific viral drugs (anti-protease or inhibitors of RNA/DNA polymerases) or by use of general antiviral strategies (interfering RNA). Future randomized placebo-controlled trials should be based upon aetiological diagnosis (viral vs. other causes) and may provide novel treatment options and possibly a better prognosis for these selected patients.

8. References

Andréoletti, L., Wattre, P., Decoene, C., Lobert, PE., Dewilde, A., & Hober, D. (1995). Detection of enterovirus-specific RNA sequences in explanted myocardium biopsy specimens from patients with dilated or ischemic cardiomyopathy. Clin Infect Dis 21:1315-1317.

Andréoletti, L., Hober, D., Becquart, P., Belaich, S., Copin, MC., Lambert, V., & Wattré, P. (1997). Experimental CVB3-induced chronic myocarditis in two murine strains: evidence of interrelationships between virus replication and myocardial damage in persistent cardiac infection. J Med Virol 52:206-214.

Andréoletti, L., Bourlet, T., Moukassa, D., Rey, L., Hot, D., Li, Y., Lambert, V., Gosselin, B., Mosnier, JF., Stankowiak, C., & Wattré, P. (2000). Enteroviruses can persist with or without active viral replication in cardiac tissue of patients with end-stage ischemic or dilated cardiomyopathy. J Infect Dis 182:1222-1227.

Andréoletti, L., Ventéo, L., Douche-Aourik, F., Canas, F., Lorin de la Grandmaison, G., Jacques, J., Moret, H., Jovenin, N., Mosnier, JF., Matta, M., Duband, S., Pluot, M., Pozzetto, B., & Bourlet, T. (2007). Active Coxsackieviral B infection is associated with disruption of dystrophin in endomyocardial tissue of patients who died suddenly of acute myocardial infarction. J Am Coll Cardiol. 50:2207-2214.

Andréoletti, L., Lévêque, N., Boulagnon, C., Brasselet, C., & Fornes, P. (2009). *Viral causes of human myocarditis*. Arch Cardiovasc Dis. 102:559-68.

Aretz, HT., Billingham, ME., Edwards, WD., Factor, SM., Fallon, JT., Fenoglio, JJ., Olsen, EG., & Schoen, FJ. (1987). Myocarditis. With histopathologic definition and classification. Am J Cardiovasc Pathol 1:3-14.

Ayach, B., Fuse, K., Martino, T., & Liu, P. (2003). Dissecting mechanisms of innate and acquired immunity in myocarditis Curr Opin Cardiol. 18 : 175-181.

Badorff, C., Lee, GH., Lamphear, BJ., Martone, ME., Campbell, KP., Rhoads, RE., Knowlton, KU. (1999). Enteroviral protease 2A cleaves dystrophin: evidence of cytoskeletal disruption in an acquired cardiomyopathy. Nat Med. 5:320-326.

Badorff, C., Zeiher, AM., Hohnloser, SH. (2001). *Torsade de pointes tachycardia as a rare manifestation of acute enteroviral myocarditis*. Heart 86:489-490.

Baughman, KL. (2006). Diagnosis of myocarditis: death of Dallas criteria. Circulation 113 : 593-595.

Bock, CT., Klingel, K., & Kandolf, R. (2010). *Human parvovirus B19-associated myocarditis*. N Engl J Med. 362:1248-9.

Bönsch, C., Zuercher, C., Lieby, P., Kempf, C., Ros, C. (2010). The globoside receptor triggers structural changes in the B19 virus capsid that facilitate virus internalization. J Virol. 84:11737-46.

Bowles, NE., Ni, J., Kearney, DL., Pauschinger, M., Schultheiss, HP., McCarthy, R., Hare, J., Bricker, JT., Bowles, KR., & Towbin, JA. (2003). *Detection of viruses in myocardial tissues by polymerase chain reaction. evidence of adenovirus as a common cause of myocarditis in children and adults.* J Am Coll Cardiol. 42:466-72.

Bültmann, BD., Klingel, K., Sotlar, ., Bock, CT., Baba HA., Sauter, M., & Kandolf R. (2003). Fatal parvovirus B19-associated myocarditis clinically mimicking ischemic heart disease: an endothelial cell-mediated disease. Hum Pathol. 34:92-5.

Caruso, A., Rotola, A., Comar, M., Favilli, F., Galvan, M., Tosetti, M., Campello, C., Caselli, E., Alessandri, G., Grassi, M., Garrafa, E., Cassai, E., & Di Luca, D. (2002). HHV-6 infects human aortic and heart microvascular endothelial cells, increasing their ability to secrete proinflammatory chemokines. J Med Virol. 67:528 -533.

Chapman, NM., & Kim, KS. (2008a). *Persistent coxsackievirus infection: enterovirus persistence in chronic myocarditis and dilated cardiomyopathy.* Curr Top Microbiol Immunol. 323:275-92.

Chapman, NM., Kim, KS., Drescher, KM., Oka, K., & Tracy, S. (2008b). *5' terminal deletions in the genome of a coxsackievirus B2 strain occurred naturally in human heart.* Virology. 375:480-91.

Chimenti, C., Russo, A., Pieroni, M., Calabrese, F., Verardo, R., Thiene, G., Russo, MA., Maseri, A., & Frustaci, A. (2004). Intramyocyte detection of Epstein-Barr virus genome by laser capture microdissection in patients with inflammatory cardiomyopathy. Circulation. 110:3534 -3539.

Cioc, AM., & Nuovo, GJ. (2002). Histologic and in situ viral findings in the myocardium in cases of sudden, unexpected death. Mod Pathol. 15:914–922.

Cooper, LT. (2003). Myocarditis: from bench to bedside. Totowa, NJ, Humana Press.

Cooper, LT., Baughman, KL., Feldman, AM., Frustaci, A., Jessup, M., Kuhl, U., Levine, GN., Narula, J., Starling, RC., Towbin, J., & Virmani, R. (2007). *The role of endomyocardial biopsy in the management of cardiovascular disease: a scientific statement from the American Heart Association, the American College of Cardiology, and the European Society of Cardiology.* J Am Coll Cardiol. 50:1914-31.

Cooper, LT. (2009). Myocarditis. N Engl J Med 360 : 1526-1538.

Dec, GW., Palacios, IF., Fallon, JT., Aretz, HT., Mills, J., Lee, DC., & Johnson, RA. (1985). Active myocarditis in the spectrum of acute dilated cardiomyopathies. Clinical features, histologic correlates, and clinical outcome. N Engl J Med. 312:885-90.

Coyne, CB., & Bergelson, JM. (2006). *Virus-induced Abl and Fyn kinase signals permit coxsackievirus entry through epithelial tight junctions.* Cell. 124:119-31.

Dennert, R., Crijns, HJ., & Heymans, S. (2008). Acute viral myocarditis. Eur Heart J 29:2073-2082.

Domenico, C., & Gaetano, T. (2006). Arrhythmogenic right ventricular cardiomyopathy / dysplasia: clinical impact of molecular genetic studies. Circulation. 113:1634-1637.

Duechting, A., Tschöpe, C., Kaiser, H., Lamkemeyer, T., Tanaka, N., Aberle, S., Lang, F., Torresi, J., Kandolf, R., & Bock, CT. (2008). Human parvovirus B19 NS1 protein modulates inflammatory signaling by activation of STAT3/PIAS3 in human endothelial cells. J Virol. 82:7942-52.

Ecker, DJ., Sampath, R., Massire, C., Blyn, LB., Hall, TA., Eshoo, MW., & Hofstadler, SA. (2008). Ibis T5000: a universal biosensor approach for microbiology. Nat Rev Microbiol. 6:553-8.

Feire, AL., Koss, H., & Compton, T. (2004). Cellular integrins function as entry receptors for human cytomegalovirus via a highly conserved disintegrin-like domain. Proc Natl Acad Sci U S A. 101:15470-5.

Feldman, AM., & McNamara, D. (2000). Myocarditis. N Engl J Med 343:1388-1398.

Gravanis, MB., & Sternby, NH. (1991). Incidence of myocarditis. A 10-year autopsy study from Malmo, Sweden. Arch Pathol Lab Med. 115:390-392.

Grodums, EI., & Zbitnew, A. (1976). *Experimental herpes simplex virus carditis in mice.* Infect Immun. 14:1322-31.

Huber, SA. (1993). Animal models: immunological aspects. In Banatvla JE, ed, Viral Infections in the Heart. London, Edward Arnold, 82-109.

Kawai, C. (1999). From myocarditis to cardiomyopathy: mechanisms of inflammation and cell death: learning from the past for the future. Circulation. 99 : 1091-1100.

Kramer, M., Schulte, BM., Toonen, LW., de Bruijni, MA., Galama, JM., Adema, GJ., van Kuppeveld, FJ. (2007). *Echovirus infection causes rapid loss-of-function and cell death in human dendritic cells.* Cell Microbiol. 9:1507-18.

Kramer, M., Schulte, BM., Toonen, LW., Barral, PM., Fisher, PB., Lanke, KH., Galama, JM., van Kuppeveld, FJ., & Adema, GJ. (2008). *Phagocytosis of picornavirus-infected cells induces an RNA-dependent antiviral state in human dendritic cells.* J Virol. 82:2930-7.

Kühl, U., Noutsias, M., Seeberg, B., & Schultheiss, HP. (1996). *Immunohistological evidence for a chronic intramyocardial inflammatory process in dilated cardiomyopathy.* Heart 75:295-300.

Kühl U., Pauschinger M., Schwimmbeck P.L., Seeberg, B., Lober, C., Noutsias, M., Poller, W., & Schultheiss, HP. (2003). Interferon-beta treatment eliminates cardiotropic viruses and improves left ventricular function in patients with myocardial persistence of viral genomes and left ventricular dysfunction. Circulation. 107 : 2793-2798.

Kühl, U., Pauschinger, M., Noutsias, M., Seeberg, B., Bock, T., Lassner, D., Poller, W., Kandolf, R., & Schultheiss HP. (2005a). High prevalence of viral genomes and multiple viral infections in the myocardium of adults with "idiopathic" left ventricular dysfunction. Circulation. 111:887-893.

Kühl, U., Pauschinger, M., Seeberg, B., Lassner, D., Noutsias, M., Poller, W., & Schultheiss, HP. (2005b). *Viral persistence in the myocardium is associated with progressive cardiac dysfunction.* Circulation 112:1965-1970.

Kyto, V., Vuorinen, T., Saukko, P., Lautenschlager, I., Lignitz, E., Saraste, A., & Voipio-Pulkki, LM. (2005). Cytomegalovirus infection of the heart is common in patients with fatal myocarditis. Clin Infect Dis. 40:683- 688.

Lee, GH., Badorff, C., & Knowlton, KU. (2000). Dissociation of sarcoglycans and the dystrophin carboxyl terminus from the sarcolemma in enteroviral cardiomyopathy. Circ Res 87:489–495.

Lenzo, JC., Fairweather, D., Cull, V., Shellam, GR., & James Lawson, CM. (2002). *Characterisation of murine cytomegalovirus myocarditis: cellular infiltration of the heart and virus persistence.* J Mol Cell Cardiol. 34:629-40.

Li, Y., Bourlet, T., Andréoletti, L., Mosnier, JF., Peng, T., Yang, Y., Archard, LC., Pozzetto, B., & Zhang, H. (2000). Enteroviral capsid protein VP1 is present in myocardial tissues from some patients with myocarditis or dilated cardiomyopathy. Circulation 101:231-234.

Liu, PP., & Mason, JW. (2001). Advances in the understanding of myocarditis. Circulation. 104 : 1076-1082.

Mahfoud, F., Gärtner, B., Kindermann, M., Ukena, C., Gadomski, K., Klingel, K., Kandolf, R., Böhm, M., & Kindermann, I. (2011). *Virus serology in patients with suspected myocarditis: utility or futility?* Eur Heart J. 32:897-903.

Magnani, JW., & Dec, GW. (2006). Myocarditis: current trends in diagnosis and treatment. Circulation 113:876-890.

Mahrholdt, H., Goedecke, C., Wagner, A., Meinhardt, G., Athanasiadis, A., Vogelsberg, H., Fritz, P., Klingel, K., Kandolf, R., & Sechtem, U. (2004). Cardiovascular magnetic resonance assessment of human myocarditis: a comparison to histology and molecular pathology. Circulation. 109:1250-8.

Matsumori, A., & Kawai, C. (1982). *An animal model of congestive (dilated) cardiomyopathy: dilatation and hypertrophy of the heart in the chronic stage in DBA/2 mice with myocarditis caused by encephalomyocarditis virus.* Circulation 66:355-360.

Matsumori, A., Shimada, T., Chapman, NM., Tracy, SM., & Mason, JW. (2006). Myocarditis and heart failure associated with hepatitis C virus infection. J Card Fail. 12:293-298.

Matsumori, A., Yamada, T., Suzuki, H., Matoba, Y., & Sasayama, S. (1994). Increased circulating cytokines in patients with myocarditis and cardiomyopathy. Br Heart J. 72 : 561-566.

Oldstone, MB. (2006). *Viral persistence: parameters, mechanisms and future predictions.* Virology. 344:111-8.

Renois, F., Talmud, D., Huguenin, A., Moutte, L., Strady, C., Cousson, J., Lévêque, N., & Andréoletti, L. (2010). *Rapid detection of respiratory tract viral infections and coinfections in patients with influenza-like illnesses by use of reverse transcription-PCR DNA microarray systems.* J Clin Microbiol. 48:3836-42.

Santoro, F., Kennedy, PE., Locatelli, G., Malnati, MS., Berger, EA., & Lusso, P. (1999). *CD46 is a cellular receptor for human herpesvirus 6.* Cell. 99:817-27.

Schönian, U., Crombach, M., Maser, S., & Maisch, B. (1995). Cytomegalovirus-associated heart muscle disease. Eur Heart J. Suppl O:46-9.

Seko, Y., Tsuchimochi, H., Nakamura, T., Okumura, K., Naito, S., Imataka, K., Fujii, J., Takaku, F., Yazaki, Y. (1990). Expression of major histocompatibility complex class I antigen in murine ventricular myocytes infected with Coxsackievirus B3. Circ Res 67:360-367.

Shi, Y., Chen, C., Lisewski, U., Wrackmeyer, U., Radke, M., Westermann, D., Sauter, M., Tschöpe, C., Poller, W., Klingel, K., & Gotthardt, M. (2009). Cardiac deletion of the Coxsackievirus-adenovirus receptor abolishes Coxsackievirus B3 infection and prevents myocarditis in vivo. J Am Coll Cardiol. 53:1219-26.

Takano, H., Nakagawa, K., Ishio, N., Daimon, M., Kobayashi, Y., Hiroshima, K., & Komuro, I. (2008). Active myocarditis in a patient with chronic active Epstein-Barr virus infection. Int J Cardiol. 130:e11- e13.

Sudano, I., Spieker, LE., Noll, G., Corti, R., Weber, R., & Luscher, TF. (2006). Cardiovascular disease in HIV infection. Am Heart J. 151:1147-1155.

Ventéo, L., Bourlet, T., Renois, F., Douche-Aourik, F., Mosnier, JF., Maison, GL., Pluot, M., Pozzetto, B., & Andreoletti, L. (2010). Enterovirus-related activation of the cardiomyocyte mitochondrial apoptotic pathway in patients with acute myocarditis. Eur Heart J. 31:728-36.

Wickham, TJ., Mathias, P., Cheresh, DA., & Nemerow, GR.(1993). Integrins alpha v beta 3 and alpha v beta 5 promote adenovirus internalization but not virus attachment. Cell. 73:309-19.

Yajima, T., & Knowlton, KU. (2009). *Viral myocarditis: from the perspective of the virus.* Circulation. 119:2615-24.

Yilmaz, A., Kindermann, I., Kindermann, M., Mahfoud, F., Ukena, C., Athanasiadis, A., Hill, S., Mahrholdt, H., Voehringer, M., Schieber, M., Klingel, K., Kandolf, R., Böhm, M., Sechtem, U. (2010). Comparative evaluation of left and right ventricular endomyocardial biopsy: differences in complication rate and diagnostic performance. Circulation. 122:900-9.

Acute Myocarditis in Emergency Medicine

Yukihiro Ikegami and Choichiro Tase
Fukushima Medical University,
Japan

1. Introduction

Emergency doctors provide primary care to many patients with an acute-onset condition in the emergency room (ER) every day. We occasionally must address circulatory failure in patients that ranges from "acutely developing" to "severe." Usually, it is not difficult to diagnose or to choose the proper therapeutic procedures, because most of these cases are caused by heart diseases, such as ischemic heart disease or an arrhythmia. However, in some cases the causes of circulatory failure cannot be determined immediately.

It is known that cardiomyopathies account for some of those undiagnosed cases. Classically, cardiomyopathies have been regarded as idiopathic myocardial diseases because of the difficulty of detecting their etiology or the mechanisms causing the problem. Recent developments in biochemical technology have provided the option of approaching these unknown mechanisms using genetic analyses (Richardson et al., 1996). Cardiomyopathies are presently classified into several groups, defined by the cause, tissue type, and clinical course. In 2006, a committee of the American Heart Association (AHA) advocated new criteria for cardiomyopathies. With those criteria, primary cardiomyopathies are classified into a genetic type, a mixed type, and an acquired type (Maron et al., 2006).

We encounter several types of cardiomyopathy in the ER. Immediate adequate primary treatment of these cases must be prudent because circulatory insufficiency can rapidly progress to cardiac arrest.

In most cases, myocarditis is caused by an inflammatory response and is classified as an acquired type of primary cardiomyopathy. It is also categorized as either acute or chronic. The comprehensive concept of chronic myocarditis has not yet been established because cases of chronic myocarditis have not been sufficiently reported. For most cases of chronic myocarditis, the causes and developmental mechanisms remain unclear.

We have only practical guidelines for treating chronic myocarditis in Japan (JCS, 1996). These patients usually have long-term therapeutic histories. Therefore, the patients' own doctors who are familiar with their clinical histories should be responsible for treatment in the ER. On the other hand, most cases of acute myocarditis are of sudden onset, and severe cases are taken to the ER by the emergency medical service. Doctors in the ER must then be responsible for the primary treatment of these patients. Because there is the risk of sudden development of circulatory insufficiency with acute myocarditis, immediate and adequate initial treatment is necessary for survival.

In this chapter, we explain the causes, mechanisms as presently known, classification, and clinical course of myocarditis. Additionally, we outline the recommended treatment for the acute phase of myocarditis.

2. Epidemiology and prognosis

The clinical course of myocarditis varies. The symptoms range widely, from slight to severe, and it is difficult to investigate myocarditis epidemiologically. In 2002 in Japan, a large-scale investigation for cardiomyopathy was performed and reported that cardiomyopathy was found in 21.3 per 100,000 population (Miura et al., 2002). However, the subjects of this investigation were consulted patients with data provided by hospitals. It is thought that actual morbidity is higher, because there are many non-consulted persons with occult cardiomyopathy, such as early stage dilated cardiomyopathy or hypertrophic cardiomyopathy with no symptoms. Therefore, we still cannot grasp the exact morbidity of myocarditis in Japan. Okada et al. (1989) reported that among 10,000 autopsied cases during 1958–1978 there were 115 cases of myocarditis. In another report, occult myocarditis was found in 0.6% of autopsied cases in which cardiac disease had not detected while the patients were alive (Feely et al., 2000). Therefore, it should be recognized that myocarditis is not clinically infrequent and includes a mild type that displays no symptoms. The mortality rate for myocarditis has not been established. An investigative committee of the Ministry of Public Welfare and Labor in Japan reported in 1986 that 13 (4.7%) of 274 patients died within 1 month in a small-scale investigation targeting acute-phase myocarditis (Kawamura et al., 1986). Among those cases, the causes of death were cardiogenic shock in six cases (46%), congestive heart failure in five cases (38%), and complete atrioventricular block in two cases (15%). Intensive treatment for severe cardiac dysfunction and fatal arrhythmias are important to reduce mortality during the acute phase of severe myocarditis.

3. Cause of myocarditis and classification

Myocarditis is classified by cause, clinical type, and pathological picture. In clinical medicine, myocarditis presenting as a sudden development should be attended to because any delay of treatment presents a risk of fatal circulatory failure. It should be recognized that there is different prognosis depending on the clinical type of myocarditis. The classification of myocarditis is shown in Table 1.

3.1 Causes

Several causes or mechanisms of the development of myocarditis have been detected, among which infection is the most the frequent and important. In earlier years, myocarditis was often caused by rheumatic fever and diphtheria. More recently, in advanced nations it is mostly caused by viral infections. Bowles et al. (1986) reported that Coxsackie B virus was detected in patients with myocarditis using a dot blot hybridization method. Coxsackie virus, an enterovirus belonging to the picornavirus family, was extracted from patients with polio in 1982 and is particularly compatible with myocardium (Clements, 1993). Half of group A types and all of group B types of the Coxsackie virus cause myocarditis accompanied by symptoms of the common cold.

Presently, it is possible to detect many viruses with polymerase chain reaction or in situ hybridization. Therefore, we can detect myocarditis due to viral infection in most cases. In

Causes	Histological classification	Clinical classification
Infection	Lymphocytic myocarditis	Acute type
Virus	Giant cell myocarditis	Fulminant type
Bacterium	Eosinophilic myocarditis	Chronic type (including persistent symptoms type and unremarkable symptoms type)
Fungus	Granulomatous myocarditis	
Rickettsia		
Spirochete		
Parasite		
Others		
Drugs, chemical materials		
Allergy, autoimmunity		
Collagen disease		
Kawasaki disease		
Sarcoidosis		
Radiation		
Heat stroke		
Unknown (idiopathic)		

Table 1. classification of myocarditis. modified from the guideline for the diagnosis and treatment of myocarditis (JCS, 2005).

1. Nonsteroidal anti-inflammatory drugs
Indomethacin, oxyphenbutazone, phenylbutazone
2. Psychotropic drugs
(Tricyclic) antidepressant: imipramine, clomipramine, amitriptyline
Antimanic: lithium carbonate, lithium oxalic acid
Antiepileptic: phenytoin, carbamazepine
3. Diuretic: acetazolamide, hydrochlorothiazide, spironolactone, chlorthalidone
4. Depressor: methyldopa
5. Anticancer drug: adriamycin, daunorubicin, mitoxantrone
6. Antibiotics
Amphotericin B, penicillin, ampicillin, tetracycline
Chloramphenicol, streptomycin
7. Sulfaminum: sulfadiazine, sulfisoxazole
8. Antiphthisic: isoniazid (INH), para-aminosalicylic acid (PAS)
9. Biological agents: tetanus toxoid, α-interferon, interleukin 2 (IL-2)
10. Antidiabetic: sulfonylurea
11. Others: catecholamines, cocaine, amphetamine, arsenic

Table 2. Drugs that cause myocarditis.

recent reports, adenovirus, sharing the same receptors as the Coxsackie virus, parvovirus B19, human herpes virus 6, and hepatitis C virus, are known to cause myocarditis (Okabe et al., 1997).

Myocarditis does not always develop in patients infected by a virus compatible with the myocardium (e.g., the Coxsackie virus). In such cases, symptoms of myocarditis are unremarkable or slight, and the mechanism of development of myocarditis remains unknown. Based on the results in experimental animal models, Cupta et al. (2008) suggested a developmental pattern of myocardial damage by an infective virus and the host's reactions as follows: (1) initial infection of virus in myocardial cells; (2) innate immune reaction; (3) defense by adaptive immunity; and (4) recovery of inflammatory reaction.

Several kinds of drugs, external physical stimulations such as exposure to irradiation or excessive heat, metabolic disorders, pregnancy, collagen diseases, sarcoidosis, and Kawasaki disease are important causes of myocarditis. It should be well noted that drug-induced myocarditis, particular in Japan, Europe, and the United States, is caused by many of the drugs that are administered or prescribed to patients in advanced countries. Drugs that cause myocarditis are shown in Table 2.

3.2 Histological classification

Histologically, myocarditis is classified as lymphocytic myocarditis, giant cell myocarditis, eosinophilic leukocyte myocarditis, and granuloma myocarditis. Most cases of lymphocytic myocarditis are caused by infection. Other types are due to materials toxic to the myocardium, a drug allergy, or an autoimmune reaction.

3.2.1 Lymphocytic myocarditis

Lymphocytic myocarditis is the most frequent histological type, and most cases are caused by a viral infection. Kodama et al. found that 85% of patients with myocarditis were diagnosed with the lymphocytic variety (Kodama et al., 2001). The primary symptoms—fever and pharyngeal pain—are not specific for myocarditis during the early phase, but symptoms of circulatory failure, such as edema, are specific and are observed during the developed phase. The severity of circulatory failure ranges widely from slight to fulminant.

3.2.2 Giant cell myocarditis

Giant cell myocarditis is encountered infrequently. Clinically, it has a poor prognosis because it can easily progress to fulminant myocarditis. After the onset, circulatory failure develops suddenly and in many cases rapidly progresses to a fatal state. It is suggested that an allergic reaction or an autoimmune reaction participates in this development. Infiltration by inflammatory cells and multinucleated cells are observed in the myocardium (Davidoff et al., 1991). Cardiac function markedly deteriorates with massive necrosis of the myocardium. Identification of multinucleated cells is necessary for a definitive diagnosis. It is difficult to decide on the timing of a biopsy because multinucleated cells are seen only during the acute phase. In patients presenting with a chronic course, cardiac sarcoidosis must be excluded (Shield et al., 2002).

3.2.3 Eosinophilic myocarditis

The clinical symptoms of eosinophilic myocarditis—fever, pharyngeal pain, cough—during the early phase are similar to those seen with myocarditis due to a viral infection. The differential diagnosis between viral myocarditis and eosinophilic myocarditis is often impossible because the eosinophil count is normal during the early phase of eosinophilic myocarditis (Morimoto et al., 2003). White blood cells (WBCs) gradually increase with the development of an inflammatory reaction; and materials toxic to the myocardium released from eosinophilic leukocytes cause severe contraction of the myocardium as the eosinophil count exceeds 500/nm^3.

In most cases, the increase in eosinophils is detected in a peripheral blood examination. However, some patients who suffer from circulatory insufficiency exhibit a delayed increase in eosinophils (Gets et al., 1991). Therefore, we should perform more frequent eosinophil counts during the acute phase. Infiltration of eosinophilic leukocytes, degranulation, and destruction of myocardium are observed in the biopsy specimen.

The main causes are an allergic reaction, drugs, and parasitic infection. Most cases, however, are treated as idiopathic myocarditis (Forrester et al., 1976). It has been reported that the mortality rate among patients with acute-phase eosinophilic myocarditis is approximately 7% (Morimot et al., 2003), (Mori et al., 2004).

3.3 Clinical classification

Myocarditis is clinically classified as acute or chronic. Since it is possible to detect the exact onset of acute myocarditis, it is easier to estimate the circulatory parameters for diagnosis and establish the strategy for treatment of acute myocarditis than for chronic myocarditis. In some cases of acute myocarditis, we treat it as fulminant myocarditis that has developed suddenly and may progress to severe circulatory failure during the acute phase (Aoyama et al., 2002). The worldwide morbidity and mortality rates associated with fulminant myocarditis are not yet clear. Cupta et al. (2008) reported that the frequency of fulminant myocarditis is 10% among all cases of acute myocarditis in the United States.

The global concept of chronic myocarditis has not been established, although several studies have suggested that viral infection (Fujioka et al., 2000) or autoimmunity (Lauer et al., 2000) play a role in its development. There are clinically two types of chronic myocarditis, and they have different clinical courses. One type has persistent, continuous symptoms, and the other has unremarkable symptoms (JCS, 1996).

In an investigation of clinical types of myocarditis in 48 patients reported by Kodama et al. (2001), nine were the acute type, 21 were the fulminant type, three were the chronic persistent symptom type, and 15 were the chronic unremarkable symptom type. The mortality rates during the first admission were 22% for the acute type, 43% for the fulminant type, 33% for the chronic persistent symptom type, and 40% for the chronic unremarkable symptom type. The long-term prognosis for patients who recovered from their cardiac dysfunction during the early phase was good. However, the long-term prognosis for patients who were diagnosed with the chronic, unremarkable symptom type was not good because they developed irreversible circulatory dysfunction, such as dilated cardiomyopathy.

4. Clinical symptoms and diagnosis

4.1 Clinical symptoms and physical symptoms

Clinically, symptoms range from slight problems—fever, pharyngeal pain, cough, vomiting, diarrhea, and arthropathies, as observed with the common cold—to severe circulatory failure. Therefore, we cannot list any symptoms characteristic of acute-phase myocarditis. In cases of established cardiac dysfunction, patients suffer from dyspnea, edema, cyanosis, palpitations due to hypoxia or arrhythmia, and other severe symptoms such as loss of consciousness and cramping. Whenever we treat acute-onset patients who present with symptoms of cardiac dysfunction in the ER, we maintain the suspicion that they are in the pre-developmental phase of severe myocarditis.

Among the physical symptoms of myocarditis, dysfunction of the heart's conduction system, which occurs in 60%-80% of patients with myocarditis, is critical. Particularly notable is the 30% incidence of severe bradycardia requiring temporary pacing in those with fulminant myocarditis (Kawamura et al., 1986). A galloping rhythm, a heart murmur caused by backflow in the atrioventricular valves, and pulmonary moist rales are found in patients who are developing heart failure. Pericardial and pleural stridulation can be auscultated in patients with pericarditis or pleuritis. Furthermore, pericardial effusion or cardiac tamponade is observed in some cases of developmental pericarditis.

4.2 Blood examinations

Inflammatory reactions such as increased WBCs, an increased erythrocyte sedimentation rate (ESR), or an increased C-reactive protein (CRP) level are detected in blood examinations during the early phase. Additionally, creatine kinase MB (CPK-MB) and cardiac troponin T assays, which are elevated in the presence of myocardial damage, are useful. Troponin T sensitivity is particularly high, and the severity of the myocardial damage can be estimated by a fixed quantity analysis (Lauer et al., 1997). Troponin T continuously increases with development of cardiac dysfunction and maintains a high peak value in those with fulminant myocarditis.

4.3 Chest radiography

Cardiac dilatation is present in 70% of chest radiography examinations, and pulmonary congestion or pleural effusion is often present in patients with severe heart failure. It should be noted that cardiac dilatation and pulmonary congestion are not remarkable in some cases of myocarditis, which causes mainly right ventricular failure (McFalls and van Suylen, 1993).

4.4 Electrocardiography

Various abnormal changes are revealed by electrocardiography (ECG), although none of the changes are specific for myocarditis. ECG is not an invasive procedure, and it has the benefit of simplicity of performance. The sensitivity is high, and any changes on the ECG tracing probably enhance with the development of myocarditis even if only slight changes are detected during the early phase. ECG should be repeated in the case of suspected myocarditis. Limited elevation of ST-T, mainly observed with acute myocardial infarction (AMI), is present in some patient with myocarditis. Elevation of ST-T in all leads is present in cases complicated by pericarditis. Bundle branch block or atrioventricular block is present in cases complicated by dysfunction of the heart's conduction system. It should be noted that the change to a wide QRS complex on the ECG tracing suggests the development of cardiac dysfunction. Because there is the risk of sudden changes with fatal ventricular tachycardia (VT) or ventricular fibrillation (VF) in the case of frequent arrhythmias, continuous ECG monitoring is necessary.

4.5 Echocardiography

Temporal thickening of the ventricular wall and deterioration of ventricular wall motion are present at inflammatory sites. All-round centripetal thickening, diffuse deterioration of wall motion, and stenosis of the intracardiac space are present in typical cases (Hiramatsu et al., 2001). In the cases of severe circulatory failure or fulminant myocarditis, multiple left ventricular thrombi are frequently caused by the deterioration of all-round wall motion. Continuous wall motion dysfunction causes diffuse thinning of the wall and/or ventricular aneurysms, and dilatation of the left ventricle develops. Ultimately, there is no morphological difference from dilated cardiomyopathy. Diagnosis by exclusion of ischemic heart disease is necessary in patients with wall thickening or wall motion deterioration.

4.6 Cardiac magnetic resonance

Cardiac magnetic resonance (CMR) is a noninvasive, useful examination for myocarditis (JCS, 2011). It can be used to estimate the morphological changes in the ventricles, contractive function, perfusion in the myocardium, and histological characteristics in one performance. In myocarditis, hyperemia and capillary leakage in the cardiac microcirculation are caused by an inflammatory reaction. The site of inflammation in the myocardium has high signal intensity on T1-weighted magnetic resonance imaging (MRI) several minutes after gadolinium contrast enhancement during the acute phase. It is suggested that the changes of microcirculation caused by an inflammatory reaction can be directly visualized with CMR (Friedrich et al., 1998). In many cases, widespread edema in the myocardium is caused during the acute phase. High signal intensity on T2-weighted images is present in 36% of myocarditis diagnosed by the Dallas criteria (Aretz et al., 1987), (Mahrholdt et al., 2004). In those patients, follow-up CMR, performed a year later, shows reduced left ventricular capacity (Zagrosesek et al., 2008). We can predict the histological changes and prognosis for cardiac function using CMR.

4.7 Radioisotope examination

Gallium-67 (^{67}Ga) is specific for infiltration of large monocytes, but it does not have high sensitivity (O'Connel et al., 1984). Pyrophosphate scintigraphy using technetium-99m (^{99m}Tc) is sensitive and accumulates at the inflammatory site in the myocardium (Morguet et al., 1994).

4.8 Cardiac catheterization and endomyocardial biopsy

We perform cardiac catheterization for the differential diagnosis during the acute phase if the patient's circulatory condition can tolerate it. We first exclude significant coronary stenosis by coronary angiography and then perform endomyocardial biopsy (Sekiguchi et al., 1980). The endomyocardial biopsy is now the most important and reliable technique for a definitive diagnosis. However, we often cannot obtain samples of the lesion site because the inflammatory reaction in the myocardium occurs inhomogeneously in most cases (Baughman, 2006). Cooper et al. (2007) reported that cardiac tamponade or ventricular perforation occurs at the time of sampling with a 0.1%–0.5% frequency.

4.9 Detection of viruses

In cases of suspected viral myocarditis, we measure the antibody titer using paired sera collected at a more than a 2-week interval. The reliable positive ratio is only 10%, and the capability to detect infected organs is not available. A definitive diagnosis is possible if we can directly detect the original viruses using a polymerase chain reaction or in situ hybridization. However, these techniques are not yet approved as standard examinations because their results vary widely depending on the institution in which they are performed.

4.10 Other diagnostic factors

In cases of suspected drug-induced myocarditis, we narrow down the list of causative drugs by detailed interviews with the patient regarding his or her clinical history. We can then identify the causative drug by a drug-induced lymphocyte stimulation test. Soluble Fas and Fas ligand (Fuse et al., 2000), interleukin-10 (Nishii et al., 2004), and tenascin-C (Imanaka-Yoshida et al., 2002) may be used in upcoming tests for diagnosing myocarditis.

Guidelines for diagnosis are presented in Table 3. The basic concept is to exclude ischemic heart disease and confirm an active lesion site by endomyocardial biopsy. It is currently impossible to detect the cause in most cases. Clinically, it is best to provide the primary care that is given to patients suspected of having myocarditis caused by a viral infection.

5. Development and strategy for treatment during the acute phase

Generally, the clinical conditions of patients are similar in many cases of myocarditis. A toxic protein produced by the infecting virus destroys the myocardial dystrophin complex within several days after onset of the myocarditis. It has been noted that this mechanism causes severe myocardial dysfunction accompanied by widespread myocardial cell death (Bandorff et al., 1999). Silver and Kowaldzuk (1989) reported that viral infection directly causes widespread myocardial ischemia by microvascular spasm.

After the viral infection is established, the immune response produces inflammatory cytokines in large quantities (Fairweather et al., 2005). This cytokine network originally plays a role in prophylaxis against the viral infection. Inflammatory cytokines such as interleukins 1 and 2 and tumor necrosis factor-α eliminate infected viruses by activating macrophages, lymphocytes, and endothelial cells. However, excessive cytokine release damages myocardial cells and causes myocardial dysfunction (Kawai, 1999). Additionally, inducible nitric oxide (NO) synthase (iNOS) induced by activated macrophages acts to encourage NO to eliminate infected viruses. It has been reported that excessive release of NO strongly damages myocardial cells (Mikami et al., 1996).

Infiltration by inflammatory cells, including T cells and natural killer cells, peaks 7–14 days after viral infection and causes widespread necrosis of myocardial cells (Seko et al., 1993). As already noted, infected virus and released inflammatory cytokines are the main mechanisms in the development of myocardial dysfunction during the acute phase. Severe deciduation of myocardial cells causes pump failure, which progresses to fatal circulatory collapse.

It is important to remember that cardiac dysfunction associated with myocarditis is reversible in many cases. Full recovery of cardiopulmonary function can be expected if the patient's life support is adequately performed. Therefore, we compress the strategy for treatment into three stages to give patients suffering from myocarditis the best chance for survival.

In most cases, the first strategic issue is intervention regarding the cause. Unfortunately, it is impossible to provide antibiotic therapy because effective antiviral drugs to address viral myocarditis have not been developed. There is a risk of further viral propagation when

1. Primary symptoms (nonspecific symptoms in most cases)
- Symptoms that appear with the common cold (fever, headache, cough, pharyngeal pain)
- Digestive symptoms (nausea, vomiting, diarrhea, abdominal pain)
- Others (eruption, arthralgia, myalgia)
    - *Note*: Some patients are found in sudden cardiac arrest
2. Physical findings
- Tachycardia, bradycardia, arrhythmia, weak heart sounds
- Galloping rhythm (III, IV sounds), pericardial friction murmur
- Systolic murmur
3. Abnormality of ECG: various changes
- Atrioventricular block, wide QRS complex, reduction of height in R wave, abnormal Q wave
- Change of ST-T level, low-voltage wave, frequent premature contractions
- Supraventricular tachycardia, atrial fibrillation, sinus arrest
- Ventricular tachycardia, ventricular fibrillation, asystole
4. Echocardiography
- Focal or diffuse thickening of the ventricular wall
- Focal or diffuse deterioration of ventricular wall motion
- Stenosis of intracardiac space
- Pericardial effusion
5. Blood examinations
- Detection of creatine kinase MB (CPK-MB)
- Detection troponin T
- Inflammatory reaction (increased WBCs, CRP level)
    - *Note*: Troponin T is sensitive using whole blood during the acute phase
6. Items 2–5 (above) change within several hours. Therefore, continuous observation is necessary. Bradycardia, wide QRS complex, frequent premature contractions, enhanced thickening of the ventricular wall and deterioration of ventricular wall motion, and continuous high troponin T levels are dangerous symptoms of fatal circulatory crisis.
7. A differential diagnosis of acute myocardial infarction (AMI) is necessary.
8. Endocardial biopsy provides a definitive diagnosis, but AMI cannot be excluded if tissue images are not obtained.
- Diagnostic criteria in tissue image:
- Infiltration of large and small monocytes
- Rupture, fusion, or disappearance of myocardial cells
- Edema or fibrotic changes in interstitial tissue
9. More than four-fold change of viral antibody titer in paired sera is adequate for viral detection. Polymerase chain reaction is effective for diagnosing a viral infection. Additionally, virus isolation or detection of viral antigen from a throat swab, urine, feces, blood, or particularly pericardial effusion or myocardial tissue are direct evidence of the diagnosis.

Table 3. Guidelines for diagnosing myocarditis. Modified from the guideline for diagnosis and treatment of myocarditis (JCS, 2005).

administering anti-inflammatory drugs such as immunosuppressants and steroids. On the other hand, we can expect to reverse cardiac dysfunction by initially giving anti-inflammatory drugs because it has been reported that allergic and autoimmune reactions strongly participate in the development of the giant cell myocarditis and eosinophilic myocarditis, both unusual forms. Therefore, early and adequate ascertainment of the cause is the maximum priority. Presently, the performance of myocardial biopsy is limited. Steroids should not be selected as a first choice even if the patient is in a shock state.

The second issue is to provide cardiopulmonary support during continuing fatal circulatory failure. During the acute phase of severe myocarditis, there is the risk of cardiogenic shock, complete atrioventricular block, fatal arrhythmia, and/or sudden cardiac arrest at any time. Therefore, most patients require intensive care. Drug therapy for myocarditis is no different from that for usual heart failure. Catecholamines, a diuretic, or both are administered following Forrester's classification. Mechanical cardiopulmonary life support should be immediately introduced when the circulatory insufficiency cannot be reversed with drugs. Full recovery of cardiac function is expected by advanced life support within several days in patients with acute myocarditis.

The third issue is to control the inflammatory reaction. If the actions of excessive inflammatory cytokines and NO are reduced, cardiac dysfunction is expected to be reversed during the acute phase. Although treatment using high doses of steroid, high doses of γ-globulin, and plasma exchange have been tried and evaluated, we have no evidence of their effectiveness.

5.1 Cardiopulmonary support

Immediate cardiac resuscitative support must be provided if the patients with fulminant myocarditis are to survive. Delay of treatment results in fatal circulatory collapse. Although the short-term mortality rate for fulminant myocarditis is generally high, the long-term functional prognosis for patients who survive the acute circulatory crisis is good compared with that for dilated cardiomyopathy (McCarthy et al., 2000).

The Scientific Committee of the Japanese Circulation performed a retrospective follow-up survey on severe fulminant myocarditis (Aoyama et al., 2002). The cases of 52 patients who required percutaneous cardiopulmonary support (PCPS) because of severe circulatory failure were investigated. The mortality rate for the acute phase was 40.4% (21/52). Among the 31 surviving patients, 30 (96.8%) had fully recovered from their cardiac dysfunction. McCarthy et al. (2000) noted that cardiac function had been maintained in good condition for a long time in more than 90% of patients who had recovered from fulminant myocarditis. Therefore, the "bridge" treatment of using mechanical cardiopulmonary support to avoid multiple organ dysfunction caused by hypoperfusion is an important treatment strategy during the acute phase of fulminant myocarditis. Patients who have survived on mechanical support, such as percutaneous cardiopulmonary support or a ventricular assist system, have also been reported (Chen et al, 2005), (Topkara et al., 2006).

5.1.1 Percutaneous cardiopulmonary support

A guideline for the use of percutaneous cardiopulmonary support (PCPS) has been formulated in Japan (Fig. 1) (Aoyama et al., 2002). In suspected cases of low cardiac output due to pump dysfunction, we may apply PCPS in accordance with continuous monitoring of the circulatory condition. Important clinical parameters to examine when making the decision of whether to use PCS include the urinary volume, SvO_2 (< 60%), development of

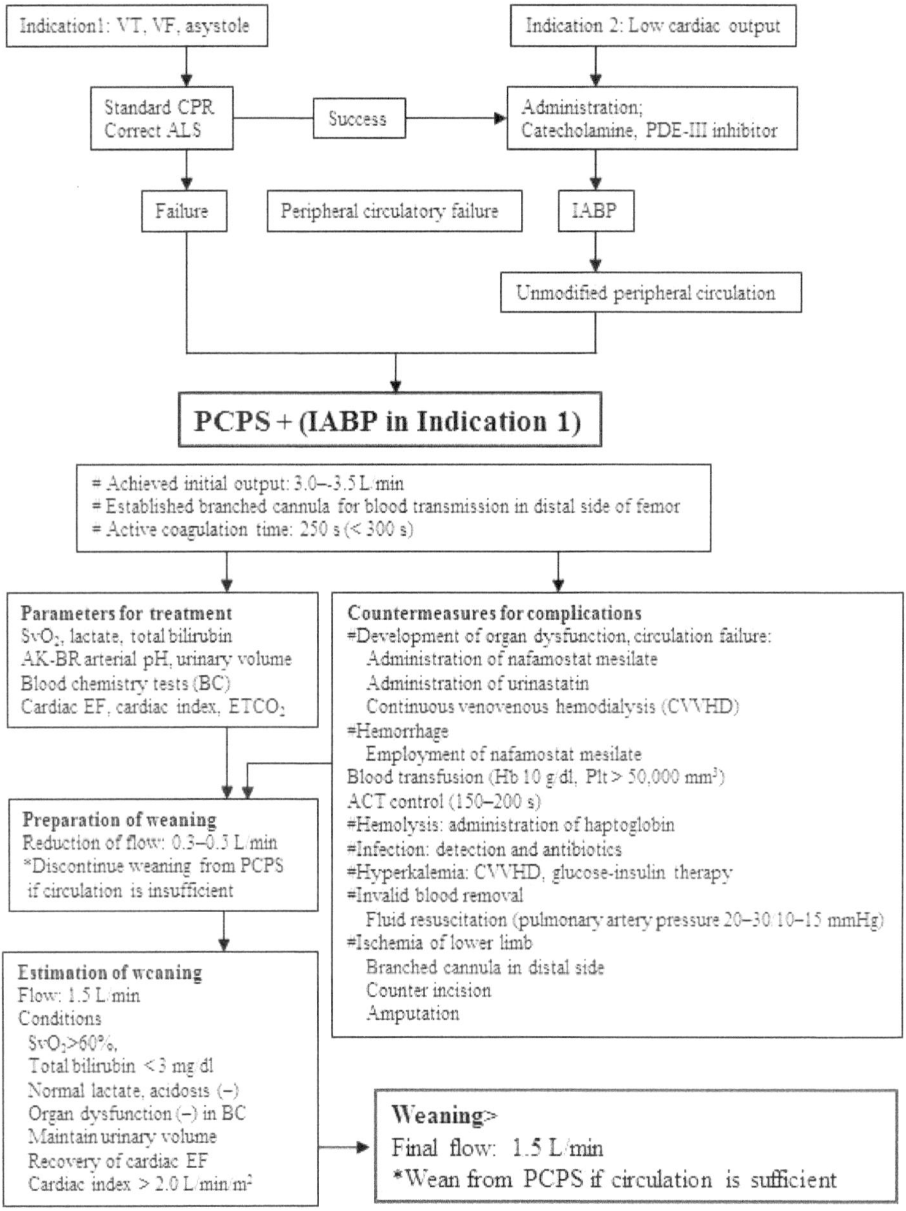

Fig. 1. Modified algorithm of PCPS for fulminant myocarditis (Aoyama et al, 2002).

metabolic acidosis, and multiple organ dysfunction suggested by blood chemistry examinations. The initial flow of PCPS should be established at 3.0–3.5 L/min. Concomitant use of intra-aortic balloon pumping (IABP) provides the benefits of reduced afterload, improved peripheral circulation by pulsatile flow, and backup support at the completion of PCPS. It is recommended that a branched cannula be established in the distal side of the femoral artery for blood transfusion because there is a risk of ischemia in the lower limb.

Unfortunately, we occasionally experience patients in severe situations in whom sufficient organ perfusion cannot be provided even if PCPS is fully operative. Aoyama et al. (2002) reported that 40% of patients supported by PCPS died during the acute phase. Among them, multiple organ dysfunction due to hypoperfusion was found in 25% and ischemia in the lower limb in 23%. Because the prognosis of fulminant myocarditis depends on the outcome of radical treatment of the circulation, we discuss early exchange via a ventricular assist system when sufficient organ perfusion cannot be provided by PCPS.

Case report: We treated a patient with severe fulminant myocarditis who survived owing to emergency PCPS. The young woman consulted her family doctor because of fever and was prescribed anti-inflammatory drugs with a diagnosis of pharyngitis. She was admitted to our hospital because of sudden severe circulatory failure that required high-flow oxygenation and high doses of catecholamine. Blood examination showed an elevation in troponin I, CPK, and other cardiac enzymes. Chest radiography showed marked cardiac dilatation and pleural effusion (Fig. 2). Echocardiography revealed pericardial effusion and deterioration of all-round wall motion of the left ventricle (Fig. 3). No significant coronary stenosis was detected by coronary angiography. We introduced emergency PCPS with IABP because her left ventricular ejection fraction was decreased by less than 20%. Her circulatory condition dramatically recovered, and she was weaned from PCPS on the 10th day. She obtained full recovery of her circulatory function. We could not detect any viruses when measuring the antibody titer using paired sera.

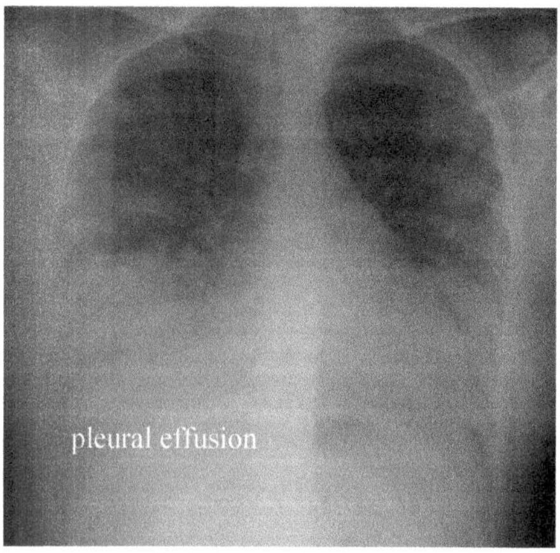

Fig. 2. Chest radiography shows marked cardiac dilatation and pleural effusion.

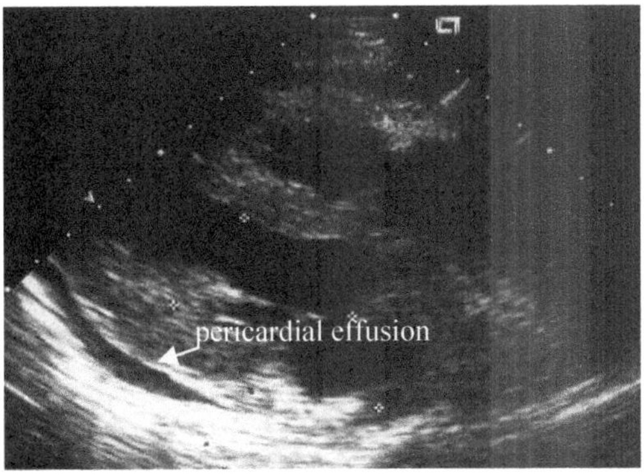

Fig. 3. Echocardiography shows pericardial effusion and deterioration of the all-round wall motion of the left ventricle.

5.1.2 Ventricular assist system

There is the risk of severe pulmonary congestion due to PCPS in cases of extreme deterioration of left ventricular function. In such cases, the patient should be switched to a ventricular assist system (VAS) before organ dysfunction develops. Grinda et al. (2004) reported that they introduced VAS in five cases of severe fulminant myocarditis and obtained good outcomes. Recently, the clinical effectiveness of modified VAS using an extracorporeally established centrifugal pump was advocated by John et al. (2007) in the United States. Modified VAS has combined the advantages of minimally invasive extracorporeal membrane oxygenation and high efficiency.

5.2 Immunoregulation therapy

Generally, the time limit for continuous mechanical circulatory support, including PCPS or VAS, is approximately 1 week. We withdraw the system even if recovery from circulatory failure is incomplete. In such cases, introduction of immunoregulation therapy is discussed. Many case reports have asserted the effectiveness of immunoregulation therapy. Although there is no established evidence, we believe that immunoregulation is acceptable in intractable cases because no radical treatments are presently available.

5.2.1 High-dose γ-globulin

The effectiveness of high-dose γ-globulin was reported by Takada et al. (1995). It is expected that γ-globulin counteracts the actions of the infective viruses and reduces suppression of cardiac function by inflammatory cytokines during the acute phase. γ-Globulin intensifies patients' immune competence, and therefore complications, such as an infection compromised by steroid administration, do not take hold. The mechanisms of high-dose administration have not been completely clarified, although several hypotheses have been suggested: (1) it functions as a neutralizing antibody; (2) it has an anti-inflammatory effect, reducing the release of inflammatory cytokines induced by a combination of the Fc part of γ-globulin and the suppressive Fc receptor of macrophages; and (3) it has the effect of anti-activation on activated complement (Rosen, 1993). However, it is not strongly recommended because there is no evidence that has been confirmed by large clinical trials. Finally, cardiac function has not recovered in several cases with its use.

5.2.2 High-dose steroids

The effectiveness of steroids as anti-inflammatory and immunosuppressant drugs has been widely accepted. Its effectiveness when treating patients with fulminant myocarditis has been also reported in many studies (Ino et al., 1995). However, administration of steroid was not proved effective in patients with lymphocytic myocarditis in a clinical trial (Mason et al., 1995). We would not hastily administer steroids to patients with acute-phase myocarditis with a suspected viral infection. On the other hand, it is expected that administration of steroids alleviates cardiac dysfunction in patients with giant cell myocarditis and eosinophilic myocarditis (Cooper et al., 1997). Particularly, high-dose steroids should be given prior to other treatments in patients with the fulminant type of giant cell myocarditis.

6. Conclusions

It is not easy to explain myocarditis concisely and clearly because there are varieties of causes, clinical types, clinical courses, and the severity of circulatory failure. Some patients present with common cold-like symptoms, whereas others require mechanical circulatory support in the ER because of a suddenly developing circulatory crisis. Information of the patient's background and clinical history is essential when deciding on a treatment plan for myocarditis in most cases, although we are sometimes unexpectedly confronted with emergency conditions regarding these patients in the ER.

Currently, the most troublesome issue in the course of treating myocarditis is when to perform a myocardial biopsy for a definitive diagnosis. Although noninvasive diagnostic methods such as CMR have been developed to reduce the risk of serious complications and physical strain on the patient, an effective diagnosis cannot be established during the acute phase. Regarding the treatment for myocarditis, we cannot presently exclude original causes in many cases and can only provide unpredictable "bridge" support, such as PCPS or VAS.

Many patients with myocarditis can survive if we remember the possibility of myocarditis in the differential diagnosis and provide immediate, adequate treatment. When we face illness of unknown origin in patients with a severe arrhythmia or circulatory failure, we should immediately assemble the medical staff and prepare cardiac support. Any delay in treatment can allow abrupt deterioration of the circulation. Additionally, we should establish a system of simultaneous processing of the histological diagnosis to decide on the propriety of immunoregulation therapy.

7. References

Aoyama, N., Izumi, T., Hiramori, K., et al. (2002). Japanese investigations of fulminant myocarditis: national survey of fulminant myocarditis in Japan: therapeutic guidelines and long-term prognosis of using percutaneous cardiopulmonary support for fulminant myocarditis (special report from a scientific committee). *Circ J*, 66, 133-144.

Aretz, H.T., Billingham, M.E., Edwards, W.D., et al. (1987). Myocarditis: a histopathologic definition and classification. *Am J Cardiovasc Pathol*, 1, 3-14.

Bandorff, C., Lee, G.H., Lamphear, B.J., et al. (1999). Enteroviral protease 2A cleaves dystrophin: evidence of cytoskeletal disruption in an acquired cardiomyopathy. *Nat Med*, 5, 320-326.

Baughman, K.L. (2006). Diagnosis of myocarditis: death of Dallas criteria. *Circulation,* 113, 593-595.

Bowles, N.E., Richardson, P.J., Olsen, E.G., et al. (1986). Detection of Coxsackie-B-virus-specific RNA sequences in myocardial biopsy samples from patients with myocarditis and dilated cardiomyopathy. *Lancet,* 17, 1120-1123.

Chen, Y.S., & Yu, H.Y. (2005). Choice of mechanical support for fulminant myocarditis: ECMO vs. VAD? *Eur J Cardiothorac Surg,* 27, 921-932.

Clements, G.B. (1993). Characteristics of viruses inducing cardiac disease, In: *Viral Infection of the Heart,* J.E. Banatvala (Ed.), l-21, Hodder & Stoughton, London.

Cooper, L.T., Berry, G.J., & Shabetai, R. (1997). Idiopathic giant-cell myocarditis: natural history and treatment. *N Engl J Med,* 336, 1860-1866.

Cooper, L.T., Baughman, K.L., Feldman, A.M., et al. (2007). The role of endomyocardial biopsy in the management of cardiovascular disease: a scientific statement from the American Heart Association, the American College of Cardiology, and the European Society of Cardiology; endorsed by the Heart Failure Society of America and the Heart Failure Association of the European Society of Cardiology. *J Am Coll Cardiol,* 50, 1914-1931.

Cupta, S., Markham, D.W., & Drazner, M.H. (2008). Mammen fulminant myocarditis. *Nat Clin Pract Cardiovasc,* 11, 693-706.

Davidoff, R., Palacios, I., Southern, J., et al. (1991). Giant cell versus lymphocytic myocarditis: a comparison of their clinical features and long-term outcomes. *Circulation,* 83, 953-961.

Fairweather, D., Frisancho-Kiss, S., & Rose, N.R. (2005). Viruses as adjuvants for autoimmunity: evidence from Coxsackie-virus-induced myocarditis. *Rev Med Virol,*15, 17-27.

Feely, K.M., Harris, J., & Suvarna, S.K. (2000). Necropsy diagnosis of myocarditis: a retrospective study using CD45RO immunohistochemistry. *J Clin Pathol,* 53, 147-149.

Felker, G.M., Thompson, R.E., Hare, J.M., et al. (2000). Underlying causes and long-term survival in patients with initially unexplained cardiomyopathy. *N Engl J Med,* 342, 1077-1084.

Forrester, J.S., Diamond, G., Chatterjee, K., et al. (1976). Medical therapy of acute myocardial infarction by application hemodynamic subsets (second of two parts). *N Engl J Med,* 295, 1404-1413.

Friedrich, M.G., Strohm, O., Schulz-Menger, J., et al. (1998). Contrast media-enhanced magnetic resonance imaging visualizes myocardial changes in the course of viral myocarditis. *Circulation,* 97, 1802-1809.

Fujioka, S., Kitaura, Y., Ukimura, A., et al. (2000). Evaluation of viral infection in the myocardium of patients with idiopathic dilated cardiomyopathy. *J Am Coll Cardiol,* 36, 1920-1926.

Fuse, K., Kodama, M., Okura, Y., et al. (2000). Predictors of disease course in patients with acute myocarditis. *Circulation,* 102, 2829-2835.

Getz, M. A., Subramanian, R., Logemann, T., et al. (1991). Acute necrotizing eosinophilic myocarditis as a manifestation of severe hypersensitivity myocarditis. Antemortem diagnosis and successful treatment. *Ann Intern Med,* 201-202.

Grinda, J.M., Chevalier, P., D'Attellis, N., et al. (2004). Fulminant myocarditis in adults and children: bi-ventricular assist device for recovery. *Eur J Cardiothorac Surg,* 26, 1169-1173.

Hiramitsu, S., Morimoto, S., Kato, S., et al. (2001). Transient ventricular wall thickening in acute myocarditis: a serial echocardiographic and histological study. *Jpn Circ J,* 65, 2001.

Imanaka-Yoshida, K., Hiroe, M., Yasutomi, Y., et al. (2002). Tenascin-C is a useful marker for disease activity in myocarditis. *J Pathol,* 197, 388-394.

Ino, T., Okubo, M., Akimoto, K., et al. (1995). Corticosteroid therapy for ventricular tachycardia in children with silent lymphocytic myocarditis. *J Pediatr,* 126, 304-308.

Japanese Circulation Society (JCS) Task Force Committee on Chronic Myocarditis. (1996). Guideline for diagnosing chronic myocarditis. *Jpn Circ J,* 60, 263-264.

Japanese Circulation Society; Joint Working Group for Guidelines for Diagnosis and Treatment of Cardiovascular Diseases. (2005). Guidelines for diagnosis and treatment for myocarditis (JCS 2004). *J Cardiol,* 45, 377-384.

Japanese Circulation Society joint working group. (2011). Guidelines for Diagnosis and Treatment of Myocarditis (JCS 2009). *Circ J,* 75, 734-743.

John, R., Liao, K., Lietz, K., et al. (2007). Experience with the Levitronix CentriMag circulatory support system as a bridge to decision in patients with refractory acute cardiogenic shock and multisystem organ failure. *J Thorac Cardiovasc Surg,* 134, 351-358.

Kawai, C. (1999). From myocarditis to cardiomyopathy: mechanisms of inflammation and cell death: learning from the past for the future. *Circulation,* 99, 1091-1100.

Kawamura, K., Kitaura, Y., Deguchi H., et al. (1986). National questionnaire survey of viral or idiopathic myocarditis: 3rd report (Japanese), pp 23-26.

Kodama, M., Oda, H., Okabe, M., et al. (2001). Early and long-term mortality of the clinical subtypes of myocarditis. *Jpn Circ J,* 65, 961-964.

Lauer, B., Niederau, C., Kuhl, U., et al. (1997). Cardiac troponin T in patients with clinically suspected myocarditis. *J Am Coll Cardiol,* 30, 1354-1359.

Lauer, B., Schannwell, M., Kuhl, U., et al. Antimyosin autoantibodies are associated with deterioration of systolic and diastolic left ventricular function in patients with chronic myocarditis. *J Am Coll Cardiol,* 35, 11-18.

Mahrholdt, H., Goedecke, C., Wagner, A., et al. (2004). Cardiovascular magnetic resonance assessment of human myocarditis: a comparison to histology and molecular pathology. *Circulation,* 109, 1250-1258.

Maron, B.J., Towbin, J. A., Thiene, G., et al (2006). Contemporary definitions and classification of the cardiomyopathies: an American Heart Association Scientific Statement from the Council on Clinical Cardiology, Heart Failure and Transplantation Committee; Quality of Care and Outcomes Research and Functional Genomics and Translational Biology Interdisciplinary Working Groups; and Council on Epidemiology and Prevention. *Circulation,* 113, 1807-1816.

Mason, J.W., O'Connell, J.B., Herskowitz, A., et al. (1995). A clinical trial of immunosuppressive therapy for myocarditis. *N Engl J Med,* 333, 269-275.

McCarthy, R., 3rd, Boehmer, J.P., Hruban, R.H., et al. (2000). Long-term outcome of fulminant myocarditis as compared with acute (nonfluminant) myocarditis. *N Engl J Med,* 342, 690-695.

McFalls, E.O., van Suylen, R.J. (1993). Myocarditis as a cause of primary right ventricular failure. *Chest,* 103, 1607-1608.
McNamara, D.M., Holubkov, R., Starling, R.C., et al. (2001). Controlled trial of intravenous immune globulin in recent-onset dilated cardiomyopathy. *Circulation,* 103, 2254-2259.
Mikami, S., Kawashima, S., Kanazawa, K., et al. (1996). Expression of nitric oxide synthase in a murine model of viral myocarditis induced by coxsackievirus B3. *Biochem Biophys Res Commun,* 220, 983-989.
Miura, K., Nakagawa, H., Morikawa, Y., et al. (2002). Epidemiology of idiopathic cardiomyopathy in Japan: results from a nationwide survey. *Heart,* 87, 126-130.
Mori, N., Morimoto, S., Hiramatsu, S., et al. (2004). Clinical pictures of 35 cases with eosinophilic myocarditis. *Circ J,* 68(suppl), 244.
Morimoto, S., Kubo, N., Hiramatsu, S., et al. (2003). Changes in the peripheral eosinophil count in patients with acute eosinophilic myocarditis. *Heart Vessels,* 18, 193-196.
Morguet, A.J., Munz, D.L., Kreuzer, H., et al. (1994). Scintigraphic detection of inflammatory heart disease. *Eur J Nucl Med,* 21, 666-674.
Nishii, M., Inomata, T., Takehana, H., et al. (2004). Serum levels of interleukin-10 on admission as a prognostic predictor of human fulminant myocarditis. *J Am Coll Cardiol,* 44, 1292-1297.
O'Connel, J.B., Henkin, R.E., Robinson, J.A., et al. (1984). Gallium-67 imaging in patients with dilated cardiomyopathy and biopsy-proven myocarditis. *Circulation,* 70, 58-62.
Okabe, M., Fukuda, K., Arakawa, K., et al. (1997). Chronic variant of myocarditis associated with hepatitis C virus infection. *Circulation,* 96, 22-24.
Okada, R., Kawai, S., & Kasuya, R. (1989). Nonspecific myocarditis: a statistical and clinicopathological study of autopsy cases. *Jpn Circ J,* 53, 40-48.
Richardson, P., McKenna, W., Bristow, M., et al (1996). Report of the 1995 World Health Organization/International Society and Federation of Cardiology Task Force on the Definition and Classification of Cardiomyopathies. *Circulation,* 93, 841-842.
Rosen, F.S. (1993). Putative mechanisms of the effect of intravenous gamma-globulin. *Clin Immunol Immunopathol,* 67, S41-S43.
Sekiguchi, M., Hiroe, M., Take, M., et al. (1980). Clinical and histopathological profile of sarcoidosis of the heart and acute idiopathic myocarditis: concepts through a study employing endomyocardial biopsy. II. Myocarditis. *Jpn Circ J,* 44, 264-273.
Seko, Y., Matsuda, H., Kato, K., et al. (1993). Expression of intercellular adhesion molecule-1 in murine hearts with acute myocarditis caused by coxsackievirus B3. *J Clin Invest,* 91, 1327-1336.
Shields, R.C., Tazelaar H.D., Berry, G.J., et al. (2002). The role of right ventricular endomyocardial biopsy for idiopathic giant cell myocarditis. *J Cardiac Fail,* 8, 74-78.
Silver, M.A., Kowalczyk, D. (1989). Coronary microvascular narrowing in acute murine coxsackie B3 myocarditis. *Am Heart J,* 118, 173-174.
Takada, H., Kishimoto, C., & Hiraoka, Y. (1995). Therapy with immunoglobulin suppresses myocarditis in a murine coxsakievirus B3 model: antiviral and anti-inflammatory effects. *Circulation,* 92, 1604-1611.
Topkara V.K., Dang, N.C., Barili, F., et al. (2006). Ventricular assist device use for the treatment of acute viral myocarditis. *J Thorac Cardiovasc Surg,* 131, 1190-1191.

Zagrosek, A., Wassmuth, R., Abdel-Aty, H., et al. (2008). Relation between myocardial edema and myocardial mass during the acute and convalescent phase of myocarditis: a CMR study. *J Cardiovasc Magn Reson,* 10,19.

5

Perimyocarditis

Hesham R. Omar[1], Hany Abdelmalak[1], Engy Helal[2], Yara Mikhaeil[3] and Ahmed Fathy[4]

[1]*Internal Medicine Department. Mercy Hospital and Medical Center, Chicago, Illinois,*
[2]*Emergency Department, Agouza Police Hospital, Cairo, Egypt*
[3]*Northwestern University, Feinberg School of Medicine.*
[4]*Cardiology Department. National Heart institute. Cairo, Egypt*
[1,3]*USA*
[2,4]*Egypt*

1. Introduction

Perimyocarditis is an acute inflammation of the pericardium and the underlying myocardium resulting in myocellular damage. It can simply be considered as acute pericarditis with elevated cardiac biomarkers. The coexistence of acute myocarditis and pericarditis is not uncommon since both are commonly caused by cardiotropic viruses. The 2 terms "perimyocarditis" and "myopericarditis" are used to describe the disease. While perimyocarditis implies predominant myocardial involvement and myopericarditis implies predominant pericardial involvement, both terms are used interchangeably without specific reference to the type of cardiac involvement. There is a wide spectrum of clinical presentations reflecting the extent of myocardial involvement ranging from asymptomatic cases with spontaneous recovery, to mild cases where symptoms are masked by the existing illness, to more severe cases complicated with heart failure necessitating inotropic support or even cardiac transplantation. Due to detrimental complications of acute myocarditis including left ventricular dysfunction and ventricular arrhythmias the diagnosis of myocarditis is more important and should be thoroughly looked for. Monitoring of the cardiac biomarkers is therefore mandatory in every patient presenting with clinical picture and electrocardiographic (EKG) evidence of acute pericarditis to exclude an underlying myocarditis. Acute pericarditis can present with ST segment elevation which can sometimes be focal rather than diffuse. In this scenario, chest pain associated with focal ST segment elevation and elevated cardiac biomarkers (if myocarditis co-existed) can mimic transmural myocardial infarction. Differentiation between both entities is of utmost importance to avert the un-necessary utilization of thrombolytic therapy which can be deleterious in perimyocarditis or to avoid missing a more serious diagnosis of ST segment elevation myocardial infarction (STEMI). After hospital discharge, patients should be followed for several weeks to exclude the development of heart failure or subclinical left ventricular dysfunction.

2. Etiology

Similar to myocarditis, perimyocarditis is most commonly of viral aetiology and less likely due to bacterial infection. Viral etiologies are predominately due to the coxsackie B virus, however, other viruses have been incriminated including cytomegalovirus [1], parvovirus B 19 [2], Epestein-Barr virus [3], Rubella [4], influenza A virus [5] and during hepatitis A virus infection [6]. The most famous bacterial pathogens associated with perimyocarditis are Borrelia burgderferi [7] and Campylobacter jejuni [8]. Others include Mycoplasma pneumonia [9], Chlamydia pneumonia, [10], Brucella [11], Rickettsia Helvetica [12], Yersinia enterocolitica [13], rickettsial Q fever [14], Shigella boydii [15], Shigella sonnei [16], tuberculosis [17], following Streptococcal tonsillitis [18] and Meningococcal septicemia[19]. The protozoan Toxoplasma gondii has also been described as a cause [20]. Immunizations have also been linked with perimyocarditis. The Smallpox vaccine has received great attention especially after its reinstitution for military personnel in 2002 and the report of 50 cases of perimyocarditis [21, 22]. There are several reported cases of perimyocarditis that developed hours after Diphtheria-Tetanus-acellular Pertussis (DTaP) vaccination [23, 24]. Perimyocarditis has also been linked to the administration of certain drugs including meselazine used in the treatment of inflammatory bowel disease [25]. Table 1 represents a compilation of reported etiologies of perimyocarditis.

Etiology of perimyocarditis	
Viral pathogens	Coxsackie B virus Cytomegalovirus Parvovirus B19 Epestein barr virus Rubella Influenza A virus Hepatitis A virus
Bacterial pathogens	Borrelia burgderferi Campylobacter jejuni Mycoplasma pneumonia Chlamydia pneumonia Brucella Rickettsia Helvetica Yersinia enterocolitica Rickettsial q fever shigella boydii Shigella sonnei Tuberculosis Following streptococcal tonsiliitis Following meningococcal septicemia
Protozoa	Toxoplasma gondii
Immunizations	Smallpox vaccine Diphtheria-tetanus-acellular pertussis (DTaP) vaccination tetanus vaccination alone
Immunologic/Connective tissue disease	Sarcoidosis Rheumatoid arthritis Systemic lupus erythematosus Acute rheumatic fever
Drug induced	Meselazine Methydolpa Sulphonamide Cocaine

Table 1. Causes of perimyocarditis.

3. Clinical picture

Perimyocarditis has a wide spectrum of presentation with some cases being asymptomatic, some suffering from symptoms of the preceding viral illness and some presenting with acute heart failure and cardiogenic shock as in cases with fulminant myocarditis. 60% of the cases have constitutional symptoms including fever, arthralgia, malaise and chills. In 35% of the cases, there is chest pain which is usually mild, persistent, stitching, worsens with deep inspiration or coughing and radiates specifically to the trapezius ridge. Chest pain can sometimes be severe raising the suspicion of myocardial infarction which is always in the differential. Patients may also present with palpitations, syncope, Stokes-Adams attacks or sudden death due to arrhythmias including ventricular tachycardia and variable degrees of conduction abnormalities. Careful history taking is mandatory with specific reference to the patient's age, underlying medical problems including diabetes mellitus, hypertension, dyslipidemia, smoking history, positive family history of coronary artery disease and cocaine abuse that can place the patient at risk for myocardial ischemia. Clinical examination may be irrelevant with non-specific features as fever and tachycardia being the only positive clinical findings. Other clues in examination include a pericardial friction rub, however, only a minority of patients have pericardial rub on exam which tends to be transient and variable [26, 27]. A study of a cohort of patients with acute pericarditis confirmed poor sensitivity of a pericardial friction rub, which was found in only 35% of the cases [26]. Signs of decompensated heart failure (e.g. S3 gallop, elevated jugular venous pressure, lower limb edema and pulmonary congestion) can be detected in patients with fulminant myocarditis.

4. Cardiac biomarkers and other laboratory tests

Laboratory investigations in perimyocarditis can reveal elevated white blood cell count (WBC), erythrocyte sedimentation rate (ESR), C-reactive protein (CRP) and Brain natriuretic peptide (BNP) levels. Cardiac biomarkers are also elevated due to myocarditis. The incidence of elevated cardiac troponin I in patients with viral or idiopathic acute pericarditis has been reported to be 32.2%; of these patients 23.7% had a troponin I level at admission higher than those seen in myocardial infarction [28]. Elevated cardiac biomarkers in pericardial disease are not unusual and further complicate the diagnosis, raising suspicion for alternative diagnoses including myocardial infarction [29]. A study by Machdo et. al. concluded that perimyocarditis has a higher cardiac mortality than pericarditis [30]. This illustrates the importance of checking cardiac markers in all patients presenting with pericarditis. Studies also showed that elevated troponin is more common than elevated CKMB [31, 32]. The sole increase in troponin without other cardiac markers might represent a mild degree of myocardial injury.

5. Electrocardiography

Because the pericardium is electrically inert, EKG changes found in patients with acute pericarditis are suggestive of an underlying myocardial involvement. The typical EKG evolution is seen in up to 60 % of cases of acute pericarditis [26]. EKG may reveal sinus tachycardia, diffuse ST segment elevation that is concave upwards involving any lead except aVR and V1. In pericarditis, T wave inversion occurs only after the elevated ST segment returns to baseline. ST-segment elevation associated with pericarditis should not result in the reciprocal depressions in aVL that accompany inferior MI, although this may not apply in some cases of localized pericarditis [33]. The most specific EKG finding for acute pericarditis is PR segment depression (PR segment elevation in aVR) which is considered an early EKG marker in the evolution of acute pericarditis. PR segment depression is due to subepicardial atrial injury and is present in more than 60 % of the patients. Acute pericarditis causes characteristic EKG changes that typically evolve through 4 stages as demonstrated in table 2.

Stage 1	Occurs during the first few days of pericardial inflammation and may last up to 2 weeks	- Widespread concave upward ST segment elevation except in leads aVR and V1 - Ratio of ST segment elevation to the T-wave amplitude in lead V5 or V6 is ≥ 0.25 - PR segment depression - Absence of reciprocal ST changes
Stage 2	Occurs hours to days after initial symptoms and may last from days to several weeks	- ST segment returns to baseline - In the early phase, the J point returns to baseline while T waves are still upright and in the late phase T waves becomes flattened or even inverted
Stage 3	Begins between the second and third week and may continue for several weeks	- Diffuse T wave inversion
Stage 4	May last from days up to 3 months	- Resolution of T wave inversion and EKG returns back to baseline. - Rarely T wave in nversions may persist indefinitely (chronic pericarditis).

Table 2. The 4 Electrocardiographic stages of acute pericarditis.

Nevertheless, perimyocarditis can present with focal instead of diffuse ST segment elevation mimicking transmural myocardial infarction. This, in addition to the presence of chest pain and elevated cardiac biomarkers can make the differentiation of increasing difficulty. This is important because fatal complications can occur if thrombolytic therapy is administered for a patient with acute pericarditis, or if a diagnosis of transmural myocardial infarction is missed. Omar et al. demonstrated a similar scenario where an EKG of a patient presenting with chest pain revealed focal ST segment elevation (figure 1) and the cardiac biomarkers were elevated mimicking STEMI. [34] Careful history taking, EKG interpretation and urgent echocardiogram favored the diagnosis of acute perimyocarditis.

Previous studies have reported the use of thrombolytic therapy for what was later determined to be acute pericarditis [35, 36]. The utilization of urgent coronary angiography is not uncommon in patients with acute perimyocarditis. Salisbury and colleagues described the frequency of urgent coronary angiography in 238 patients with a final diagnosis of acute pericarditis to be 16.8 % [37].

6. Echocardiography

Echocardiography looking for pericardial effusion and regional wall motion abnormalities is mandatory to help in making the diagnosis and excluding other serious differentials. Imazio

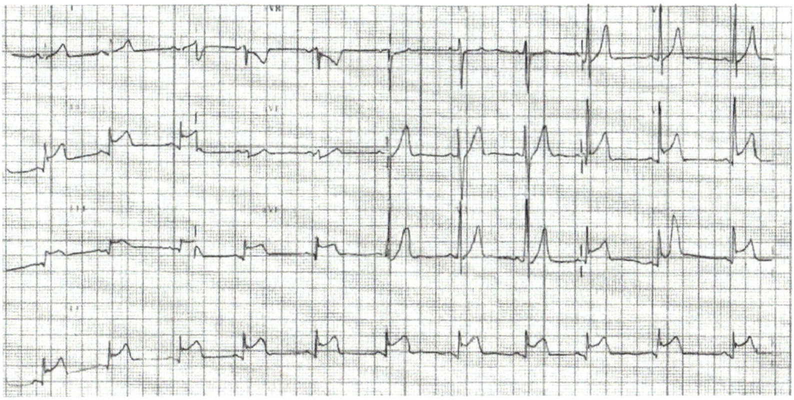

Fig. 1. Concave upward ST segment elevation in leads II, III, Avf, V5 and V6 in a patient with perimyocarditis. Notice the focal pattern of ST segment elevation (inferolateral leads) thereby mimicking transmural myocardial infarction. Adapted from Omar et. al. [34].

and collegues found that pericardial effusions are present in approximately 60% of cases of acute pericarditis, with 80% being mild, 10% being moderate, and 10% being severe [26]. Pericardial effusion was present in 38.1% of patients in the ST segment elevation group and 73.5% of the patients in the non ST segment elevation and was explained by the tendency of the larger pericardial effusions to decrease voltage including the magnitude of ST segment elevation [26]. The presence of regional wall motion abnormalities favors an ischemic process rather than acute pericarditis. Another potential echocardiographic finding in perimyocarditis is transient myocardial thickening (figure 2 and 3) which is due to interstitial edema and its presence likely predicts a poor prognosis as it has been associated with a fulminant course [38]. In a series of 25 patients with acute myocarditis who underwent echocardiogram and endomyocardial biopsy, a significant decrease in myocardial thickness was observed between the acute and the convalescent phase. The reduction of the edema shown by the biopsy was also significant [39].

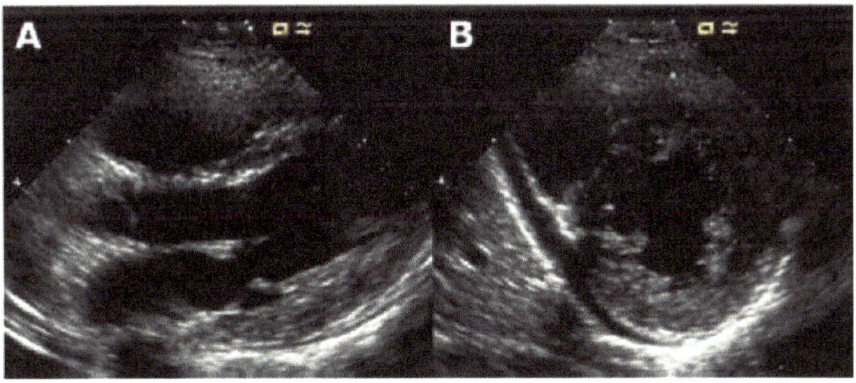

Fig. 2. Echocardiogram on admission. Parasternal long axis view (A) and short axis (B) in diastole. There is an asymmetrical thickening of the posterior wall involving the posterior papillary muscle, and slight pericardial effusion. Adapted from reference number 38 with permission.

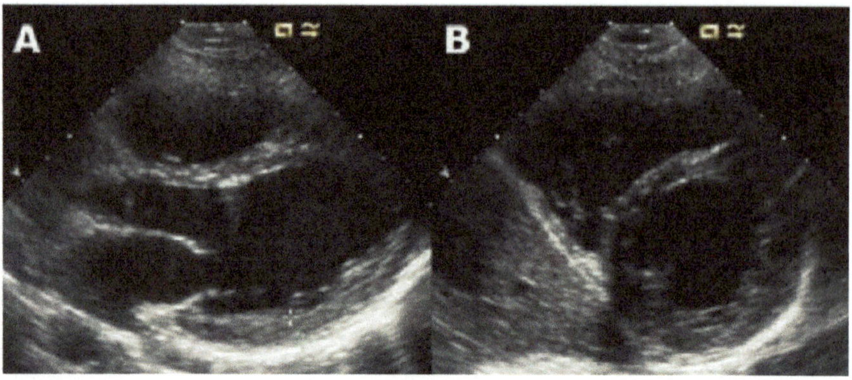

Fig. 3. Echocardiogram 5 days after admission. Parasternal long axis view (A) and short axis (B) in diastole. Normalization of the myocardial thickness in the posterior wall and posterior papillary and resolution of the pericardial effusion can be seen. Adapted from reference 38 with permission.

7. CT angiography

Another non-invasive diagnostic tool in patients presenting with chest pain, ST segment elevation and elevated cardiac biomarkers is the use of the 64-slice coronary CT angiography (CCTA) which is a reliable test that can be utilized in patients with low to intermediate pretest probability for coronary artery disease. Shturman et. al. used the 64-slice CCTA to rule out coronary artery disease in a case of perimyocarditis mimicking myocardial infarction [40]. This simple noninvasive test and can avert the unnecessary need for coronary angiography or thrombolytic therapy for a presumed STEMI. Recently, Computed tomographic angiography (CTA) "triple rule out" protocol has been utilized in the emergency department for patients presenting with acute chest pain to differentiate between pulmonary embolism, aortic dissection and acute coronary syndrome. Compared with the usual radiation dose of a standard 64-slice CCTA, the effective radiation dose of a "triple rule-out" scan is often increased by 50% which should limit its unrestricted use. Takakuwa et. al. reported the successful use of the "triple rule-out" scan in diagnosing acute perimyocarditis (figure 4) and excluding other serious etiologies as acute coronary syndrome, aortic dissection and pulmonary embolism [41].

8. Cardiac magnetic resonance imaging

In perimyocarditis, gadolinium contrast MRI is useful to confirm the diagnosis by detecting an area of delayed contrast-enhancement, to evaluate the severity of inflammation in the acute stage as well as to determine the extent of fibrosis in the pericardium and myocardium [42]. The normal pericardium is observed as an area of low intensity on T1-weighted images and T2-weighted images [43]. In acute pericarditis, the inflamed pericardium is thickened and appears as an area of medium to high intensity with delayed contrast-enhancement recognized in the swollen pericardium which extends to the subepicardial myocardium affected by myocarditis [42]. The delayed enhancement in cardiac magnetic resonance (CMR) is explained by the leaking of the contrast media into the interstitial space due to

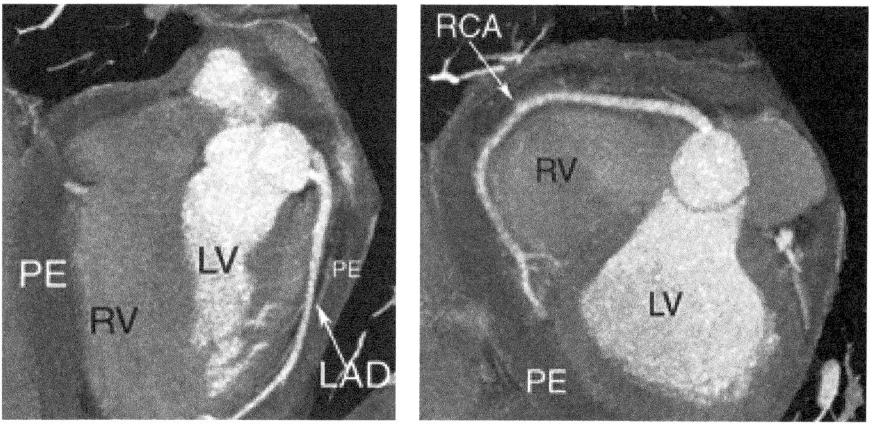

Fig. 4. Four chamber view (left). TRO study demonstrating mild-to-moderate pericardial effusion surrounding the heart. Left anterior oblique view (right) optimized to visualize the full length of the RCA. PE - pericardial effusion, RV - right ventricle, LV - left ventricle, LAD - left anterior descending coronary artery. Adapted with modification from reference number 41 with permission.

inflammation. As it stays out of the vessel, it cannot be washed away and is held for a longer time allowing it to be seen in the delayed enhancement images (figure 5) [44].

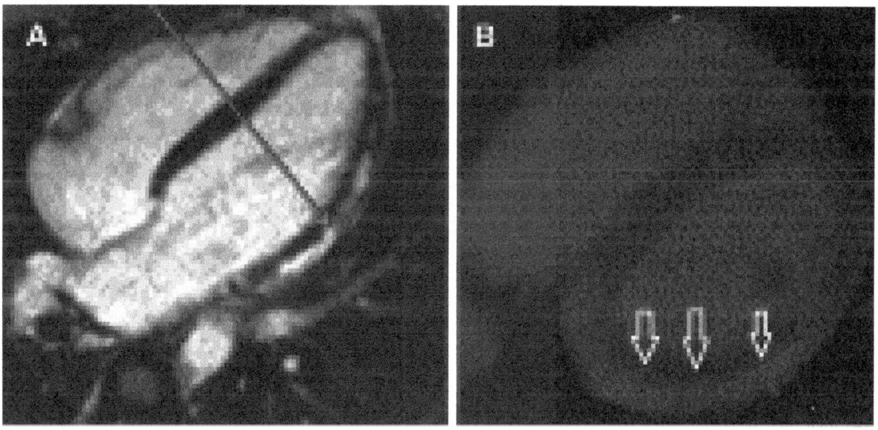

Fig. 5. Four chamber long-axis views. (A) Cardiac magnetic gadolinium delayed enhancement showing subepicardial hyperenhancement (arrow). (B) Cardiac CT delayed enhancement (arrows). Adapted from reference 44 with permission from Elsevier.

Cardiac magnetic resonance can also be a tool to differentiate between acute perimyocarditis and myocardial infarction. In acute myocarditis, myocardial late gadolinium enhancement is present in up to 88% of cases [45,46] which characteristically has patchy distribution not conforming to any particular coronary artery territory and is usually in the subepicardial and not the subendocardial layer [47] differentiating it from myocardial infarction.

9. Endomyocardial biopsy

Myocarditis may be focal or diffuse affecting any or all cardiac chambers. Although biopsy is the gold standard for the diagnosis, it is of limited utility especially in acute myocarditis, because of the patchy nature of active inflammation. In a series of over 2,000 patients with clinically suspected myocarditis, endomyocardial biopsy was only positive in 10% of the cases [48-50]. Given the potential risks of biopsy and the limited value it offers, its use should be limited to the patients with left ventricular dysfunction unresponsive to conventional therapy [51].

The various histologic patterns of myocarditis include either lymphocytic (including viral and autoimmune forms), eosinophilic (in which hypersensitivity myocarditis is the most common, followed by cases of hypereosinophilic syndrome), granulomatous (sarcoid and giant cell myocarditis), neutrophilic (bacterial, fungal, and early forms of viral myocarditis), and reperfusion type/contraction band necrosis (present in catecholamine-induced injury and reperfusion injury). Figure 6 represents the microscopic picture of acute perimyocarditis after diphtheria-tetanus vaccination.

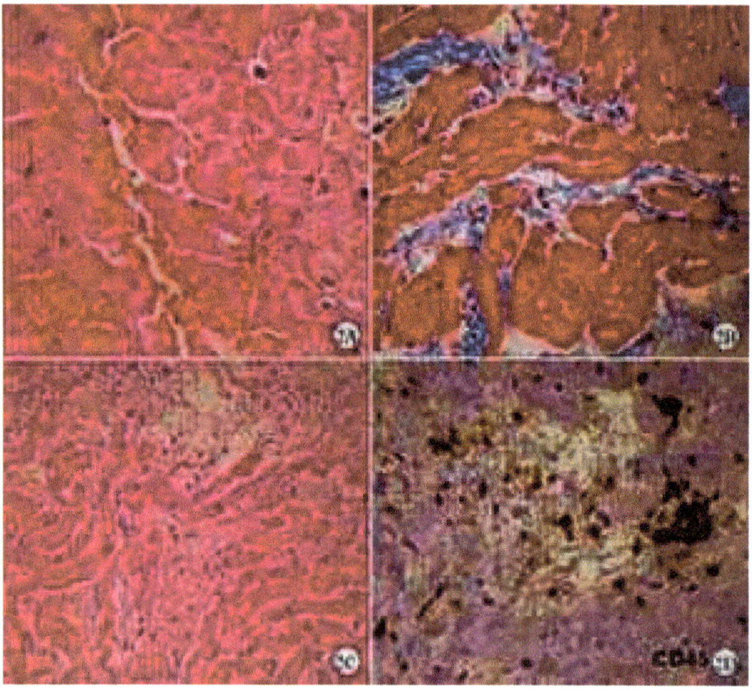

Fig. 6. Right ventricular endomyocardial biopsy. A . Haematoxylin-eosin, original magnification 200x: Diffuse interstitial oedema with scattered inflammatory cells. B. Immunohistochemical staining with anti-CD45 antibody, original magnification 400x: Lymphocyte inflammatory infiltrate associated with myocyte damage. C. Mallory triple stain, original magnification 200x: minimal interstitial fibrosis mixed with interstitial oedema. D. Haematoxylin-eosin, original magnification 200x: One focus of interstitial haemorrhage. Adapted from Journal of Chinese Clinical Medicne;2008,9;Vol.3,No.9. [24]

10. Management

As earlier described, perimyocarditis is a combination of both pericardial inflammation and myocardial damage. Treatment should therefore target both pathologies. Because myocarditis is a more serious diagnosis owing to the potential of serious ventricular arrhythmias and heart failure, the diagnosis of myocarditis is deemed more important. Acute pericarditis usually runs a smooth and benign course after empiric treatment with NSAID and routine hospitalization in most cases is not necessary. Perimyocarditis on the other hand has higher incidence of complications and is one of the indications for hospitalization. Checking the levels of cardiac biomarkers and echocardiography is therefore mandatory in any case of acute pericarditis. Imazio et. al. identified certain poor prognostic predictors that are more frequently associated with an increased risk of short term complications and therefore an indication for hospitalization [26]. Table 3 lists various indications for hospitalization of patients presenting with acute pericarditis

Indications for Hospitalization of Patients with Acute Pericarditis
1. Anticoagulation therapy
2. Body temperature greater than 100.4° F (38° C)
3. Echocardiographic findings of a large pericardial effusion
4. Findings of cardiac tamponade (i.e., hypotension and neck vein distention)
5. History of trauma and compromised immune system
6. Myopericarditis
7. Troponin I elevation

Table 3. Indications for Hospitalization of Patients with Acute Pericarditis. (adapted from reference 26)

There are certain scenarios when perimyocarditis present with focal EKG signs suggestive of STEMI. This can be challenging especially in developing countries where thrombolytic therapy is the mainstay of management of STEMI. In patients with acute pericarditis, thrombolytic therapy can be detrimental because of the risk of cardiac tamponade [52, 53].

Although the use of anticoagulants in patients with acute pericarditis is deemed unfavorable, in their study on 274 consecutive cases of idiopathic or viral acute pericarditis, Imazio and colleagues concluded that neither the use of heparin, anticoagulants nor glycoprotein IIb/IIIa inhibitors is associated with an increased risk of cardiac tamponade. [54] Risk factors for complications in that study included the lack of complete response to aspirin or NSAID (OR = 14.6, 95% CI 6.1 to 35.1; P = 0.001), or corticosteroid use (OR = 3.0, 95% CI 1.1 to 8.9; P = 0.048).

The mainstay of therapy for acute pericarditis is NSAID (class 1 recommendation in 2004 ESC guidelines). The goal of NSAID is to reduce pain and inflammation. Ibuprofen might be preferred because of its rare side effects, favorable impact on coronary artery blood flow and large dose range from 1200 to 1800 mg daily [55]. Aspirin can also be used in anti-inflammatory doses (up to 800 mg every 6 hours). Dose tapering is preferred to avoid recurrence. Gastric protection is mandatory and should be commenced in all patients. In perimyocarditis, NSAID should be used cautiously because in animal models they were shown to enhance the myocarditic process and may increase mortality [56-58]. Lower anti-inflammatory doses should therefore be considered whenever possible in perimyocarditis and its main use is to control symptoms. Failure to respond to NSAID within one week

(indicated by persistence of fever, new pericardial effusion, or continuing chest pain) indicates that a cause other than viral is responsible and should be searched for. Although colchicines can be used alone or in conjunction with NSAID in treatment and prevention of recurrent pericarditis, there is lack of data regarding its benefit in perimyocarditis [59].
The use of corticosteroids was found to be an independent risk factor for recurrence of acute pericarditis [60, 61] because of their ability to promote viral replication [62, 63]. Its use should therefore be restricted for those with autoimmune disease or in cases refractory to NSAID and colchicine and a specific cause has not been found. Despite the long list of pathogens, in most cases, a specific etiology for acute perimyocarditis can't be determined. In instances where an underlying treatable cause is confirmed, treatment of the target organism should be commenced. After hospital discharge, patient should be followed for several weeks to rule out the development of heart failure or subclinical left ventricular dysfunction. All patients should be advised to avoid strenuous exercise during the recovery phase (4-6 weeks) which can increase the risk of ventricular arrhythmias.

11. References

[1] Maisch B, Schönian U, Crombach M, Wendl I, Bethge C, Herzum M, Klein HH: Cytomegalovirus associated inflammatory heart muscle disease. Scand J Infect Dis Suppl 1993, 88:135-48.
[2] Orth T, Herr W, Spahn T, Voigtländer T, Michel D, Mertens T, Mayet WJ, Dippold W, Meyer zum Bûschenfelde KH: Human parvovirus B19 infection associated with severe acute perimyocarditis in a 34-year-old man. Eur Heart J 1997, 18(3):524-5.
[3] Roubille F, Gahide G, Moore-Morris T, Granier M, Davy JM, Vernhet H, Piot C: Epstein Barr virus (EBV) and acute myopericarditis in an immunocompetent patient: first demonstrated case and discussion. Intern Med 2008, 47(7):627-9.
[4] Harada T, Ohtaki E, Tobaru T, Kitahara K, Sumiyoshi T, Hosoda S: Rubella-associated perimyocarditis--a case report. Angiology 2002, 53(6):727-32.
[5] Franzen D, Mertens T, Waidner T, Kruppenbächer J, Höpp HW, Hilger HH: Perimyocarditis in influenza A virus infection. Klin Wochenschr 1991, 69(9):404-8.
[6] Bosson C, Lim DQ, Hadrami J, Chotard Y: Myopericarditis during hepatitis A. Presse Med 1996, 25(21):995-6.
[7] Vasiljević Z, Vujisić B, Dmitrović R, Reljić B, Smiljanić J, Perunicić J, Nikitović S, Vukcević V, Stankov S: [Clinical picture of cardioborreliosis: from AV block to perimyocarditis. Glas Srp Akad Nauka Med 1993:213-8.
[8] Turpie DF, Forbes KJ, Hannah A, Metcalfe MJ, McKenzie H, Small GR: Food-the way to a man's heart: A mini-case series of Campylobacter perimyocarditis. Scand J Infect Dis 2009, 24:1-4.
[9] Pascual Velasco F, Rodríguez Pérez JC: Primary perimyocarditis caused by Mycoplasma pneumonia. An Med Interna 1991, 8(7):360.
[10] Gnarpe H, Gnarpe J, Gästrin B, Hallander H: Chlamydia pneumonia and myocarditis. Scand J Infect Dis Suppl 1997, 104:50-2.
[11] García de Lucas MD, Castillo Domínguez JC, Martínez González MS: [Brucella myopericarditis]. Rev Esp Cardiol 2004, 57(7):709.
[12] Nilsson K, Lindquist O, Påhlson C: Association of Rickettsia Helvetica with chronic perimyocarditis in sudden cardiac death. Lancet 1999, 354(9185):1169-73.

[13] Zöllner B, Sobottka I, Lippe G von der, Boyens M, Pokahr A, Grüter L, Laufs R: [Perimyocarditis caused by Yersinia enterocolitica serotype 0:3. Dtsch Med Wochenschr 1992, 117(47):1794-7.
[14] Maisch B: Rickettsial perimyocarditis--a follow-up study. Heart Vessels 1986, 2(1):55-9.
[15] Vieira NB, Rodriguez-Vera J, Grade MJ, Santos C: Traveler's myopericarditis. Eur J Intern Med 2008, 19(2):146-7.
[16] Védrine L, Perez JP, Debien B, Petitjeans F, Bordier E, Pats B: Myopericarditis complicating severe Shigella sonnei infection. Gastroenterol Clin Biol 2003, 27(12):1176-7.
[17] Roubille F, Gahide G, Granier M, Cornillet L, Vernhet-Kovacsik H, Moore-Morris T, Macia JC, Piot C: Likely tuberculous myocarditis mimicking an acute coronary syndrome. Intern Med 2008, 47(19):1699-701.
[18] Putterman C, Caraco Y, Shalit M: Acute nonrheumatic perimyocarditis complicating streptococcal tonsillitis. Cardiology 1991, 78(2):156-60.
[19] Sipilä R, Kiilavuori K: Meningococcus septicemia accompanied by perimyocarditis. Duodecim 1997, 113(17):1702.
[20] Mroczek-Czernecka D, Rostoff P, Piwowarska W: Acute toxoplasmic perimyocarditis in a 67-year-old HIV-negative woman, a case report. Przegl Lek 2006, 63(2):100-3.
[21] Arness MK, Eckart RE, Love SS, Atwood JE, Wells TS, Engler RJ, Collins LC, Ludwig SL, Riddle JR, Grabenstein JD, Tornberg DN: Myopericarditis following smallpox vaccination. Am J Epidemiol 2004, 160(7):642-51.
[22] Cassimatis DC, Atwood JE, Engler RM, Linz PE, Grabenstein JD, Vernalis MN: Smallpox vaccination and myopericarditis: a clinical review. J Am Coll Cardiol 2004, 43(9):1503-10.
[23] Boccara F, Benhaiem-Sigaux N, Cohen A. Acute myopericarditis after diphtheria, tetanus, and polio vaccination. Chest. 2001 Aug;120(2):671-2.
[24] Taglieri N, Leone O, Ortolani P, Marzocchi A, Dallara G, Rosmini S, Baldazzi F, Rapezzi C, Branz. Acute myopericarditis after diphtheria-tetanus vaccination. Journal of Chinese Clinical Medicne;2008,9;Vol.3,No.9.
[25] García-Morán S, Sáez-Royuela F, Pérez-Alvarez JC, Gento E, Téllez J: Myopericarditis and mitral insufficiency associated with ulcerative colitis treated with mesalazine. Inflamm Bowel Dis 2006, 12(4):334-5.
[26] Imazio M, Demichelis B, Parrini I, et al. Day-hospital treatment of acute pericarditis: a management program for outpatient therapy. J Am Coll Cardiol. 2004;43(6):1042-1046.
[27] Bonnefoy E, Godon P, Kirkorian G, Fatemi M, Chevalier P, Touboul P. Serum cardiac troponin I and ST-segment elevation in patients with acute pericarditis. Eur Heart J. 2000;21(10):832-836.
[28] Imazio M, Demichelis B, Cecchi E, et al. Cardiac troponin I in acute pericarditis. J Am Coll Cardiol. 2003;42(12):2144-2148.
[29] Smith KJ, Theal M, Mulji A . Pericarditis presenting and treated as an acute anteroseptal myocardial infarction. Can J Cardiol. 2001;17(7):815-817.
[30] Machado S, Roubille F, Gahide G, Vernhet-Kovacsik H, Cornillet L, Cung TT, Sportouch-Dukhan C, Raczka F, Pasquié JL, Gervasoni R, Macia JC, Cransac F,Davy JM, Piot C, Leclercq F. Can troponin elevation predict worse prognosis in patients with acute pericarditis?

[31] Smith SC, Ladenson JH, Mason JW, Jaffe AS. Elevations of cardiac troponin I associated with myocarditis. Experimental and clinical Correlates. Circulation. 1997 Jan 7;95(1):163-8.

[32] Lauer B, Niederau C, Kühl U, Schannwell M, Pauschinger M, Strauer BE, Schultheiss HP. Cardiac troponin T in patients with clinically suspected myocarditis. J Am Coll Cardiol. 1997 Nov 1;30(5):1354-9.

[33] Wang K, Asinger RW, Marriott HJ . ST-segment elevation in conditions other than acute myocardial infarction. N Engl J Med.2003;349(22):2128-2135

[34] Omar HR, Fathy A, Rashad R, Elghonemy M. Acute perimyocarditis mimicking transmural myocardial infarction. Int Arch Med. 2009 Dec 9;2(1):37.

[35] Smith KJ, Theal M, Mulji A . Pericarditis presenting and treated as an acute anteroseptal myocardial infarction. Can J Cardiol. 2001;17(7):815-817.

[36] Millaire A, de Groote P, Decoulx E, Leroy O, Ducloux G. Outcome after thrombolytic therapy of nine cases of myopericarditis misdiagnosed as myocardial infarction. Eur Heart J. 1995;16(3):333-338.

[37] Salisbury AC, Olalla-Gómez C, Rihal CS, Bell MR, Ting HH, Casaclang-Verzosa G, Oh JK. Frequency and predictors of urgent coronary angiography in patients with acute pericarditis. Mayo Clin Proc. 2009;84(1):11-5.

[38] Fontenla Cerezuela A, Teijeiro Mestre R, Luaces Méndez M, Serrano Antolín JM. Transient myocardial thickening of the posterior wall in a patient with acute myopericarditis. Rev Esp Cardiol. 2010 Apr;63(4):497-8.

[39] Hiramitsu S, Morimoto S, Kato S, Uemura A, Kubo N, Kimura K, et al. Transient ventricular wall thickening in acute myocarditis. A serial echocardiographic and histopathologic study. Jpn Circ J. 2001;65:863-6.

[40] Shturman A, Chernihovski A, Goldfeld M, Furer A, Wishniak A, Roguin N. Usefulness of 64 multi-slice computed tomography in acute myopericarditis. Isr Med Assoc J. 2007 Apr;9(4):333-4.

[41] Takakuwa KM, Ku BS, Halpern EJ. Myopericarditis diagnosed by a 64-slice coronary CT angiography "triple rule out" protocol. Int J Emerg Med. 2010 Aug 21;3(4):447-9.

[42] Teraoka K, Hirano M, Yannbe M, Ohtaki Y, Ohkubo T, Abe K, Yamashina A. Delayed contrast enhancement in a patient with perimyocarditis on contrast-enhanced cardiac MRI: case report. Int J Cardiovasc Imaging. 2005 Apr-Jun;21(2-3):325-9.

[43] Stark DD, Higgins CB, Lanzer P, et al. Magnetic resonance imaging of the pericardium: normal and pathologic findings. Radiology 1984; 150: 469–474

[44] Ricardo Krieger Azzolini MDa, Fernando Arturo Effio Solis MDa, Paulo Cury Rezende MDa, Claudio Campi MD, PhDa, b, Henrique Lane Staniak MDa, Rodolfo Sharovsky MD, PhDa, Alexandre Volney Villa MDb, Paulo Andrade Lotufo MD, PhDa and Márcio Sommer Bittencourt MDa Acute inferolateral ST-elevation myopericarditis diagnosed by delayed enhancement cardiac computed tomography. Journal of Cardiology Cases. Volume 3, Issue 2, April 2011, Pages e90-e93.

[45] Mahrholdt H, Goedecke C, Wagner A, Meinhardt G, Athanasiadis A, Vogelsberg H, et al.: Cardiovascular magnetic resonance assessment of human myocarditis: a comparison to histology and molecular pathology. Circulation 2004, 109:1250-8.

[46] Abdel-Aty H, Boye P, Zagrosek A, Wassmuth R, Kumar A, Messroghli D, et al.: Diagnostic performance of cardiovascular magnetic resonance in patients with suspected acute myocarditis: comparison of different approaches. J Am Coll Cardiol 2005, 45:1815-22.

[47] Friedrich MG: Tissue characterization of acute myocardial infarction and myocarditis by cardiac magnetic resonance. J Am Coll Cardiol Img 2008, 1:652-62.

[48] Aretz HT, Billingham ME, Edwars WD, et al. Myocarditis. A histopathologic definition and classification. Am J Cardiovasc Pathol. 1987;1:3–14

[49] Davies MJ, Ward DE. How can myocarditis be diagnosed and should it be treated? Br Heart J. 1992;68:346–347

[50] Mason JW, O'Connell JB, Herskowitz A, et al. A clinical trial of immunosuppressive therapy for myocarditis. The Myocarditis Treatment Trial Investigators. N Engl J Med. 1995;333:269–275

[51] Cassimatis DC, Atwood JE, Engler RM, Linz PE, Grabenstein JD, Vernalis MN. Smallpox vaccination and myopericarditis: a clinical review. J Am Coll Cardiol. 2004 May 5;43(9):1503-10.

[52] Blankenship JC, Almquist AK. Cardiovascular complications of thrombolytic therapy in patients with a mistaken diagnosis of acute myocardial infarction. J Am Coll Cardiol. 1989 Nov 15;14(6):1579-82.

[53] Tilley WS, Harston WE. Inadvertent administration of streptokinase to patients with pericarditis. Am J Med. 1986 Sep;81(3):541-4.

[54] Imazio M, Cecchi E, Demichelis B, Chinaglia A, Ierna S, Demarie D, Ghisio A, Pomari F, Belli R, Trinchero R. Myopericarditis versus viral or idiopathic acute pericarditis. Heart. 2008 Apr;94(4):498-501.

[55] Maisch B, Seferović PM, Ristić AD, Erbel R, Rienmüller R, Adler Y, Tomkowski WZ, Thiene G, Yacoub MH; Task Force on the Diagnosis and Management of Pricardial Diseases of the European Society of Cardiology. Guidelines on the diagnosis and management of pericardial diseases executive summary; The Task force on the diagnosis and management of pericardial diseases of the European society of cardiology. Eur Heart J. 2004 Apr;25(7):587-610.

[56] Costanzo-Nordin MR, Reap EA, O'Connell JB, et al. A nonsteroidal antiinflammatory drug exacerbates coxsackievirus B3 murine myocarditis. J Am Coll Cardiol 1985;6:1078–82.

[57] Rezkalla S, Khatib G, Khatib R. Coxsackievirus B3 murine myocarditis. Deleterious effects of non-steroidal anti-inflammatory agents. J Lab Clin Med 1986;107:393–5.

[58] Khatib R, Reyes MP, Smith F, et al. Enhancement of coxsackievirus B4 virulence by indomethacin. J Lab Clin Med 1990;116:116–20.

[59] Imazio M, Trinchero R. Myopericarditis: Etiology, management, and prognosis. Int J Cardiol. 2008 Jun 23;127(1):17-26. Epub 2008 Jan 24.

[60] Imazio M, Bobbio M, Cecchi E, Demarie D, Demichelis B, Pomari F, Moratti M, Gaschino G, Giammaria M, Ghisio A, Belli R, Trinchero R. Colchicine in addition to conventional therapy for acute pericarditis: results of the COlchicine for acute PEricarditis (COPE) trial. Circulation. 2005 Sep 27;112(13):2012-6.

[61] Imazio M, Demichelis B, Parrini I, Cecchi E, Demarie D, Ghisio A, Belli R, Bobbio M, Trinchero R. Management, risk factors, and outcomes in recurrent pericarditis. Am J Cardiol. 2005 Sep 1;96(5):736-9.

[62] Soler-Soler J, Sagristà-Sauleda J, Permanyer-Miralda G. Relapsing pericarditis. Heart. 2004 Nov;90(11):1364-8.
[63] Imazio M, Cecchi E, Demichelis B, Ierna S, Demarie D, Ghisio A, Pomari F, Coda L, Belli R, Trinchero R. . Indicators of poor prognosis of acute pericarditis. Circulation. 2007 May 29;115(21):2739-44.

6

Pathogenesis and Pathology of Chagas' Chronic Myocarditis

Julián González, Roberto Guerri-Guttenberg,
Daniel Grana, Francisco Azzato and José Milei
Instituto de Investigaciones Cardiológicas Prof. Dr. A. Taquini - UBA - CONICET
Argentina

1. Introduction

Chronic chagasic cardiomyopathy (CCC) is the most serious manifestation of the chronic phase of Chagas' disease and constitutes the most common type of chronic myocarditis in the world (Guerri-Guttenberg, et al., 2008, Milei, et al., 1996a, Milei, et al., 2009, Milei, et al., 1992a, Storino, et al., 1992). Chagas' disease, a chronic illness caused by the flagellate parasite *Trypanosoma cruzi* (*T. cruzi*), was first described in 1909 by the Brazilian physician Carlos Chagas (Chagas C, 1909). The insect vectors of the disease are present throughout most of South and Central America, and their zone of distribution extends across the southern United States (Rassi, et al., 2010). It was estimated by year 2000, that in endemic areas 40 million people were considered to be at risk of infection, being 20 million already infected. Every year near 200,000 new cases are expected to happen, and 21,000 deaths per year occur (WHO, 2005).

Although always considered to be confined to Latin America, due to migratory movements from endemic countries to Europe and North America, Chagas' disease is being detected more frequently in developed countries. Europe is estimated to have from 24,001 to 38,708 (lower or upper limit of estimate, respectively) immigrants with *T. cruzi* infection (Guerri-Guttenberg, et al., 2008). In the United States, six autochthonous cases, five transfusion related cases and five transplant related cases have been reported, but migratory movements still remain the main source of Chagas' disease. It has been estimated that around 89,221 to 693,302 infected Latin Americans migrated to the United States in the period 1981 to 2005 (Milei, et al., 2009).

Two phases of the disease can be distinguished: (1) acute phase, with transiently high concentration of parasites in tissue and blood, nonspecific symptoms, and a 5% myocarditis incidence, lasting 4 - 8 weeks; and (2) chronic phase, lasting lifelong. Chronic phase can be presented as indeterminate form, characterized by lack of symptoms and normal ECG and normal radiographic examination of the chest, esophagus and colon. Approximately 60 - 70% of patients remain in this form for the rest of their lives. Only 20-40% of infected individuals, 10-30 years after the original acute infection, will develop cardiac, digestive or mixed form of the disease, characterized by the appearance of megavicera (dilated cardiomyopathy, megaesophagus and/or megacolon). It poses a substantial public health burden due to high morbidity and mortality (Milei, et al., 2009, Rassi, et al., 2000, Rassi, et al., 2010).

CCC is manifested by a chronic, diffuse, progressive fibrosing myocarditis that involves not only the working myocardium but also the atrioventricular (AV) conduction system, autonomic nervous system and microcirculation (Andrade, 1985, Marin-Neto, et al., 2007, Milei, et al., 1991b). This leads to cardiomegaly, cardiac failure, arrhythmias, thromboembolism, and death (Milei, et al., 1991b). Colon and esophagus are also commonly affected by Chagas' disease, being megacolon with constipation and megaesofagus with achalasia also features of the disease (Rassi, et al., 2010).

2. Pathogenesis of Chagas' myocarditis

Milei et al. proposed a combined theory that could explain the pathogenic mechanism in chronic chagasic myocarditis (Milei, et al., 1996a, Storino & Milei, 1994). This theory is based on three ingredients: the parasite, host immune system and fibrosis. These ingredients are proposed as being the primary causative agents of damage on myocardial tissue, conduction system, autonomic ganglia and nerves and microvasculature.

2.1 First ingredient: the parasite

The role of *T. cruzi* in the chronic phase has been previously underestimated due to the fact that its presence was believed to be scarce and unrelated to the inflammatory infiltrate present at this stage. Nowadays, the involvement of the parasite in the chronic phase has been well documented. Using dissimilar methods, different authors demonstrated either the persistence of *T. cruzi* or parasite antigens in mice (Younées-Chennoufi, et al., 1988), the parasite DNA sequence amplified by the polymerase chain reaction (PCR) (Jones, et al., 1993, Schijman, et al., 2004), *T. cruzi* antigens from inflammatory lesions in human chagasic cardiomyopathy (Higuchi, Brito et al. 1993), or the immunohistochemical finding of the parasite in endomyocardial biopsies with PCR confirmation (Añez, Carrasco et al. 1999). This would suggest a direct role for the parasite in the perpetuation of myocardial inflammation. In other words, the antigen stimulation would persist throughout the chronic stage, even though the parasites are not morphologically detectable by light microscopy (Andrade 1992).

The role of parasitemia is more controversial. High parasitemia correlated with severity of disease in one report (Basquiera, et al., 2003), but showed no association in another (Castro C., et al., 2005).

Interestingly, it has been observed that immunosuppression reactivates rather than ameliorates the disease, as seen in patients receiving immunosuppressive therapy to prevent transplant rejection and in AIDS patients. Accordingly, many experimental models where strains of genetically manipulated mice lacking various immune functions showed increased susceptibility to develop the disease (Tarleton & Zhang, 1999).

2.1.1 Life cycle of *Trypanosoma cruzi*

When a reduviid bug feeds from an infected mammal, it takes up circulating trypomastigotes, which reach then the bug's gut. There, they differentiate to amastigotes, which proliferate and start to differentiate into epimastigotes. In this process, when amastigote is still sphere-shaped but has developed its flagellum, some authors call this stage spheromastigotes. Then, it elongates its cell body and flagellum, taking the classical epimastigote shape. At this stage, the parasite undergoes metacyclogenesis, differentiating in metacyclic trypomastigotes, the infective form for mammals. When the bug feeds again, it excretes trypomastigotes with feces, which in turn reach blood torrent through bug's wound. Trypomastigotes can infect a wide variety of host cells, within them it differentiate into amastigotes and proliferate. Then, they can differentiate into trypomastigotes again, reach circulation and infect new cells. If an uninfected bug feeds from the animal in the moment of parasitemia, cycle starts again (Tyler & Engman, 2001).

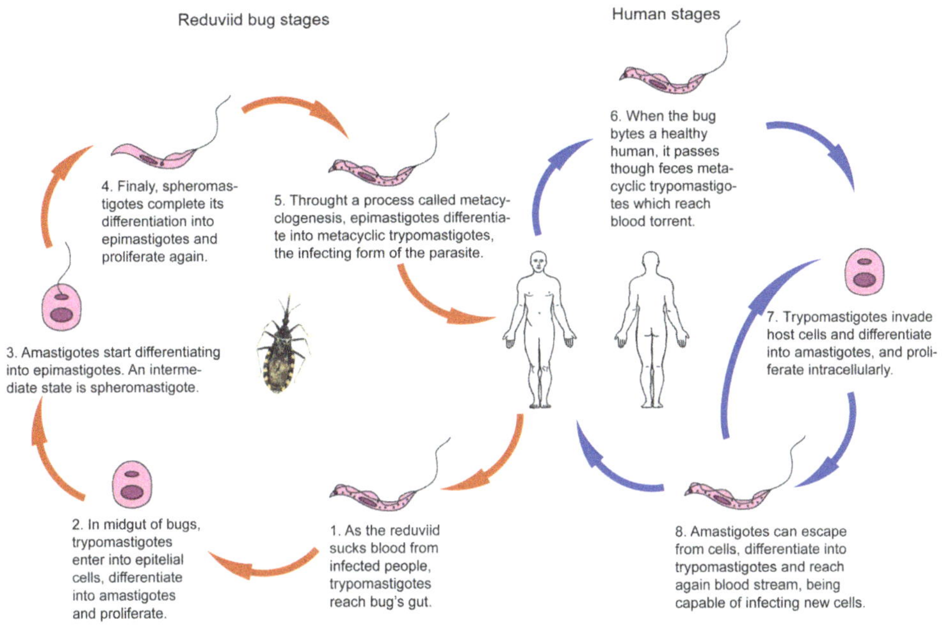

Fig. 1. Life cycle of *Trypanosoma cruzi*.

2.1.2 Genetic variability of *Trypanosoma cruzi* and its relation to its pathogenesis

The genetics of *T. cruzi* caught the attention of researchers in late 80' and early 90'. First studies on variability were performed analyzing electrophoretic variants on cellular enzymes. The groups resulting were called zymodemes and were named Z1, Z2, Z3. Only Z2 was associated with domestic transmission cycle.

The development of PCR based techniques, allowed the study of new variant regions and the characterization of multiple variants of a great number of genes. All these variants showed significant correlation with each other, suggesting the existence of two subtypes of *T. cruzi* based on these data (Macedo, et al., 2004). Moreover, *T. cruzi II* which is clearly linked to human pathology, being *T. cruzi I* mainly related to infection of wild sylvatic mammals. Even, applying LSSP-PCR to the study of the variable region of kinetoplast minicircle from *T. cruzi* provided evidence of a differential tissue distribution of genetically diverse *T. cruzi* populations in chronic Chagas' disease, suggesting that the genetic variability of the parasite is one of the determining factors of the clinical form of the disease (Vago, et al., 2000).

2.1.3 Cell host invasion and intracellular survival by *Trypanosoma cruzi*

Once *T. cruzi* reaches blood torrent, it invades a great variety of cells in the host. When parasiting non phagocytic cells, *T. cruzi* uses some surface glycoproteins to attach to cell: gp82, gp30 and gp35/50. All three glycoproteins are known to induce calcium mobilization from intracellular reservoirs. Gp82 is linked to the phospholipase C (PLC) and inositol 1,4,5 - triphosphate (IP3). Gp 35/50 is associated to increasing intracellular levels of cyclic AMP. On the other side, cruzipain, a protein known to be secreted by *T. cruzi*, acts on kininogen and produces bradykinin, which binds to its receptor, further increasing intracellular calcium. Increased intracellular calcium produces modifications in cytoskeleton that lead to parasite endocytosis (Yoshida & Cortez, 2008).

In the parasitoforous vacuole, mainly by the action of gp85/TS a glycoprotein with trans-sialidase action, and TcTox, a protease, the parasite degrades the membrane of the vacuole, escapes from it and proliferates within the cell (Alves & Colli, 2007).

2.1.4 Molecular mimicry

The induction of autoimmunity by similarities between *T. cruzi* and host epitopes has been long proposed as a mechanism that leads to tissue damage in the chronic phase of the disease. Both humoral and cellular autoimmune responses have been described, but we will discuss them in more detail in the section of immune system. The real importance of molecular mimicry in the pathogenesis of chagasic myocarditis is still a matter of debate (Girones, et al., 2005).

Although it seems that in some cases this mechanism triggers autoimmunity, in many others, autoimmunity seems to be an epiphenomenon of cellular destruction, with exposition of intracellular epitopes not normally exposed to the immune system. This, in turn may activate autoreactive lymphocytes leading to the appearance of autoantibodies that are not the cause of damage, rather a consequence (Girones, et al., 2005).

The most important cross reacting epitopes of *T. cruzi* and the correspondent epitopes in humans are listed in table 1, as well as the kind of immune response they elicit.

2.2 Second ingredient: host immune system

When the three ingredients theory was first proposed (Storino and Milei 1994, Milei, et al. 1996), second ingredients were mainly T lymphocytes and macrophages. In the subsequent years some evidence grew about the participation of humoral immune system through autoantibodies in the pathogenesis. As a consequence, the whole immune system of the host is now considered as the second ingredient.

As described earlier, mononuclear cells persist in the chronic stage of the disease, contributing to the inflammation through its products of secretion or through its own cytotoxicity (suppressor T cells) and cytolytic action (macrophages) (Storino & Milei, 1994).

As previously stated, molecular mimicry may be the main explanation of autoimmunity, triggering both cellular and humoral autoreactivity (Girones, et al., 2005). Figure 2 summarizes the most important immune events in CCC pathogenesis.

2.2.1 Innate immunity

In recent years innate immunity came to the attention of researchers of Chagas' disease pathogenesis. The role of NK cells has been particularly studied in early and late indeterminate forms of the disease and in CCC patients. In early indeterminate patients,

Parasite antigen	Human Antigen	Immune reaction
B13	Cardiac myosin heavy chain	Autoantibodies Autoreactive T cells
R13 (ribosomal protein)	Ribosomal protein β_1-adrenergic receptor M_2-muscarinic receptor 38-kDa heart antigen	Autoantibodies
Ribosomal protein PO	β_1-adrenergic receptor	Autoantibodies
FL-160	47-kDA neuron protein	Autoantibodies
Shed acute-phase antigen (SAPA)	Cha antigen	Autoreactive T cells
TENU2845/36 kDa	Cha antigen	Autoantibodies
Calcireticulin	Calcireticulin	Autoantibodies Autoreactive T cells
Galactosyl-cerebrosides	Galactosyl-cerebrosides	Autoantibodies
Unknown	Neurons, liver, kidney, testis	Autoantibodies
Sulphated glycolipids	Neurons	Autoantibodies
150-kDa protein	Smooth and striated muscle	Autoantibodies
Cruzipain	Cardiac myosin heavy chain M_2-muscarinic receptor	Autoantibodies
Microsomal fraction	Heart and skeletal muscle	Autoantibodies
Cytoskeleton	95-kDa myosin tail	Autoantibodies
SRA	Skeletal muscle Ca^{2+} dependent SRA	Autoantibodies
MAP	MAP (brain)	Autoantibodies
Soluble extract	Myelin basic protein	Autoantibodies Autoreactive T cells
55-kDa membrane protein	28-kDa Lymphocyte membrane protein	Autoantibodies

Table 1. Examples of cross-reacting epitopes (Girones, et al., 2005, Marin-Neto, et al., 2007).

compared to non infected people, increased values of pre-natural killer (NK)-cells ($CD3^-$ $CD16^+$ $CD56^-$), and higher values of proinflammatory monocytes ($CD14^+$ $CD16^+$ HLA-DR^{++}) were found. The higher values of activated B lymphocytes ($CD19^+$ $CD23^+$) contrasted with impaired T cell activation, indicated by lower values of $CD4^+$ $CD38^+$ and $CD4^+$ HLA-DR^+ lymphocytes, a lower frequency of $CD8^+$ $CD38^+$ and $CD8^+$ HLA DR$^+$ cells; a decreased frequency of $CD4^+$ $CD25^{HIGH}$ regulatory T cells was also observed. All these data suggest a rather proinflammatory profile (Vitelli-Avelar, et al., 2006). This profile may be useful to limit parasitemia and confine infection to tissues. In fact, it has been demonstrated that NK cells are important in defense against the spread of parasitic infection (Brener & Gazzinelli, 1997), and are an important source of INF-γ, a key cytokine to activate macrophages and help with parasite clearance (Camargo, et al., 1997).

In late indeterminate form, $CD3^-CD16^+CD56^+$ and $CD3^-CD16^+CD56^{DIM}$ NK cells are increased but are in normal range in CCC patients, suggesting a protective role for them (Vitelli-Avelar, et al., 2005). NK cells showing $CD56^{DIM}$ may play a role in the down

modulation of cytotoxic deleterious T CD8+ response reported in CCC patients (Sathler-Avelar, et al., 2009).
Monocytes display different cytokine profile. In indeterminate patients they produce more IL-10 (Gomes, et al., 2003) while in CCC patients they produce more TNF-α (Vitelli-Avelar, et al., 2008), leading to a proinflammatory profile that could be responsible for chronic myocarditis.
Toll-like receptors (TLR) are also implied in the response to acute infection with *T. cruzi*. TLR-2 has been shown to recognize GPI surface molecules from the parasite. In vitro and in vivo studies have demonstrated that macrophages stimulated with GPIs through TLR-2/CD14 receptors produce NO, TNF-α and IL-12 (Campos & Gazzinelli, 2004).

2.2.2 Cellular adaptative immunity

The role of immune cells in the pathogenesis of Chagas' heart disease has been the dominant hypothesis for many years. The paucity of parasite cells in the inflamed myocardium and the presence throughout the evolution of the disease of macrophages and lymphocytes in patched infiltrates lead to this hypothesis. As early as in 1929, Magariños Torres, observing those infiltrates postulated an "allergic" mechanism for CCC. Further, Mazza and Jörg followed this thought and supported the "allergic" theory (Storino & Milei, 1994).
The study of circulating lymphocytes in peripheral blood of chagasic patients showed an increase in the percentages and actual numbers of double-positive cells of the phenotype CD3+/HLA-DR+, as well as decrease in the percentage of CD45RA+/CD4+ and CD45RA+/CD8+ T cells, indicating greater numbers of activated T cells circulating. Consistent parallel increases were seen also in the B lymphocyte subset which stained double-positive for CD19/CD5 (Dutra W. O., et al., 1994). These results were similar for both indeterminate and CCC patients. Moreover, activated T cells lacking the co-stimulatory molecule CD28 are increased in chagasic patients (Menezes, et al., 2004) and express high levels of HLA-DR molecules (Dutra, et al., 2000). Some interesting differences were demonstrated between indeterminate and CCC patients. CD28- T cells in indeterminate patients showed expression of CTLA-4, which recognizes the same ligands as CD28, but instead of inducing cell activation it causes down modulation of T cells. On the contrary, T cells in CCC patients do not up-regulate CTLA-4 (Souza P. E. A., et al., 2007). It is particularly interesting that CD8+CD28- cells are increased in CCC patients compared to indeterminate patients, and that these cells do not require co-stimulation to exert their cytotoxic functions. More strikingly, CD4+CD28- cells behave differently in indeterminate and CCC patients. In the formers, they are closely related to IL-10 levels, while in CCC patients they correlate with INF-γ levels (Menezes, et al., 2004).
Another interesting difference has been found in cellular response between indeterminate and CCC patients. CD4+ cells from CCC patients had an increased expression of Vβ5+-TCR, not found in indeterminate patients. When CCC patients mononuclear cells from peripheral blood were cultured in the presence of trypomastigotes antigens, a selective expansion of CD4+ Vβ5+ cells was obtained; while when cultured in the presence of epimastigotes antigens, an expansion of CD8+ Vβ5+ cells was also noted. These findings could not be repeated in indeterminate patients. Trypomastigote stimulation led to the expansion of CD4+ Vβ17+ in indeterminate patients, not seen in CCC patients. This suggests that CCC patients and indeterminate patients respond to different antigen repertoires (Costa, et al., 2000).

Monocytes from indeterminate patients, when infected *in vitro* with *T. cruzi*, express low levels of HLA-DR and high levels of CD80, a ligand for CTLA-4 (Souza P. E., et al., 2004). The interaction of these monocytes with CTLA-4$^+$ T cells leads to the expression of IL-10, a cytokine known to down-modulate inflammatory responses (Gomes, et al., 2003). This is not observed in CCC patients. CD28$^-$ T cells, not expressing CTLA-4, express TNF-α and INF-γ (Menezes, et al., 2004).

In the same direction, CD4$^-$CD8$^-$ $\gamma\delta$ T cells are found to be increased in indeterminate patients compared with CCC ones. These cells are also linked to the production of IL-10 and a down modulator effect on inflammation (Villani, et al., 2010).

Cells infiltrating myocardium have also been studied. As demonstrated with immunostaining of endomyocardial biopsies by our group, leukocytes infiltrating myocardium in Chagas' disease were approximately 50% macrophages, and 50% lymphocytes, mainly T lymphocytes (Milei, et al., 1992b). Further immunohistochemical characterization of these cells with CD45R for lymphocytes, CD20 and lambda and kappa light chains for B lymphocytes, CD45R0 for T lymphocytes and CD68 for macrophages, confirmed these findings (Milei, et al., 1996a).

Autoreactive T cells have caught the attention of many investigators. In experimental models, CD4$^+$ T cells from infected mice showed a proliferative response to the exposition to human cardiac myosin heavy chain and to *T. cruzi* B13 protein. They also arrested the beating of fetal heart cells and, more importantly, induced myocarditis in immunized mice and promoted rejection of transplanted normal hearts in the absence of *T. cruzi* (Ribeiro-Dos-Santos, et al., 2001). Also, it has been described that T cells infiltrating the myocardium of chagasic patients cross react with human cardiac myosin heavy chain and to *T. cruzi* B13 protein and express high levels of INF-γ and low levels of IL-4, switching to a Th1 profile (Cunha-Neto Edecio & Kalilf, 2001).

In recent years, Treg cells have come to attention in relation to Chagas' disease pathogenesis. These cells are characterized by the expression of CD4, CD25 and FOXP3 (Ziegler & Buckner, 2009). Treg cells are increased in indeterminate patients compared to CCC, which correlates negatively with levels of activated CD8$^+$ (Vitelli-Avelar, et al., 2005). A second subset of T CD4+ cells, recently described, the Th17 cells, resulted important in Chagas' disease pathogenesis. These cells, mainly linked to autoimmune pathology, are characterized by the expression of CD4+, RORγt, and secrete IL-17 (Di Jin, et al., 2008). They were increased in a murine model of acute myocarditis induced by *T. cruzi* infection, as well as by immunization with heat-killed *T. cruzi* antigens (Bonney, et al., 2011). Both cell subsets seem to be related, as they require TGF-β to differentiate. In the presence of proinflammatory cytokines, differentiation to Th17 cell prevails and a pro-autoimmune profile develops (Ziegler & Buckner, 2009).

An additional mechanism is the bystander activation. This is the activation of autoreactive lymphocytes by antigen presenting cells in a proinflammatory environment (Fujinami, et al., 2006). This kind of autoreactive T cells activation has been described in Chagas'disease (Fedoseyeva, et al., 1999).

2.2.3 Humoral adaptative immunity

The importance of humoral immunity in controlling *T. cruzi* acute infection has been clearly established. Mice lacking B lymphocytes rapidly succumb to infection (Kumar & Tarleton, 1998). But the fact that attracted most attention is the production of autoantibodies.

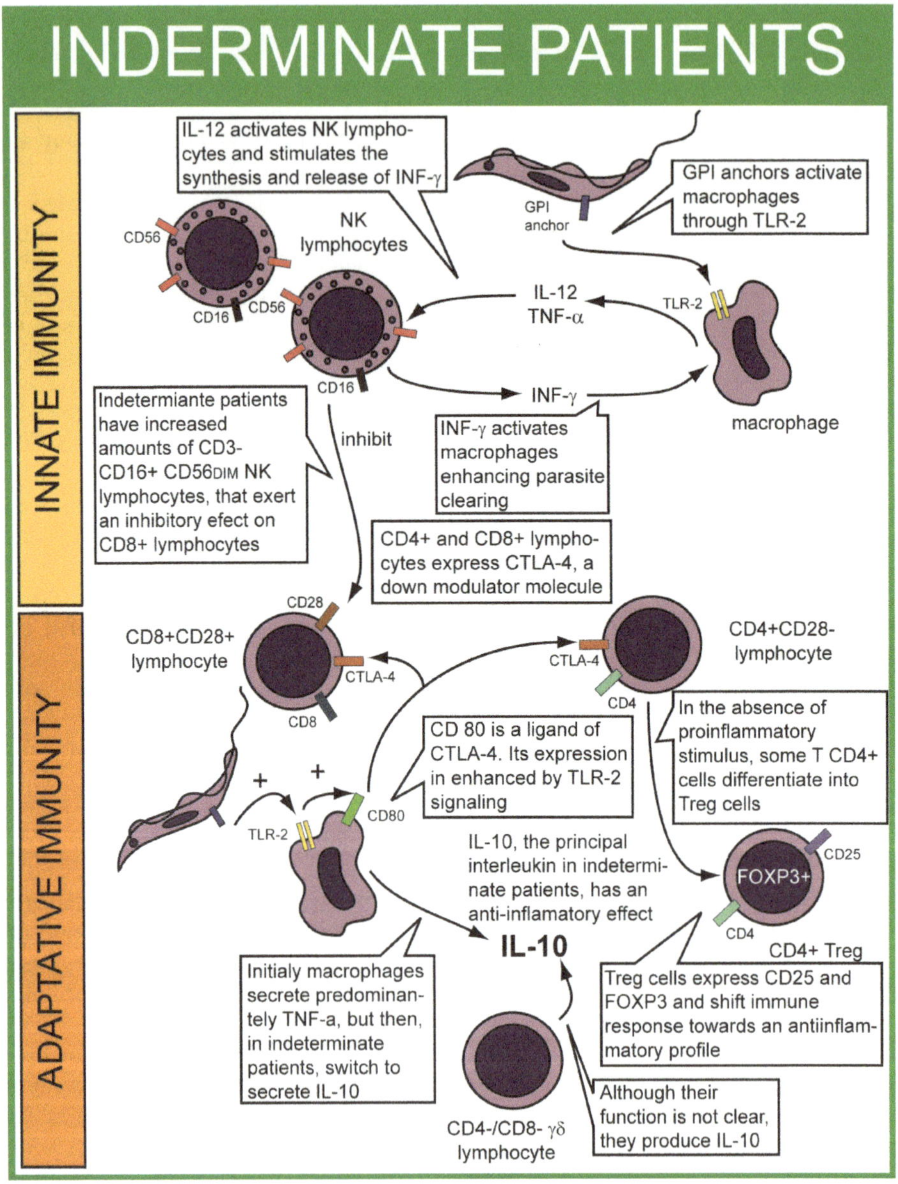

Fig. 2A. The immune pathogenesis of Chagas disease in indeterminate patients. The presence on numerous down regulating mechanisms shift the response towards an anti-inflammatory profile.

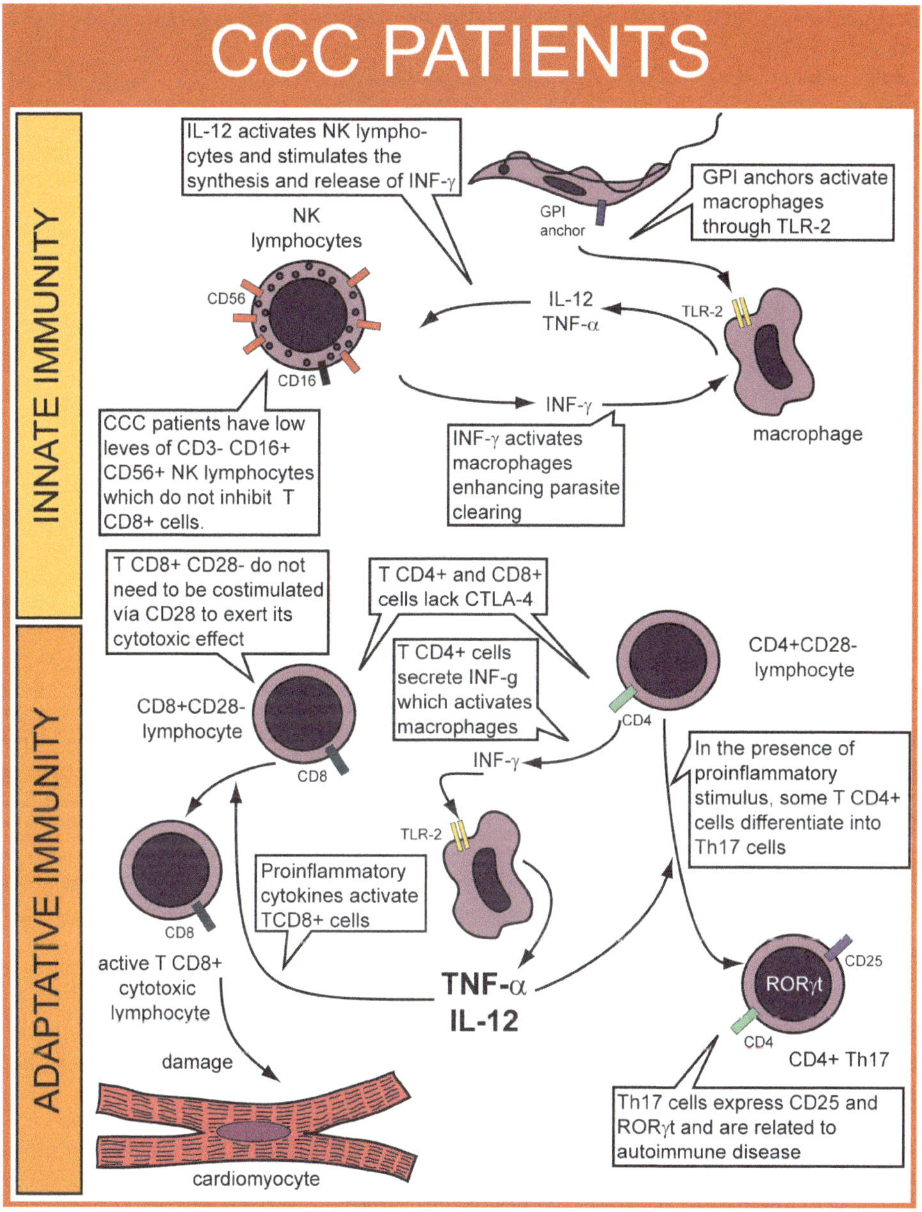

Fig. 2B. The immune pathogenesis of Chagas disease in CCC patients. Cells evolve towards a proinflammatory profile, with development of autoimmunity.

The first autoantibody to be described was one that reacted to endocardium, blood vessels and interstitium of skeletal muscle (EVI) (Cossio, et al., 1974), but was the same group of investigators who recognized the heterophil nature of the antibody and realized that had no pathogenic role (Khoury, et al., 1983).

Another autoantibody, studied by our group, was anti-laminin antibody (Sanchez, Milei et al. 1993, (Milei, et al., 1993). These antibodies were shown to react against *T. cruzi* amastigotes and trypomastigotes and human laminin (Szarfman, et al., 1982) and deposition of this antibody in marked thickened basement membranes of myocytes, endothelial cells, and vascular smooth muscle cells was shown by us with light microscopy, electron microscopy and immunohistochemical techniques in endomyocardial biopsies of chagasic patients (Sanchez, et al., 1993) but then we found that only 50% of patients had the antibody on their sera and no correlation with disease severity could be established (Milei, et al., 1993).

Anti-myosin antibodies were postulated by some authors to be generated through molecular mimicry with two *T. cruzi* antigens: B13 protein (Gruber & Zingales, 1993) and cruzipain (Giordanengo Laura, et al., 2000a, Giordanengo Laura, et al., 2000b). Although cruzipain antibodies mainly react to skeletal muscle myosin, they can cause conduction disturbances when transferred to uninfected mice and, when transferred to pregnant animals, they caused conduction disturbances in pups (Giordanengo Laura, et al., 2000b). On the other hand, immunossuppresed mice did not mount any humoral response when immunized with myosin but still develop myocarditis (Neu, et al., 1990). This fact made some authors doubt on the molecular mimicry hypothesis and rather consider antibodies to myosin a consequence of myocyte damage (Kierszenbaum, 2003).

Antibodies that react with muscarinic receptors were intensely studied. In early 1990's IgG from chagasic patients was observed to bind to muscarinic M2 receptors and activate them (Sterin-Borda L, et al., 1991). These anti-muscarinic antibodies were found to increase intracellular cGMP and decrease cAMP (Goin J., et al., 1997) and were positively related to the presence of dysautonomia (Goin J. C., et al., 1994). These antibodies also caused accumulation of inositol phosphate and nitric oxide synthase stimulation, with a negative inotropic effect on myocardium (Sterin-Borda Leonor, et al., 1997). As mentioned before, anti-muscarinic autoantibodies are positively related to the presence of dysautonomia (Goin J. C., et al., 1994), the presence of achalasia in chagasic patients (Goin J. C., et al., 1999), sinus node dysfunction (Altschuller, et al., 2007), but are not related with the degree of myocardial dysfunction (Altschuller, et al., 2007, Talvani Andre, et al., 2006), nor with the presence of brain lesions (Py, et al., 2009). In fact, patients with cardiomyopathy and left ventricular dysfunction but without autonomic dysfunction show low levels of anti-muscarinic antibodies (Sterin-Borda Leonor & Borda, 2000).

Antibodies against β_1-adrenergic receptors were also deeply studied. Described in early 1980's (Borda E., et al., 1984) these antibodies increased cAMP in mouse atrial fibers, increasing the release of PGE_2 and TXB_2 causing diminished contractility (Gorelik, et al., 1990). Increased cAMP activates PKA and then increases the intracellular calcium concentration. This causes in turn inhibition of the Na^+/K^+-ATPase and stimulates Ca^{2+}-ATPase activity leading to intracellular depletion of K^+ and further increase in Ca^{2+}. These alteration alter contractility and electric impulse generation and conduction (Borda E. S. & Sterin-Borda, 1996). Antiadrenergic autoantibodies titers could not be related to the severity of left ventricular dysfunction (Talvani Andre, et al., 2006) and patients with overt cardiomyopathy but without autonomic dysfunction show low levels of these antibodies (Sterin-Borda Leonor & Borda, 2000). Antibodies against β_2-adrenergic receptors have also been described but are mainly related to megacolon (Wallukat, et al., 2010).

Autoantibody	Hypothetic pathogenic role	Reference
Anti-Cerebroside	Probably related to neurologial symptoms	(Avila & Rojas, 1990)
Anti-Gal	Apparently protective	(Gazzinelli, 1991)
Anti-Brain Microtubules	Unknown	(Kerner, et al., 1991)
Anti-Ribosome	Unknown	(Levitus, et al., 1991, Skeiky, et al., 1992)
Anti- UsnRNPs	Unkwnown	(Bach-Elias, et al., 1998)
Anti-Sulfatides	May cause myocarditis and induce arrhythmias	(Garcia, et al., 1998)
Anti-Galectin-1	Increased in CCC patients	(Giordanengo L., et al., 2001)
Anti-Cha R3	Specific of CCC	(Girones, et al., 2001a)
Anti-Desmoglein-1	Related to Penphigus foliaceum	(Diaz, et al., 2004)
Anticardiolipin	Unknown	(Pereira De Godoy, et al., 2005)
Anti- TrkA, TrkB and TrkC	Prevents apoptosis of neurons and helps cellular invasion	(Lu, et al., 2010)
Anti-MBP	Related to gastrointestinal form	(Oliveira E. C., et al., 2009)

Table 2. Less studied autoantibodies in Chagas' disease.

Antibodies against AV node and sinus auricular node tissues have been studied as markers of CCC. When compared in chronic chagasic cardiopathy patients, non-chagasic cardiopathy patients, indeterminate chagasic subjects and healthy blood donors as controls, they more frequently found in chronic chagasic cardiopathy, but not enough to be good markers for chagasic cardiopathy group. Besides, no clear association with complex rhythm or conduction alterations was found (Arce-Fonseca, et al., 2005).

Many other autoantibodies have been described (table 2) but are not so widely studied and their role in pathogenesis of chagasic myocarditis is not clear.

2.2.4 Genetic factors

Human leukocyte antigens (HLA) have shown some relation to the development of CCC. HLA-B40 and Cw3 combination was protective for CCC (Llop, et al., 1991), as resulted DRB1*14, DQB1*0303 (Fernandez-Mestre, et al., 1998), HLA-DQB1*06 (Deghaide, et al., 1998) and HLA-A68 (Cruz-Robles, et al., 2004). On the other hand, HLA-C*03 (Layrisse, et al., 2000), DRB1*1503 (Garcia Borras, et al., 2009), DRB1*01, DRB1*08, DQB1*0501 (Fernandez-Mestre, et al., 1998) and HLA-DR16 alelles (Cruz-Robles, et al., 2004) were positively related to the development of CCC.

A number of other genes related to immune system have been studied in order to determine their relation to a predisposition to develop CCC. In table 3 we list those positively related to the appearance of CCC (Cunha-Neto E., et al., 2009).

Gene	**Polymorphism**
CCL2/MCPI	- 2518
CCR5	+ 53029
TNF-α	- 308
LTA	+ 80, + 252
BAT-1	- 22, - 348
NFkBIL-1	- 62, - 262
IL-1B	- 31, + 3954, + 5810
IL-10	- 1082
IL-12B	+ 1188
MAL/TRIAP	S180L

Table 3. Genetic polymorphisms related to CCC. Adapted from (Cunha-Neto E., et al., 2009).

2.2.5 The cytokines and chemokines

Although proinflammatory cytokines seem to be necessary for controlling parasitemia during acute phase of the disease (Cunha-Neto E., et al., 2009), CCC patients display a rather proinflammatory cytokine while indeterminate patients display a down modulator one. CCC patients had higher levels of TNF-α and CCL2 than indeterminate patients (Ferreira, et al., 2003, Talvani A., et al., 2004). Infiltrating macrophages from CCC patients expressed INF-γ, TNF-α and IL-6 but showed low levels of IL-2, IL-4 and IL-10 (Abel, et al., 2001, Reis D. D., et al., 1993, Reis M. M., et al., 1997). Also CCR5, CXCR3 and CCR7 and their ligands were increased in hearts of CCC patients, as well as monocytes expressing CXCR3, CCR5, CXCL9 and CCL5 (Cunha-Neto E., et al., 2009). It has been shown that INF-γ and CCL2 induceed myocytes to secrete arial natriuretic factor and caused hypertrophy (Cunha-Neto E., et al., 2005), and IL-18 and CCR7 ligands, which are increased in CCC, caused cardiomyocyte hypertrophy and fibrosis (Reddy, et al., 2008, Riol-Blanco, et al., 2005, Sakai, et al., 2006).

2.3 The third ingredient: fibrosis

Fibrosis is one of the most striking characteristics of CCC. In our patients with CCC in endomyocardial biopsies, fibrosis had replaced between 8.2 and 49% of contractile myocardium, with only one patient having less than 10% (Milei, et al., 1992b). While in autopsies, fibrosis was more extensive reaching in the conduction system than in the contracting myocardium ($51.5 \pm 18\%$ vs $43.4 \pm 8\%$, $p < 0.05$) (Milei, et al., 1996a).

The deposition of laminin in extracellular and basement membranes has been implicated in the pathogenesis of inflammatory process, as laminin is able to bind proinflammatory citokines (Savino, et al., 2007). The inflammatory infiltrate in CCC was related to the production of citokines such as INF-γ, TNF-α, IL-18, CCL2 and CCL21, that may have modulator actions on fibrotic process (Cunha-Neto E., et al., 2009).

3. A combined theory that could explain the pathogenic mechanism in chronic chagasic myocarditis

With the perpetuation of inflammation, necrosis and scarring fibrosis, damage to all histological components of myocardium occurs. Damage to contracting myocardial fibers determines contractile failure as well as electrophysiological disturbances. Conduction system, nervous autonomic system and microvasculature are also damaged and as a consequence they cause further damage to contractile myocardium and produce electrical instability. Figure 3 illustrates with a flow chart the interactive network of different elements in the pathogenesis of CCC.

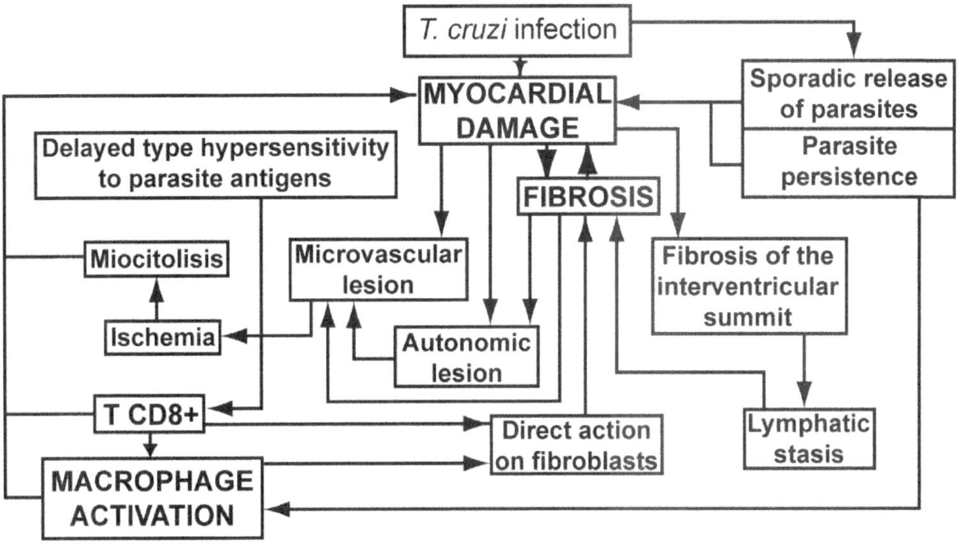

Fig. 3. Schematic representation of the integrated theory of multiple factors that determine myocardial damage in CCC.

4. Pathophysiological consequences of organ damage

4.1 Dysautonomia

As early as 1922 Carlos Chagas noted that the chronotropic response to atropine was altered in chagasic patients (Chagas C. & Vilella, 1922), but it was not until late 1950's that Köberle published his works showing impressive neuronal depopulation in microscopic sections obtained from the intercaval atrial strip in chagasic patients using a standardized technique of cardiac intramural neuronal counting developed by himself (Köberle, 1956a, 1956b). These findings led to the "neurogenic hypothesis" (Köberle, 1959), which explained all megas in Chagas' disease as a consequence of neuronal depletion.

Although many other authors claimed to have confirmed this finding (Mott & Hagstrom, 1965, Oliveira J. S., 1985), other authors called to attention about the criteria used to diagnose neuronal depletion because of the great variability in the number of neurons in autonomic ganglia (Rossi L., et al., 1994) and they also remarked that the only right criterion to establish neuronal depletion is the presence of proliferation of satellite cells, with the formation of Terplan's nodules, a characteristic lesion described as proliferating satellite cells which replace degenerating neurons, forming nodular structures. These lesions, once considered patognomonic, can be found in other cardiomyopathies (Rossi L., et al., 1994). The same author could not confirm the loss of neurons or denervation in CCC (Rossi L., 1988). Finally, it was demonstrated that, using Terplan's nodules as diagnostic criterion,

CCC patients with heart failure had more neuronal depletion than patients with dilated cardiomyopathy of other causes (Oliveira J. S., 1985). In our experience the neuroganglionic involvement was variable in autopsies of chagasic hearts (Milei, et al., 1991b).
According to pioneer neurogenic hypothesis (Köberle, 1959), early and irreversible damage to the parasympathetic system during acute phase of the disease causes a cathecolaminergic cardiomyopathy, but this point of view has been debated and evidence is contradictory. Functional test performed in CCC patients demonstrated impaired parasympathetic heart rate regulation (metaraminol, phenylephrine and atropine intravenous injections, facial immersion, Valsalva maneuver, head-up and head-down tilt tests, respiratory sinus arrhythmia, handgrip, graded dynamic exercise, and spectral analysis of Holter recordings) (Amorim, et al., 1968, Amorim, et al., 1973, Gallo, et al., 1975, Guzzetti, et al., 1991, Junqueira Junior, et al., 1985, Manço, et al., 1969, Marin-Neto, et al., 1975, Sousa, et al., 1987). However, a careful analysis of these data showed that many patients had normal autonomic function and most patients had heart failure, that could explain autonomic dysfunction *per se* (Davila, et al., 1998).
On the other hand, the study of indeterminate patients has shown conflicting results. While some authors could demonstrate impaired autonomic function (Molina, et al., 2006, Vasconcelos & Junqueira, 2009) others could demonstrate that autonomic function was normal in patients without myocardial damage and that abnormalities in autonomic dysfunction was proportional to heart dysfunction, leading these authors to propose that these abnormalities arise as a compensating mechanism for the progressive left ventricular dilatation (Davila, et al., 1991, Davila Spinetti, et al., 1999). These findings led to a new "neurogenic theory", which considers autonomic dysfunction as secondary to ventricular dilatation and hemodynamic alterations, but once installed, acts synergistically with parasitism and inflammation to cause further myocardial damage (Davila, et al., 2004).

4.2 Microvascular damage

Microcirculation abnormalities in CCC have been firstly pointed out by Jorg as an angiographic anarchy due to capillary loss (Jörg, 1974) and furtherly demonstrated in experimental models as well as in clinical practice (Rossi M. A., et al., 2010).
Many investigators have found abnormal myocardial perfusion using isonitrile-99m-technetium (Castro R., et al., 1988) and thallium-201 (Hagar & Rahimtoola, 1991, Marin-Neto, et al., 1992) scintigraphy in chagasic patients with normal epicardial coronary arteries. Furthermore, the progression of left ventricular systolic dysfunction is associated with both, the presence of reversible perfusion defects and the increase in perfusion defects at rest (Hiss, et al., 2009, Schwartz & Wexler, 2009). Anatomopathological studies in humans also provided evidence of microvascular damage in CCC. In late 1950's first reports showing collapse of arterioles and intimal proliferation (Torres, 1960) caught the attention of investigators. Also, microthrombi have been described (Rossi M. A., et al., 1984). As said, in endomyocardial biopsies thickening of capillary basement membranes was also found (Milei, et al., 1992b).
Additional evidence of microvascular damage was obtained from experimental models. Vascular constriction, microaneurysms, dilatation and proliferation of microvessels has been demonstrated (Factor & Sonnenblick, 1982, Morris, et al., 1989, Tanowitz H. B., et al., 1996, Tanowitz Herbert B., et al., 1992b).
Many factors have been advocated in the genesis of these lesions. First, the parasite itself. It was shown that *T. cruzi* produces a neuraminidase that removes sialic acid from de surface

of endothelial cells. This results in thrombin binding and platelet aggregation (Libby, et al., 1986). *T. cruzi* also produces tromboxane A_2 (TXA_2), specially during amastigote state (Ashton, et al., 2007), also favouring platelet aggregation and vascular spasm. Direct parasitism of endothelial cells by *T. cruzi* has also been demonstrated, and this causes the activation of the NF-κB pathway increasing the expression af adhesion molecules (Huang, et al., 1999a), and secreting proinflammatory citokines (Tanowitz Herbert B., et al., 1992a) and iNOS (Huang, et al., 1999b).

Endothelin-1 (ET-1) is another proposed pathogenic element. Elevated levels of mRNA for preproendothelin-1, endothelin converting enzyme and endothelin-1 were observed in the infected myocardium (Petkova Stefka B., et al., 2000), and elevated levels of ET-1 have been found in CCC patients (Salomone, et al., 2001). Mitogen-activated protein kinases and the transcription factor activator-protein-1 regulate the expression of endothelin-1, and both are shown to be increased in myocardium, interstitial cells and vascular and endocardial endothelial cells (Petkova S. B., et al., 2001). Besides, treatment with phosphoramidon, an inhibitor of endothelin converting enzyme, decreases heart size and severity of lesions in an experimental model of Chagas' disease (Jelicks, et al., 2002).

Inflammation also produces dysfunction of endothelial cells. Macrophages secrete TXA_2 and platelet activating factor (PAF) act on endothelium causing vasoconstriction (Rossi M. A. & Carobrez, 1985). Endothelial cells infected *in vitro* with *T. cruzi* lose their antithrombotic properties in response to interleukin 1 β (IL-1β) (Bevilacqua, et al., 1984, Nachman, et al., 1986).

It is remarkable that, although the data presented, endothelial function seems to be normal in CCC patients without heart failure, as measured by increases in blood flow in response to acetylcholine and sodium nitroprusside (Consolim-Colombo, et al., 2004). Further, in our concept, microvascular damage found in CCC, seems to be secondary to fibrosis and distortion of myocardial fiber arrangement by necrosis and chronic infiltrates, but as once established, may contribute to the perpetuation of myocardial damage.

5. Pathology

Pathological findings are described mostly according to our own findings.

5.1 Macroscopic features

The most striking characteristic of CCC is enlargement of heart with variable degrees of dilatation of chambers (Andrade, 1985) (Figure 4A). In autopsy series, hearts were overweighted (Andrade, 1985, Baroldi, et al., 1997, Bestetti, et al., 1993, Lopes, et al., 1981) compared with indeterminate chagasic patients and non-chagasic subjects. Marked cardiomegalies reached up to 500 grams. Right ventricle (RV) and atrium (RA) were generally more compromised than left chambers, being RV the most dilated in one paper (Laranja, et al., 1956) but RA was in other (Andrade, 1985).

A second remarkable feature is the thinning of the left ventricular apical wall, resulting in apical aneurysm, a very characteristic lesion in CCC (Figure 4B) (Moia, et al., 1955).

Other lesions described are flattening of the papillary muscles and a marked subendocardial sclerosis, parietal and/or aneurismal thrombosis and fibrotic plaques in pericardium (Milei, et al., 1996a, Milei, et al., 1991b, Storino & Milei, 1994).

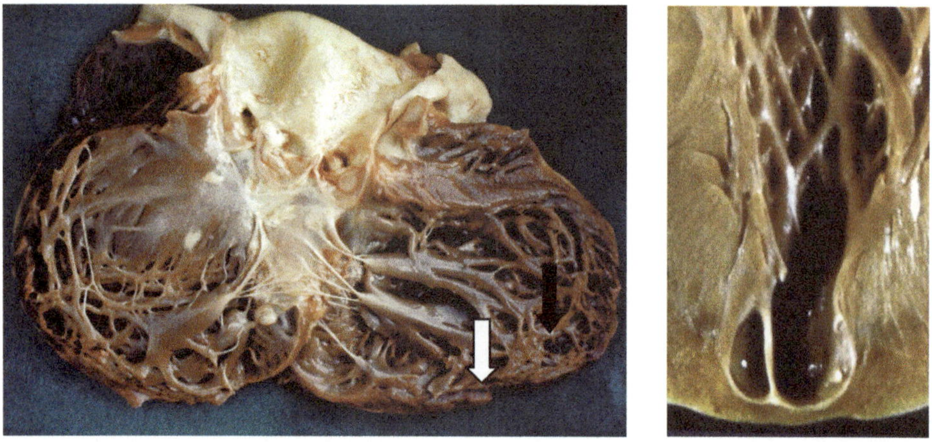

Fig. 4. A. High grade heart dilatation. Thining of the apical wall of the left ventricle (white arrow) and cavitary thrombus (black arrow). B. Characteristic apical aneurysm. A from Milei, et al., 1996b, B from Milei, et al., 2008.

5.2 Histological features

Microscopically, myocardial lesions consisted of a chronic inflammatory process with fibrotic scars and extensive mononuclear infiltrates. Such infiltrates were more prominent in the working myocardium and in the specialized cells of the left branch of the His bundle than in the AV node and in the right hisian branch, showing a microfocal disposition (Figure 5A). The percentage of fibrosis was variable and ranged between 8.2 to 49% (Milei, et al., 1996a, Milei, et al., 1992b) (Figure 5B).

Extensive myocytolysis and spotty contraction band necrosis were observed. Cell hypertrophy in the apparently preserved myocytes was revealed by hypertrophic bizarre nuclei. Dilated lymphatic channels widespread in the ventricular septum and in the AV node, His bundle, and in the root of the right and left bundles branches were observed. In the case of apical aneurysm of the left ventricle, dilated lymphatic were distributed subepicardically (Milei, et al., 1996a).

The serial sectioning of the conducting system showed prominent lesions. Sino-atrial node presented mononuclear infiltrates, necrosis of specialized fibers, and intense fibrosis (Milei, et al., 1991b). In the remaining specialized system lesions consisted of mild to moderate diffuse fibrosis of the AV node and of the penetrating and branching portions of the His bundle, complete destruction of the proximal segments of the right and left bundles branch by varying degrees of replacement by dense collagen tissue (Figure 5A). The remaining specialized fibers presented atrophy and mild fatty infiltration and were surrounded in most cases by infiltrates consisting mainly of lymphocytes and macrophages. The subendocardial Purkinje fibers were usually damaged by chronic inflammation and fibrosis (Milei, et al., 1991b) (Figure 5B). These vast fibrosis in the conduction system (Figure 5C) showed severe conduction alterations in electrocardiograms, although curiously in one revision, there were needed sophisticated electrophysiological studies to demonstrate electrical abnormalities in these patients (Andrade, et al., 1988)

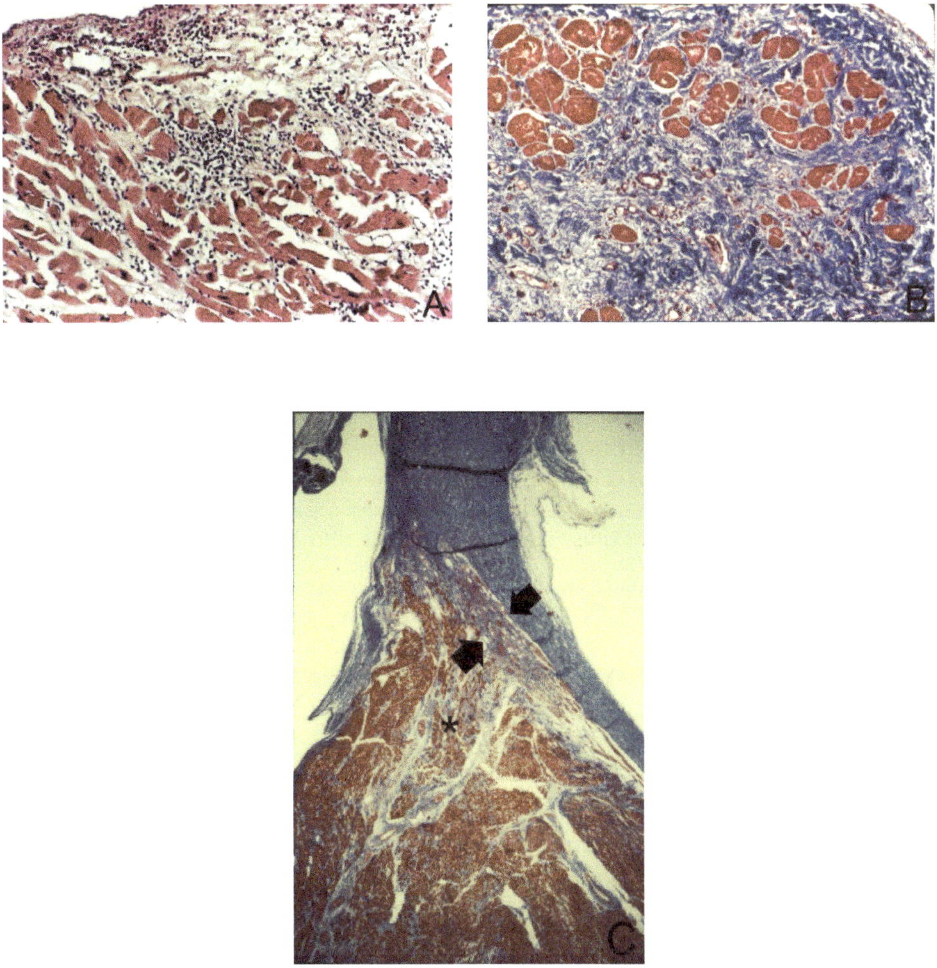

Fig. 5. A. Extensive mononuclear infiltrates, myocytes loss, and subendocardial fibrosis. Hematoxylin and eosin stain, X25. B. Atrophic myocardial fibres (red) separated by thick bands of fibrous tissue (blue). Mallory trichrome, X 25. C. Bifurcating His bundle showing severe fibrosis at the left branch (between arrows). The right branch (asterisk) is intramyocardial and surrounded by connective tissue. Mallory trichrome, X25. A and C from Milei, 1996a. B from Milei, 2008.

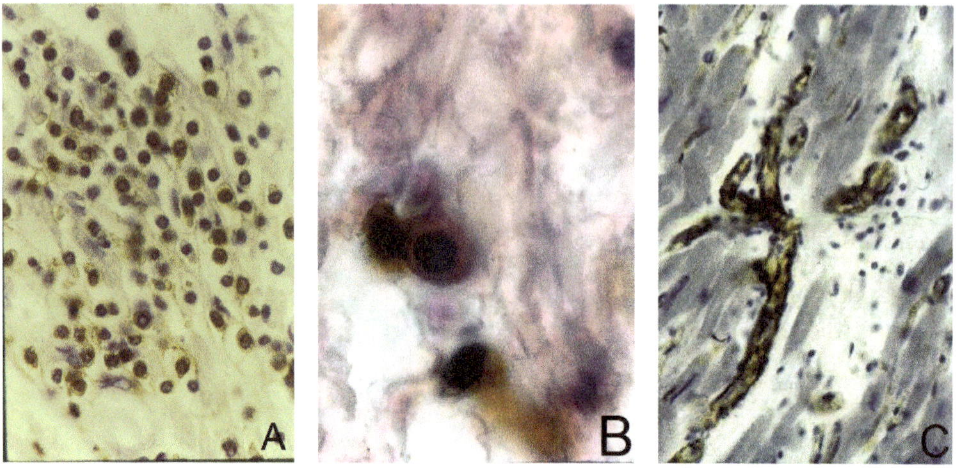

Fig. 6. A. Detail of the left bundle of His is shown. Immunostaining for T lymphocyte. Positive cells express CD45R0 antigen (brown); specialized myocardial cells have almost disappeared. Extensive mononuclear infiltrate, the majority of them being T lymphocytes. X20. B. Double immunostaining for the simultaneous demonstration of T lymphocytes (CD45RO) and macrophages (CD68). T lymphocytes (brown) in close contact with a macrophage (pinky cytoplasm). X1000. C. Immunostaining to show endothelial cells. Capillaries and small vessels are clearly showed by the expression of CD31. Vessels are midly or moderately disorted because of the surrounding fibrosis. X100. From Milei, 1996a.

In our studies in endomyocardial biopsies, infiltrates were approximately 50% lymphocytes and 50% macrophages. Almost 80% of lymphocytic population were T lymphocytes, being only 20% B lymphocytes. Eosinophils were scarce in infiltrates reaching 5%, and were associated with areas of necrotic myocardium. Mast cells also were scarce or absent in specialized and in contracting myocardium. (Milei, et al., 1996a, Milei, et al., 1992b)

Histological study of aneurisms showed a thinned wall 2-4 mm, with sclerotic plaques of thickened endocardium of up to 92% of total tissue and extensive mononuclear chronic inflammatory infiltrates and widespread fibrosis in myocardium. Myocytes were organized in thin bands or atrophic units surrounded by fibrotic tissue (Figure 5B) (Milei, et al., 1991a).

Autonomic ganglia showed above described Terplan's nodules, with satellite cell proliferation replacing degenerated autonomic neurons. As stated, these lesions, once considered patognomonic, can be found in other cardiomyopathies (Rossi L., et al., 1994).

5.3 Immunohistochemical findings

Immunophenotyping of infiltrates allowed a better characterization of the cells participating in the inflammatory infiltrates, mainly macrophages ($CD68^+$) and lymphocytes ($CD45R^+$). In our works 26.5% percent of them were T lymphocytes ($CD45R^+$, $CD45R0^{+)}$ and 10.5% were B lymphocytes ($CD20^+$, light chains kappa and/or lambda$^+$) (Figure 6A). Thirty percent of the infiltrate was composed of macrophages ($CD68^+$). The remaining infiltrate was composed of mononuclear cells resembling macrophages and CLA-negative mononuclear cells. Contacts between CD68 positive cells and T lymphocytes were frequently found

(Figure 6B). CD31 antibodies clearly pointed out normal endothelial cells, in either normal or damaged vessels (Figure 6C) (Milei, et al., 1996a).

5.4 Ultrastructural features

Myocardial fibers showed nuclear enlargement, nuclear membrane invaginations, lipofuscin deposits, myofibrils derangements and loss, swelling, mitochondrial atrophy, dilatation of sarcotubular system, and interstitial fibrosis (Carrasco, et al., 1982, Palacios-Prü, et al., 1982). These findings have been confirmed by our group in endomyocardial biopsies (Ferrans, et al., 1988, Milei, et al., 1992b). Platelet thrombi can be demonstrated within capillaries (Figure 7B).

Other striking alteration in these specimens was the thickening of the basement membranes of cardiac myocytes (Figures 7A, 7C), endothelium Figure 7C) and vascular smooth muscle up to 20 times their normal thickness of 500 Å (Ferrans, et al., 1988). The thickened basement membranes appeared structurally homogeneous, without being multilayered or subdivided into a lamina rara and a lamina densa. They were of relatively low electron density, had a finely fibrillar appearance at high magnification and measured up to 1 μm in thickness. Using gold-conjugated antibodies, we could demonstrate the presence of laminin in the thickened basal membranes of myocytes and endothelium (Sanchez, et al., 1993).

Regarding the ultrastructure of aneurysms resected from chagasic patients we observed, hypertrophy of myocytes, with swelling, partial or complete loss of myofibrils, swelling of mitochondria, disruption of mitochondrial cristae, lipofuscin granules, and intact sarcolemmas . Basement membranes were thickened, as previously described (Milei, et al., 1991a)

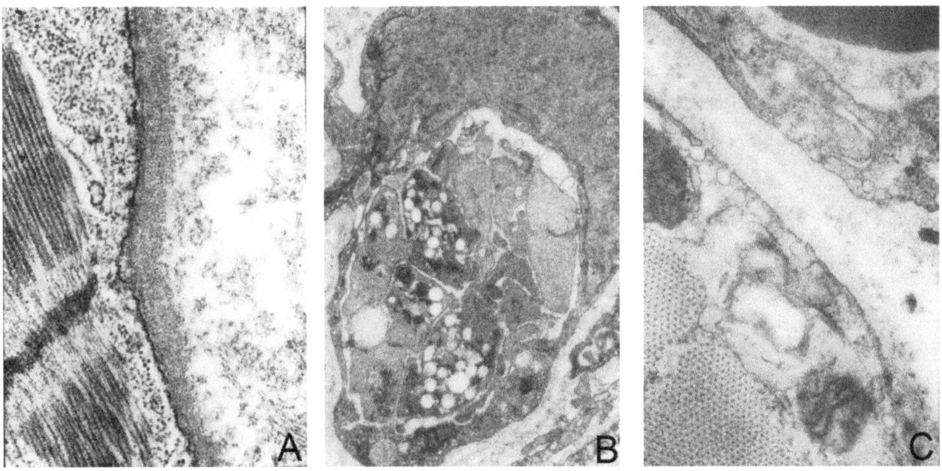

Fig. 7. A. Myocardial fibre with thickened basement membrane. B. Platelet thrombus within a capillary. C. Thickened basement membranes in a myocardial fibre and a capillary. From Milei, et al., 2008.

6. Conclusions

As shown across the sections of this chapter, the numerous hypothesis about pathogenic pathways of CCC have supporting data and pitfalls. Finally all proposals interact with each other, giving us the idea that none of these theories explains the very complex development of CCC by itself. Rather, it seems more feasible that all these hypothesis conform a network of damaging elements, and that all ingredients cause and/or enhances each other. The triggering factor is obviously the interaction between parasite and host's immune system. Cell parasitism, the inflammatory process and consequent necrosis and fibrosis cause damage to contracting myocardium, autonomic system, conduction system and microcirculation. Autonomic damage causes impaired regulation of microvasculature and further alterations in blood flow. Ischemia causes more myocardial damage. Necrosis exposes intracellular epitopes and causes autoantibodies production with more necrosis, fibrosis and so on. It seems that, if adequate down modulator immune mechanisms work properly, this vicious circle stops and patients do not develop cardiomyopathy, rather they remain in the indeterminate form lifelong.

7. References

Abel L. C., Rizzo L. V., Ianni B., Albuquerque F., Bacal F., Carrara D., Bocchi E. A., Teixeira H. C., Mady C., Kalil J. & Cunha-Neto E. (2001). Chronic Chagas' disease cardiomyopathy patients display an increased IFN-gamma response to Trypanosoma cruzi infection. *Journal of Autoimmunity.* Vol. 17, No. 1, pp. 99-107, ISSN 0896-8411

Altschuller M. B., Pedrosa R. C., Pereira Bde B., Correa Filho W. B., Medeiros A. S., Costa P. C. & de Carvalho A. C. (2007). Chronic Chagas disease patients with sinus node dysfunction: is the presence of IgG antibodies with muscarinic agonist action independent of left ventricular dysfunction? *Revista da Sociedade Brasileira de Medicina Tropical.* Vol. 40, No. 6, pp. 665 - 671, ISSN 0037-8682

Alves M. J. M. & Colli W. (2007). Trypanosoma cruzi: Adhesion to the Host Cell and Intracellular Survival. *IUBMB Life.* Vol. 59, No. 4 - 5, pp. 274 - 279, ISSN 1521-6551

Amorim D. S., Godoy R. A., Manco J. C., Tanaka A. & Gallo L., Jr. (1968). Effects of acute elevation in blood pressure and of atropine on heart rate in Chagas' disease. A preliminary report. *Circulation.* Vol. 38, No. 2, pp. 289-294, ISSN 0009-7322

Amorim D. S., Mello de Oliveira J. A., Manco J. C., Gallo L., Jr. & Meira de Oliveira J. S. (1973). Chagas' heart disease. First demonstrable correlation between neuronal degeneration and autonomic impairment. *Acta Cardiologica.* Vol. 28, No. 4, pp. 431-440, ISSN 0001-5385

Andrade Z. A. (1985). A patologia da doenca de Chagas no honen. *Annales de la Societe Belge de Medecine Tropicale.* Vol. 65, No. 1, pp. 15-30

Andrade Z. A., Cámara E. J. N., Sadigursky M. & Andrade S. G. (1988). Envolvimento do nodulo sinusal na doença de Chagas. *Arquivos Brasileiros de Cardiologia.* Vol. 50, No. pp. 153

Arce-Fonseca M., Ballinas-Verdugo M. A., Reyes P. A., Aranda-Fraustro A. & Monteon V. M. (2005). Autoantibodies to human heart conduction system in Chagas' disease. *Vector Borne and Zoonotic Diseases.* Vol. 5, No. 3, pp. 233-236, ISSN 1530-3667

Ashton A. W., Mukherjee S., Nagajyothi F., Huang H., Braunstein V. L., Desruisseaux M. S., Factor S. M., Lopez L., Berman J. W., Wittner M., Scherer P. E., Capra V., Coffman

T. M., Serhan C. N., Gotlinger K., Wu K. K., Weiss L. M. & Tanowitz H. B. (2007). Thromboxane A2 is a key regulator of pathogenesis during Trypanosoma cruzi infection. *The Journal of Experimental Medicine.* Vol. 204, No. 4, pp. 929-940

Avila J. L. & Rojas M. (1990). Elevated cerebroside antibody levels in human visceral and cutaneous leishmaniasis, Trypanosoma rangeli infection, and chronic Chagas' disease. *The American Journal of Tropical Medicine and Hygiene.* Vol. 43, No. 1, pp. 52-60, ISSN 0002-9637

Bach-Elias M., Bahia D., Teixeira D. C. & Cicarelli R. M. (1998). Presence of autoantibodies against small nuclear ribonucleoprotein epitopes in Chagas' patients' sera. *Parasitology Research.* Vol. 84, No. 10, pp. 796-799, ISSN 0932-0113

Baroldi G., Oliveira S. J. M. & Silver M. D. (1997). Sudden and unexpected death in clinically silent' Chagas' disease. A hypothesis. *International Journal of Cardiology.* Vol. 58, No. 3, pp. 263-268, ISSN 0167-5273

Basquiera A. L., Sembaj A., Aguerri A. M., Omelianiuk M., Guzman S., Moreno Barral J., Caeiro T. F., Madoery R. J. & Salomone O. A. (2003). Risk progression to chronic Chagas cardiomyopathy: influence of male sex and of parasitaemia detected by polymerase chain reaction. *Heart.* Vol. 89, No. 10, pp. 1186-1190, ISSN 1468-201X

Bestetti R. B., Freitas O. C., Muccillo G. & Oliveira J. S. (1993). Clinical and morphological characteristics associated with sudden cardiac death in patients with Chagas' disease. *European Heart Journal.* Vol. 14, No. 12, pp. 1610-1614, ISSN 0195-668X

Bevilacqua M. P., Pober J. S., Majeau G. R., Cotran R. S. & Gimbrone M. A. (1984). Interleukin 1 (IL-1) induces biosynthesis and cell surface expression of procoagulant activity in human vascular endothelial cells. *The Journal of Experimental Medicine.* Vol. 160, No. 2, pp. 618-623

Borda E., Pascual J., Cossio P., De La Vega M., Arana R. & Sterin-Borda L. (1984). A circulating IgG in Chagas' disease which binds to beta-adrenoceptors of myocardium and modulates their activity. *Clinical & Experimental Immunology.* Vol. 57, No. 3, pp. 679 - 686

Borda E. S. & Sterin-Borda L. (1996). Antiadrenergic and mucarinic receptor antibodies in Chagas' cardiomyopathy. *International Journal of Cardiology.* Vol. 54, No. pp. 149-156

Brener Z. & Gazzinelli R. T. (1997). Immunological control of Trypanosoma cruzi infection and pathogenesis of Chagas' disease. *International Archives of Allergy and Immunology.* Vol. 114, No. 2, pp. 103-110, ISSN 1018-2438

Camargo M. M., Andrade A. C., Almeida I. C., Travassos L. R. & Gazzinelli R. T. (1997). Glycoconjugates isolated from Trypanosoma cruzi but not from Leishmania species membranes trigger nitric oxide synthesis as well as microbicidal activity in IFN-gamma-primed macrophages. *The Journal of Immunology.* Vol. 159, No. 12, pp. 6131-6139

Campos M. & Gazzinelli R. (2004). Trypanosoma cruzi and its components as exogenous mediators of inflammation recognized through Toll-like receptors. *Mediators of Inflammation.* Vol. 13, No. 3, pp. 139-143, ISSN 0962-9351

Carrasco G. H. A., Palacios-Prü E., Scorza C., Rangel A., Inglessis G., Sanoja C. L., Molina C. & Fuenmayor A. (1982). La biopsia endomiocárdica: ¿un recurso diagnóstico? Experiencia clínica en pacientes chagásicos y con otras miocardiopatías. *Revista Latinoamericana de Cardiología.* Vol. 3, No. 105, pp. 105

Castro C., Prata A. & Macedo V. (2005). The influence of the parasitemia on the evolution of the chronic Chagas' disease. *Revista da Sociedade Brasileira de Medicina Tropical.* Vol. 38, No. 1, pp. 1-6, ISSN 0037-8682

Castro R., Kuschnir E. & Sgammini H. (1988). Evaluación de la performance cardíaca y perfusión miocárdica con radiotrazadores en la cardiopatía chagásica crónica. *Revista de la Federación Argentina de Cardiología.* Vol. 17, No. pp. 226 - 231

Chagas C. (1909). Nova tripanozomiaze humana. Estudos sobre a morfolojia e o ciclo evolutivo do Schizotripannum cruzi n. gen., n. sp., ajente etiolojico de nova entidade mobida do homem. *Memorias do Instituto Oswaldo Cruz.* Vol. 1, No. 2, pp. 159 - 218

Chagas C. & Vilella E. (1922). Cardiac form of American trypanosomiasis. . *Memorias do Instituto Oswaldo Cruz.* Vol. 14, No. 1, pp. 5 - 61

Consolim-Colombo F. M., Lopes H. F., Rosetto E. A., Rubira M. C., Barreto-Filho J. A. S., Baruzzi A. C. A., Rocha N. N., Mady C., Irigoyen M. C. & Krieger E. M. (2004). Endothelial Function Is Preserved in Chagas' Heart Disease Patients Without Heart Failure. *Endothelium.* Vol. 11, No. 5-6, pp. 241-246

Cossio P. M., Diez C., Szarfman A., Kreutzer E., Candiolo B. & Arana R. M. (1974). Chagasic Cardiopathy: Demonstration of a Serum Gamma Globulin Factor Which Reacts with Endocardium and Vascular Structures. *Circulation.* Vol. 49, No. 1, pp. 13-21

Cruz-Robles D., Reyes P. A., Monteon-Padilla V. M., Ortiz-Muniz A. R. & Vargas-Alarcon G. (2004). MHC class I and class II genes in Mexican patients with Chagas disease. *Human Immunology.* Vol. 65, No. 1, pp. 60-65, ISSN 0198-8859

Cunha-Neto E., Dzau V. J., Allen P. D., Stamatiou D., Benvenutti L., Higuchi M. L., Koyama N. S., Silva J. S., Kalil J. & Liew C. C. (2005). Cardiac gene expression profiling provides evidence for cytokinopathy as a molecular mechanism in Chagas' disease cardiomyopathy. *The American Journal of Pathology.* Vol. 167, No. 2, pp. 305-313, ISSN 0002-9440

Cunha-Neto E. & Kalilf J. (2001). Heart-infiltrating and Peripheral T Cells in the Pathogenesis of Human Chagas' Disease Cardiomyopathy. *Autoimmunity.* Vol. 34, No. 3, pp. 187-192

Cunha-Neto E., Nogueira L. G., Teixeira P. C., Ramasawmy R., Drigo S. A., Goldberg A. C., Fonseca S. G., Bilate A. M. & Kalil J. (2009). Immunological and non-immunological effects of cytokines and chemokines in the pathogenesis of chronic Chagas disease cardiomyopathy. *Memorias do Instituto Oswaldo Cruz.* Vol. 104 Suppl 1, No. pp. 252-258, ISSN 1678-8060

Davila D. F., Donis J. H., Torres A. & Ferrer J. A. (2004). A modified and unifying neurogenic hypothesis can explain the natural history of chronic Chagas heart disease. *International Journal of Cardiology.* Vol. 96, No. 2, pp. 191-195, ISSN 0167-5273

Davila D. F., Donis J. H., Torres A., Gottberg C. F. & Rossell O. (1991). Cardiac parasympathetic innervation in Chagas' heart disease. *Medical Hypotheses.* Vol. 35, No. 2, pp. 80-84, ISSN 0306-9877

Davila D. F., Inglessis G. & Mazzei de Davila C. A. (1998). Chagas' heart disease and the autonomic nervous system. *International Journal of Cardiology.* Vol. 66, No. 2, pp. 123-127, ISSN 0167-5273

Davila Spinetti D. F., Inglessis G. & Mazzei de Davila C. A. (1999). Chagas cardiomyopathy and the autonomic nervous system. Clinical studies. *Archivos del Instituto de Cardiologia de Mexico*. Vol. 69, No. 1, pp. 35-39, ISSN 0020-3785

Deghaide N. H., Dantas R. O. & Donadi E. A. (1998). HLA class I and II profiles of patients presenting with Chagas' disease. *Digestive Diseases and Sciences*. Vol. 43, No. 2, pp. 246-252, ISSN 0163-2116

Diaz L. A., Arteaga L. A., Hilario-Vargas J., Valenzuela J. G., Li N., Warren S., Aoki V., Hans-Filho G., Eaton D., dos Santos V., Nutman T. B., de Mayolo A. A., Qaqish B. F., Sampaio S. A. & Rivitti E. A. (2004). Anti-desmoglein-1 antibodies in onchocerciasis, leishmaniasis and Chagas disease suggest a possible etiological link to Fogo selvagem. *The Journal of Investigative Dermatology*. Vol. 123, No. 6, pp. 1045-1051, ISSN 0022-202X

Dutra, Colley, Pinto D., Gazzinelli, Brener, Pereira, Coffman, Correa O. & Carvalho P. (2000). Self and Nonself Stimulatory Molecules Induce Preferential Expansion of CD5+ B Cells or Activated T Cells of Chagasic Patients, Respectively. *Scandinavian Journal of Immunology*. Vol. 51, No. 1, pp. 91-97, ISSN 1365-3083

Dutra W. O., Martins-Filho O. A., Cancado J. R., Pinto-Dias J. C., Brener Z., Freeman Junior G. L., Colley D. G., Gazzinelli G. & Parra J. C. (1994). Activated T and B lymphocytes in peripheral blood of patients with Chagas' disease. *International Immunology*. Vol. 6, No. 4, pp. 499-506, ISSN 0953-8178

Factor S. M. & Sonnenblick E. H. (1982). Hypothesis: Is congestive cardiomyopathy caused by a hyperreactive myocardial microcirculation (Microvascular spasm)? *The American Journal of Cardiology*. Vol. 50, No. 5, pp. 1149-1152, ISSN 0002-9149

Fedoseyeva E. V., Zhang F., Orr P. L., Levin D., Buncke H. J. & Benichou G. (1999). De Novo Autoimmunity to Cardiac Myosin After Heart Transplantation and Its Contribution to the Rejection Process. *The Journal of Immunology*. Vol. 162, No. 11, pp. 6836-6842

Fernandez-Mestre M. T., Layrisse Z., Montagnani S., Acquatella H., Catalioti F., Matos M., Balbas O., Makhatadze N., Dominguez E., Herrera F. & Madrigal A. (1998). Influence of the HLA class II polymorphism in chronic Chagas' disease. *Parasite immunology*. Vol. 20, No. 4, pp. 197-203, 0141-9838

Ferrans V. J., Milei J., Tomita Y. & Storino R. A. (1988). Basement membrane thickening in cardiac myocytes and capillaries in chronic Chagas' Disease. *American Journal of Cardiology*. Vol. 61, No. pp. 1137-1140

Ferreira R. C., Ianni B. M., Abel L. C., Buck P., Mady C., Kalil J. & Cunha-Neto E. (2003). Increased plasma levels of tumor necrosis factor-alpha in asymptomatic/"indeterminate" and Chagas disease cardiomyopathy patients. *Memorias do Instituto Oswaldo Cruz*. Vol. 98, No. 3, pp. 407-411, ISSN 0074-0276

Fujinami R. S., von Herrath M. G., Christen U. & Whitton J. L. (2006). Molecular Mimicry, Bystander Activation, or Viral Persistence: Infections and Autoimmune Disease. *Clinical Microbiological Reviews*. Vol. 19, No. 1, pp. 80-94

Gallo L., Jr., Neto J. A., Manco J. C., Rassi A. & Amorim D. S. (1975). Abnormal heart rate responses during exercise in patients with Chagas' disease. *Cardiology*. Vol. 60, No. 3, pp. 147-162, ISSN 0008-6312

Garcia Borras S., Racca L., Cotorruelo C., Biondi C., Beloscar J. & Racca A. (2009). Distribution of HLA-DRB1 alleles in Argentinean patients with Chagas' disease cardiomyopathy. *Immunological Investigations.* Vol. 38, No. 3-4, pp. 268-275, ISSN 1532-4311

Garcia R., Avila J. L., Rojas M., Martinez A., Garcia W. & Bergel P. (1998). Anti-sulfatide antibody titers in patients with chronic Chagas disease and other forms of cardiopathy. *Revista Panamericana de Salud Publica.* Vol. 3, No. 4, pp. 249-256, ISSN 1020-4989

Gazzinelli R. T. (1991). Natural anti-Gal antibodies prevent, rather than cause, autoimmunity in human Chagas' disease. *Research in Immunology.* Vol. 142, No. 2, pp. 164-167, ISSN 0923-2494

Giordanengo L., Fretes R., Díaz H., Cano R., Bacile A., Vottero-Cima E. & Gea S. (2000a). Cruzipain induces autoimmune response against skeletal muscle and tissue damage in mice. *Muscle & Nerve.* Vol. 23, No. 9, pp. 1407-1413, ISSN 1097-4598

Giordanengo L., Gea S., Barbieri G. & Rabinovich G. A. (2001). Anti-galectin-1 autoantibodies in human Trypanosoma cruzi infection: differential expression of this beta-galactoside-binding protein in cardiac Chagas' disease. *Clinical and Experimental Immunology.* Vol. 124, No. 2, pp. 266-273, ISSN 0009-9104

Giordanengo L., Maldonado C., Rivarola H. W., Iosa D., Girones N., Fresno M. & Gea S. (2000b). Induction of antibodies reactive to cardiac myosin and development of heart alterations in cruzipain-immunized mice and their offspring. *European Journal of Immunology.* Vol. 30, No. 11, pp. 3181-3189, ISSN 1521-4141

Girones N., Cuervo H. & Fresno M. (2005). Trypanosoma cruzi-induced molecular mimicry and Chagas' disease. *Current Topics in Microbiology and Immunology.* Vol. 296, No. pp. 89-123, ISSN 0070-217X

Girones N., Rodriguez C. I., Basso B., Bellon J. M., Resino S., Munoz-Fernandez M. A., Gea S., Moretti E. & Fresno M. (2001a). Antibodies to an epitope from the Cha human autoantigen are markers of Chagas' disease. *Clinical and Diagnostic Laboratory Immunology.* Vol. 8, No. 6, pp. 1039-1043, ISSN 1071-412X

Girones N., Rodriguez C. I., Carrasco-Marin E., Hernaez R. F., de Rego J. L. & Fresno M. (2001b). Dominant T- and B-cell epitopes in an autoantigen linked to Chagas' disease. *The Journal of Clinical Investigation.* Vol. 107, No. 8, pp. 985-993, ISSN 0021-9738

Goin J., Leiros C., Borda E. & Sterin-Borda L. (1997). Interaction of human chagasic IgG with the second extracellular loop of the human heart muscarinic acetylcholine receptor: functional and pathological implications. *The FASEB Journal.* Vol. 11, No. 1, pp. 77-83

Goin J. C., Borda E., Leiros C. P., Storino R. & Sterin-Borda L. (1994). Identification of antibodies with muscarinic cholinergic activity in human Chagas' disease: pathological implications. *Journal of the Autonomic Nervous System.* Vol. 47, No. 1-2, pp. 45-52, ISSN 0165-1838

Goin J. C., Sterin-Borda L., Bilder C. R., Varrica L. M., Iantorno G., Ríos M. C. & Borda E. (1999). Functional implications of circulating muscarinic cholinergic receptor autoantibodies in chagasic patients with achalasia. *Gastroenterology.* Vol. 117, No. 4, pp. 798-805, ISSN 0016-5085

Gomes J. A., Bahia-Oliveira L. M., Rocha M. O., Martins-Filho O. A., Gazzinelli G. & Correa-Oliveira R. (2003). Evidence that development of severe cardiomyopathy in human

Chagas' disease is due to a Th1-specific immune response. *Infection and Immunity*. Vol. 71, No. 3, pp. 1185-1193, ISSN 0019-9567

Gorelik G., Genaro A. M., Sterin-Borda L., Gonzalez Cappa S. & Borda E. S. (1990). Antibodies bind and activate beta adrenergic and cholinergic lymphocyte receptors in Chagas' disease. *Clinical Immunology and Immunopathology*. Vol. 55, No. 2, pp. 221-236, ISSN 0090-1229

Gruber A. & Zingales B. (1993). Trypanosoma cruzi: characterization of two recombinant antigens with potential application in the diagnosis of Chagas' disease. *Experimental Parasitology*. Vol. 76, No. 1, pp. 1-12, ISSN 0014-4894

Guerri-Guttenberg R. A., Grana D. R., Ambrosio G. & Milei J. (2008). Chagas cardiomyopathy: Europe is not spared!†. *European Heart Journal*. Vol. 29, No. 21, pp. 2587-2591

Guzzetti S., Iosa D., Pecis M., Bonura L., Prosdocimi M. & Malliani A. (1991). Impaired heart rate variability in patients with chronic Chagas' disease. *American Heart Journal*. Vol. 121, No. 6 Pt 1, pp. 1727-1734, ISSN 0002-8703

Hagar J. M. & Rahimtoola S. H. (1991). Chagas' Heart Disease in the United States. *New England Journal of Medicine*. Vol. 325, No. 11, pp. 763-768

Hiss F. C., Lascala T. F., Maciel B. C., Marin-Neto J. A. & Simoes M. V. (2009). Changes in myocardial perfusion correlate with deterioration of left ventricular systolic function in chronic Chagas' cardiomyopathy. *JACC. Cardiovascular Imaging*. Vol. 2, No. 2, pp. 164-172, ISSN 1876-7591

Huang H., Calderon T. M., Berman J. W., Braunstein V. L., Weiss L. M., Wittner M. & Tanowitz H. B. (1999a). Infection of Endothelial Cells with Trypanosoma cruzi Activates NF-kappa B and Induces Vascular Adhesion Molecule Expression. *Infection and Immunity*. Vol. 67, No. 10, pp. 5434-5440

Huang H., Chan J., Wittner M., Jelicks L. A., Morris S. A., Factor S. M., Weiss L. M., Braunstein V. L., Bacchi C. J., Yarlett N., Chandra M., Shirani J. & Tanowitz H. B. (1999b). Expression of Cardiac Cytokines and Inducible Form of Nitric Oxide Synthase (NOS2) inTrypanosoma cruzi-infected Mice. *Journal of Molecular and Cellular Cardiology*. Vol. 31, No. 1, pp. 75-88, ISSN 0022-2828

Jelicks L. A., Chandra M., Shirani J., Shtutin V., Tang B., Christ G. J., Factor S. M., Wittner M., Huang H., Weiss L. M., Mukherjee S., Bouzahzah B., Petkova S. B., Teixeira M. M., Douglas S. A., Loredo M. L., D'Orleans-Juste P. & Tanowitz H. B. (2002). Cardioprotective effects of phosphoramidon on myocardial structure and function in murine Chagas' disease. *International Journal for Parasitology*. Vol. 32, No. 12, pp. 1497-1506, ISSN 0020-7519

Jones E. M., Colley D. G., Tostes S., Reis Lopez E., Vnencak-Jones C. L. & McCurley T. L. (1993). Amplification of Trypanosoma cruzi DNA sequence from inflammatory lesions in human chagasic cardiomyopathy. *American Journal of Tropical Medicine and Hygiene*. Vol. 48, pp. 348-357

Jorg M. E. (1974). Tripanosomiasis cruzi: anarquía angiotopográfica por descapilarización mesenquimorreactiva, cofactor patogénico de la miocardiopatía crónica. *Prensa Médica Argentina*. Vol. 61, pp. 94.

Junqueira Junior L. F., Gallo Junior L., Manco J. C., Marin-Neto J. A. & Amorim D. S. (1985). Subtle cardiac autonomic impairment in Chagas' disease detected by baroreflex sensitivity testing. *Brazilian Journal of Medical and Biologival Research.* Vol. 18, No. 2, pp. 171-178, ISSN 0100-879X

Kerner N., Liegeard P., Levin M. J. & Hontebeyrie-Joskowicz M. (1991). Trypanosoma cruzi: antibodies to a MAP-like protein in chronic Chagas' disease cross-react with mammalian cytoskeleton. *Experimental Parasitology.* Vol. 73, No. 4, pp. 451-459, ISSN 0014-4894

Khoury E. L., Diez C., Cossio P. M. & Arana R. M. (1983). Heterophil nature of EVI antibody in Trypanosoma cruzi infection. *Clinical Immunology and Immunopathology.* Vol. 27, No. 2, pp. 283-288, ISSN 0090-1229

Kierszenbaum F. (2003). Views on the autoimmunity hypothesis for Chagas disease pathogenesis. *FEMS Immunology and Medical Microbiology.* Vol. 37, No. 1, pp. 1-11, ISSN 0928-8244

Köberle F. (1956a). Chagas disease: a disease of the peripheral autonomic nervous system. *Wien Klin Woschenschr.* Vol. 68, No. 17, pp. 333 - 339,

Köberle F. (1956b). Pathological findings in muscular hollow organs in experimental Chagas disease. *Zentralbl Allg Pathol.* Vol. 95, No. 7 - 8, pp. 321 - 329,

Köberle F. (1959). Cardiopathia parasympathicopriva. *Münch Med Wochenschr.* Vol. 101, No. pp. 1308-1310, ISSN 0027-2973

Kumar S. & Tarleton R. L. (1998). The relative contribution of antibody production and CD8+ T cell function to immune control of Trypanosoma cruzi. *Parasite Immunology.* Vol. 20, No. 5, pp. 207-216, ISSN 1365-3024

Laranja F. S., Dias E., Nobrega G. & Miranda A. (1956). Chagas' Disease: A Clinical, Epidemiologic, and Pathologic Study. *Circulation.* Vol. 14, No. 6, pp. 1035-1060

Layrisse Z., Fernandez M. T., Montagnani S., Matos M., Balbas O., Herrera F., Colorado I. A., Catalioti F. & Acquatella H. (2000). HLA-C(*)03 is a risk factor for cardiomyopathy in Chagas disease. *Human Immunology.* Vol. 61, No. 9, pp. 925-929, ISSN 0198-8859

Levitus G., Hontebeyrie-Joskowicz M., Van Regenmortel M. H. & Levin M. J. (1991). Humoral autoimmune response to ribosomal P proteins in chronic Chagas heart disease. *Clinical and Experimental Immunology.* Vol. 85, No. 3, pp. 413-417, ISSN 0009-9104

Libby P., Alroy J. & Pereira M. E. (1986). A neuraminidase from Trypanosoma cruzi removes sialic acid from the surface of mammalian myocardial and endothelial cells. *The Journal of Clinical Investigation.* Vol. 77, No. 1, pp. 127-135, ISSN 0021-9738

Llop E., Rothhammer F., Acuna M., Apt W. & Arribada A. (1991). HLA antigens in Chagas cardiomyopathy: new evidence based on a case-control study. *Revista Médica de Chile.* Vol. 119, No. 6, pp. 633-636, ISSN 0034-9887

Lopes E. R., Chapadeiro E., Andrade Z. A., Almeida Hde O. & Rocha A. (1981). Pathological anatomy of hearts from asymptomatic Chagas disease patients dying in a violent manner. *Memorias do Instituto Oswaldo Cruz.* Vol. 75, No. 2, pp. 189 - 197

Lu B., Luquetti A. O., Rassi A. & PereiraPerrin M. (2010). Autoantibodies to neurotrophic receptors TrkA, TrkB and TrkC in patients with acute Chagas' disease. *Scandinavian Journal of Immunology.* Vol. 71, No. 3, pp. 220-225, ISSN 1365-3083

Macedo A. M., Machado C. R., Oliveira R. P. & Pena S. D. J. (2004). Trypanosoma cruzi: Genetic Structure of Populations and Relevance of Genetic Variability to the Pathogenesis of Chagas Disease. *Memorias do Instituto Oswaldo Cruz.* Vol. 99, No. 1, pp. 1 - 12

Manço J. C., Gallo L., Jr., Godoy R. A., Fernandes R. G. & Amorim D. S. (1969). Degeneration of the cardiac nerves in Chagas' disease. Further studies. *Circulation*. Vol. 40, No. 6, pp. 879-885, ISSN 0009-7322

Marin-Neto J. A., Cunha-Neto E., Maciel B. C. & Simoes M. V. (2007). Pathogenesis of Chronic Chagas Heart Disease. *Circulation*. Vol. 115, No. 9, pp. 1109-1123

Marin-Neto J. A., Gallo L., Jr., Manço J. C., Rassi A. & Amorim D. S. (1975). Postural reflexes in chronic Chagas's heart disease. Heart rate and arterial pressure responses. *Cardiology*. Vol. 60, No. 6, pp. 343-357, 0008-6312

Marin-Neto J. A., Marzullo P., Marcassa C., Gallo Junior L., Maciel B. C., Bellina C. R. & L'Abbate A. (1992). Myocardial perfusion abnormalities in chronic Chagas' disease as detected by thallium-201 scintigraphy. *The American Journal of Cardiology*. Vol. 69, No. 8, pp. 780-784, ISSN 0002-9149

Menezes C. A. S., Rocha M. O. C., Souza P. E. A., Chaves A. C. L., Gollob K. J. & Dutra W. O. (2004). Phenotypic and functional characteristics of CD28+ and CD28− cells from chagasic patients: distinct repertoire and cytokine expression. *Clinical & Experimental Immunology*. Vol. 137, No. 1, pp. 129-138, ISSN 1365-2249

Milei J., Fernandez Alonso G., Vanzulli S., Storino R. A., Maturri L. & Rossi L. (1996a). Myocardial Inflammatory infiltrate in human chronic Chagasic cardiomyopathy: Immunohistochemical findings. *Cardiovascular Pathology*. Vol. 5, No. 4, pp. 209-219

Milei J., Storino R.A., Matturri L., Rossi L. (1996b). Studio anatomo-clinico ed epidemiologico della malattia di Chagas. *Pathologica*. Vol. 88, pp. 117, 127

Milei J., Guerri-Guttenberg R. A., Grana D. R. & Storino R. (2009). Prognostic impact of Chagas disease in the United States. *American Heart Journal*. Vol. 157, No. 1, pp. 22-29, ISSN 0002-8703

Milei J., Mautner B., Storino R. A., Sanchez J. A. & Ferrans V. J. (1992a). Does Chagas' disease exist as an undiagnosd form of cardiomyopathy in the United States? *American Heart Journal*. Vol. 123, No. 6, pp. 1732-1735

Milei J., Pesce R., Valero E., Muratore C., Beigelman R. & Ferrans V. J. (1991a). Electrophysiologic-structural correlations in chagasic aneurysms causing malignant arrhythmias. *International Journal of Cardiology*. Vol. 32, No. 1, pp. 65-73, ISSN 0167-5273

Milei J., Sánchez J., Storino R., Yu Z.-X., Denduchis B. & Ferrans V. J. (1993). Antibodies to laminin and immunohistochemical localization of laminin in chronic chagasic cardiomyopathy: a review. *Molecular and Cellular Biochemistry*. Vol. 129, No. 2, pp. 161-170, ISSN 0300-8177

Milei J., Storino R. A., Beigelman R., Fernandez Alonso G., Maturri L. & Rossi L. (1991b). Histopathology of specialized and ordinary myocardium and nerves in chronic Chagas disease, with a morphometric study of inflammation and fibrosis. *Cardiologia*. Vol. 36, No. 2, pp. 107-115

Milei J., Storino R. A., Fernandez Alonso G., Beigelman R., Vanzulli S. & Ferrans V. J. (1992b). Endomyocardial biopsies in chronic chagasic cardiomyopathy. Immunohistochemical and ultrastructural findings. *Cardiology*. Vol. 80, No. 5-6, pp. 424-437

Milei J., Guerri-Guttenberg R. A., Azzato F. & Storino R. (2008). Chagasic Cardiomyopathy: New trends for an old burden, Nova Science Publishers, 978-1-60692-193-7

Moia B., Rosenbaum M. & Hojman D. (1955). Aneurismas ventriculares en la miocarditis crónica chagásica. *Revista Argentina de Cardiología*. Vol. 22, No. pp.

Molina R. B. G., Matsubara B. B., Hueb J. C., Zanati S. G., Meira D. A., Cassolato J. L., Paiva S. A. R. & Zornoff L. A. M. (2006). Dysautonomia and ventricular dysfunction in the indeterminate form of Chagas disease. *International Journal of Cardiology*. Vol. 113, No. 2, pp. 188-193, ISSN 0167-5273

Morris S. A., Weiss L. M., Factor S., Bilezikian J. P., Tanowitz H. & Wittner M. (1989). Verapamil ameliorates clinical, pathologic and biochemical manifestations of experimental chagasic cardiomyopathy in mice. *Journal of the American College of Cardiology*. Vol. 14, No. 3, pp. 782-789, ISSN 0735-1097

Mott K. E. & Hagstrom J. W. C. (1965). The Pathologic Lesions of the Cardiac Autonomic Nervous System in Chronic Chagas' Myocarditis. *Circulation*. Vol. 31, No. 2, pp. 273-286

Nachman R. L., Hajjar K. A., Silverstein R. L. & Dinarello C. A. (1986). Interleukin 1 induces endothelial cell synthesis of plasminogen activator inhibitor. *The Journal of Experimental Medicine*. Vol. 163, No. 6, pp. 1595-1600

Neu N., Ploier B. & Ofner C. (1990). Cardiac myosin-induced myocarditis. Heart autoantibodies are not involved in the induction of the disease. *The Journal of Immunology*. Vol. 145, No. 12, pp. 4094-4100

Oliveira E. C., Fujisawa M. M., Hallal Longo D. E., Farias A. S., Contin Moraes J., Guariento M. E., de Almeida E. A., Saad M. J., Langone F., Toyama M. H., Andreollo N. A. & Santos L. M. (2009). Neuropathy of gastrointestinal Chagas' disease: immune response to myelin antigens. *Neuroimmunomodulation*. Vol. 16, No. 1, pp. 54-62, 1423-0216

Oliveira J. S. (1985). A natural human model of intrinsic heart nervous system denervation: Chagas' cardiopathy. *American heart journal*. Vol. 110, No. 5, pp. 1092 - 1098

Palacios-Prü E., Carrasco G. H. A., Scorza C. & Espinosa R. (1982). Ultraestructura miocárdica en la enfermedad de Chagas. Diagnóstico diferencial con la miocardiopatía dilatada o congestiva y con las miocardiopatías arrítmicas. *Revista Latinoamericana de Cardiología*. Vol. 3, No. pp. 115

Pereira de Godoy M. R., Cacao J. C., Pereira de Godoy J. M., Brandao A. C. & Silva Rossi Souza D. (2005). Chagas disease and anticardiolipin antibodies in older adults. *Archives of Gerontology and Geriatrics*. Vol. 41, No. 3, pp. 235-238, ISSN 0167-4943

Petkova S. B., Huang H., Factor S. M., Pestell R. G., Bouzahzah B., Jelicks L. A., Weiss L. M., Douglas S. A., Wittner M. & Tanowitz H. B. (2001). The role of endothelin in the pathogenesis of Chagas' disease. *International Journal for Parasitology*. Vol. 31, No. 5-6, pp. 499-511, ISSN 0020-7519

Petkova S. B., Tanowitz H. B., Magazine H. I., Factor S. M., Chan J., Pestell R. G., Bouzahzah B., Douglas S. A., Shtutin V., Morris S. A., Tsang E., Weiss L. M., Christ G. J., Wittner M. & Huang H. (2000). Myocardial Expression of Endothelin-1 in Murine Trypanosoma cruzi Infection. *Cardiovascular Pathology*. Vol. 9, No. 5, pp. 257-265, ISSN 1054-8807

Py M. O., Maciel L., Pedrosa R. C., Nascimento J. H. & Medei E. (2009). The presence of antiautonomic membrane receptor antibodies do not correlate with brain lesions in Chagas' disease. *Arquivos Brasileiros de Cardiologia*. Vol. 67, No. 3A, pp. 633 - 638

Rassi A., Jr., Rassi A. & Little W. C. (2000). Chagas' heart disease. *Clinical cardiology*. Vol. 23, No. 12, pp. 883-889, ISSN 0160-9289

Rassi A., Jr., Rassi A. & Marin-Neto J. A. (2010). Chagas disease. *Lancet*. Vol. 375, No. 9723, pp. 1388-1402, 1474-547X

Reddy V. S., Harskamp R. E., van Ginkel M. W., Calhoon J., Baisden C. E., Kim I. S., Valente A. J. & Chandrasekar B. (2008). Interleukin-18 stimulates fibronectin expression in primary human cardiac fibroblasts via PI3K-Akt-dependent NF-kappaB activation. *Journal of Cell Physiology*. Vol. 215, No. 3, pp. 697-707, ISSN 1097-4652

Reis D. D., Jones E. M., Tostes S., Jr., Lopes E. R., Gazzinelli G., Colley D. G. & McCurley T. L. (1993). Characterization of inflammatory infiltrates in chronic chagasic myocardial lesions: presence of tumor necrosis factor-alpha+ cells and dominance of granzyme A+, CD8+ lymphocytes. *The American Journal of Tropical Medicine and Hygiene*. Vol. 48, No. 5, pp. 637-644, ISSN 0002-9637

Reis M. M., Higuchi Mde L., Benvenuti L. A., Aiello V. D., Gutierrez P. S., Bellotti G. & Pileggi F. (1997). An in situ quantitative immunohistochemical study of cytokines and IL-2R+ in chronic human chagasic myocarditis: correlation with the presence of myocardial Trypanosoma cruzi antigens. *Clinical Immunology and Immunopathology*. Vol. 83, No. 2, pp. 165-172, ISSN 0090-1229

Ribeiro-Dos-Santos R., Mengel J. O., Postol E., Soares R. A. O., Ferreira-Fernandez E., Soares M. B. P. & Pontes-De-Carvalho L. C. (2001). A heart-specific CD4+ T-cell line obtained from a chronic chagasic mouse induces carditis in heart-immunized mice and rejection of normal heart transplants in the absence of Trypanosoma cruzi. *Parasite Immunology*. Vol. 23, No. 2, pp. 93-101, ISSN 1365-3024

Riol-Blanco L., Sanchez-Sanchez N., Torres A., Tejedor A., Narumiya S., Corbi A. L., Sanchez-Mateos P. & Rodriguez-Fernandez J. L. (2005). The chemokine receptor CCR7 activates in dendritic cells two signaling modules that independently regulate chemotaxis and migratory speed. *Journal of Immunology*. Vol. 174, No. 7, pp. 4070-4080, ISSN 0022-1767

Rossi L. (1988). Neuroanatomopathology of the cardiovascular system., In: *Neurocardiology.*, Kulbertus, H. E. and Franck, G., pp. Futura Publishing Co. Inc., Mount Kisco, N.Y.

Rossi L., Storino R., Milei J. & Matturri L. (1994). Depleción neuronal en la enfermedad de Chagas: todo debería revisarse. *Revista Argentina de Cardiología*. Vol. 62, No. 3, pp. 239 - 246

Rossi M. A. & Carobrez S. G. (1985). Experimental Trypanosoma cruzi cardiomyopathy in BALB/c mice: histochemical evidence of hypoxic changes in the myocardium. *British Journal of Experimental Pathology*. Vol. 66, No. 2, pp. 155 - 160

Rossi M. A., Gonçalves S. & Ribeiro-dos-Santos R. (1984). Experimental Trypanosoma cruzi Cardiomyopathy in BA4LB/c Mice. The Potential Role of Intravascular Platelet Aggregation in its Genesis. *American Journal of Pathology*. Vol. 114, No. 2, pp. 209 - 216

Rossi M. A., Tanowitz H., Malvestio L. M., Celes M. R., Campos E. C., Blefari V. & Prado C. M. (2010). Coronary Microvascular Disease in Chronic Chagas Cardiomyopathy Including an Overview on History, Pathology, and Other Proposed Pathogenic Mechanisms. *PLoS Neglected Tropical Diseases*. Vol. 4, No. 8, pp. e674

Sakai N., Wada T., Yokoyama H., Lipp M., Ueha S., Matsushima K. & Kaneko S. (2006). Secondary lymphoid tissue chemokine (SLC/CCL21)/CCR7 signaling regulates fibrocytes in renal fibrosis. *Proceedings of the National Academy Science U S A.* Vol. 103, No. 38, pp. 14098-14103, ISSN 0027-8424

Salomone O. A., Caeiro T. F., Madoery R. J., Amuchástegui M., Omelinauk M., Juri D. & Kaski J. C. (2001). High plasma immunoreactive endothelin levels in patients with Chagas' cardiomyopathy. *The American Journal of Cardiology.* Vol. 87, No. 10, pp. 1217-1220, ISSN 0002-9149

Sanchez J. A., Milei J., Yu Z. X., Storino R., Wenthold R. J. & Ferrans V. J. (1993). Immunohistochemical localization of laminin in the hearts of patients with chronic chagasic cardiomyopathy: relationship to thickening of basement membranes. *American Heart Journal.* Vol. 126, No. 6, pp. 1392 - 1401

Sathler-Avelar R., Vitelli-Avelar D. M., Teixeira-Carvalho A. & Martins-Filho O. A. (2009). Innate immunity and regulatory T-cells in human Chagas disease: what must be understood? *Memorias do Instituto Oswaldo Cruz.* Vol. 104 Suppl 1, No. pp. 246-251, ISSN 1678-8060

Savino W., Villa-Verde D. M., Mendes-da-Cruz D. A., Silva-Monteiro E., Perez A. R., Aoki M. d. P., Bottasso O., Guiñazú N., Silva-Barbosa S. D. & Gea S. (2007). Cytokines and cell adhesion receptors in the regulation of Immunity to Trypanosoma cruzi. *Cytokine & Growth Factor Reviews.* Vol. 18, No. pp. 107 - 124

Schijman A. G., Vigliano C. A., Viotti R. J., Burgos J. M., Brandariz S., Lococo B. E., Leze M. I., Armenti H. A. & Levin M. J. (2004). Trypanosoma cruzi DNA in cardiac lesions of Argentinean patients with end-stage chronic chagas heart disease. *The American Journal of Tropical Medicine and Hygiene.* Vol. 70, No. 2, pp. 210-220, ISSN 0002-9637

Schwartz R. G. & Wexler O. (2009). Early Identification and Monitoring Progression of Chagas' Cardiomyopathy With SPECT Myocardial Perfusion Imaging. *JACC: Cardiovascular Imaging.* Vol. 2, No. 2, pp. 173-175, ISSN 1936-878X

Skeiky Y. A., Benson D. R., Parsons M., Elkon K. B. & Reed S. G. (1992). Cloning and expression of Trypanosoma cruzi ribosomal protein P0 and epitope analysis of anti-P0 autoantibodies in Chagas' disease patients. *The Journal of Experimental Medicine.* Vol. 176, No. 1, pp. 201-211, ISSN 0022-1007

Sousa A. C., Marin-Neto J. A., Maciel B. C., Gallo L., Jr. & Amorim D. S. (1987). Cardiac parasympathetic impairment in gastrointestinal Chagas' disease. *Lancet.* Vol. 1, No. 8539, pp. 985, ISSN 0140-6736

Souza P. E., Rocha M. O., Rocha-Vieira E., Menezes C. A., Chaves A. C., Gollob K. J. & Dutra W. O. (2004). Monocytes from patients with indeterminate and cardiac forms of Chagas' disease display distinct phenotypic and functional characteristics associated with morbidity. *Infection and immunity.* Vol. 72, No. 9, pp. 5283-5291, ISSN 0019-9567

Souza P. E. A., Rocha M. O. C., Menezes C. A. S., Coelho J. S., Chaves A. C. L., Gollob K. J. & Dutra W. O. (2007). Trypanosoma cruzi Infection Induces Differential Modulation of Costimulatory Molecules and Cytokines by Monocytes and T Cells from Patients with Indeterminate and Cardiac Chagas' Disease. *Infection and. Immunity.* Vol. 75, No. 4, pp. 1886 - 1894

Sterin-Borda L. & Borda E. (2000). Role of Neurotransmitter Autoantibodies in the Pathogenesis of Chagasic Peripheral Dysautonomia. *Annals of the New York Academy of Sciences.* Vol. 917, No. 1, pp. 273-280, ISSN 1749-6632

Sterin-Borda L., Gorelik G. & Borda E. S. (1991). Chagasic IgG binding with cardiac muscarinic cholinergic receptors modifies cholinergic-mediated cellular transmembrane signals. *Clin Immnol Immunopathol.* Vol. 61, No. pp. 387-397

Sterin-Borda L., Leiros C. P., Goin J. C., Cremaschi G., Genaro A., Echagüe A. V. & Borda E. (1997). Participation of Nitric Oxide Signaling System in the Cardiac Muscarinic Cholinergic Effect of Human Chagasic IgG. *Journal of Molecular and Cellular Cardiology.* Vol. 29, No. 7, pp. 1851-1865, ISSN 0022-2828

Storino R. A., Barragan H. & Milei J. (1992). Aspectos epidemiologicos de la enfermedad de Chagas en la Argentina y America Latina. *Revista Federación Argentina de Cardiología.* Vol. 21, No. 3, pp. 239-246

Storino R. A. & Milei J. (1994). *Enfermedad de Chagas*, Mosby-Doyma, Buenos Aires

Szarfman A., Terranova V. P., Rennard S. I., Foidart J. M., de Fatima Lima M., Scheinman J. I. & Martin G. R. (1982). Antibodies to laminin in Chagas' disease. *The Journal of Experimental Medicine.* Vol. 155, No. 4, pp. ISSN 1161-1171

Talvani A., Rocha M. O., Barcelos L. S., Gomes Y. M., Ribeiro A. L. & Teixeira M. M. (2004). Elevated concentrations of CCL2 and tumor necrosis factor-alpha in chagasic cardiomyopathy. *Clinical Infectious Disease.* Vol. 38, No. 7, pp. 943-950, ISSN 1537-6591

Talvani A., Rocha M. O. C., Ribeiro A. L., Borda E., Sterin-Borda L. & Teixeira M. M. (2006). Levels of anti-M2 and anti-[beta]1 autoantibodies do not correlate with the degree of heart dysfunction in Chagas' heart disease. *Microbes and Infection.* Vol. 8, No. 9-10, pp. 2459-2464, 1286-4579

Tanowitz H. B., Gumprecht J. P., Spurr D., Calderon T. M., Ventura M. C., Raventos-Suarez C., Kellie S., Factor S. M., Hatcher V. B., Wittner M. & Berman J. (1992a). Cytokine Gene Expression of Endothelial Cells Infected with Trypanosoma cruzi. *Journal of Infectious Diseases.* Vol. 166, No. 3, pp. 598-603

Tanowitz H. B., Kaul D. K., Chen B., Morris S. A., Factor S. M., Weiss L. M. & Wittner M. (1996). Compromised Microcirculation in Acute Murine Trypanosoma cruzi Infection. *The Journal of Parasitology.* Vol. 82, No. 1, pp. 124 - 130

Tanowitz H. B., Morris S. A., Factor S. M., Weiss L. M. & Wittner M. (1992b). Parasitic diseases of the heart I: Acute and chronic Chagas' disease. *Cardiovascular Pathology.* Vol. 1, No. 1, pp. 7-15, ISSN 1054-8807

Tarleton R. & Zhang L. (1999). Chagas Disease Etiology: Autoimmunity or Parasite Persistence? *Parasitology Today.* Vol. 15, No. 3, pp. 94 - 99

Torres C. M. (1960). Miocitólise e fibrose do miocárdio na doença de Chagas. *Memorias do Instituto Oswaldo Cruz.* Vol. 58, No. 2, pp. 161 - 182

Tyler K. M. & Engman D. M. (2001). The life cycle of Trypanosoma cruzi revisited. *International Journal for Parasitology.* Vol. 31, No. pp. 472 - 481

Vago A. R., Andrade L. O., Leite A. A., d'Avila Reis D., Macedo A. M., Adad S. J., Tostes S., Jr., Moreira M. C., Filho G. B. & Pena S. D. (2000). Genetic characterization of Trypanosoma cruzi directly from tissues of patients with chronic Chagas disease: differential distribution of genetic types into diverse organs. *The American Journal of Pathology.* Vol. 156, No. 5, pp. 1805-1809, ISSN 0002-9440

Vasconcelos D. F. & Junqueira L. F., Jr. (2009). Distinctive impaired cardiac autonomic modulation of heart rate variability in chronic Chagas' indeterminate and heart diseases. *Journal of Electrocardiology.* Vol. 42, No. 3, pp. 281-289, ISSN 1532-8430

Villani F. N., Rocha M. O., Nunes Mdo C., Antonelli L. R., Magalhaes L. M., dos Santos J. S., Gollob K. J. & Dutra W. O. (2010). Trypanosoma cruzi-induced activation of functionally distinct alphabeta and gammadelta CD4- CD8- T cells in individuals with polar forms of Chagas' disease. *Infection and Immunity*. Vol. 78, No. 10, pp. 4421-4430, ISSN 1098-5522

Vitelli-Avelar D. M., Sathler-Avelar R., Dias J. C. P., Pascoal V. P. M., Teixeira-Carvalho A., Lage P. S., Elói-Santos S. M., Corrêa-Oliveira R. & Martins-Filho O. A. (2005). Chagasic Patients with Indeterminate Clinical Form of the Disease have High Frequencies of Circulating CD3+CD16–CD56+ Natural Killer T Cells and CD4+CD25High Regulatory T Lymphocytes. *Scandinavian Journal of Immunology*. Vol. 62, No. 3, pp. 297-308, ISSN 1365-3083

Vitelli-Avelar D. M., Sathler-Avelar R., Massara R. L., Borges J. D., Lage P. S., Lana M., Teixeira-Carvalho A., Dias J. C., Eloi-Santos S. M. & Martins-Filho O. A. (2006). Are increased frequency of macrophage-like and natural killer (NK) cells, together with high levels of NKT and CD4+CD25high T cells balancing activated CD8+ T cells, the key to control Chagas' disease morbidity? *Clinical and Experimental Immunology*. Vol. 145, No. 1, pp. 81-92, ISSN 0009-9104

Vitelli-Avelar D. M., Sathler-Avelar R., Teixeira-Carvalho A., Pinto Dias J. C., Gontijo E. D., Faria A. M., Eloi-Santos S. M. & Martins-Filho O. A. (2008). Strategy to assess the overall cytokine profile of circulating leukocytes and its association with distinct clinical forms of human Chagas disease. *Scandinavian Journal of Immunology*. Vol. 68, No. 5, pp. 516-525, ISSN 1365-3083

Wallukat G., Munoz Saravia S. G., Haberland A., Bartel S., Araujo R., Valda G., Duchen D., Diaz Ramirez I., Borges A. C. & Schimke I. (2010). Distinct patterns of autoantibodies against G-protein-coupled receptors in Chagas' cardiomyopathy and megacolon. Their potential impact for early risk assessment in asymptomatic Chagas' patients. *Journal of the American College of Cardiology*. Vol. 55, No. 5, pp. 463-468, ISSN 1558-3597

Yoshida N. & Cortez M. R. (2008). *Trypanosoma cruzi: parasite and host cell signaling during the invasion process*, Springer Science, Houton

Younées-Chennoufi A. B., Hontebeyre-Joskowicz M., Tricottet V., Eisen H., Reynes M. & Said G. (1988). Persistence of Trypanosoma cruzi antigens in the inflammatory lesions of chronically infected mice. *Trans Roy Soc Trop Med Hyg*. Vol. 82, No. pp. 77

7

Exacerbation of Viral Myocarditis by Tobacco Smoke: The Catecholamine Hypothesis

Nicolas Hanabergh and James P. Morgan
Steward Carney Hospital, Dorchester, Steward St. Elizabeth's Medical Center, Boston and Tufts University School of Medicine, Boston, United States of America

1. Introduction

1.1 Tobacco smoke exposure and cardiovascular disease

More than 1 in every 10 cardiovascular deaths in the world during the year 2000 were attributable to smoking, demonstrating that it is an important preventable cause of cardiovascular mortality (Ezzati et al., 2005). It has been clearly established that exposure to environmental tobacco smoke increases the risk of cardiovascular disease among persons who have never smoked (Steenland, 1992). The cardiovascular effects of secondhand smoke are nearly as large as those confronting the principal smoker (Barnoya & Glantz, 2005). Non-smokers living with smokers have about a 25% increase in risk of death from heart disease and are more likely to suffer a stroke. Exposure to secondhand smoke may increase the risk of heart disease by non-smokers as much as 60% (Whincup et al., 2004). In 2004, Ong & Glantz estimated that only about 69% of U.S. indoor workers were covered by a smoke-free workplace policy. Making all workplaces smoke free as been accomplished for the commercial aircraft industry (Repace, 2004) would in one year prevent about 1500 myocardial infarctions and 350 strokes, and result in nearly 49 million dollars in savings in direct medical costs. These estimates are supported by reports of reduced incidence of admissions for myocardial infarction associated with smoking bans (Sargent et al., 2004).

The cardiovascular effects of tobacco smoke exposure have been summarized in several excellent reviews (for example, see Barnoya and Glantz, 2005). Among the strongest pathophysiological correlates of tobacco smoking are accelerated endothelial dysfunction (Puranik & Celermajer, 2003) and acute clinical events, the latter being largely thrombotic (Ambrose & Barus, 2004). Recent studies indicate that increased oxidative stress is a potential mechanism for initiating cardiovascular dysfunction (Yang et al., 2004; Talukder et al, 2011). Tobacco smoke has also been demonstrated to increase inflammatory markers in patients exposed to secondhand smoke, including homocysteine, C-reactive protein, fibrinogen, and oxidized LDL cholesterol, (Panagiotakos et al., 2004) suggesting that an increased inflammatory response may contribute to accelerated atherosclerosis. Clearly, the incidence of ischemic coronary and peripheral vascular disease is increased in patients exposed to tobacco smoke, either as smokers or through exposure to secondhand tobacco smoke (Ambrose & Barus, 2004; Benowitz, 2003; Law & Wald, 2003; Burns, 2003; Leone et al., 2004). The cardiovascular effects of tobacco smoke exposure are summarized in Table l.

MECHANISMS OF CARDIAC AND VASCULAR INJURY FROM TOBACCO SMOKE EXPOSURE

Initiates inflammatory response
Enhanced platelet activation and thrombosis
Increased oxidative stress
Increased insulin resistance
Endothelial cell dysfunction
Accelerates atherosclerosis

Table 1. Cardiovascular effects of tobacco smoke exposure.

1.2 Tobacco smoke exposure and heart failure

National hospital discharge surveys estimate that 4.8 million Americans have heart failure, which has become an increasingly frequent reason for inpatient admission (Ho et al., 1993). One recent study estimated that among individuals aged 55 and older almost 1 in 3 will develop heart failure during their remaining lifespan. Heart failure is a fatal disease, with only 35% surviving 5 years after diagnosis (Bleumink et al., 2004). Coronary disease and diabetes mellitus along with hypertension are the leading causes of heart failure in the United States and it is therefore not surprising that tobacco smoke exposure has been identified as an independent risk factor for developing heart failure (Kannel et al., 1994; He et al., 2001). However, in at least 5% of patients, the cause of heart failure is initially unknown (Baldasseroni et al., 2002) and it has been estimated that myocarditis or inflammation of the heart muscle, may account for some 9% of these cases (Felker et al., 2000). Although estimates vary, these figures indicate that hundreds of thousands of Americans and millions of patients worldwide with heart failure may have myocarditis as a primary or exacerbating cause. The true incidence of myocarditis from any cause among the general population is unknown and most patients do not develop clinical manifestations of heart failure (Olinde & O'Connell, 1994). However, the Myocarditis Treatment Trial in which endomyocardial biopsy was performed in over 2,200 patients with unexplained heart failure of less than two years duration indicated a prevalence of 10%, implicating myocarditis as a potential cause of heart failure in hundreds of thousands of patients (Mason et al., 1995). Since only around 5% of patients systemically infected with a cardiotropic virus (Coxsakie β) may develop cardiac involvement, it is important to determine what factors may increase the risk of cardiac involvement (Grist & Bell, 1969; Gerzen et al., 1972; Rodeheffer & Gersh, 1996).

1.3 Catecholamines exacerbate myocarditis

Evidence from several different sources indicates that catecholamines may exacerbate viral myocarditis in animals and patients. A variety of sympathomimetic agents have been reported to induce or exacerbate myocarditis (Table 2). It is also important to note that nicotine has been shown to increase catecholamine levels in the blood (Wong et al, 2007). The most direct evidence arises from carefully controlled studies of murine myocarditis indicting that hypercatecholaminergeic states, secondary to pheochromocytoma and during infusion with sympathomimetic drugs, can cause or significantly exacerbate myocarditis (Cho et al., 1987; Van Vliet et al., 1966; Bindoli et al., 1992; Kammermeier & Grobecker, 1995; Davila et al., 1995; Prichard et al., 1991; Brown & O'Connell, 1995; Siltanen et al., l982; Haft, 1974; Noda, 1970; Morin & Cote, 1972; Seta et al., 1997; Nash & Carter, 1967; Karch, 1987; Krentz et al., 2001; Rezkalla et al., 1988). Reports of a prospective study by Karch (Karch, 1987) showed significantly elevated levels of epinephrine and norepinephrine in a group of patients who presented with cardiac symptoms immediately after using cocaine. Moreover, sympatholytic agents and states may ameliorate the manifestations of myocarditis and decrease mortality, although this effect is controversial (Rezkalla et al., 1988; Anandasabapathy & Frishman, 1998; Mehes et al., 1966; Dunn & Vickers, 1994). We have shown a beneficial effect of beta blockade, ameliorating cocaine and catecholamine exacerbation of myocarditis in a murine model (Wang et al., 2005). It is provocative to consider that many of the interventions shown to ameliorate viral myocarditic pathgenicity, including calcium channel blockers, act predominantly to attenuate sympathomimetic effects on the heart (Dong et al., 1992; Hiraoka et al., 1996; Lowenstein et al., 1996; Wang et al., 1997; Keaney et al., 1996). Additional evidence includes the observation that, among commonly abused substances in the general population (alcohol, nicotine, caffeine, marijuana, and cocaine), cocaine has been most strongly associated with an increased incidence of myocarditis, suggesting that its unique sympathomimetic properties, not shared with these other agents, may be the causative factor. Moreover, in the clinical area, it has been accepted clinical practice for many years to restrict the activities of patients with myocarditis, primarily based on animal studies and circumstantial clinical evidence in man that exercise exacerbates the disease (Abelmann, 1966; Cabinian et al., 1990; Gatmaitan et al., 1970; Friman et al., 1983; Kiel et al., 1989; Tilles et al., 1964; Elson & Abelmann, 1965; Hosenpud et al., 1987). In addition to directly increasing the work of the heart, normal exercise is associated with a marked increase in circulating catecholamine levels (Cabinian et al., 1990; Gatmaitan et al., 1970; Friman et al., 1983; Kiel et al., 1989). While the cardiac effects of sympathomimetic drugs and interventions using sympatholytic agents require additional testing in animal models of myocarditis and in man, the available evidence points to catecholaminergic effects in the development of myocarditis.

1.4 Adrenergic activation by cigarette smoke

It has been estimated that there are over 4,000 chemical constituents in cigarette smoke. Of these, about 400 have been measured or estimated in mainstream or sidestream smoke; of the 400, a significant amount of toxicology data exists for less than 100 (Fowles & Bates, 2000). Nicotine is the most comprehensively studied constituent of cigarette smoke, and has been shown to act primarily on nicotinic acetylcholine receptors in autonomic ganglia and in the brain (Benowitz, 2008; Mobascher & Winterer, 2008). This results in activation of the sympathetic nervous system, increasing the release of epinephrine (EPI) and norepinephrine (NE) from adrenergic nerve endings and the adrenal medulla, both systemically and into the local milieu of adrenergically innervated organs, including the heart (Haass & Kübler, 1997; Adamopoulos, et al., 2008; Shinozaki et al., 2008). Cigarette smoke also contains monoamine oxidase inhibitors (Cooper & Magwere, 2008; Fowles & Bates, 2000; Herraiz et al., 2005). Cigarette smoke has been shown to increase norepinephrine and epinephrine levels with

SYMPATHOMIMETIC AGENTS WITH THE POTENTIAL TO CAUSE MYOCARDITIS

Catecholamines	(Wang et al, 2005)
Ephedrine	(Naik & Freudenberger, 2004)
Cocaine	(Wang et al, 2002a)
Amphetamine	(Smith et al, 1976)
Terbutaline	(Sykes et al, 1991)
Clozapine	(Wang et al, 2008)
Methylxanthines	(Nino et al, 1987)

Table 2. Sympathomimetic agents that may initiate or exacerbate myocarditis.

associated increases in heart rate, blood pressure and coronary vasoconstriction (Haass & Kübler, 1997, Adamopoulos et al., 2008, Shinozaki et al., 2008). Nicotine may also potentiate catecholamine actions, perhaps via effects on nitric oxide synthesis or release (Haass & Kübler, 1997). The adrenergic actions of nicotine can be attenuated or blocked by administration of beta-adrenergic antagonists, although it has been proposed that the drug may act by additional mechanisms to activate the beta-adrenergic pathway (Haas & Kübler, 1997; Sofuoglu et al., 2006; Marano et al., 1999, Wang et al., 2005).

2. Experimental evidence

2.1 Overview

Our previous studies indicated that catecholamines exacerbate the severity of viral myocarditis in a murine model (Soodini & Morgan, 2001; Wang & Morgan, 2003; Wang et al., 2002a, 2002b, 2005). We performed studies with a variety of agents known to enhance the adrenergic tone, all of which exacerbated myocarditis in our viral model; in contrast, treatment with propranolol ameliorated the severity of myocarditis. Tobacco smoke has also been demonstrated to increase adrenergic activation in animals and patients, in part due to its content of nicotine (Cavarra et al., 2001; Pomerleau, 1992; Su, 1982) which in turn may exacerbate the severity of viral myocarditis in a murine model through adrenergically mediated mechanisms (Bae et al., 2010). As a more generalized hypothesis, exposure to tobacco smoke may be an important and as yet underappreciated cause of heart failure in patients receiving treatments with pro-inflammatory drugs (i.e. clozapine) or who are exposed to pathogens (i.e. viruses) or physical factors (i.e. radiotherapy) that can produce a level of myocarditis susceptible to exacerbation.

Sympathomimetic agents have the potential to produce toxic effects on the heart through a variety of mechanisms that are summarized in Figure 1. Note the overlap with mechanisms attributed to tobacco smoke exposure in Table 1, most notably with regard to myocarditis, their effects on inflammation, immune function, and factors associated with cardiac and vascular dysfunction. Although multiple factors undoubtedly contribute to the exacerbation of myocarditis we have observed with tobacco smoke exposure, it is reasonable to propose that catecholamine-related effects play a central role.

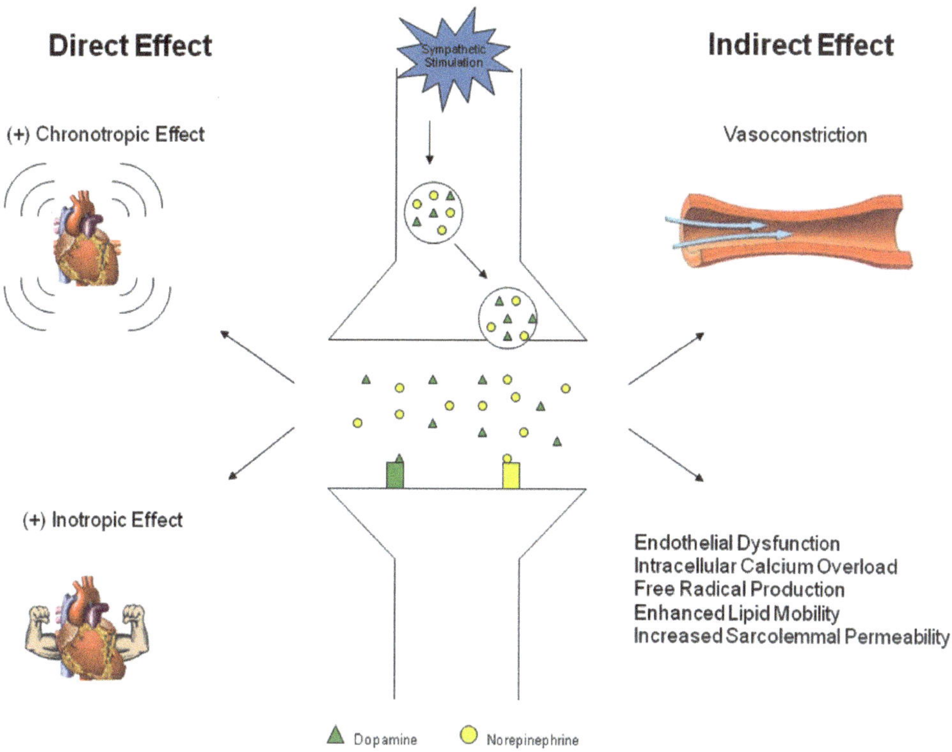

Fig. 1. Direct and indirect effects of catecholamines and related sympathomimetic agents on the heart.

2.2 Propranolol ameliorates and epinephrine exacerbates progression of acute and chronic viral myocarditis

Recent studies point to important interactions between proinflammatory cytokines and neurohumoral mediators in heart failure. We investigated the influence of the β-adrenergic system on cytokines and neurohumoral factors and the sequelae of viral myocarditis (Wang et al., 2005). In an experimental model with virus-infected BALB/c mice, we studied the acute and chronic effects of epinephrine and propranolol on myocardial morphology, cytokine gene expression, and survival. BALB/c mice were inoculated with the encephalomyocarditis virus (EMCV) or sham inoculated with saline and followed for 30 days. Epinephrine increased the severity of inflammatory cell infiltration and myocardial necrosis induced by EMCV-inoculated mice. Survival rate after 30 days was reduced to 40% in epinephrine-treated EMCV-inoculated mice compared with 70% in untreated EMCV-inoculated mice ($P<0.05$). Treatment with the β-blocker propranolol significantly decreased mortality, myocardial necrosis and infiltration of inflammatory cells in EMCV-inoculated mice. Propranolol also suppressed gene expression of the cytokines TNF-α, IL-6 and IL-10 involved in inflammation. A single dose of epinephrine 120 days after EMCV inoculation caused death in 70% of infected mice; propranolol significantly reduced the incidence of death to 33%. These results indicate that acute and chronic stages of viral myocarditis are modulated by the β-adrenergic system and its interactions with proinflammatory factors.

2.3 Cocaine enhances myocarditis induced by encephalomyocarditis virus in murine models

This study (Wang et al., 2002a) was designed to investigate whether cocaine can exacerbate viral myocarditis and increase its incidence. Clinical evidence suggests that cocaine abuse increases the incidence of myocarditis. However, it had not been directly demonstrated that cocaine exposure enhances murine myocarditis. BALB/c mice were divided into eight groups saline control, encephalomyocarditis virus (EMCV), 10 mg/kg cocaine (Coc-10), 30 mg/kg cocaine (Coc-30), 50 mg/kg cocaine (Coc-30), EMCV+Coc-50. After inoculation with EMCV, the mice were daily treated with either cocaine or saline for 90 days. Mice were euthanized at different days after EMCV inoculation. Mortality was recorded and myocarditis severity was evaluated. The mortality of the myocarditis mice treated with cocaine increased significantly from 22% (EMCV) to 25.7% (Coc-10+ EMCV), 41.4% 9 (Coc-30+EMCV) and 51.4% (Coc-50+EMCV) ($P<0.05$) respectively. The incidence and severity of inflammatory cell infiltration and myocardial lesions was higher in infected mice exposed to cocaine. Cocaine administered only before infection did not exacerbate myocarditis. Norepinephrine assay showed that cocaine exposure significantly increased myocardial norepinephrine concentration, but this increase was partially inhibited in infected animals. Adrenalectomy abolished the effect of cocaine on mortality. Furthermore, propranolol, a β-blocker, significantly decreased the enhancing effects of cocaine on myocarditis mice. In conclusion, cocaine increases the severity and mortality of viral myocarditis in mice. Increased catecholamines may be a major factor in this effect.

A variety of viruses have been reported as causative agents of myocarditis in man, including Coxsackie, echo and influenza viruses, cytomegalovirus, poliomyelitis virus, Epstein Barr virus, herpes simplex virus, adenovirus and several others (Rodeheffer & Gersh, 2001; Ensley et al., 1995; Abelmann, 1966). Our laboratory has demonstrated that cocaine can exacerbate viral myocarditis in a murine model (Wang et al., 2002a). Possible mechanisms of such an interaction include, (a) cocaine-induced damage to the endothelial/endocardial cells in the extracellular matrix or to the myocytes themselves, thereby reducing structural and immunological barriers to cellular penetration of the virus and increasing the myocardial and vascular permeability and infectivity of viral particles. Evidence supporting "possibility (a)" includes reports suggesting that cocaine can damage the endothelial lining of cells after even a single exposure, thereby accelerating atherosclerosis in animal models (Egashira et al., 1991; Bacharach et al., 1992). Cocaine has also been reported to increase natural killer cell activity (Van Dyke et al., 1986). Both lymphocytic and eosinophilic myocarditis have been reported in cocaine abusers (Virmani et al., 1988; Tazelaar et al., 1987) and heart failure is a common finding (Weiner et al., 1986; Duell, 1987). Alternatively, "possibility (b)", cocaine may exacerbate viral myocarditis by permitting enhanced viral replication of the viral agent once it has penetrated the cell membrane. Such an effect may occur through a direct or catecholamine-mediated alteration in the cellular milieu that in turn could alter viral transcription and replication. Enhanced viral replication could occur through a change in cellular pH, shift in osmolarity, or likely depletion of high-energy stores necessary for protective proteolytic enzyme activity. Of course, it is likely that the effects of cocaine on the animal or a patient with myocarditis are complex and involve several mechanisms or conditioning factors, including drug diluents with intrinsic pharmacological activity or sensitizing effects (Ensing, 1985; Wolf and Blum, 1983). However, the observation that exacerbation of myocarditis seems to occur with cocaine but not other commonly abused drugs without prominent cardiac effects, including heroin and phencyclidine, suggests that cocaine may have a unique combination of properties that make its use in patients exposed or infected with viral pathogens likely to enhance development of myocarditis and its sequelae. Our data indicate that the unique ability of cocaine to increase local release and circulating levels of catecholamines is the primary factor responsible for exacerbation of myocarditis (Ensing, 1985).

2.4 Clozapine-induced myocarditis: role of catecholamines in a murine model

Clozapine, an atypical neuroleptic agent, is very effective in the treatment of resistant schizophrenia. However, cardiotoxicity of clozapine, particularly in young patients, has raised concerns about its its safety and smoking may have a significant effect on serum concentrations of clozapine (Seppala et al., 1999). A particularly high incidence of myocarditis has been reported among patients treated with atypical neuroleptic drugs, including clozapine and risperidone. Clozapine has been shown to markedly increase circulating levels of catecholamines (Coulter et al., 2001; Elman et al., 2002). Increased catecholamines have been postulated to trigger an inflammatory response resulting in myocarditis, dilated cardiomyopathy, and death, although this has not yet been thoroughly studied. Here (Wang et al., 2008), we used the mouse to study whether clozapine administration could caused adverse myocarditis associated with an increase in catecholamines. Male BALB/c mice, age ~6 weeks, were administered 5, 10 or 25 mg/kg clozapine daily for 7 and 14 days; one group was administered 25 mg/kg clozapine plus 2 mg/kg propranolol for 14 days. Saline-treated mice served as controls. Heart sections were stained with hematoxylin and eosin for histopathological examination. Plasma catecholamines were measured with HPLC. Myocardial TNF-α concentrations were determined by ELISA. Histopathologic examination of clozapine-treated mice showed a significant dose-related increase in myocardial inflammation that correlated with plasma catecholamine levels and release of TNF-α. Propranolol significantly attenuated these effects. A hypercatecholaminergic state induced by clozapine could explain the occurrence of myocarditis in some patients. Our data suggest that β-adrenergic blocking agents may be effective in reducing the incidence and severity of clozapine-induced myocarditis.

3. Tobacco smoke

3.1 Exacerbation of viral myocarditis by tobacco smoke as a cause of heart failure

In this study (Bae et al. 2010), we determined whether exposure to tobacco smoke will exacerbate the severity of viral myocarditis in mice. Viral myocarditis was generated n 4-week old male BALB/c mice by i.p. injection of encephalomyocarditis virus (EMCV). Mice were exposed to cigarette smoke for 90 minutes/day 5x/week. Four groups were studied: 1) Control (C, no smoke and no virus), 2) Smoke (S) only, and 3) Virus only (V), and 4) Pre-exposure to smoke for 1 week prior to virus injection (S+V). We observed an over 2-fold increase in mortality among mice that were pre-exposed to smoke compared to the virus alone. Tobacco smoke alone did not affect mortality. There was a significant increase in virus load among hearts from mice exposed to S+V compared to V alone.

In this study, we also investigated the rate of apoptosis 5 days after i.p. injection of virus. Viral exposure alone significantly increased the number of apoptotic cells. The number of apoptotic cells was increased further by smoke exposure prior to viral injection. Viral injection increased the translocation of apoptosis-inducing factor from mitochondria, a hallmark of caspace-independent apoptosis activation. Exposure to tobacco smoke exacerbated these effects without changing the total expression of apoptosis-inducing factor suggesting activation of caspace-independent apoptotic pathways as well.

Apoptosis has been shown to play an important role in human and animal heart failure (Kang et al., 2000; Kang & Izumo, 2003). Other investigators have demonstrated EMCV-induced apoptosis in the hearts of mice and pigs (for example, see Mizutani et al., 1996 and Brewer et al., 2001). Activation of caspaces may be a critical facilitator of viral infection in cardiomyocytes (DeBiasi et al., 2004, Kyoto et al., 2004). In fact, DeBiasi et al., have shown that inhibition of caspaces effectively blocks virus-induced apoptosis in vitro, although caspace-independent factors also appeared to be involved. Apoptosis-inducing factor release from mitochondria is one important caspace-independent factor, and appears to play an important role in EMCV-infection related apoptosis, as shown in our study. These data were later to show that viral infection induced a significant increase in apoptosis, through caspace-independent apoptosis, and that preexposure to tobacco smoke exacerbated this effect.

Several studies have shown a relationship between myocyte apoptosis and increased sympathetic activity in patients with underlying heart disease, most commonly heart failure (Singh et al., 2001). Communal et al., 1998 showed that over-stimulation by norepinephrine produced apoptosis in ventricular myocytes of adult rats and blocking the beta-receptor decreased apoptosis. These data are consistent with our hypotheses that catecholamines are a major factor inducing inflammation and cell death in tobacco smoke exposed animals.

4. Conclusions

Evidence from our laboratory and elsewhere (summarized above) indicates that both mainstream and secondhand tobacco smoke exposure can exacerbate viral myocarditis. Induction of a systemic inflammatory response appears to be a central initiating mechanism responsible for myocarditis, an effect that can be mediated by a cardiotropic viral infection itself and exacerbated by additional factors, most notably, catecholamines and other sympathomimetic agents, (Figure 2).

There appears to be an additive or synergistic effect of factors producing inflammation, which in turn can enhance viral load in the myocytes and exacerbate the extent and severity of myocarditis. Severe cardiac dysfunction and clinical heart failure may result. Our data suggest that disruption of gap junctions plays an important role in this regard (Figure 1). Moreover, to the extent that catecholamines are responsible, beta-adrenergic antagonists can attenuate the effect. Although the results presented in this review are consistent with a primary pathogenic role of catecholamines in the exacerbation of myocarditis by tobacco smoke, they do not exclude other factors that may operate through different mechanisms.

Additional animal and human studies will be necessary to further elucidate the several factors that may be involved. However, taken together, the available data indicate that tobacco smoke can exacerbate myocarditis which in turn may result in irreversible cardiac dysfunction and failure. Even in the absence of additional data, these results provide another example of the adverse effects of tobacco smoke and strengthen the argument for minimizing exposure to this agent in our environment.

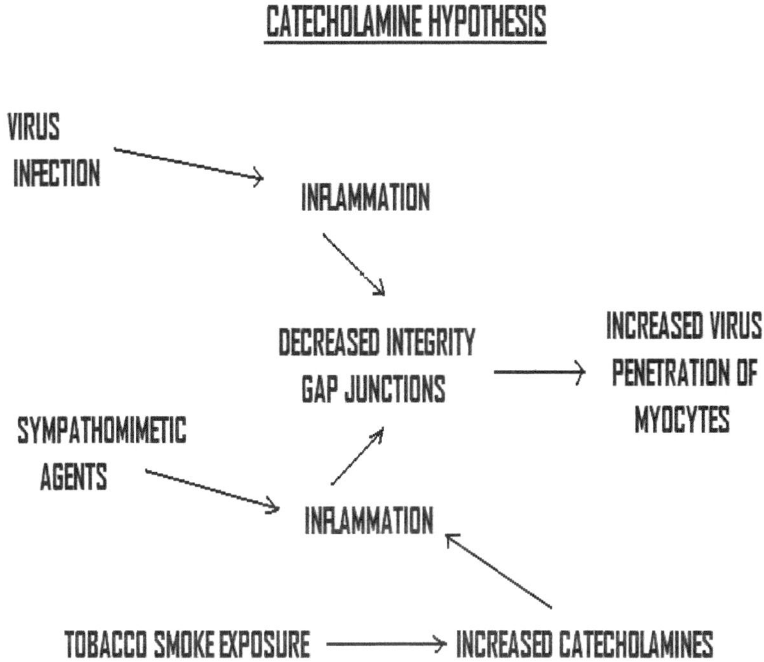

Fig. 2. Proposed primary mechanism for exacerbation of viral myocarditis by tobacco smoke exposure: the catecholamine hypothesis.

5. Acknowledgement

This manuscript is dedicated to the memory of Dr. Walter H. Abelmann (1921-2011) who made many contributions to our understanding of myocarditis in the laboratory and clinic. We acknowledge the generous support provided by the Flight Attendant Medical Research Institute (FAMRI) for tobacco smoke related studies in our laboratory. We also express our appreciation to Ms. Patricia Crilley for her expert assistance in manuscript preparation.

6. References

Abelmann, W.H. Myocarditis. *N Engl J Med,* (1966), 275:944-945.

Adamopoulos, D., van de Borne, P. & Argacha, J.F. New insights into the sympathetic, endothelial, and coronary effects of nicotine. *Clin Exp Pharmacol Physiol,* (2008), 35:458-63.

Ambrose, J.A., & Barus, R.S. The pathophysiology of cigarette smoking and cardiovascular disease: an update. *J Am Coll Cardiol*, (2004), 43:1731-1737.

Anandasabapathy, S., & Frishman, W.H. Innovative drug treatments for viral and autoimmune myocarditis. *J Clin Pharmacol, (1998), 38:295-308.*

Bacharach, J.M., Colville, D.S., & Lie, J.T. Accelerated atherosclerosis, aneurismal disease, and aortitis possible pathogenetic association with cocaine abuse. *Int Angiol*, (1992), 11:83-86.

Bae, S., Ke, Q., & Koh, Y.Y., et al. Exacerbation of acute viral myocarditis by tobacco smoke is associated with increased viral load and cardiac apoptosis. *Can J Physiol Pharmacol, (*2010), 88:568-575.

Baldasseroni, SA., Opasich, C. & Gorini M., et al.,. Left bundle-branch block is associated with increased 1-year sudden and total mortality rate in 5517 outpatients with congestive heart failure: a report from the Italian network on congestive heart failure. *Am Heart J*, (2002), 143:398-405.

Barnoya J., & Glantz, S.A. Cardiovascular effects of secondhand smoke: nearly as large as smoking. *Circulation*, (2005), 111:2684-2698.

Benowitz, N.L. Cigarette smoking and cardiovascular disease: pathophysiology and implications for treatment. *Prog Cardiovasc Dis*, (2003), 46:91-111.

Benowitz, N.L. Pharmacology of nicotine: addiction, smoking-induced disease, and therapeutics. *Annu Rev Pharmacol Toxicol*, (2008), 49:57-71.

Bindoli, A., Rigobello, M.P., & Deeble, D.J. Biochemical and toxicological properties of the oxidation products of catecholamines. *Free Radic Biol Med*, (1992), 13:391-405.

Bleumink, G. S.; Knesch, A.M. & Sturkenbom, M.D., et al. Quantifying the heart failure epidemic: prevalence, incidence rate, lifetime risk and prognosis of heart failure in The Rotterdam Study. *Eur Heart J*, (2004), 25:1614-1619.

Brewer, L.A., Lwamba, H.C., & Murtaugh, M.P., et al. Porcine encephloamyocarditis virus persists in pig myocardium and infects human myocardial cells. *J Virol*, (2001), 75(23), 11621-11629.

Brown, C.A, & O'Connell, J.B. Myocarditis and idiopathic dilated cardiomyopathy. *Am J Med*, (1995), 99 : 309-314.

Burns, D.M. Epidemiology of smoking-induced cardiovascular disease. *Prog Cardiovasc Dis*, (2003), 46 :11-29.

Cabinian, A.E., Kiel, R., & Smith, F., et al. Modification of exercise-aggravated Coxsackie virus B3 murine myocarditis by T-lymphocyte suppression in an inbred model. *J Lab Clin Med*, (1990), 115, 454-462.

Cavarra, E., Bartalesi, B. & Lucattelli, M., et al. Effects of cigarette smoke in mice with different levels of α_1 proteinase inhibitor and sensitivity to oxidants *Amer J Respir Crit Care Med*, (2001), 164:886-890.

Cho, T., Tanimura, A., & Saito Y. Catecholamine-induced cardiopathy accompanied with pheochromocytoma. *Acta Pathol Jpn*, (1987), 37 :123-132.

Communal, C., Singh, K., & Pimetal, D., et al. Norepinephrine stimulates apoptosis in adult rat ventricular myocytes by activation of the *B*-adrenergic pathway. *Circulation*, (1998), 98:1329-1334.

Cooper, R.G. & Magwere, T. Nitric oxide-mediated pathogenesis during nicotine and alcohol consumption. *Indian J Physiol Pharmacol*, (2008), 52: 11-18.

Coulter, D.M., Bare, A., & Meyboom, R.H.B., et al. Antipsychotic drugs and heart muscle disorder in international pharmacovigilance: data mining study. *BMJ*, (2001), 322:1207-1209.

Davila, D.F., & Gottberg, C.F., & Torres, A., et al. Cardiac sympathetic-parasympathetic balance in rats with experimentally-induced acute chagasic myocarditis. *Rev Inst Med Trop Sao Paulo*, (1995), 37:155-159.
DeBiasi, R.I., Robinson, B.A., & Sherry, B., et al. Caspase inhibition protects against reovirus-induced myocardial injury in vitro and in vivo. *J Virol*, (2004), 78:11040-11050.
Dong, R., Liu, P., & Wee, L., et al. Verapamil ameliorates the clinical and pathological course of murine myocarditis. *J Clin* Invest, *(1992), 90:2022-2030.*
Duell, F.B. Chronic cocaine abuse and dilated cardiomyopathy. *Am J Med*, (1987), 83:601 (Letter).
Dunn, A.J., & Vickers, S.L. Neurochemical and neuroendocrine responses to Newcastle disease virus administration in mice. *Brain Res*, (1994), 645:103-112.
Egashira, K., Pipers, F.S., & Morgan, J.P. Effects of cocaine on epicardial coronary artery reactivity in miniature swine after endothelial injury and high cholesterol feeding; In vivo and in vitro analysis. *J Clin Invest*, (1991), 88, 1307-1314.
Elman, I., Goldstein, D.S., & Green, A.I., et al. Effects of risperidone on the peripheral noradrenergic system in patients with schizophrenia: a comparison with Clozapine and placebo. *Neuropsychopharmacology*, (2002), 27:293-300.
Elson, S.H., & Abelmann, W.A. Effects of muscular activity upon the acute myocarditis of C3H mice infected with Trypanosoma cruzi. *Am H J*, 1965, 69:348-50.
Ensing, J.G. Bazooka: cocaine-base and manganese carbonate. *J Anal Toxicol*, (1985), 9:45-46
Ensley, R.D., Renlund, D.G., & Mason, J.W. Myocarditis. In: *Cardiovascular Medicine*, Edited by Willerson & Cohn, J.N., New York, NY, Churchill Livingstone, (1995), pp 894-923.
Ezzati, M, Henley S.J., & Thun, M.J., et al. Role of smoking in global and regional cardiovascular mortality. *Circulation*, (2005), 112, 489-497.
Felker, G.M.,Thompson, R.E. & Hare, J.M., et al. Underlying causes and long-term survival in patients with initially unexplained cardiomyopathy. *N Engl J Med*, (2000), 342:1077-1084.
Fowles, J.A., & Bates, M.A. The chemical constituents in cigarettes and cigarette smoke: priorities for harm reduction. *A report to the New Zealand Ministry of Health. Epidemiology and Toxicology Group, Kenepuru Science Center, Porirua, New Zealand*, (2000), pp 1-65.
Friman, G., Larsson, E., & Rolf, C. Interaction between infection and exercise. *Annu Rev Physiol*, (1983), 45:139-53.
Gatmaitan, B.G., Chason, J.L., & Lerner, A.M. Augmentation of the virulence of murine Coxsackie virus B-3 myocardiopathy by exercise. *J Exp Med*, (1970), 131:1121-1136.
Gerzen, P. ,Branath, A., & Holmgren, B., et al. Acute myocarditis, a follow-up study. *Br Heart J*, (1972), 34:575-583.
Grist, N.R. & Bell E.J. Coxsackie viruses and the heart. *Am Heart J*, (1969), 77:295-300.
Haass, M., & Kübler, W. Nicotine and sympathetic neurotransmission. *Cardiovasc Drugs Ther*, (1997), 10: 657-665.
Haft, J.L. Cardiovascular injury induced by sympathetic catecholamines. *Prog Cardiovas Dis*, (1974), 17:73-86.
He, J. Ogden, L.G., & Bazzano, L.A., et al. Risk factors for congestive heart failure in US men and women, NHANES I epidemiologic follow-up study. *Arch Intern Med*, (2001), 161:996-1002.
Herraiz, T., & Chaparro, C. Human monoamine oxidase is inhibited by tobacco smoke: beta-carboline alkaloids act as potent and reversible inhibitors. *Biochem Biophys Res Commun*, (2005), 326:378-386.
Hiraoka, Y., Kishimoto, C., & Takada, H., et al. Nitric oxide and murine coxsackievirus B3 myocarditis: aggravation of myocarditis by inhibition of nitric oxide synthase. *J Am Coll Cardiol*, (1996), 28:1610-1615.

Ho, K.K., Pinsky, J.L., & Kannel, W.B., et al. The epidemiology of heart failure: the Framingham study. *J Am Coll Cardiol*, (1993), 22:6A-13A.

Hosenpud, J.D., Campbell, S.M., & Niles, N.R., et al. Exercise induced augmentation of cellular and humoral autoimmunity associated with increased cardiac dilation in experimental autoimmune myocarditis. *Cardiovas Res*, (1987), 21:217-22.

Kammermeier, M., & Grobecker, H.F. Cardiotoxicity of catecholamines after application of L-DOPA in Wistar-Kyoto (WKY) and spontaneously hypertensive rats (SHR). *Hypertens Res*, (1995), 18 (Suppl 1):S165-168.

Kang, P.M. & Izumo, S. Apoptosis in heart: basic mechanisms and implications in cardiovascular diseases. *Trends Mol Med*, (2003) 9:177-182.

Kang, P.M., Haunstetter, A., & Aoki, H., et al. Morphological and molecular characterization of adult cardiomyocyte apoptosis during hypoxia and reoxygenation. *Circ Res*, (2000), 87: 118-125.

Kannel, W.B., Ho K.K., & Thom, T. Changing epidemiological features of cardiac failure. *Br Heart J*, (1994), 72:S3-9.

Karch, S.B. Serum catecholamines in cocaine intoxicated patients with cardiac symptoms. *Annals of Emer Med*, (1987), 16:481.

Keaney, J.F., Hare, J.M., & Balligand, J.L., et al. Inhibition of nitric oxide synthase augments myocardial contractile responses to beta-adrenergic stimulation. *Am J Physiol*, (1996), 271:H2646-2652.

Kiel, R.J., Smith, F.E., Khatib, R., et al. Coxsackie virus B3 myocarditis in C3HeJ mide: description of an inbred model of the effect of exercise on virulence. *Eur J Epidemiol*, (1989), 5:348-350.

Krentz, A.J., Mikhail, S., & Cantrell, P., et al. Pseudopheochromocytoma syndrome associated with clozapine. *BMJ*, (2001), 322:1213.

Kyotö, V., Saraste, A., & Saukko, P., et al. Apoptotic cardiomyocyte death in fatal myocarditis. *Am J Cardiol*, (2004), 94: 746-730.

Law, M.R. & Wald, N.J. Environmental tobacco smoke and ischemic heart disease. *Prog. Cardiovasc Dis*, (2003), 46: 31-38.

Leone, A., Giannini, D., & Bellotto, C., et al. Passive smoking and heart disease. *Curr Vasc Pharmacol*, (2004), 2:175-182.

Lowenstein, C.J., Hill, S.L,& Lafonde-Walker, A., et al. Nitric oxide inhibits viral replication in murine myocarditis. *J Clin Invest*, (1996), 97:1837-1843.

Mason, J.W., O'Connell, J.B. & Herskowitz, A., et al. A clinical trial of immunosuppressive therapy for myocarditis, *The Myocarditis Treatment Trial Investigators. N Engl J Med*, (1995), 333:269-265.

Marano, G., Ramirez, A., & Mori, I., et al. Sympathectomy inhibits the vasoactive effects of nicotine in conscious rats. *Cardiovasc Res, (1999), 42:201-205.*

Mehes, G., Rajkovits, K.,& Papp, G. Effect of various types of sympathicolytics on isoproterenol-induced myocardial lesions. *Acta Physiol Acad Sci Hung, (1966), 29:75-85.*

Mizutani, M.; Hirasawa, K.; & Takeda, et al. Variation in serum creatinine phosphokinase activity as indicated in two-phase EMC-D virus induced myocarditis. *Exp Anim*, (1996), 45: 333-338.

Mobascher, A. & Winterer, G. The molecular and cellular neurobiology of nicotine abuse in schizophrenia. *Pharmacopsychiatry*, (2008), 41 (Suppl 1): S51-59.

Morin, Y., & Cote, G. Toxic agents and cardiomyopathies. *Cardiovasc Clinic*, 1972, 4:245-67.

Naik, S.D., & Freudenberger, R.S. Ephedra-associated cardiomyopathy. *Ann Pharmacother*, (2004), 38, 400-3.

Nash, C.B.., & Carter, J.R. Hemorrhagic myocarditis and cardiovascular collapse induced by catecholamine infusion. *Arch Int Pharmacodyn Ther*, (1967), 166:172-180.

Nino, A.F., Berman, M.M., & Gluck E.H., et al. Drug-induced left ventricular failure in patients with pulmonary disease. Endomyocardial biopsy demonstration of catecholamine myocarditis. *Chest*, (1987), 92:732-736.

Noda, M., Kawano, O., & Uchida, O., et al. Myocarditis induced by sympathomimetic amines, 1. *Jpn Circ J*, (1970), 34 :7-12.

Olinde, K.D., & O'Connell, J.B. Inflammatory heart disease: pathogenesis, clinical manifestations and treatment of myocarditis. *Annu Rev Med*, (1994), 45:481-490.

Ong, M.K., & Glantz, S.A. Cardiovascular health and economic effects of smoke-free workplaces. *Am J Med*, (2004), 117:32-38.

Panagiotakos, D.B., Pitsavos, C., & Chrysohoou, C., et al. Effect of exposure to secondhand smoke on markers of inflammation: the ATTICA study. *Am J Med*, (2004), 116:145-150.

Pomerleau, O.F. Nicotine and the central nervous system: biobehavioral effects of cigarette smoking. *Am J Med*, (1992), 93:2s-7s.

Prichard, B.N., Owens, C.W., & Smith, C.C., et al. Heart and catecholamines. *Acta Cardiol, (1991), 46: 309-322.*

Puranik, R., & Celermajer, D.S. Smoking and endothelial function. *Prog Cardiovasc Dis*, (2003), 45:443-458.

Repace, J. Flying the smoky skies: secondhand smoke exposure of flight attendants. *Tob Control*, (2004), 13:18-19.

Rezkalla, S., Kloner, R.A., & Khatib, G., et al. Effect of metoprolol in acute coxsackievirus B3 murine myocarditis. *J Am Coll Cardiol*, (1988), 12:412-414.

Rodeheffer, R.J., & Gersh, B.J. Cardiomyopathy and biopsy, A. Dilated cardiomyopathy and the myocarditidies. In: *Mayo Clinic Practice of Cardiology*, Edited by Giuliani, E.R., Gersh, B.J., McGoon, M.D., Hayes, D.L. & Schaff, H.U.,St. Louis, Mo, Mosby, (1996), pp. 636-671.

Sargent, R.P., Shepard, R.M, & Glantz, S.A. Reduced incidence of admissions for myocardial infarction associated with public smoking ban: before and after study. *BMJ*, (2004), 328:977-980.

Seppala, N.H., Leinonen, E.V.J., & Lehtonen, M.L., et al. Clozapine serum concentrations are lower in smoking than in non-smoking schizophrenic patients. *Therapeutic Drug Monitoring*, (1999), 85:244-246.

Seta, Y., Kanda, T.,& Yokoyama, T., et al. Effect of amrinone on murine viral myocarditis. *Res Commun Mol Pathol Pharmacol*, (1997), 95: 57-66.

Shinozaki, N., Yuasa, T., & Takata, S. Cigarette smoking augments sympathetic nerve activity in patients with coronary heart disease. *Int Heart J*, (2008), 49:201-72.

Siltanen, P., Pentitila, O.,& Merikallio, E., et al. Myocardial catecholamines and their biosynthetic enzymes in various human heart diseases. *Acta Med Scan (Suppl), (*1982), 660:24-33.

Singh, K., Xiao, L., & Remondino, A., et al. Adrenergic regulation of cardiac myocyte apoptosis. *J Cell Physiol*, (2001), 189: 257-265.

Smith, H.J., Roche, A.H., & Janusch, M.M., et al. Cardiomyopathy associated with amphetamine administration. *Am Heart J*, (1976), 16:792-7.

Sofuoglu, M., Mouratidis, M., & Yoo, S., et al. Adrenergic blocker carvedilol attenuates the cardiovascular and adversive effects of nicotine in abstinent smokers. *Behav Pharmacol, (2006), 17:731-735.*

Soodini, G. & Morgan J.P. Can cocaine abuse exacerbate the cardiac toxicity of human immunodeficiency virus? *Clin Cardiol*, (2001), 24:177-181.

Steenland, K. Passive smoking and the risk of heart disease. *JAMA*, (1992), 267:94-99.

Su, C. Actions of nicotine and smoking on circulation. *Pharmacol Ther*, (1982), 17:129-141.

Sykes, A.P., Lawson, N., & Finnegan, J.A., et al. Creatinine kinase activity in patients with brittle asthma treated with long term subcutaneous terbutaline. *Thorax*, (1991), 46:580-583.

Talukder, M.A., Johnson, W.M., & Varadharaj, S., et al. Chronic cigarette smoking causes hypertension, increased oxidative stress, impaired NO bioavailability, endothelial dysfunction and cardiac remodeling in mice. *Am J Physiol Heart Circ Physiol*, (2011), 3000:H388-96.

Tazelaar, H.D., Karch, S.B., & Stephens, B.G., et al. Cocaine and the heart. *Human Path*, (1987), 18:195-199.

Tilles, J.G., Elson, S.H., & Shaka, J.A., et al. Effects of exercise on coxsackie A9 myocarditis in adult mice. *Proc Soc Exp Bio Med*, (1964), 117:77-82.

Van Dyke, G.., Stesin, A.,& Jones, R., et al. Cocaine increases natural killer cell activity. *J Clin Invest*, (1986), 77:1387-1390.

Van Vliet, P.D., Burchel, H.B., & Titus, J.L. Focal myocarditis associated with pheochromocytoma. *N Engl J Med*, (1966), 274:1102-1108.

Virmani, R., Robinowitz, M., & Smialek, J.E., et al. Cardiovascular effects of cocaine: an autopsy study of 40 patients. *Am Heart J*, (1988), 115:1068-1076.

Wang, J.F. & Morgan, J.P. Cocaine-induced exacerbation of viral myocarditis. *In: Watson RR, ed. AIDS and Heart Disease, New York: Marcel Dekker, Inc.*, (2003) pp *265-280.*

Wang, J.F., Min, J.Y., & Hampton, T.G., et al. Clozapine-induced myocarditis: role of catecholamines in a murine model. *Eur J Pharmacol*, (2008), 592:123-7.

Wang, J.F., Zhang, J, & Min, J.Y., et al. Cocaine enhances myocarditis induced by encephalomyocarditis virus in murine model. *Am J Physiol Heart Circ Physiol*, (2002a), 282:H956-H963.

Wang, J.F.; Yang, Y. & Wang G.K., et al. Embryonic stem cells attenuate viral myocarditis in a murine model. *Cell Transpl*, (2002b), 11:753-58.

Wang, J.F., Meissner, A., & Malek, S., et al. Propranolol ameliorates and epinephrine exacerbates progression of acute and chronic viral myocarditis. *Am J Physiol Heart Circ Physiol*, (2005), 289: H1577-H1583.

Wang, W.Z., Matsumori, A., & Yamada, T., et al. Beneficial effects of amlodipine in a murine model of congestive heart failure induced by viral myocarditis. A possible mechanism through inhibition of nitric oxide production. *Circulation*, (1997), 95:245-251.

Weiner, R.S., Lockhart, J.T., & Schwartz, R.G. Dilated cardiomyopathy and cocaine abuse: report of two cases. *Am J Med*, (1986), 81:699-701.

Whincup, P.H., Gilg, J.A., & Emberson, J.R., et al. Passive smoking and risk of coronary heart disease and stroke: prospective study with cotinine measurement. BMJ, (2004), 329: 200-205.

Wolf, G.L., & Blum L. Cardiovascular toxicity and tissue proton tl response to manganese injection in the dog and rabbit. *AJR*, (1983), 141:193-197.

Wong, H.P., Yu, L., & Lam, E.K., et al. Nicotine promotes colon tumor growth and angiogenesis through beta-adrenergic activation. *Toxicol Sci*, (2007), 97:279-87.

Yang, Z., Knight, C.A., & Mamerow, M.M., et al. Prenatal environmental tobacco smoke exposure promotes adult atherogenesis and mitochondrial damage in apolipoprotein E -/- mice. *Circulation*, (2004), 110:3715-3720.

8

Myocarditis in HIV Positive Patients

Simona Claudia Cambrea
"Ovidius" University, Faculty of Medicine
Romania

1. Introduction

Myocarditis is an acute or chronic inflammatory process that affects the myocardium in response to the action of various infectious, chemical or physical agents. In most patients the disease is self-limiting. The natural course of myocarditis varies greatly, ranging from an asymptomatic state secondary to local inflammation, through development of dilated cardiomyopathy with a variable course, to fatal heart failure due to disseminated myocarditis [Subinas et al., 2005].

In patients infected with human immunodeficiency virus (HIV) cardiovascular abnormalities are frequent but clinically discrete. Cardiologists and physicians throughout the world are increasingly reporting cardiac muscle disease in association with HIV. With current advances in HIV and acquired immunodeficiency syndrome (AIDS) management and increased survival, cardiac manifestations of HIV disease including HIV related myocardial disease will become more important and will be encountered more frequently. Because cardiac complications in HIV positive patients are often clinically inapparent, periodic screening of these patients is recommended, especially in those with low CD4 counts or receiving treatment with cardiotoxic drugs. The heart may be a marker of the HIV infected patient's overall health, and a decline in cardiac function should trigger more comprehensive evaluation. As the role of infection and inflammation in many other cardiovascular diseases is now recognized, identification of the molecular mechanisms of HIV related myocaditis might have broader implications for a wide range of patients [Azis F et al., 2010].

The diagnosis of myocarditis in HIV positive patients during an acute episode may prove difficult, due to the lack of diagnostic techniques with acceptable degrees of specificity and sensitivity. For these patients although endomyocardial biopsy is still considered the diagnostic gold standard, the developments of new imaging techniques, such as cardiac magnetic resonance imaging (CMR), and nuclear imaging by antimyosin scintigraphy have contributed greatly to the diagnosis of myocarditis.

2. Myocarditis in HIV positive patients

HIV infection and AIDS have a well-recognized association with myocarditis and dilated cardiomyopathy [Azis F et al., 2010]. This increased predisposition is multifactorial and may include the direct effects of HIV itself, co-infection by opportunistic organisms, toxic effects of commonly used medications or illicit drugs, and nutritional deficiencies [Azis F et al., 2010]. Further, autoimmunity can be an important contributor to the pathogenesis of cardiomyopathy in these patients as many studies demonstrated the presence of cardiac-specific antibodies in HIV positive patients when compared with HIV negative controls [Currie & Boon 2003, Currie et al., 1998]. Thus, although the precise mechanisms are poorly understood, alterations in the immune system likely play an important role in the pathogenesis of heart muscle disease in HIV-infected patients. The prevalence of myocarditis in HIV infected patients has been difficult to establish with estimates ranging from 6% [Barbaro et al., 1998b] to 52% [Levy et al., 1989]. In other studies about 10 percent of people with HIV develop myocarditis, either because HIV directly invades the heart muscle or because the patient's weakened immune system makes the heart muscle more susceptible to attack by other infectious agents, especially toxoplasmosis [Grange et al., 1990, Matturi et al., 1990].

HIV deserves special mention because it seems to function differently than other viruses. HIV-1 glycoprotein 120 can directly disrupt cardiac contractility without any inflammatory response [Currie & Boon, 2003]. This may explain why HIV genomes can be amplified from patients without histologic signs of inflammation. Myocarditis is the most commonly cardiac abnormality found on biopsy tissue, present in some degree, in more than 50% of HIV patients [Howes et al., 2010]. In addition, in patients who are infected with HIV, T-cell – mediated immune suppression increases the risk of contracting myocarditis due to other infectious causes [Howes et al., 2010].

2.1 Etiology

The actual pathogenesis of cardiac injury in HIV infection is not clear. It is however generally agreed that several factors come into play either singly or in combination to produce cardiac pathology [Aziz 2010]. There is a wide range of hypotheses regarding the pathogenesis of HIV associated heart muscle disease. These include myocardial invasion with HIV itself, opportunistic infections, viral infections, and autoimmune response to viral infection, drug-related cardiac toxicity, nutritional deficiencies, endothelial dysfunction, autonomic dysfunction, and prolonged immunosuppression. Zidovudine (AZT), an antiretroviral drug used in treatment of HIV, has also been associated with myocarditis [Herskowitz et al., 1992a].

Opportunistic infections are common complications of AIDS and the most frequent cause of morbidity and mortality. However, relatively few pathogens have been isolated from the myocardium of AIDS patients [Olson 2003]. Myocardial involvement is usually associated with disseminated disease and multiple foci of infection. Typically, infectious organisms are identified in patients dying of noncardiac causes, and the findings of myocardial abnormalities are regarded as incidental. Opportunistic pathogens represent diverse causes of infectious disease, including bacteria, fungi, protozoa, and viruses [Olson 2003].

Toxoplasma gondii (T gondii) is the most frequently documented infectious cause of myocarditis associated with AIDS, and the heart is the second most common site of infection after the brain. Autopsy series have described T gondii myocarditis (myocardial toxoplasmosis) in 1% to 16% of patients dying of AIDS [Baroldi et al., 1988, Anderson et al., 1988, Matturi et al., 1990]. Evidence of myocardial toxoplasmosis includes trophozoites or pseudocysts in myocardial fibers. A minority of cases has associated myocarditis with focal areas of necrosis and lymphocytic infiltrates [Jautzke 1993]. Antemortem diagnosis of toxoplasma myocarditis associated with left ventricular (LV) dysfunction has been described, including its successful treatment [Grange et al., 1990, Albrecht et al., 1994].

Pericardial tuberculosis has been reported in association with AIDS, typically in the setting of widespread disease. However, myocardial tuberculosis appears rare [Miller-Catchpole et al., 1989, Kinney et al., 1989].

Fungal myocarditis is an unusual complication of disseminated infection that is identified most often at autopsy [Olson 2003]. Various fungal organisms identified in the myocardium at autopsy with associated myocarditis have included *Aspergillus fumigatus, Candida albicans, Histoplasma capsulatum, Coccidioides immitis,* and *Cryptococcus neoformans.* Cardiac cryptococcus has been diagnosed in association with congestive heart failure and shown to resolve after therapy with amphotericin B and flucytosine [Kinney et al., 1989, Lewis et al., 1985, Lafont et al., 1987].

Several viruses have been implicated in myocarditis associated with AIDS. Cytomegalovirus (CMV) is a common opportunistic pathogen in AIDS, but it is associated less frequently with myocarditis [Michaels et al., 1997]. When inclusion bodies are the criterion for the detection and diagnosis of solid organ involvement by CMV, the rate of infection is underestimated compared to in situ DNA hybridization techniques [Wu et al., 1992, Myerson et al., 1984].

Other viruses identified by culture or polymerase chain reaction (PCR) within the myocardium of HIV-infected or AIDS patients, either at antemortem endomyocardial biopsy or from autopsy material, have included Epstein-Barr and coxsackie B virus in adults [Barbaro et al., 1988a] and adenovirus in children [Bowles et al., 1999]. These viruses may be present as either primary infection or as coinfection and can occur with or without associated myocarditis and with or without associated LV dysfunction.

2.2 Pathogenesis

The first clinical report to suggest a relationship between nonspecific myocarditis and dilated cardiomyopathy in AIDS patients appeared in 1986 [Cohen et al., 1986]; 3 patients had clinical, echocardiographic, and pathologic findings of dilated cardiomyopathy and 2 of the patients had focal lymphocytic infiltration associated with myocyte necrosis. Subsequent reports suggested an association between focal nonspecific myocarditis at autopsy and clinical cardiomyopathy [Barbaro et al., 1998a, Reilly et al., 1988]. Numerous hypotheses have been suggested to account for the etiology of nonspecific myocarditis and cardiomyopathy observed in HIV-infected patients, including direct HIV-1 infection of myocardial cells or coinfection with other cardiotropic viruses, [Olson 2003] cytokine cardiotoxicity [Suffredini et al., 1989, Lahdevirta et al., 1988, Levine et al., 1990], postviral cardiac autoimmunity [Herskowitz et al., 1989, 1993], nutritional deficiencies [Olson 2003], and cardiotoxicity due to illicit drugs [Olson 2003] or pharmacologic agents [Herskowitz et al., 1992a, Olson 2003].

The histologic findings of a monoclonal or oligoclonal inflammatory cellular infiltrate suggest a viral or autoimmune cause for the myocarditis associated with HIV infection. Myocarditis is more likely in individuals with more profound immunosuppression because CD4 < 400 cells/μL is more frequently observed in patients with dilated cardiomyopathy [Barbaro et al., 1998b]. In this same series, inflammatory myocardial cellular infiltrates were predominantly CD3 lymphocytes in 12 patients and CD8 lymphocytes in 64 patients. A separate report [Herskowitz et al., 1992b] described 35 HIV-infected patients with global LV dysfunction who underwent endomyocardial biopsy in which active or borderline myocarditis was observed in 55% of patients. For those patients with biopsy-proven myocarditis, mean LV ejection fraction was 28% whereas for patients without myocarditis it was 48%. The cellular infiltrate was primarily composed of CD8 T lymphocytes.

Although it has been suspected that myocarditis and cardiomyopathy associated with HIV-1 infection may be caused by direct viral infection of myocytes, definite evidence for this is lacking. Difficulty in demonstration of a link among HIV-1 infection, myocarditis, and cardiomyopathy in AIDS is related, in part, to lack of a suitable in vivo model of the disease. Because of the limited host range of HIV-1 and the difficulty in handling nonhuman primates infected with simian immunodeficiency virus-1, little investigation has been reported of myocarditis or cardiomyopathy associated with AIDS in animal models [Lewis et al., 2000].

What is the potential for direct myocardial infection? HIV-1 invades T cells by attachment to a CD4 surface-membrane receptor. However, there are no CD4 receptors on myocyte surface membranes. It is possible that the virus gains access to myocytes by other mechanisms, although the evidence to support this concept is limited. It is also possible that injury to myocytes may facilitate entry of the HIV virion; Epstein-Barr virus (EBV) promotes entry of HIV into CD4 receptor negative cells, with subsequent replication [Olson 2003].

The presence of viral genomic material within the myocytes of HIV-infected patients with myocarditis and cardiomyopathy does not definitely establish viral infection as causal. Furthermore, the significance of the finding of viral transcripts within cells is uncertain because patients may or may not have LV dysfunction [Herskowitz et al., 1993]. HIV-1 genomic material reportedly was detected within the genome of myocardial cells, although typically the findings have been sparse and may not have represented myocyte infection because the HIV nucleic acid sequence may actually have been located in endothelial cells or macrophages [Grody et al., 1990, Lipshultz et al., 1990, Flomenbaum et al., 1989, Cenacchi et al., 1990].

In one study, in 58 of 63 patients with AIDS, LV dysfunction, and biopsy-proven nonspecific lymphocytic myocarditis, a positive hybridization signal was observed but staining was weak and affected myocytes were generally not surrounded by inflammatory cells [Barbaro et al., 1998a].

In adults with AIDS-associated myocarditis, non-HIV viruses or viral genomic material identified in myocardial tissue has included CMV, Coxsackie virus group B, and EBV [Barbaro et al., 1998b, Wu et al., 1992]. In an autopsy study of 32 children who died with advanced HIV disease, including 23 with histologic evidence of myocarditis, viral sequences detected by polymerase chain reaction included adenovirus in 6, CMV in 3, and both adenovirus and CMV in 2. No other viruses were detected by polymerase chain reaction, including HIV [Bowles et al., 1999].

A high proportion of HIV-seropositive patients with LV dysfunction have evidence of latent infection of myocytes with CMV immediate-early genes [Wu et al., 1992]. Although observation of the intranuclear inclusions of active, lytic CMV infection is unusual, it has been suggested that latent viral infection may promote enhanced major histocompatibility complex expression, thereby provoking immune-mediated injury typical of animal models of myocarditis [Wu et al., 1992].

Immune-mediated mechanisms other than direct myocardial viral infection may account for the cellular infiltrates and cardiomyopathy observed in AIDS patients. Studies performed by Herskowitz demonstrated circulating autoantibodies in 4 of 6 AIDS patients with cardiomyopathy, whereas AIDS patients without cardiomyopathy did not have these antibodies [Herskowitz et al., 1989]. In the patients with autoantibodies, antimyosin antibodies were identified. In these same individuals, no evidence of HIV-1 or other viruses was identified from myocardial biopsy specimens evaluated by in situ hybridization, lending support to an autoimmune mechanism of disease. A study by Gu et al. [Gu et al., 1992] used monoclonal antibodies to HIV core proteins that reacted with myocyte antigens in 38 of 42 AIDS patients (and 11 of 28 non-AIDS patients), suggesting antibodies occurring in AIDS patients may react with antigenic epitopes of myocytes, thereby promoting autoimmune-mediated heart muscle disease.

Multiple cytokines are suspected of having a role in the mediation of myocardial inflammation, myocyte necrosis and ventricular dysfunction in myocarditis, although specifics are incompletely understood in human disease [Liu et al., 2001]. The mononuclear cells characteristic of lymphocytic myocarditis, including the focal nonspecific myocarditis of AIDS, are a likely source of cytokines that promote inflammation and maintenance of immune response, which may lead to impaired contractile function and fibrosis. Matsumori et al. 1994 showed that patients with myocarditis have markedly increased concentrations of cytokines, including tumor necrosis factor alfa (TNF-α) and interleukin -1 and -6. In animal models of myocarditis, similar profiles of cytokine activation have been described and have been demonstrated directly in cardiac tissue [Yamada et al., 1994]. TNF-α has been demonstrated to be a negative inotrope [Suffredini et al., 1989] and is increased in patients with congestive heart failure [Sharma et al., 2000], AIDS [Odeh et al., 1990, Yamamoto et al., 1995], and myocarditis [Matsumori et al., 1994]. HIV may cause myocyte injury by an "innocent bystander destruction" mechanism, as may occur in AIDS-associated encephalitis [Ho et al., 1987]. However, whether these mechanisms operate in the myocarditis and dilated cardiomyopathy of AIDS is unknown.

Three histological patterns of myocarditis have been described in patients with AIDS:

- lymphocytic infiltration with myocyte necrosis [Anderson et al., 1988], which meets the Dallas criteria;
- lymphocytic infiltration without inflammation [Lewis et al., 1992];
- myocyte damage without evidence of inflammatory infiltrate [Lafontet al., 1987].

2.3 Clinical manifestation

Clinical presentation of HIV associated myocarditis in symptomatic patients is generally similar to myocarditis due to other causes. The absence of symptoms and signs of heart disease does not however exclude cardiac involvement, as occurrence of sub-clinical cardiac abnormalities with possible fatal consequences in this population has been described [Kaminski et al., 1990]. Diagnosis requires the possibility of cardiac involvement to be constantly in mind and symptoms associated with myocarditis are varied, and relate either to the actual inflammation of the myocardium, or the weakness of the heart muscle that is secondary to the inflammation. Signs and symptoms of myocarditis include: **chest pain** (often described as "stabbing" in character); **congestive heart failure** (leading to edema, breathlessness and hepatic congestion); **palpitations** (due to arrhythmias); **sudden death** (in young adults, myocarditis causes up to 20% of all cases of sudden death); **fever** (especially when infectious); symptoms in infants and toddlers tend to be more non-specific with generalized malaise, poor appetite, abdominal pain, chronic cough. Later stages of the illness will present with respiratory symptoms with increased work of breathing and is often mistaken for asthma.

Since myocarditis is often due to a viral illness, many patients give a history of symptoms consistent with a recent viral infection, including fever, rash, diarrhea, joint pains, and frequent fatigue.

Myocarditis is often associated with pericarditis, and many patients present with signs (pericardial friction rub) and symptoms that suggest concurrent myocarditis and pericarditis.

2.4 Diagnostic

Myocarditis refers to an underlying process that causes inflammation and injury of the heart. It does not refer to inflammation of the heart as a consequence of some other insult. Many secondary causes, such as a heart attack, can lead to inflammation of the myocardium and therefore the diagnosis of myocarditis cannot be made by evidence of inflammation of the myocardium alone.

Myocardial inflammation can be suspected on the basis of electrocardiographic (ECG) results, elevated C-reactive protein (CRP) and/or erythrocyte sedimentation rate (ESR) and increased IgM (serology) against viruses known to affect the myocardium. Markers of myocardial damage (troponin or creatine kinase cardiac isoenzymes) are elevated.

The difficulty in diagnosing myocarditis lies in the known absence of specificity and sensitivity of the various diagnostic techniques used. Systematic biochemical measurements are not diagnostic and an increase in cardiotropic virus antibodies only reflects the response to a recent viral infection, but does not indicate active myocarditis. Endomyocardial biopsy, considered to be the diagnostic gold standard, is associated with a not inconsiderable risk of injury, as well as with sampling errors due to the focal involvement of the myocardium, which therefore reduces its diagnostic sensitivity. Radioactive isotope studies, widely used for the diagnosis of myocarditis, are limited by their low specificity, the exposure to radiation, and their cost [Subinas et al. 2005].

2.4.1 Physical examination

Physical findings of myocarditis can range from a normal examination, through all classes of congestive heart failure (CHF) to cardiovascular collapse and shock. Patients with mild cases of myocarditis have a nontoxic appearance and simply may appear to have a viral syndrome. Tachypnea and tachycardia are common. Tachycardia is often out of proportion to fever [Howes 2010].

More acutely ill patients have signs of circulatory impairment due to left ventricular failure. A widely inflamed heart shows the classic signs of ventricular dysfunction including the following: jugular venous distention, bibasilar crackles, ascites and peripheral edema.

Third heart sound (S_3) or a summation gallop may be noted with significant biventricular involvement. Intensity of the first heart sound (S_1) may be diminished. S_3 generally occur between 0.12 and 0.24 second after the aortic component of the second heart sound. Clinically, the third heart sound (S_3 gallop) may be a physiologic sound in children and young adults. It may be produced by factors that generate increased rate or volume of flow with high cardiac output or by conditions associated with cardiac dilatation and altered ventricular compliance, as in CHF [Smiterman TC and Willerson JT, 2007].

Cyanosis may occur. Murmurs of mitral or tricuspid regurgitation may be present due to ventricular dilation [Howes 2010].

In cases where a dilated cardiomyopathy has developed, signs of peripheral or pulmonary thromboembolism may be found [Howes 2010].

Diffuse inflammation may develop leading to pericardial effusion, without tamponade, and pericardial and pleural friction rub as the inflammatory process involves surrounding structures [Howes 2010].

2.4.2 Invasive techniques

Cardiac angiography: This is often indicated to rule out coronary ischemia as a cause of new-onset heart failure, especially when clinical presentation mimics acute myocardial infarction. It usually shows high filling pressures and reduced cardiac outputs [Tang et al., 2009].

The gold standard is still **biopsy of the myocardium**, generally done in the setting of angiography. A small tissue sample of the endocardium and myocardium is taken, and investigated by a pathologist by light microscopy and—if necessary—immunochemistry and special staining methods [Cunningham et al., 2006]. Histopathological features are: a myocardial interstitium with abundant edema and inflammatory infiltrate, rich in lymphocytes and macrophages. Focal destruction of myocytes explains the myocardial pump failure. The need for routine myocardial biopsy in patients with HIV is controversial and associated risks are significant - sensitivity is low, especially in patchy lesions, and beyond research protocols, its use is limited to patients with extensive cardiac damage with no identifiable cause [Wu et al., 1990].

Myocarditis identified at autopsy or on endomyocardial biopsy in HIV-infected patients is most often nonspecific and manifested as focal, inflammatory lymphocytic infiltrates without myocyte necrosis. Other reported histopathologic findings include lymphocytic infiltration with myocyte necrosis fulfilling the Dallas criteria or myocyte damage without associated cellular inflammatory infiltrate [Anderson et al., 1988, Barbaro et al., 1998]. The autopsy finding of focal myocarditis in many patients who die of AIDS-related complications, but have no known premortem heart disease, suggests that focal lymphocytic infiltration may have no clinical significance. By comparison, diffuse lymphocytic myocarditis meeting the Dallas criteria appears rare [Anderson et al., 1988].

The prevalence of nonspecific myocarditis is related to the stage of HIV infection and the presence of structural heart disease. In one study of HIV-infected patients with a pre-mortem diagnosis of dilated cardiomyopathy, histologic findings consistent with lymphocytic myocarditis by the Dallas criteria were identified in 63 of 76 patients (83%) [Barbaro et al., 1998].

2.4.3 Non-invasive techniques

Electrocardiography (ECG) is a useful screening tool in patients with HIV infection, and ECG changes may precede echocardiographic abnormalities. Patients with abnormal ECG patterns should be further investigated [Tang et al., 2009].

Electrocardiography is often nonspecific (eg, sinus tachycardia, nonspecific ST or T-wave changes). Occasionally, heart block (atrioventricular block or intraventricular conduction delay), ventricular arrhythmia, or injury patterns with ST- or T-wave changes mimicking myocardial ischemia or pericarditis (pseudoinfarction pattern) may indicate poorer prognosis [Gorgels 2007].

A chest X- ray can offer data about the size and shape of hart, as well as identification of fluid in or around the heart that might indicate heart failure [Round 2007].

Echocardiography has been shown to be extremely useful for the diagnosis and monitoring of HIV associated myocardial disease. Echocardiography is performed to exclude other causes of heart failure (eg, valvular, amyloidosis, congenital) and to evaluate the degree of cardiac dysfunction (usually diffuse hypokinesis and diastolic dysfunction). It also may allow gross localization of the extent of inflammation (ie, wall motion abnormalities, wall thickening, and pericardial effusion). In addition, echocardiography may distinguish between fulminant and acute myocarditis by identifying near-normal left ventricular diastolic dimensions and increased septal thickness in fulminant myocarditis (versus increased left ventricular diastolic dimensions and normal septal thickness in acute myocarditis), with marked improvement in systolic function in time [Tang et al., 2009].

De Castro et al., in 1994 performed a study of 136 HIV-infected patients without clinical, electrocardiographic or echocardiographic evidence of cardiovascular dysfunction on admission who were prospectively studied with serial echocardiograms; 93 of these patients had AIDS. During a mean follow-up period of 415 days, seven patients, all in the AIDS subgroup, developed clinical and echocardiographic findings of acute global left ventricular dysfunction; six of these seven patients died of congestive heart failure. Necropsy findings in five of these patients revealed acute lymphocytic myocarditis in three, cryptococcal myocarditis in one, and interstitial edema and fibrosis in one.

Cardiac computed tomography (CT) can have a role in the management of the undifferentiated heart failure patient, principally in excluding the presence of significant obstructive epicardial disease using CT angiography. Current generation 64-slice scanners demonstrate excellent diagnostic accuracy for both proximal coronary vessels and smaller distal vessels [Leber et al., 2005, Raff et al., 2005, Fine et al., 2006]. These recent studies especially demonstrate a high (greater than 95%) negative predictive value for the exclusion of significant epicardial stenosis.

Hence, although it has not been prospectively evaluated in the newly diagnosed heart failure population, the data would indicate that this modality can be used to stratify the patient with heart failure into an ischemic or non-ischemic etiology group.

Cardiac MRI (CMR) shows the accumulation of contrast in the myocardium as a consequence of the breakdown of the myocyte membrane resulting from the inflammatory process. The uptake of contrast usually has a characteristic patchy pattern for about the first 2 weeks after the acute event, later becoming progressively more disseminated. [Friedrich 1998] Moreover, this pattern of contrast uptake is easily distinguished from the subendocardial pattern of uptake seen in acute myocardial infarction.

CMR with contrast in association with cine-MRI is a useful tool for the diagnosis of myocarditis and provides an alternative to endomyocardial biopsy.

The availability of this diagnostic technique in the context of an acute episode might obviate the use of other, invasive diagnostic techniques which are not exempt from associated disease.

Roditi et al., in 2000 evaluated 20 patients with T1 spin-echo cine MR angiography and gadolinium-enhanced spin-echo imaging. Focal myocardial enhancement was associated with regional wall motion abnormalities in 10 of the 12 patients with suspected or proven myocarditis. The authors concluded that focal myocardial enhancement combined with regional wall motion abnormalities (hypokinesis, akinesis, or dyskinesis) strongly supported a diagnosis of myocarditis.

A combined CMR approach using T2-weighted imaging and contrast-enhanced T1-weighted images yields high diagnostic accuracy and thus, is a useful tool in the diagnosis and assessment of patients with suspected acute myocarditis [Abdel-Aty et al., 2005]. Friedrich et al. in 1998 were the first to propose CMR for the noninvasive diagnosis of acute myocarditis. Using T1-weighted images, they found that the myocardium in patients with suspected myocarditis has greater signal intensity relative to skeletal muscle [Friedrich et al., 1998]. T2-weighted images early after symptom onset can show focal increases of subepicardial and mid-wall myocardial signal, defining areas of myocardial edema [Abdel-

Aty et al., 2005]. Late gadolinium enhancement (LGE) - CMR has been shown to have additional value in the detection of active myocarditis as defined by histopathology [Mahrholdt et al., 2004].

LGE in the setting of myocarditis has a "nonischemic" pattern, typically affecting the subepicardium and the midmyocardial wall. This focal enhancement becomes diffuse over a period of days to weeks, then decreases during healing and may become invisible after recovery [Mahrholdt et al., 2004]. Alternatively, large areas of scarring might still be visible after healing, causing distinctive enhancing linear mid-wall striae. CMR-guided endomyocardial biopsy can result in a greater yield of positive findings than routine right ventricular biopsy [Mahrholdt et al., 2004].

This technique has not yet been fully evaluating in asymptomatic HIV infected subjects to establish the prevalence of unrecognized myocarditis.

Nuclear imaging: Antimyosin scintigraphy (using antimyosin antibody injections) can identify myocardial inflammation with high sensitivity (91-100%) and negative predictive power (93-100%) but has low specificity (31-44%) and low positive predictive power (28-33%). In contrast, gallium scanning is used to reflect severe myocardial cellular infiltration and has a good negative predictive value, although specificity is low [Tang et al., 2009].

In preliminary studies, a positive gallium scan improved the diagnostic yield of biopsy fourfold (baseline incidence of myocarditis - 8%; incidence associated with a positive scan - 36%). Gallium is an inflammatory avid isotope, whereas antimyosin antibodies are capable of labeling myocytes. Because histologic myocarditis consists of active inflammation in the presence of myocyte necrosis, indium 111 antimyosin antibodies may be useful in detecting this condition [O'Connell 1987].

Specific outcome data in HIV infected patients are missing.

2.5 Personal contribution

In Romania as in many other developing countries over the world cardiac MRI cannot be used widely for diagnosis. In the last several years within our cohort of adolescents and young adults HIV infected since their childhood we have noticed an increased number of patients with symptoms that suggest cardiac involvement. Dilative cardiomyopathy noticed more often in children infected by HIV was diagnosed especially postmortem at necropsy. As long as these patients present an increased rate of survival we are challenged to perform accurate diagnosis of cardiac involvement during their life.

During the last 2 years we have the opportunity to evaluate 10 patients with HIV and symptoms of cardiac involvement by performing: ECG, echocardiography, and nuclear imaging using technetium 99 (^{99}Tc). The 10 patients, 5 women and 5 men, were aged between 17 and 55 years. Echocardiography demonstrated in 4 cases normal left ventricular diastolic dimensions and small increases in septal thickness and in other 6 cases increased left ventricular diastolic dimensions and normal septal thickness. From the 4 patients with minimal echocardiography changes, nuclear imaging using technetium 99 showed no wall motions disorders and no changes in myocardial perfusions in 3 patients. In one patient we found no changes in echocardiography and ECG, while myocardial scintigraphy with ^{99}Tc showed changes in wall motility (akinesia) at rest and on stress and ischemic areas at the antero-septal wall and myocardial apex (4%), while at rest the affected area by myocardial scintigraphy was about 2%, as we can noticed in figure no. 1 [Cambrea et al., 2009]. From those 6 patients who presented changes on echocardiography, nuclear imaging with ^{99}Tc 2 patients demonstrated dilatative cardiomyopathy with no ischemic area, as shown in figure no. 2. The other 4 patients presented with dilative cardiomyopathy and ischemic areas on stress, as demonstrated in figure no. 3. All 10 patients had received HAART including protease inhibitors for at least 5 years and significant changes in lipid profile.

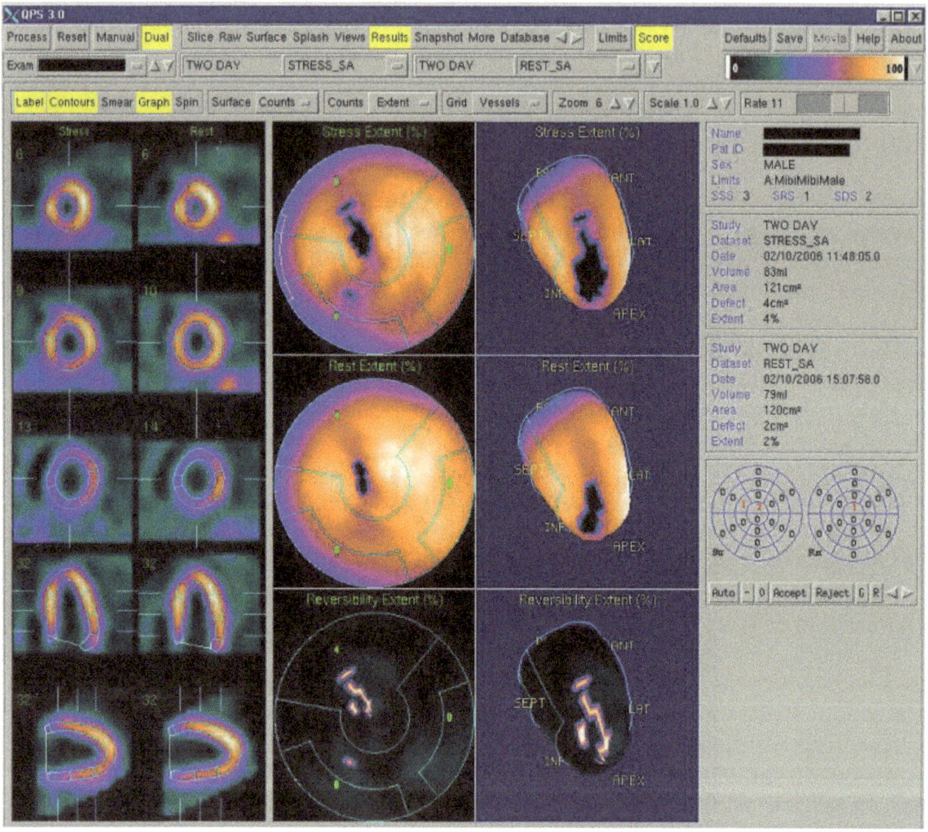

Fig. 1. Myocardic scintigraphy - ischemic areas at the antero-septal wall and myocardial apex.

2.6 Differential diagnosis of myocarditis in HIV

It is difficult to assess the clinical significance of viral infection of the myocardium in HIV-infected patients. AIDS or HIV-infected patients with myocarditis most often present with signs and symptoms of congestive heart failure or asymptomatic left ventricular dysfunction. The diagnosis of dilatative cardiomyopathy in this setting is best established by echocardiography. More specific diagnosis can be established by endomyocardial biopsy, as clinically indicated. However, in the vast majority of cases endomyocardial biopsy will not identify a specific cause that will modify therapy. In a minority of patients, biopsy may establish a treatable cause of myocarditis. Therefore, the clinician should consider the specifics of each case before making a recommendation regarding whether endomyocardial biopsy is necessary [Olson 2003].

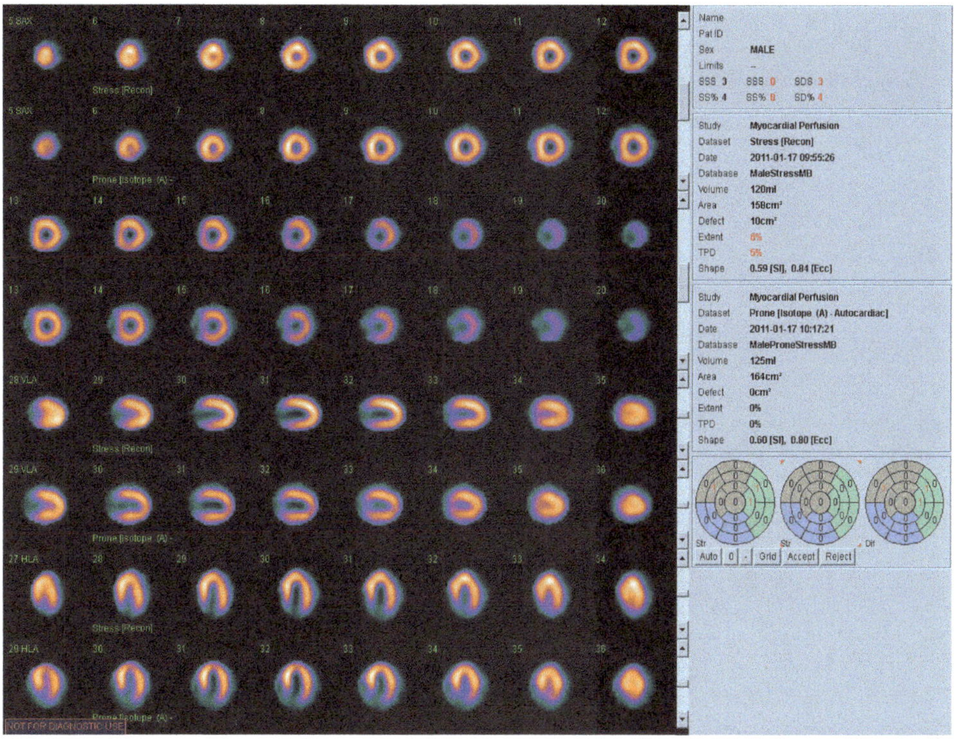

Fig. 2. Myocardic scintigraphy - dilatative cardiomyopathy with no ischemic area.

Aside from nonspecific or infectious myocarditis, the differential diagnosis of LV dysfunction in the AIDS patient includes drug toxicity from either abuse of illicit substances or iatrogenic disease from agents used in the therapy for AIDS. AIDS patients often take a great variety of prescription and nonprescription drugs and use illicit drugs. Alcohol, cocaine, or heroin may contribute to LV dysfunction in many cases [Virmani et al., 1988; Regan et al., 1990; Soodini et al., 1991]. Pharmacotherapy is also potentially associated with LV dysfunction in AIDS patients. Therapeutic agents implicated as potential cardiac toxins include zidovudine [Herskowitz et al., 1992b; d'Amati et al., 1992], and interferon alfa-2 [Deyton et al., 1989; Zimmerman et al., 1994].

If neoplastic infiltration is suspected as a cause of LV dysfunction, cardiac computed tomography or magnetic resonance imaging may be a useful adjunct to echocardiography for characterizing cardiac involvement. Neoplastic infiltration of the heart by Kaposi sarcoma is frequently seen at autopsy and usually associated with widespread disease in the terminal phases of AIDS [Silver et al., 1984]. Non-Hodgkin lymphoma is also observed in this setting and also associated with widespread disease [Holladay et al., 1992].

In addition to HIV-related cardiac conditions, differential diagnosis also includes non-HIV disease, because the latency of HIV disease may be long and patients are at risk for development of hypertensive heart disease, coronary artery disease, or other causes of left ventricular dysfunction [Olson 2003].

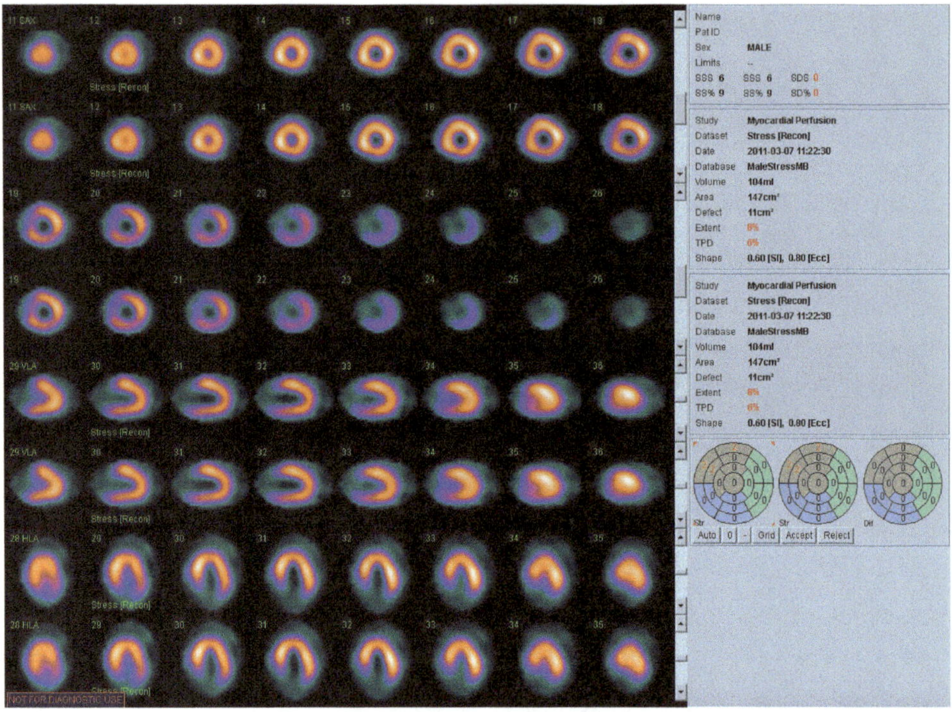

Fig. 3. Myocardic scintigraphy - dilative cardiomyopathy and ischemic areas on stress.

2.7 Treatment

Treatment for HIV related myocarditis is generally similar to that for non-HIV related myocarditis. Symptomatic treatment is the only form of therapy for HIV positive patients with myocarditis. In the acute phase, supportive therapy including bed rest is indicated. For symptomatic patients, digoxin and diuretics provide clinical improvement. For patients with moderate to severe dysfunction, cardiac function can be supported by use of inotropes such as Milrinone in the acute phase followed by oral therapy with ACE inhibitors (Captopril, Lisinopril) when tolerated. Patients who do not respond to conventional therapy are candidates for bridge therapy with left ventricular assist devices. Heart transplantation is reserved for patients who fail to improve with conventional therapy. Patients with HIV and myocarditis have enhanced sensitivity to digoxin and anticoagulation presents risks to patients with cerebral vasculopathy and possible aneurysm formation [Howes et al., 2010].

The use of immunosuppressive regimens in these patients is controversial and no convincing benefits have been reported other than with intravenous immunoglobulin [Lipshultz et al., 1995], whose efficacy may reflect inhibition of cardiac auto antibodies by competition with Fc receptors or dampened effects of cytokines and cellular growth factors.

The introduction of highly active antiretroviral therapy (HAART) regimens has substantially modified the course of HIV disease by lengthening survival and improving quality of life of HIV-infected patients [Zareba & Lipshultz 2003]. There is also good evidence that HAART significantly reduces the incidence of cardiovascular manifestations of HIV infection. By preventing opportunistic infections and reducing the incidence of myocarditis, HAART regimens have reduced the prevalence of HIV-associated myocarditis to about 30% [Barbaro 2005]. One Italian study reported an almost 7-fold reduction of the prevalence of HIV-associated myocarditis from the pre-HAART era [Pugliese et al., 2000]. In that study there is no conclusive evidence that HAART reverses cardiomyopathy, but it does appear that by preventing profound immunosuppression and the development of AIDS, heart muscle remains healthier [Pugliese et al., 2000].

3. Conclusions

Cardiac dysfunction should be considered in the differential diagnosis of any HIV-infected patient with dyspnea or cardiomegaly. In the setting of AIDS or HIV infection, the diagnosis of dilated cardiomyopathy is established by echocardiography. A significant proportion, perhaps exceeding 80%, of patients with dilated cardiomyopathy may have focal, non-specific lymphocytic myocarditis [Barbaro et al., 1998a].

Although viruses, in general, are well established as a cause of acute myocarditis, a causal role for viruses in the pathogenesis of dilated cardiomyopathy has not been demonstrated conclusively, including HIV infection.

A low CD4 count is an excellent predictor of the presence of LV dysfunction. The risk of dilated cardiomyopathy may also be increased with a history of illicit drug use [Soodini et al., 2001].

Myocarditis due to HIV-1 myocyte infection does not seem to be the most likely cause of LV dysfunction in patients with AIDS. It is more likely that the cause of LV dysfunction and congestive heart failure in this setting is multifactorial, related to drug toxicity, non-HIV viral infection, poor nutrition, or cytokines. Another situation in HIV positive patients that can cause myocarditis with or without ischemia is dyslipidemia as a consequence of highly active antiretroviral therapy that included protease inhibitor for a long period of time.

The evaluation and management of HIV positive patients with myocarditis and specific dilated cardiomyopathies remains clinically challenging. Essential to the appropriate care of these patients is not only an understanding of the patient's cardiac morphology and function but also identification of pathologic and modifiable substrate.

The ultimate proof that the patient has myocarditis is provided by endomyocardial biopsy, but the patchy nature of the disease limits its diagnostic role [Karamitsos et al., 2009].

Computed tomography or magnetic resonance imaging may help but are not widely used for diagnosis. Gadolinium-enhanced magnetic resonance imaging is used for assessment of the extent of inflammation and cellular edema, although it is still nonspecific. Delayed-enhanced MRI has also been used to quantify the amount of scarring that occurred following acute myocarditis [Al-Mallah & Kwong 2009].

By virtue of its safety, high degree of accuracy and reproducibility, and multiparametric nature, cardiac MRI represents the principal imaging modality that potentially addresses each of these points of care for heart failure patients. However, coronary CT angiography can aid in ruling out epicardial coronary artery stenosis as the cause of LV dysfunction in selected patients presenting with congestive heart failure.

In addition to clinical examination and biological evaluation, in the absence of cardiac MRI, a combination of ultrasound and scintigraphic investigations of the heart can provide sufficient data to establish myocardial dysfunction with or without ischemia.

Because cardiac CT, CMR and cardiac scintigraphy were not widely used in patients with myocarditis and in HIV cases are only sporadic presentations, to identify particular aspects of myocarditis in HIV positive patients is necessary to extend these new investigational noninvasive methods to a large number of patients.

4. References

Abdel-Aty H., et al., (2005) Diagnostic performance of cardiovascular magnetic resonance in patients with suspected acute myocarditis: comparison of different approaches. *J Am Coll Cardiol* Vol. 45, No, 11 (June 2005) pp: 1815–1822, ISSN: 0735-1097.

Albrecht H., et al., (1994) Successful treatment of Toxoplasma gondii myocarditis in an AIDS patient. *Eur J Clin Microbiol Infect Dis* 1994; Vol. 13, No. 6 (June 1994) pp: 500-504, ISSN: 0934-9723.

d'Amati G., Kwan W. & Lewis W. (1992) Dilated cardiomyopathy in a zidovudine-treated AIDS patient. *Cardiovasc Pathol;* Vol.1 No. 4 (October - December, 1992), pp: 317-320, ISSN: 1054-8807.

Anderson D.W., et al., (1988) Prevalent myocarditis at necropsy in the acquired immunodeficiency syndrome. *J Am Coll Cardiol;* Vol. 11, No. 4, (April 1988), pp: 792-799, ISSN: 0934-9723.

Aziz F., Doddi S. & Penupolu S. (2010) Human Immunodeficiency Virus–Associated Myocarditis. *The Internet Journal of Internal Medicine.* Vol. 8, No. 2, (2010), ISSN: 1528-8382

Barbaro G., et al., (1998a) Cardiac involvement in the acquired immunodeficiency syndrome: a multicenter clinical-pathological study. Gruppo Italiano per lo Studio Cardiologico dei pazienti affetti da AIDS Investigators. *AIDS Res Hum Retroviruses;* Vol. 14, No. 12, (August 1998), pp: 1071–1077, ISSN: 0889-2229

Barbaro G., et al., (1998b) Incidence of dilated cardiomyopathy and detection of HIV in myocardial cells of HIV-positive patients. Gruppo Italiano per lo Studio Cardiologico dei Pazienti Affetti da AIDS. *N Engl J Med;* Vol. 339, no. 16, (October 1998), pp: 1093-1099, ISSN: 0028-4793.

Barbaro G. (2005) Reviewing the cardiovascular complications of HIV Infection after the introduction of highly active antiretroviral therapy. *Curr Drug Targets Cardiovasc Haematol Disord;* Vol. 5, No. 4 (August 2005), pp: 337–343, ISSN: 1568-0061.

Baroldi G., et al., (1988) Focal lymphocytic myocarditis in acquired immunodeficiency syndrome (AIDS): a correlative morphologic and clinical study in 26 consecutive fatal cases. *J Am Coll Cardiol;* Vol. 12, No. 2 (August 1988), pp: 463-469, ISSN: 0934-9723.

Bowles N.E., et al., (1991) The detection of viral genomes by polymerase chain reaction in the myocardium of pediatric patients with advanced HIV disease. *J Am Coll Cardiol;* Vol. 34, No. 3, (September 1999), pp: 857-865, ISSN: 0934-9723.

De Castro S., et al., (1994) Frequency of development of acute global left ventricular dysfunction in human immunodeficiency virus infection. *J Am Coll Cardiol* Vol. 24, No. 4 (October 1994), pp: 1018-1024, ISSN: 0934-9723.

Cambrea S.C., et al., (2009) Coronary artery disease in an HIV+ adolescent. *Archives of the Balkan Medical Union;* Vol. 44, No.2, (June 2009), pp: 157-160, ISSN: 0041-6940.

Cenacchi G., et al., (1990). Human immunodeficiency virus type 1 antigen detection in endomyocardial biopsy: an immunomorphological study. *Microbiologica;* Vol. 13, No. 2, (April 1990); pp: 145-149, ISSN: 0391-5352.

Cohen I.S., et al., (1986). Congestive cardiomyopathy in association with the acquired immunodeficiency syndrome. *N Engl J Med*; Vol. 315, No. 10, (September 1986), pp: 628-630, ISSN: 0028-4793.

Cunningham K.S., Veinot J.P. & Butany J. (2006). An approach to endomyocardial biopsy interpretation, *J Clin Pathol*; Vol. 59, No. 2, (February 2006), pp:121-129, ISSN: 0021-9746.

Currie P.F. & Boon N.A. (2003) Immunopathogenesis of HIV-related heart muscle disease: current perspectives. *AIDS*; Vol 17, Suppl. 1, (April 2003), pp:S21-S28, ISSN: 0269-9370.

Currie P.F., et al., (1998) Cardiac autoimmunity in HIV related heart muscle disease. *Heart*; Vol. 79, No. 6, (June 1998), pp: 599-604, ISSN: 1468-201X.

Deyton L.R., et al., (1989) Reversible cardiac dysfunction associated with interferon alfa therapy in AIDS patients with Kaposi's sarcoma. *N Engl J Med*; Vol. 321, No. 18, (November 1989), pp: 1246-1249, ISSN: 0028-4793.

Fine J.J., et al., (2006) Comparison of accuracy of 64-slice cardiovascular computed tomography with coronary angiography in patients with suspected coronary artery disease. *Am J Cardiol*; Vol. 97, No. 2, (January 2006), pp: 173–174, ISSN: 0002-9149.

Flomenbaum M., et al., (1989) Proliferative membranopathy and human immunodeficiency virus in AIDS hearts. *J Acquir Immune Defic Syndr*; Vol.2, No. 2, (April 1989), pp: 129-135, ISSN: 1525-4135.

Friedrich, M.G., et al., (1998) Contrast media-enhanced magnetic resonance imaging visualizes myocardial changes in the course of viral myocarditis. *Circulation*; Vol. 97, No. 18, (May 1998), pp: 1802–1809, ISSN: 0009-7322.

Gorgels A.P.M. (2007) - Electrocardiography in *Cardiovascular Medicine* - Willerson et al., pp: 43- 78, Springer 2007; ISBN-10: 1-84628-188-1 3rd edition, London 2007.

Grody W.W., Cheng L. & Lewis W. (1990) Infection of the heart by the human immunodeficiency virus. *Am J Cardiol*; Vol. 66, No. 2, (July 1990), pp: 203-206, ISSN: 0002-9149.

Gu J., et al., (1992) Evidence for an autoimmune mechanism of the cardiac pathology in AIDS patients (abstract). *Circulation*; Vol. 86, Suppl 1, (1992), pp: I-795, ISSN: 0009-7322.

Grange F., et al., (1990) Successful therapy for *Toxoplasma gondii* myocarditis in acquired immunodeficiency syndrome. *Am Heart J*; Vol. 120, No. 2 (August 1990), pp: 443-444, ISSN: 0002-8703.

Herskowitz A., et al., (1989) Cardiomyopathy in acquired immunodeficiency syndrome: evidence for autoimmunity (abstract). *Circulation*; Vol. 80, Suppl 2, (1989), pp: II-322, ISSN: 0009-7322.

Herskowitz A., et al., (1993) Immunopathogenesis of HIV-1-associated cardiomyopathy. *Clin Immunol Immunopathol*; Vol. 68, No. 2 (August 1993), pp: 234-241, ISSN: 0014-2980.

Herskowitz A., et al., (1992a) Cardiomyopathy associated with antiretroviral therapy in patients with HIV infection: a report of six cases. *Ann Intern Med*; Vol. 116, No. 4, (February 1992) pp: 311-313, ISSN: 0003-4819.

Herskowitz A., et al., (1992b) Myocarditis associated with severe left ventricular dysfunction in late stage HIV infection (abstract). *Circulation*; Vol. 86, Suppl 1, (1992), pp:I-6, ISSN: 0009-7322.

Cunningham K., et al., (2005) Pathologic quiz case: a young woman with eosinophilia and heart failure. Primary hypereosinophilic syndrome with Loeffler endocarditis. *Arch Pathol Lab Med;* Vol. 129, No.1, (January 2005), pp: e29–30. ISSN: 1543-2165 [Medline].

Ho D.D., Pomerantz R.J. & Kaplan J.C. (1987) Pathogenesis of infection with human immunodeficiency virus. *N Engl J Med* Vol. 317, No. 5, (July 1987), pp: 278-286, ISSN: 0028-4793.

Holladay A.O., Siegel R.J. & Schwartz D.A. (1992) Cardiac malignant lymphoma in acquired immune deficiency syndrome. *Cancer;* Vol. 70, No. 8, (October 1992) pp: 2203-2207, ISSN: 1097-0142.

Howes D.S., et al., (2010) Myocarditis in Emergency Medicine Clinical Presentation Updated: Dec 8, 2010 http://emedicine.medscape.com/article/759212-clinical

Jautzke G., et al., (1993) Extracerebral toxoplasmosis in AIDS. (1993) Histological and immunohistological findings based on 80 autopsy cases. *Pathol Res Pract;* Vol. 189, No. 6, (July 1993), pp: 428-436, ISSN: 0344-0338.

Kaminski H.J., et al., (1988) Cardiomyopathy associated with the acquired immune deficiency syndrome. *J Acquir Immune Defic Syndr;* Vol. 1, No. 2, (April 1988), pp: 105-110, ISSN: 1525-4135.

Karamitsos T.D., et al., (2009) The Role of Cardiovascular Magnetic Resonance Imaging in Heart Failure. *J Am Coll Cardiol;* Vol. 54, No. 15, (October 2009), pp: 1407–1424, ISSN: 0934-9723.

Kinney E.L., et al., (1989) Treatment of AIDS-associated heart disease. *Angiology;* Vol. 40, No. 11, (November 1989) pp: 970-976, ISSN: 0003-3197.

Lafont A., et al., (1987) Overwhelming myocarditis due to Cryptococcus neoformans in an AIDS patients. *Lancet;* Vol. 330, No. 8568 (November 14, 1987) pp: 1145–1146, ISSN: 0140-6736.

Lahdevirta J., et al., (1988) Elevated levels of circulating cachectin/tumor necrosis factor in patients with acquired immunodeficiency syndrome. *Am J Med;* Vol. 85 complete, (1988), pp :289-291, ISSN: 0002-9343.

Leber A.W., et al., (2005) Quantification of obstructive and nonobstructive coronary lesions by 64-slice computed tomography: a comparative study with quantitative coronary angiography and intravascular ultrasound. *J Am Coll Cardiol;* Vol. 46, No. 1 (July 2005), pp: 147–154, ISSN: 0934-9723.

Levine B., et al., (1990) Elevated circulating levels of tumor necrosis factor in severe chronic heart failure. *N Engl J Med;* Vol. 323, No. 4, (July 1990) pp: 236-241, ISSN: 0028-4793.

Levy W.S., et al., (1989) Prevalence of cardiac abnormalities in human immunodeficiency virus infection. *Am J Cardiol* Vol. 63, No. 1, (January 1989) pp: 86–89, ISSN: 0002-9149.

Lewis W. & Grody W.N. (1992) AIDS and the heart: review and consideration of pathogenic mechanisms. *Cardiovasc Pathol* Vol. 1, No. 1 (Jan- March 1992), pp: 53–64, ISSN: 1054-8807.

Lewis W., Lipsick J. & Cammarosano C. (1985) Cryptococcal myocarditis in acquired immune deficiency syndrome. *Am J Cardiol;* Vol. 55, No. 9, (April 1985), pp:1240, ISSN: 0002-9149.

Lewis W. (2000) Cardiomyopathy in AIDS: a pathophysiological perspective. *Prog Cardiovasc Dis;* Vol. 43, No. 2 (October 2000), pp: 151-170, ISSN: 0033- 0620.

Lipshultz SE, et al., (1990) Identification of human immunodeficiency virus-1 RNA and DNA in the heart of a child with cardiovascular abnormalities and congenital acquired immune deficiency syndrome. *Am J Cardiol*; Vol. 66, No. 2, (July 1990), pp: 246-250, ISSN: 0002-9149.

Lipshultz S.E., et al., (1995) Immunoglobulins and left ventricular structure and function in pediatric HIV infection. *Circulation;* Vol. 92, No. 8, (October 1995) pp: 2220–2225, ISSN: 0009-7322.

Liu P.P. & Mason J.W. (2001) Advances in the understanding of myocarditis. *Circulation;* Vol. 104, No. 9, (August 2001), pp: 1076-1082, ISSN: 0009-7322.

Mahrholdt H., et al., (2004) Cardiovascular magnetic resonance assessment of human myocarditis: a comparison to histology and molecular pathology. *Circulation;* Vol. 109, No. 10, (March 2004), pp: 1250–1258, ISSN: 0009-7322.

Al-Mallah M. & Kwong R.Y. (2009) Clinical application of cardiac CMR. *Rev Cardiovasc Med;* Vol. 10, No. 3 (Summer 2009), pp: 134-141, ISSN: 1530-6550.

Matsumori A., et al., (1994) Increased circulating cytokines in patients with myocarditis and cardiomyopathy. *Br Heart J*; Vol. 72, No. 6, (December 1994), pp: 561-566, ISSN: 0007-0769.

Matturri L., et al., (1990) Cardiac toxoplasmosis in pathology of acquired immunodeficiency syndrome. *Panminerva Med;* Vol. 32, No. 3, (September 1990) pp: 194-196, ISSN: 0031-0808.

Michaels A.D., et al., (1997) Cardiovascular involvement in AIDS. *Curr Probl Cardiol;* Vol. 22, No. 3, (March 1997), pp: 115-148, ISSN: 0146-2806.

Miller-Catchpole R., et al., (1989) The Chicago AIDS autopsy study: opportunistic infections, neoplasms, and findings from selected organ systems with a comparison to national data. Chicago Associated Pathologists. *Mod Pathol;* Vol. 2, No. 4 (July 1989), pp:277-294, ISSN: 0893-3952.

Myerson D., et al. (1984) Widespread presence of histologically occult cytomegalovirus. *Hum Pathol;* Vol. 15, No. 5, (May 1984), pp: 430-439, ISSN: 0046-8177.

Odeh M. (1990) The role of tumour necrosis factor-alpha in acquired immunodeficiency syndrome. *J Intern Med;* Vol. 228, No. 6, (December 1990), pp: 549-556, ISSN: 0955-7873.

Olson L.J. - Myocarditis Associated With Human Immunodeficiency Virus Infection and Acquired Immunodeficiency Syndrome Humana Press, Totowa, New Jersey 2003 pp: 545 – 558 in Myocarditis: From Bench to Bedside Leslie T. Cooper ISBN 1-58829-112-X/03.

Pugliese A., et al., (2000) Impact of highly active antiretroviral therapy in HIV-positive patients with cardiac involve- ment. *J Infect;* Vol. 40, No. 3, (May 2000), pp: 282–284, ISSN: 0163-4453.

Raff, G.L., et al., (2005) Diagnostic accuracy of noninvasive coronary angiography using 64-slice spiral computed tomography. *J Am Coll Cardiol;* Vol. 46, No. 3, (August 2005), pp: 552–557, ISSN: 0934-9723.

Regan T.J. (1990) Alcohol and the cardiovascular system. *JAMA;* Vol. 264, No. 3, (July 18, 1990), pp: 377-381, ISSN: 0098-7484.

Reilly J.M., et al., (1988) Frequency of myocarditis, left ventricular dysfunction and ventricular tachycardia in the acquired immune deficiency syndrome. *Am J Cardiol*; Vol. 62, No. 10, Part 1, (October 1988), pp: 789-793, ISSN: 0002-9149.

Roditi G.H., Hartnell G.G. & Cohen M.C. (2000) MRI changes in myocarditis: evaluation with spin echo, cine MR angiography and contrast enhanced spin echo imaging. *Clin Radiol.* Vol. 55, No. 10, (October 2000), pp: 752–758, ISSN: 0009-9260.

Round M.E. (2007) - Chest X- ray in *Cardiovascular Medicine* - Willerson et al., pp: 79-92, Springer, ISBN-10: 1-84628-188-1 3rd edition, London 2007.

Silver M.A., et al., (1984) Cardiac involvement by Kaposi's sarcoma in acquired immune deficiency syndrome (AIDS). *Am J Cardiol;* Vol. 53, No. 7, (March 1984), pp: 983-985, ISSN: 0002-9149.

Sharma R., Coats A.J. & Anker S.D. (2000) The role of inflammatory mediators in chronic heart failure: cytokines, nitric oxide, and endothelin-1. *Int J Cardiol;* Vol. 72, No. 2, (January 2000), pp: 175-186, ISSN: 0167-5273.

Smiterman T.C. & Willerson J.T. (2007) - The history and Physical examination in *Cardiovasciular Medicine* - Willerson et al., pp: 19-42, Springer, ISBN-10: 1-84628-188-1 3rd edition, London 2007.

Soodini G. & Morgan J.P. (2001) Can cocaine abuse exacerbate the cardiac toxicity of human immunodeficiency virus? *Clin Cardiol;* Vol. 24, No. 3, (March 2001), pp: 177-181, ISSN: 0160-9289.

Subinas A., et al., (2005) Diagnosis of Acute Myocarditis by Contrast-Enhanced Cardiac Magnetic Resonance Imaging *Rev Esp Cardiol.* Vol. 58, No. 6, (June 2005), pp: 753-755, ISSN: 0300-8932.

Suffredini A.F., et al., (1989) The cardiovascular response of normal humans to the administration of endotoxin. *N Engl J Med;* Vol. 321, No. 5, (August 1989), pp: 280-287, ISSN: 0028-4793.

Tang W.H.W., et al., (2009) - Myocarditis Workup, Updated: Dec 7, 2009; http://emedicine.medscape.com/article/156330-workup.

Virmani R., et al., (1988) Cardiovascular effects of cocaine: an autopsy study of 40 patients. *Am Heart J;* Vol. 115, No. 9, (May 1988), pp: 1068-1076, ISSN: 0002-8703.

Yamada T., Matsumori A. & Sasayama S. (1994) Therapeutic effect of anti-tumor necrosis factor-alpha antibody on the murine model of viral myocarditis induced by encephalomyocarditis virus. *Circulation;* Vol. 89, No. 2, (February 1994), pp: 846-851, ISSN: ISSN: 0009-7322.

Yamamoto N. (1995) The role of cytokines in the acquired immunodeficiency syndrome. *Int J Clin Lab Res;* Vol. 25, No. 1, (March 1995), pp: 29-34, ISSN: 0940-5437.

Wu T.C., et al., (1992) In situ detection of human cytomegalovirus immediate-early gene transcripts within cardiac myocytes of patients with HIV-associated cardiomyopathy. *AIDS;* Vol. 6, No. 8, (August 1992), pp: 777-785, ISSN: 0269-9370.

Zareba K.M. & Lipshultz S.E. (2003) Cardiovascular complications in patients with HIV infection. *Curr Infect Dis Rep;* Vol. 5, No. 6, (December 2003), pp: 513–520, ISSN: 1523-3847.

Zimmerman S., et al., (1994) Irreversible, severe congestive cardiomyopathy occurring in association with interferon alpha therapy. *Cancer Biother* Vol. 9, No. 4, (Winter 1994), pp: 291-299, ISSN: 1062-8401.

9

Angiopoietin-1 for Myocardial Angiogenesis

Vien Khach Lai, Muhammad Zeeshan Afzal,
Muhammad Ashraf and Khawaja Husnain Haider
Department of Pathology
University of Cincinnati, Cincinnati, OH,
USA

1. Introduction

In response to ischemic damage, the heart undergoes vicious process of remodeling wherein the damaged myocardium is replaced by scar tissue and as compensatory mechanism, its existing collateral vessels and neovascularization with concomitant changes in cell recruitment, multiplication and cytokine/growth factor action. Angiogenesis is a complex process which involves an interplay between multiple pro- and anti-angiogenic factors and a harmonized interaction between endothelial progenitor cells, smooth muscle cells, pericytes and supportive environment. Besides Vegf/ Vegf receptor system, angiopoietin family of pro-angiogenic growth factors in conjunction with their receptor system are critical for vascular protection, remodeling, proliferation and maturation beside preservation of the integrity of newly formed vascular structures for functional activity (Thurston et al. 2000; Saharinen et al. 2005; Brindle, Saharinen et al. 2006).

An outside intervention to support the inefficient intrinsic myocardial repair processes by administration of stem/ progenitor cells has emerged as a promising strategy for the treatment of ischemic heart diseases. The transplanted stem cells have shown both myogenic as well as vasculogenic differentiation potential and participate in the myocardial regeneration *via* angiomyogenesis (Chen et al. 2010; Uemura et al. 2006; Eguchi et al. 2007). In addition to differentiation, stem cells can also ameliorate inflammation, migrate to ischemic regions and secrete bioactive molecules as a part of their paracrine activity and significantly contribute myocardial protection and angiogenesis. Alternatively, multimodal therapeutic strategies have also been adopted to accentuate the angiomyogenic potential of stem cells. This includes preconditioning of stem cells with growth factor treatment, their genetic modification with plasmids encoding for various angiogenic growth factors and concomitant administration of recombinant angiogenic growth factor proteins (Jiang et al. 2006; Haider et al. 2008; Kim et al. 2009; Lu et al. 2009). Such multimodal treatment strategies have elicited beneficial effects in terms of improving stem cell survival and enhancing their paracrine behavior besides stimulation of angiogenesis through direct recruitment, proliferation and maturation of precursor cells such as endothelial progenitor cells, mesenchymal stem cells and monocytes to the ischemic heart (Banai et al. 1994; Hiasa et al. 2004; Elmadbouh et al. 2007; Haider et al. 2008). We discuss here the biological regulation of angiopoietin-1 expression, its interaction with specific receptor system and the advantages of transgenic over expression of angiopoietin-1 either alone or in combination with Vegf to support angiogenesis as a therapeutic option for the treatment of ischemic heart disease.

2. Angiopoietin-1

2.1 Angiopoietin-1 and Tie2 ligand/receptor interaction in angiogenesis

The angiopoietin family of proteins consists of four members, all of which interact with the endothelial receptor tyrosine kinase, (tunica intima endothelial kinase 2, Tie2) (Thomas & Augustin 2009). Whereas two of these factors, angiopoietin-1 and angiopoietin-4, are constitutive agonists and Tie2 receptor activators (Davis et al. 1996), angiopoietin-2 and angiopoietin-3 have different effector functions and may activate or antagonize angiopoietin-1 induced Tie2 phosphorylation (Suri et al. 1996; Valenzuela et al. 1999; Fiedler et al. 2003). The essential role of angiopoietin-1 in the expansion and stabilization of newly formed vessels has been widely demonstrated (Suri et al. 1998). The process of vasculogenesis consists of differentiation, proliferation, and coalescence of vascular endothelial cells to establish a primitive vascular network in the early stage. This is followed by maturation of the neovasculature through the process of angiogenic remodeling that involves sprouting, branching, pruning, differential growth of vessels, and the recruitment of supporting cells (Suri et al. 1998; Hattori et al. 2001).

Both angiopoietin-1 and angiopoietin-2 have discrete participation in the occurrence of angiogenic cascade wherein angiopoietin-2 accumulates at the leading edge of proliferating vessels and angiopoietin-1 shows diffused localization behind the leading edge (Suri et al. 1998). Based on this distinct pattern of expression, it is suggested that angiopoietin-2 negatively mediates Tie2 activation and destabilizes the vessels to make these responsive to other angiogenic growth factors including Vegf, Pdgf and Fgf. On the contrary, angiopoietin-1 activates Tie2 and triggers remodeling and stabilization of the newly formed vasculature which leads to its maturation (Suri et al. 1998; Huang et al. 2009). The antagonizing activity of angiopoietin-2 is imperative for normal vascular maturation and spatial configuration (Feng et al. 2009). Over expression of angiopoietin-1 results in increased number, size and branches of the blood vessels without affecting the association among endothelial cells and with no evidence of plasma leakage, edema, or erythrocyte extravasation unlike Vegf (Suri et al. 1998; Thurston et al. 1999; Thurston et al. 2000; Kim et al. 2002). Angiopoietin-1 also contributes to attenuation of inflammatory response by mediating anti-permeability effects to counter Vegf and tumor necrosis factor (TNF)-induced inflammatory molecules in the endothelial cells such as vascular adhesion molecule-1 (VCAM-1), intercellular adhesion molecule-1 (ICAM-1) and endothelin-1 which control cell-cell interaction, maintain vascular quiescence and prevent leakiness (Kim et al. 2002; Hughes et al. 2003; Jeon et al. 2003; McCarter et al. 2006).

Tie2 receptor, a member of receptor tyrosine kinase family, consists of an extracellular domain, a trans-membrane domain and a split intracellular kinase domain (Takahara et al. 2004). This receptor is more specifically expressed on vascular endothelium in both quiescence and active states although it is also found on some other cell types such as smooth muscle cells, fibroblasts, mural cells, ganglion cells and carcinoma cells (Dumont et al. 1992; Takahara et al. 2004; Kosacka et al. 2005; Nakayama et al. 2005; Hamaguchi et al. 2006). Tie2 is highly conserved from zebra fish to mammals with the greatest amino acid homology occurring in the kinase domain, indicating the importance of its biological function (Lyons et al. 1998). Disrupting the function of Tie2 in transgenic mice was lethal and resulted in early embryonic death due to failure of vascular branching and differentiation. Homozygous mutated embryos also displayed abnormalities in the development of the heart (Dumont et al. 1994; Sato et al. 1995). Lack of Tie2 also resulted in angiogenic defects in term of vessel branching and remodeling, and displayed defects in the developing vessels to have scarce peri-endothelial cells and thinner collagen-like fibers (Suri et al. 1996). Dysregulated expression of Tie2 have also been observed in several clinical diseases including venous malformations, intramuscular hemangiomas, pulmonary hypertension and infantile hemangiomas (Yu et al. 2001; Wang et al. 2004; Morris et al. 2005). On the contrary, overexpression of angiopoietin-1 in the skin of experimental animal models led to the formation of highly branched and larger vessels, and resulted in reduction of microvascular leakage (Suri et al. 1998; Thurston et al. 1999). Tie2 over expression in the skin caused psoriasis-like phenotype after birth and persisted throughout adulthood, and was featured by epidermal hyperplasia, accumulation of inflammatory cells and altered dermal angiogenesis (Voskas et al. 2005). These findings clearly suggested that a delicate level of Tie2 receptor was required for physiological functioning and any unregulated induction or loss of Tie2 resulted in potentially worsened effects. Despite considerable similarity with Tie1, experiments with Tie1- or Tie2-deficient mice have provided evidence of their distinct functions in response to different members of angiopoietin family (Seegar et al. 2011).

2.2 Angiopoietin-1, Tie2 receptor and intracellular signaling

It is interesting to note that angiopoietin-1 and angiopoietin-2 have different effects on vascular formation and development, however, they bind to Tie2 receptor with distinct kinetics of release following binding thus indicating that activation of Tie2 receptor is regulated independently by these two molecules. In fact, angiopoietin-2, a natural antagonist of angiopoietin-1 (Maisonpierre et al. 1997), binds to Tie2 receptor without its activation (Davis et al. 2003). Similarly, structural characteristics and distinguishable interaction with other molecules in the extracellular environment of the ligands may also essentially contribute to their counteractive properties (Kim et al. 2005). More recent studies have shown that the effects of angiopoietin-1 and angiopoietin-2 on the receptor tyrosine kinase Tie2 are differentially regulated at the endothelial cell surface (Hansen et al. 2010) and a critical balance is maintained between angiopoietin-1 and angiopoietin-2 expression by sonic hedgehog and fibroblast growth factor-2 during angiogenesis (Fujii & Kuwano, 2010). Phosphorylation of tyrosine residues of Tie2 occurs subsequent to binding with angiopoietin-1 and activates kinase domain of the receptor to initiate various downstream intracellular signaling cascades (Murray et al. 2001). The phosphorylation of tyrosine residues on the intracellular domain of Tie2 receptor interacts with the p85 subunit of PI3K *via* Src homology 2 or phosphotyrosine binding domain. These molecular changes result in activation of PI3K and its downstream Akt in the endothelial cells and ultimately lead to multiple responses such as cell survival, differentiation and chemotaxis (Witzenbichler et al. 1998; Fujikawa et al. 1999; Abdel-Malak et al. 2009; Bai et al. 2009). Although some studies have already demonstrated that angiopoietin-1 mediated activation of Tie2 does not cause mitogenesis of endothelial cells, the others have reported a pro-proliferative effect of angiopoietin-1 on vascular cells (Kanda et al. 2005; Abdel-Malak et al. 2009). These contradictions in the data may be explained on the basis of the observation that angiopoietin-1 may induce various effects on endothelial cells depending on the tissue type and conditional environments.

Angiopoietin-1 activity also involves Forkhead box O-1 (FOXO1) transcription factor which principally acts as a regulator of cell cycle and endothelial cell functions in vascular destabilization and remodeling (Kanda et al. 2005; Evans-Anderson et al. 2008). Angiopoietin-1 is known to inhibit the activity of FOXO1 *via* phosphorylation and promotes cell proliferation in the cultured endothelial cells by upregulation of cyclin D1 downstream of FOXO1 (Kanda et al. 2005; Huang & Tindall 2007). Phosphorylation of FOXO1 by Akt in the endothelial cells occurs at three conserved sites which results in the inhibition of FOXO1 by promoting its translocation from the nucleus to the cytoplasm (Daly et al. 2004; Huang & Tindall 2007). In addition to interaction with FOXO1, GATA3 which is highly expressed in human endothelial cells especially in the large vessels, plays a significant role in the expression of angiogenesis related genes and endothelial cell functions subsequent to stimulation with angiopoietin-1 (Song et al. 2009). Knock down of GATA3 significantly abrogated these effects of angiopoietin-1. Besides these transcription factors, angiopoietin-1 can activate MAPK in the cultured endothelial cells (Fujikawa et al. 1999; Kim et al. 2002; Zhu et al. 2002). Pharmacological inhibition of ERK1/2 abolishes Tie2 phosphorylation and its downstream signaling for morphogenesis of capillary endothelium and suppresses endothelial cell proliferation which are involved in angiogenesis (Kim et al. 2002). However, inhibition of ERK1/2 activity in endothelial cells does not effect angiopoietin-1-induced survival and migration (Fujikawa et al. 1999). Hence, it is suggested that MAPK activity as a consequence of Tie2 activation during angiogenesis is more important for endothelial sprouting and branching than for endothelial recruitment and maintenance. On the other hand, angiopoietin-1 mediated activation of p38 MAPK signaling promoted mural cell recruitment during angiogenesis (Zhu et al. 2003). Angiopoietin-1 also has the ability to directly bind to the monocytes without interacting with Tie2 and promote their transendothelial migration by directly activating PI3K for its role in inflammatory angiogenesis (Ahmad et al. 2010).

2.3 Angiopoietin-1, Tie2 receptor and extracellular response

Under physiological conditions, endothelial cells of the vasculature remain quiescent in the inner layer of vessels. However, during active vascular remodeling in response to pathological conditions like vascular occlusion, myocardial infarction or *de-novo* vascular formation, circulating endothelial progenitors and local endothelial cells migrate to the ischemic areas. More so, some of these cells penetrate and traverse to distant sites of the occluded vessels to participate in the repair process. Angiopoietin-2, which is mainly released by endothelial cells and localized at the site of vascular remodeling, functions as a Tie2 blocker and promotes the destabilization of pericytes from existing vessels and increases vascular permeability. This in turn allows the infiltration of proteases, cytokines and angiogenic cells to support robust angiogenic response. The blood vessels are thus formed by the complex contribution of an intricate network of smooth muscle layer that surrounds endothelial cells in arteries, arterioles and veins resulting from migration, proliferation and interaction of different cell types like pericytes, smooth muscle cells and fibroblasts (Asahara et al. 1999; Carmeliet 2000; Bentley et al. 2009). It is suggested that interaction between angiopoietin-1 and Tie2 also regulates cross-talk between endothelial cells and pericytes (Davis et al. 1996; Sundberg et al. 2002). Angiopoietin-1 is a pericyte derived signal that mediates maturation and quiescence of the microvascular endothelium (Armulik et al. 2005). In addition to its role as an effector for the secondary step of vascular formation, angiopoietin-1 can stimulate endothelial cell migration and induce angiogenesis independent of its interaction with angiopoietin-2 or Vegf (Koblizek et al. 1998; Hayes et al. 1999; Babaei et al. 2003). The pro-angiogenic activity of angiopoietin-1 independent of Vegf involves phosphorylation of Tie2 and activation of PI3K/Akt signaling. These observations have been substantiated by *in-vivo* experimental evidence which showed that the angiogenic efficacy of angiopoietin-1 alone was comparable to that of Vegf stimulation (Babaei et al. 2003). More recent studies have shown that angiopoietin-1 also regulate the functions of hematopoietic stem cells in the bone marrow. Treatment of ckit+ cells with angiopoietin-1 helped the cells to maintain their functional activity *in vitro* on long term basis, however, with little influence on their colony forming potential (Gomei et al. 2010).

2.4 Angiopoietin-1, Tie2 and anti-apoptotic effect

Angiopoietin-1 is critical for cell survival and proliferation and functions *via* PI3K/Akt and MAPK/ERK signaling pathway (Daly et al. 2004; Kanda et al. 2005). ERK1/2 kinases have important role in regulation of apoptosis in various cells including endothelial cells wherein ERK1/2 have been consistently shown to mediate the anti-apoptotic effects of VEGF and angiopoietin-1 by targeting caspase-9, -3 and -7. Angiopoietin-1 also induces p38 MAPK phosphorylation as a part of its anti-apoptotic activity in the endothelial cells (Gratton et al. 2001; Harfouche et al. 2003). The pro-survival effects of angiopoietin-1 have been extensively studied in variety of cells against pro-apoptotic stimuli (Tuo et al. 2010; Lee et al. 2008; Liu et al. 2008; Bai et al. 2009). In most cases, angiopoietin-1 treatment phosphorylated Tie2 receptors leading to activation of Akt signaling. Treatment of neuronal progenitor cells with angiopoietin-1 protected the cells against oxygen-glucose deprivation induced apoptosis by activation of PI3K/Akt to inhibit pro-apoptotic signaling (Bai et al. 2009). Similarly, activation of pro-apoptotic signaling was reversed in myocardial endothelial cells in high glucose culture conditions upon treatment with angiopoietin-1 which incidentally also increased angiogenesis (Tuo et al. 2010). These salutary effects of angiopoietin-1 were however, antagonized and blunted by angiopoietin-2. Treatment with angiopoietin-1 protein or its transgenic expression in endothelial cells also induces some secondary mediators such as interleukin-8 through ERK1/2, SAPK/JNK, and PI3K pathways, which trigger c-Jun phosphorylation on Ser63 and Ser73 (Abdel-Malak et al. 2008). Interleukin-8 then acts in autocrine fashion to suppress apoptosis and facilitate cell proliferation and migration (Abdel-Malak et al. 2008).

3. Angiopoietin-1 gene delivery in combination with Vegf

Whereas Vegf is one of the most potent vasoactive growth factors which is involved in angiogenesis and regulates vascular permeability, angiopoietin-1 is also being recognized for its angiogenic potential besides its role as a vascular stability factor. Both of these growth factors are discretely produced in a succession during the development of mature blood vessels (Thurston, 2002). Angiopoietin-1 acts as a mitogen for endothelial cells and synergistically induces sprout formation with Vegf (Koblizek et al. 1998). The regulatory mechanism of angiopoietin-1 induced neovascularization involves pro-survival effects on the endothelial cells by activation of PI3K/Akt signaling and stabilization of nascent blood vessels to become leak resistant (Thurston et al. 2000).

Both Vegf and angiopoietin-1 have been extensively used for angiogenic protein or gene therapy to exploit complementarities between their functional relationship (Zhu et al. 2002; Cheng et al. 2007). Given a coordinated role of angiopoietin-1 and Vegf during both physiologic and pathologic development of blood vessels, simultaneous use of the two growth factors have been reported for the treatment of tissue ischemia (Gale et al. 2002; Ye et al. 2007). The application of this combinatorial growth factor therapy approach is not only for induction of angiogenesis; it is also intended to involve circulating endothelial progenitor cells. These progenitors then home into the ischemic tissues in response to the concentration gradient for participation in the ongoing repair process of vasculogenesis (Kalka et al. 2000; Wang et al. 2006). We have already reported the feasibility of combining stem cell mobilization from bone marrow in combination with Vegf gene delivery to the infarcted heart to show that the mobilized stem cells homed into the heart and participated in myocardial angiogenesis (Wang et al. 2006). Although the use of recombinant growth factors has given encouraging results with both Vegf and angiopoietin-1, the very short biological half-life of these growth factors warrants alternative treatment strategies. A more recent study has reported covalent immobilization of Vegf and angiopoietin-1 onto three-dimensional porous collagen scaffolds using 1-ethyl-3-[3-dimethylaminopropyl] carbodiimide hydrochloride (EDC) chemistry to enhance the duration of the growth factors availability and effectiveness (Chiu & Radisic, 2011).

As an alternative to recombinant protein administration, transgenic expression of angiopoietin-1 and Vegf gene therapy is being assessed to achieve arteriogenesis and angiogenesis for the treatment of myocardial ischemia (Samuel et al. 2010; Siddiqui et al. 2003; Ye et al. 2007). The efficacy of Vegf and angiopoietin-1 gene delivery to the heart has been extensively studied to promote angiogenesis and improve regional blood flow et al. 2007; Haider, Ye et al. 2004). The authors reported the first bi-cistronic adenoviral vector encoding for Vegf and angiopoietin-1 for co-expression of the two angiogenic growth factors. The vector was used to genetically modify stem cells for overexpression of angiopoietin-1 and Vegf. Transplantation of genetically modified skeletal myoblasts demonstrated development of functionally mature blood vessels in the infarcted heart and in the hind limb ischemia model in rabbits (Niagara et al. 2004; Ye et al. 2007). These observations were in harmony with the previously published data suggesting enhanced perfusion accompanied by the development of stable and mature blood vessels with combined Vegf and angiopoietin-1 administration (Arsic et al. 2004; Gurunluoglu et al. 2002; Shyu et al. 2003). In a recently reported study, Tao *et al.* co-expressed Vegf/angiopoietin-1 using adeno-associated viral vectors (AAVs) expressing cardiac-specific and hypoxia-inducible Vegf and Ang1 into the porcine infarcted heart immediately after ligation of the left descending coronary artery (Tao et al. 2010). Vegf and Ang1 were predominantly expressed in the heart in the infarct and border of the infarct. Gated single-photon emission computed tomography showed improved cardiac function and myocardial perfusion at 8 weeks after vector injection which corresponded well with higher vascular density. They also observed higher level activation of Akt and Bcl-xL, less Caspase-3 and Bad, and reduced TUNEL positivity in angiopoietin-1/ Vegf treated animal hearts. These results showed that simultaneous expression of angiopoietin-1/ Vegf in the infarcted heart stimulated pro-survival pathways besides improved regional blood flow. Although the authors claimed to have observed significant change in the number of cycling cardiomyocytes subsequent to angiopoietin-1/ Vegf overexpression, this may be insufficient to replace the massive loss of the functioning cardiomyocytes in the infarcted heart. Although direct injection of angiopoietin-1 and Vegf growth factors has been shown to significantly improve the regional blood flow in the ischemic heart, this strategy if combined with stem cell therapy would be more effective in addressing the core issue of myocardial regeneration which requires neomyogenesis for replacement of the scar tissue.

4. Combining stem cell transplantation and Angiopoietin-1 delivery

Gene delivery strategy has developed over the years from direct plasmid injection to stem cell based ex-vivo delivery strategy. Stem cells are excellent carriers of therapeutic genes for delivery to the various body tissues and organs including the heart (Suzuki et al. 2001; Yau et al. 2007; Ye et al. 2007; Haider et al. 2008). Despite all the progress made, it remains to be defined whether cell based gene therapy can overcome several potential impediments such as poor transfection efficiency, unregulated transgene expression, low survival rate of transplanted cells into ischemic zones etc. On the same note, there are a number of parameters which require optimization including cell type, number of transfected cells to be transplanted, time of cell transplantation after infarction, and route of cell transplantation.

Angiopoietin-1 is one of the many angiogenic growth factors which have been extensively studied for pro-angiogenic activity in the ischemic tissues. We performed a comparative assessment of the methods to deliver angiopoietin-1 gene delivery for angiogenic repair of the infarcted heart using an experimental porcine heart model of chronic infarction (Ye et al. 2007). Our results showed that skeletal myoblast based delivery of angiopoietin-1 transgene was more effective as compared to the approach of direct injection of adenoviral vector encoding for angiopoietin-1. The genetically modified skeletal myoblasts carrying angiopoietin-1 transgene served as a reservoir of the transgene product and ensured localized release of angiopoietin-1 at the site of the cell graft without safety concerns associated with the use of direct injection of adenoviral vector (Ye et al. 2007). Besides we observed extensive survival of the transplanted skeletal myoblasts which underwent myogenic differentiation to repopulate the infarcted myocardium.

Given that the development of stable and functional blood vessels is regulated by a critical balance between several pro- and anti-angiogenic factors which also co-ordinate with various vasculogenic cells, we hypothesized that a single angiogenic factor may be insufficient to achieve the desired outcome. We therefore opted to combine angiopoietin-1 and Vegf for co-expression to achieve angiogenic synergism between the two growth factors (Ye et al. 2007). We developed a bicistronic adenoviral vector which encoded for human $Vegf_{165}$ and angiopoietin-1 driven by the same promoter. The vector was used to genetically modify human skeletal myoblasts which were later transplanted in a porcine heart model of coronary artery ligation. We observed excellent survival of the transplanted skeletal myoblasts for up to 12 weeks using transient immunosuppression. Immunohistological studies showed myogenic differentiation of the skeletal myoblasts and increased blood vessel density in the infarct as well as peri-infarct regions with highest maturation index in the animal heart treated with skeletal myoblasts co-expressing Vegf and angiopoietin-1. Regional blood flow, measured with fluorescent microspheres, was significantly improved which revealed the functional competence of the newly formed blood vessels. These findings signified the feasibility of multimodal therapeutic approach based on simultaneous delivery of angiopoietin-1 and Vegf combined with cell transplantation.

Although skeletal myoblasts showed excellent ability as transgene carriers, one of the major drawbacks is their failure to develop gap junctions with the host cardiomyocytes and arrhythmogenicity (Fouts et al. 2006). We therefore hypothesized that the use of bone marrow derived mesenchymal stem cells might be a better option. Mesenchymal stem cells have been extensively studied for their cardiac reparability and regenerative potential (Chen et al. 2010; Kim et al 2010.; Labovsky et al. 2010; Haider et al. 2009) besides having superior transgene carrying capability (Chen et al. 2010; Huang et al. 2010; Tang et al. 2010; Haider et al. 2008). Besides, we also opted to replace Vegf with survival signaling molecule Akt to support survival of the genetically modified mesenchymal stem cells (Jiang et al. 2006). Our choice of transgene combination of angiopoietin-1 and Akt achieved maximum beneficial effects in terms of donor stem cell survival and angiomyogenic repair of the infarcted heart. More importantly, the therapeutic benefits in terms of cell graft survival, stability of newly formed blood vessels and global cardiac function were stable for up to 3 months (Shujia et al. 2008). A more recent study has used sendai viral vector for transduction of mesenchymal stem cells, however, it remains difficult to see the advantages of mesenchymal stem cells modified with sendai vector harboring human angiopoietin-1 gene (Piao, Wang et al.)

5. Conclusions

Genetic modification increases the therapeutic efficacy of stem cells by improving their survival, enhancement of paracrine activity and by supporting their angiomyogenic differentiation (Tang et al. 2004). A combined cell and gene therapy approach reverses the deteriorating function of the infarcted heart (Mangi et al. 2003; Matsumoto et al. 2005) and offers an extended and localized expression of the transgene product. From the clinical standpoint, the strength of stem cell therapy and gene therapy approaches lies in their combined application to achieve stable therapeutic benefits. The viability and persistence of the genetically modified stem cells and their derivative graft in the heart can be significantly enhanced by restoration of regional blood flow *via* biological bypass surgery which is achieved by neovascularization of the infarcted heart. The new emerging pro-angiogenic role of angiopoietin-1 independent of VEGF, in addition to its well recognized participation in the angiogenic cascade as a maturation factor, makes angiopoietin-1 as a growth factor of choice for ex-vivo stem cell based gene therapy which can be used independently or in combination with VEGF to support angiomyogenic recovery of the infarcted heart.

6. Acknowledgements

This work was supported by National Institutes of Health Grants #R37-HL074272;HL-080686;HL-087246(M.A) and HL-087288;HL-089535; HL106190-01 (Kh.H.H).

7. References

Abdel-Malak NA, Mofarrahi M, Mayaki D, Khachigian LM, Hussain SN. (2009). Early growth response-1 regulates angiopoietin-1-induced endothelial cell proliferation, migration, and differentiation. *Arterioscler Thromb Vasc Biol* 29(2): 209-16.

Abdel-Malak NA, Srikant CB, Kristof AS, Magder SA, Di Battista JA, Hussain SN. (2008). Angiopoietin-1 promotes endothelial cell proliferation and migration through AP-1-dependent autocrine production of interleukin-8. *Blood* 111(8): 4145-54.

Ahmad S, Cudmore MJ, Wang K, Hewett P, Potluri R, Fujisawa T, Ahmed A. (2010). Angiopoietin-1 induces migration of monocytes in a tie-2 and integrin-independent manner. *Hypertension* 56(3): 477-83.

Armulik A, Abramsson A, Betsholtz C. (2005). Endothelial/pericyte interactions. *Circ Res* 97(6): 512-23.

Arsic N, Zacchigna S, Zentilin L, Ramirez-Correa G, Pattarini L, Salvi A, Sinagra G, Giacca M. (2004). Vascular endothelial growth factor stimulates skeletal muscle regeneration in vivo. *Mol Ther* 10(5): 844-54.

Asahara T, Masuda H, Takahashi T, Kalka C, Pastore C, Silver M, Kearne M, Magner M, Isner JM. (1999). Bone marrow origin of endothelial progenitor cells responsible for postnatal vasculogenesis in physiological and pathological neovascularization. *Circ Res* 85(3): 221-8.

Babaei S, Teichert-Kuliszewska K, Zhang Q, Jones N, Dumont DJ, Stewart DJ. (2003). Angiogenic actions of angiopoietin-1 require endothelium-derived nitric oxide. *Am J Pathol* 162(6): 1927-36.

Bai Y, Cui M, Meng Z, Shen L, He Q, Zhang X, Chen F, Xiao J. (2009). Ectopic expression of angiopoietin-1 promotes neuronal differentiation in neural progenitor cells through the Akt pathway. *Biochem Biophys Res Commun* 378(2): 296-301.

Bai Y, Meng Z, Cui M, Zhang X, Chen F, Xiao J, Shen L, Zhang Y. (2009). An Ang1-Tie2-PI3K axis in neural progenitor cells initiates survival responses against oxygen and glucose deprivation. *Neuroscience* 160(2): 371-81.

Banai S, Jaklitsch MT, Shou M, Lazarous DF, Scheinowitz M, Biro S, Epstein SE, Unger EF. (1994). Angiogenic-induced enhancement of collateral blood flow to ischemic myocardium by VEGF in dogs. *Circulation* 89(5): 2183-9.

Bentley K, Mariggi G, Gerhardt H, Bates PA. (2009). Tipping the balance: robustness of tip cell selection, migration and fusion in angiogenesis. *PLoS Comput Biol* 5(10): e1000549.

Brindle NP, Saharinen P, Alitalo K. (2006). Signaling and functions of angiopoietin-1 in vascular protection. *Circ Res* 98(8): 1014-23.

Carmeliet, P. (2000). Mechanisms of angiogenesis and arteriogenesis. *Nat Med* 6(4): 389-95.

Chen Y, Liu W, Li W, Gao C. (2010). Autologous bone marrow mesenchymal cell transplantation improves left ventricular function in a rabbit model of dilated cardiomyopathy. *Exp Mol Pathol* 88(2): 311-5.

Cheng M, Park H, Engelmayr GC, Moretti M, Freed LE. (2007). Effects of regulatory factors on engineered cardiac tissue in vitro. *Tissue Eng* 13(11): 2709-19.

Chiu LL, & Radisic M. Scaffolds with covalently immobilized VEGF and Angiopoietin-1 for vascularization of engineered tissues. *Biomaterials* 31(2): 226-41.

Davis S, Papadopoulos N, Aldrich TH, Maisonpierre PC, Huang T, Kovac L, Xu A, Leidich R, Radziejewska E, Rafique A, Goldberg J, Jain V, Bailey K, Karow M, Fandl J, Samuelsson SJ, Ioffe E, Rudge JS, Daly TJ, Radziejewski C, Yancopoulos GD. (2004). Angiopoictin-1 modulates endothelial cell function and gene expression via the transcription factor FKHR (FOXO1). *Genes Dev* 18(9): 1060-71.

Davis S, Aldrich TH, Jones PF, Acheson A, Compton DL, Jain V, Ryan TE, Bruno J, Radziejewski C, Maisonpierre PC, Yancopoulos GD. (1996). Isolation of angiopoietin-1, a ligand for the TIE2 receptor, by secretion-trap expression cloning. *Cell* 87(7): 1161-9.

Davis, S., N. Papadopoulos, et al. (2003). Angiopoietins have distinct modular domains essential for receptor binding, dimerization and superclustering. *Nat Struct Biol* 10(1): 38-44.

Dumont DJ, Gradwohl G, Fong GH, Puri MC, Gertsenstein M, Auerbach A, Breitman ML. (1994). "Dominant-negative and targeted null mutations in the endothelial receptor tyrosine kinase, tek, reveal a critical role in vasculogenesis of the embryo. *Genes Dev* 8(16): 1897-909.

Dumont DJ, Yamaguchi TP, Conlon RA, Rossant J, Breitman ML. (1992). tek, a novel tyrosine kinase gene located on mouse chromosome 4, is expressed in endothelial cells and their presumptive precursors. *Oncogene* 7(8): 1471-80.

Eguchi M, Masuda H, Asahara T. (2007). Endothelial progenitor cells for postnatal vasculogenesis. *Clin Exp Nephrol* 11(1): 18-25.

Elmadbouh I, Haider H, Jiang S, Idris NM, Lu G, Ashraf M. (2007). Ex vivo delivered stromal cell-derived factor-1alpha promotes stem cell homing and induces angiomyogenesis in the infarcted myocardium. *J Mol Cell Cardiol* 42(4): 792-803.

Evans-Anderson HJ, Alfieri CM, Yutzey KE. (2008). Regulation of cardiomyocyte proliferation and myocardial growth during development by FOXO transcription factors. *Circ Res* 102(6): 686-94.

Feng Y, Vom Hagen F, Wang Y, Beck S, Schreiter K, Pfister F, Hoffmann S, Wagner P, Seeliger M, Molema G, Deutsch U, Hammes HP. (2009). The absence of angiopoietin-2 leads to abnormal vascular maturation and persistent proliferative retinopathy. *Thromb Haemost* 102(1): 120-30.

Fiedler U, Krissl T, Koidl S, Weiss C, Koblizek T, Deutsch U, Martiny-Baron G, Marme D, Augustin HG. (2003). Angiopoietin-1 and angiopoietin-2 share the same binding domains in the Tie-2 receptor involving the first Ig-like loop and the epidermal growth factor-like repeats. *J Biol Chem* 278(3): 1721-7.

Fouts K, Fernandes B, Mal N, Liu J, Laurita KR. (2006). Electrophysiological consequence of skeletal myoblast transplantation in normal and infarcted canine myocardium. *Heart Rhythm* 3(4): 452-61.

Fujii, T. & H. Kuwano Regulation of the expression balance of angiopoietin-1 and angiopoietin-2 by Shh and FGF-2. *In Vitro Cell Dev Biol Anim* 46(6): 487-91.

Fujikawa K, de Aos Scherpenseel I, Jain SK, Presman E, Christensen RA, Varticovski L. (1999). Role of PI 3-kinase in angiopoietin-1-mediated migration and attachment-dependent survival of endothelial cells. *Exp Cell Res* 253(2): 663-72.

Gale NW, Thurston G, Davis S, Wiegand SJ, Holash J, Rudge JS, Yancopoulos GD. (2002). Complementary and coordinated roles of the VEGFs and angiopoietins during normal and pathologic vascular formation. *Cold Spring Harb Symp Quant Biol* 67: 267-73.

Gomei Y, Nakamura Y, Yoshihara H, Hosokawa K, Iwasaki H, Suda T, Arai F. (2010) Functional differences between two Tie2 ligands, angiopoietin-1 and -2, in regulation of adult bone marrow hematopoietic stem cells." *Exp Hematol* 38(2): 82-9.

Gratton JP, Morales-Ruiz M, Kureishi Y, Fulton D, Walsh K, Sessa WC. (2001). Akt down-regulation of p38 signaling provides a novel mechanism of vascular endothelial growth factor-mediated cytoprotection in endothelial cells. *J Biol Chem* 276(32): 30359-65.

Gurunluoglu R, Ozer K, Skugor B, Lubiatowski P, Carnevale K, Siemionow M. (2002). Effect of transfection time on the survival of epigastric skin flaps pretreated with adenovirus encoding the VEGF gene. *Ann Plast Surg* 49(2): 161-9.

Haider H, Jiang S, Idris NM, Ashraf M. (2008). IGF-1-overexpressing mesenchymal stem cells accelerate bone marrow stem cell mobilization via paracrine activation of SDF-1alpha/CXCR4 signaling to promote myocardial repair. *Circ Res* 103(11): 1300-8.

Haider H, Ye L, Jiang S, Ge R, Law PK, Chua T, Wong P, Sim EK. Angiomyogenesis for cardiac repair using human myoblasts as carriers of human vascular endothelial growth factor. *J Mol Med* 82(8): 539-49.

Haider KH, Kim HW, Ashraf M. (2009). Hypoxia-inducible factor-1alpha in stem cell preconditioning: mechanistic role of hypoxia-related micro-RNAs. *J Thorac Cardiovasc Surg* 138(1): 257.

Hamaguchi I, Morisada T, Azuma M, Murakami K, Kuramitsu M, Mizukami T, Ohbo K, Yamaguchi K, Oike Y, Dumont DJ, Suda T. (2006). Loss of Tie2 receptor compromises embryonic stem cell-derived endothelial but not hematopoietic cell survival. *Blood* 107(3): 1207-13.

Hansen TM, Singh H, Tahir TA, Brindle NP. (2010). Effects of angiopoietins-1 and -2 on the receptor tyrosine kinase Tie2 are differentially regulated at the endothelial cell surface. *Cell Signal* 22(3): 527-32.

Harfouche R, Gratton JP, Yancopoulos GD, Noseda M, Karsan A, Hussain SN. (2003). Angiopoietin-1 activates both anti- and proapoptotic mitogen-activated protein kinases. *Faseb J* 17(11): 1523-5.

Hattori K, Dias S, Heissig B, Hackett NR, Lyden D, Tateno M, Hicklin DJ, Zhu Z, Witte L, Crystal RG, Moore MA, Rafii S. (2001). Vascular endothelial growth factor and angiopoietin-1 stimulate postnatal hematopoiesis by recruitment of vasculogenic and hematopoietic stem cells. *J Exp Med* 193(9): 1005-14.

Hayes AJ, Huang WQ, Mallah J, Yang D, Lippman ME, Li LY. (1999). Angiopoietin-1 and its receptor Tie-2 participate in the regulation of capillary-like tubule formation and survival of endothelial cells. *Microvasc Res* 58(3): 224-37.

Hiasa K, Ishibashi M, Ohtani K, Inoue S, Zhao Q, Kitamoto S, Sata M, Ichiki T, Takeshita A, Egashira K. (2004). Gene transfer of stromal cell-derived factor-1alpha enhances ischemic vasculogenesis and angiogenesis via vascular endothelial growth factor/endothelial nitric oxide synthase-related pathway: next-generation chemokine therapy for therapeutic neovascularization. *Circulation* 109(20): 2454-61.

Huang H, & Tindall DJ. (2007). Dynamic FoxO transcription factors. *J Cell Sci* 120(Pt 15): 2479-87.

Huang J, Bae JO, Tsai JP, Kadenhe-Chiweshe A, Papa J, Lee A, Zeng S, Kornfeld ZN, Ullner P, Zaghloul N, Ioffe E, Nandor S, Burova E, Holash J, Thurston G, Rudge J, Yancopoulos GD, Yamashiro DJ, Kandel JJ. (2009). Angiopoietin-1/Tie-2 activation contributes to vascular survival and tumor growth during VEGF blockade. *Int J Oncol* 34(1): 79-87.

Huang J, Zhang Z, Guo J, Ni A, Deb A, Zhang L, Mirotsou M, Pratt RE, Dzau VJ. (2010) Genetic modification of mesenchymal stem cells overexpressing CCR1 increases cell viability, migration, engraftment, and capillary density in the injured myocardium. *Circ Res* 106(11): 1753-62.

Hughes DP, Marron MB, Brindle NP. (2003). The antiinflammatory endothelial tyrosine kinase Tie2 interacts with a novel nuclear factor-kappaB inhibitor ABIN-2. *Circ Res* 92(6): 630-6.

Jeon BH, Khanday F, Deshpande S, Haile A, Ozaki M, Irani K. (2003). Tie-ing the antiinflammatory effect of angiopoietin-1 to inhibition of NF-kappaB. *Circ Res* 92(6): 586-8.

Jiang S, Haider H, Idris NM, Salim A, Ashraf M. (2006). Supportive interaction between cell survival signaling and angiocompetent factors enhances donor cell survival and promotes angiomyogenesis for cardiac repair. *Circ Res* 99(7): 776-84.

Kalka C, Masuda H, Takahashi T, Gordon R, Tepper O, Gravereaux E, Pieczek A, Iwaguro H, Hayashi SI, Isner JM, Asahara T. (2000). Vascular endothelial growth factor(165) gene transfer augments circulating endothelial progenitor cells in human subjects. *Circ Res* 86(12): 1198-202.

Kanda S, Miyata Y, Mochizuki Y, Matsuyama T, Kanetake H. (2005). Angiopoietin 1 is mitogenic for cultured endothelial cells. *Cancer Res* 65(15): 6820-7.

Kim HW, Haider HK, Jiang S, Ashraf M. (2009). Ischemic preconditioning augments survival of stem cells via miR-210 expression by targeting caspase-8-associated protein 2. *J Biol Chem* 284(48): 33161-8.

Kim I, Oh JL, Ryu YS, So JN, Sessa WC, Walsh K, Koh GY. (2002). Angiopoietin-1 negatively regulates expression and activity of tissue factor in endothelial cells. *Faseb J* 16(1): 126-8.

Kim I, Ryu YS, Kwak HJ, Ahn SY, Oh JL, Yancopoulos GD, Gale NW, Koh GY. (2002). EphB ligand, ephrinB2, suppresses the VEGF- and angiopoietin 1-induced Ras/mitogen-activated protein kinase pathway in venous endothelial cells. *Faseb J* 16(9): 1126-8.

Kim KT, Choi HH, Steinmetz MO, Maco B, Kammerer RA, Ahn SY, Kim HZ, Lee GM, Koh GY. (2005). Oligomerization and multimerization are critical for angiopoietin-1 to bind and phosphorylate Tie2. *J Biol Chem* 280(20): 20126-31.

Kim SK, Pak HN, Park JH, Fang YF, Kim GI, Park YD, Hwang C, Kim YH, Kim BS. Cardiac cell therapy with mesenchymal stem cell induces cardiac nerve sprouting, angiogenesis, and reduced connexin43-positive gap junctions, but concomitant electrical pacing increases connexin43-positive gap junctions in canine heart. *Cardiol Young* 20(3): 308-17.

Koblizek TI, Weiss C, Yancopoulos GD, Deutsch U, Risau W. (1998). Angiopoietin-1 induces sprouting angiogenesis in vitro. *Curr Biol* 8(9): 529-32.

Kosacka J, Figiel M, Engele J, Hilbig H, Majewski M, Spanel-Borowski K. (2005). Angiopoietin-1 promotes neurite outgrowth from dorsal root ganglion cells positive for Tie-2 receptor. *Cell Tissue Res* 320(1): 11-9.

Labovsky V, Hofer EL, Feldman L, Fernandez Vallone V, Garcia Rivello H, Bayes-Genis A, Hernando Insua A, Levin MJ, Chasseing NA. (2010). Cardiomyogenic differentiation of human bone marrow mesenchymal cells: Role of cardiac extract from neonatal rat cardiomyocytes. *Differentiation* 79(2): 93-101.

Lee S, Kim W, Kim DH, Moon SO, Jung YJ, Lee AS, Kang KP, Jang KY, Lee SY, Sung MJ, Koh GY, Park SK. (2008). Protective effect of COMP-angiopoietin-1 on cyclosporine-induced renal injury in mice. *Nephrol Dial Transplant* 23(9): 2784-94.

Liu XB, Jiang J, Gui C, Hu XY, Xiang MX, Wang JA. (2008). Angiopoietin-1 protects mesenchymal stem cells against serum deprivation and hypoxia-induced apoptosis through the PI3K/Akt pathway. *Acta Pharmacol Sin* 29(7): 815-22.

Lu G, Haider HK, Jiang S, Ashraf M. (2009). Sca-1+ stem cell survival and engraftment in the infarcted heart: dual role for preconditioning-induced connexin-43. *Circulation* 119(19): 2587-96.

Lyons MS, Bell B, Stainier D, Peters KG. (1998). Isolation of zebrafish homologues for the tie-1 and tie-2 endothelium-specific receptor tyrosine kinases. *Dev Dyn* 212(1): 133-40.

Maisonpierre PC, Suri C, Jones PF, Bartunkova S, Wiegand SJ, Radziejewski C, Compton D, McClain J, Aldrich TH, Papadopoulos N, Daly TJ, Davis S, Sato TN, Yancopoulos GD. (1997). Angiopoietin-2, a natural antagonist for Tie2 that disrupts in vivo angiogenesis. *Science* 277(5322): 55-60.

Mangi AA, Noiseux N, Kong D, He H, Rezvani M, Ingwall JS, Dzau VJ. (2003). Mesenchymal stem cells modified with Akt prevent remodeling and restore performance of infarcted hearts. *Nat Med* 9(9): 1195-201.

Matsumoto R, Omura T, Yoshiyama M, Hayashi T, Inamoto S, Koh KR, Ohta K, Izumi Y, Nakamura Y, Akioka K, Kitaura Y, Takeuchi K, Yoshikawa J. (2005). Vascular endothelial growth factor-expressing MSC transplantation for the treatment of acute myocardial infarction. *Arterioscler Thromb Vasc Biol* 25(6): 1168-73.

McCarter SD, Lai PF, Suen RS, Stewart DJ. (2006). Regulation of endothelin-1 by Ang-1: implications for inflammation. *Exp Biol Med (Maywood)* 231(6): 985-91.

Morris PN, Dunmore BJ, Tadros A, Marchuk DA, Darland DC, D'Amore PA, Brindle NP. (2005). Functional analysis of a mutant form of the receptor tyrosine kinase Tie2 causing venous malformations. *J Mol Med* 83(1): 58-63.

Murray BW, Padrique ES, Pinko C, McTigue MA. (2001). Mechanistic effects of autophosphorylation on receptor tyrosine kinase catalysis: enzymatic characterization of Tie2 and phospho-Tie2. *Biochemistry* 40(34): 10243-53.

Nakayama T, Hatachi G, Wen CY, Yoshizaki A, Yamazumi K, Niino D, Sekine I. (2005). Expression and significance of Tie-1 and Tie-2 receptors, and angiopoietins-1, 2 and 4 in colorectal adenocarcinoma: Immunohistochemical analysis and correlation with clinicopathological factors. *World J Gastroenterol* 11(7): 964-9.

Niagara MI, Haider H, Ye L, Koh VS, Lim YT, Poh KK, Ge R, Sim EK. (2004). Autologous skeletal myoblasts transduced with a new adenoviral bicistronic vector for treatment of hind limb ischemia. *J Vasc Surg* 40(4): 774-85.

Piao W, Wang H, Inoue M, Hasegawa M, Hamada H, Huang J. (2010). Transplantation of sendai viral angiopoietin-1-modified mesenchymal stem cells for ischemic limb disease." *Angiogenesis* 13(3): 203-10.

Saharinen P, Kerkela K, Ekman N, Marron M, Brindle N, Lee GM, Augustin H, Koh GY, Alitalo K. (2005). Multiple angiopoietin recombinant proteins activate Tie1 receptor tyrosine kinase and promote its interaction with Tie2.*J Cell Biol* 169(2): 239-43.

Samuel SM, Akita Y, Paul D, Thirunavukkarasu M, Zhan L, Sudhakaran PR, Li C, Maulik N. Coadministration of adenoviral vascular endothelial growth factor and angiopoietin-1 enhances vascularization and reduces ventricular remodeling in the infarcted myocardium of type 1 diabetic rats. *Diabetes* 59(1): 51-60.

Sato TN, Tozawa Y, Deutsch U, Wolburg-Buchholz K, Fujiwara Y, Gendron-Maguire M, Gridley T, Wolburg H, Risau W, Qin Y. (1995). Distinct roles of the receptor tyrosine kinases Tie-1 and Tie-2 in blood vessel formation. *Nature* 376(6535): 70-4.

Seegar TC, Eller B, Tzvetkova-Robev D, Kolev MV, Henderson SC, Nikolov DB, Barton WA. (2010). Tie1-Tie2 interactions mediate functional differences between angiopoietin ligands. *Mol Cell* 37(5): 643-55.

Shujia J, Haider HK, Idris NM, Lu G, Ashraf M. (2008). Stable therapeutic effects of mesenchymal stem cell-based multiple gene delivery for cardiac repair. *Cardiovasc Res* 77(3): 525-33.

Shyu KG, Chang H, Isner JM. (2003). Synergistic effect of angiopoietin-1 and vascular endothelial growth factor on neoangiogenesis in hypercholesterolemic rabbit model with acute hindlimb ischemia. *Life Sci* 73(5): 563-79.

Siddiqui AJ, Blomberg P, Wardell E, Hellgren I, Eskandarpour M, Islam KB, Sylven C. (2003). Combination of Ang-1 and VEGF gene therapy enhances arteriogenesis in the ischemic myocardium. *Biochem Biophys Res Commun* 310(3): 1002-9.

Song H, Suehiro J, Kanki Y, Kawai Y, Inoue K, Daida H, Yano K, Ohhashi T, Oettgen P, Aird WC, Kodama T, Minami T. (2009). Critical role for GATA3 in mediating Tie2 expression and function in large vessel endothelial cells. *J Biol Chem* 284(42): 29109-24.

Sundberg C, Kowanetz M, Brown LF, Detmar M, Dvorak HF. (2002). Stable expression of angiopoietin-1 and other markers by cultured pericytes: phenotypic similarities to a subpopulation of cells in maturing vessels during later stages of angiogenesis in vivo. *Lab Invest* 82(4): 387-401.

Suri C, Jones PF, Patan S, Bartunkova S, Maisonpierre PC, Davis S, Sato TN, Yancopoulos GD. (1996). Requisite role of angiopoietin-1, a ligand for the TIE2 receptor, during embryonic angiogenesis. *Cell* 87(7): 1171-80.

Suri C, McClain J, Thurston G, McDonald DM, Zhou H, Oldmixon EH, Sato TN, Yancopoulos GD. (1998). Increased vascularization in mice overexpressing angiopoietin-1. *Science* 282(5388): 468-71.

Suzuki K, Murtuza B, Smolenski RT, Sammut IA, Suzuki N, Kaneda Y, Yacoub MH. (2001). Cell transplantation for the treatment of acute myocardial infarction using vascular endothelial growth factor-expressing skeletal myoblasts. *Circulation* 104(12 Suppl 1): I207-12.

Takahara K, Iioka T, Furukawa K, Uchida T, Nakashima M, Tsukazaki T, Shindo H. (2004). Autocrine/paracrine role of the angiopoietin-1 and -2/Tie2 system in cell proliferation and chemotaxis of cultured fibroblastic synoviocytes in rheumatoid arthritis. *Hum Pathol* 35(2): 150-8.

Tang J, Wang J, Guo L, Kong X, Yang J, Zheng F, Zhang L, Huang Y. (2010). Mesenchymal stem cells modified with stromal cell-derived factor 1 alpha improve cardiac remodeling via paracrine activation of hepatocyte growth factor in a rat model of myocardial infarction." *Mol Cells* 29(1): 9-19.

Tang YL, Zhao Q, Zhang YC, Cheng L, Liu M, Shi J, Yang YZ, Pan C, Ge J, Phillips MI. (2004). Autologous mesenchymal stem cell transplantation induce VEGF and neovascularization in ischemic myocardium. *Regul Pept* 117(1): 3-10.

Tao Z, Chen B, Tan X, Zhao Y, Wang L, Zhu T, Cao K, Yang Z, Kan YW, Su H. Coexpression of VEGF and angiopoietin-1 promotes angiogenesis and cardiomyocyte proliferation reduces apoptosis in porcine myocardial infarction (MI) heart. *Proc Natl Acad Sci U S A* 108(5): 2064-9.

Thomas M, Augustin HG. (2009). The role of the Angiopoietins in vascular morphogenesis. *Angiogenesis* 12(2): 125-37.

Thurston, G. (2002). "Complementary actions of VEGF and angiopoietin-1 on blood vessel growth and leakage. *J Anat* 200(6): 575-80.

Thurston G, Rudge JS, Ioffe E, Zhou H, Ross L, Croll SD, Glazer N, Holash J, McDonald DM, Yancopoulos GD. (2000). Angiopoietin-1 protects the adult vasculature against plasma leakage. *Nat Med* 6(4): 460-3.

Thurston G, Suri C, Smith K, McClain J, Sato TN, Yancopoulos GD, McDonald DM. (1999). Leakage-resistant blood vessels in mice transgenically overexpressing angiopoietin-1. *Science* 286(5449): 2511-4.

Tuo QH, Xiong GZ, Zeng H, Yu HD, Sun SW, Ling HY, Zhu BY, Liao DF, Chen JX. (2010). Angiopoietin-1 protects myocardial endothelial cell function blunted by angiopoietin-2 and high glucose condition. *Acta Pharmacol Sin* 32(1): 45-51.

Uemura R, Xu M, Ahmad N, Ashraf M. (2006). BM stem cells prevent left ventricular remodeling of ischemic heart through paracrine signaling." *Circ Res* 98(11): 1414-21.

Valenzuela DM, Griffiths JA, Rojas J, Aldrich TH, Jones PF, Zhou H, McClain J, Copeland NG, Gilbert DJ, Jenkins NA, Huang T, Papadopoulos N, Maisonpierre PC, Davis S, Yancopoulos GD. (1999). Angiopoietins 3 and 4: diverging gene counterparts in mice and humans. *Proc Natl Acad Sci U S A* 96(5): 1904-9.

Voskas D, Jones N, Van Slyke P, Sturk C, Chang W, Haninec A, Babichev YO, Tran J, Master Z, Chen S, Ward N, Cruz M, Jones J, Kerbel RS, Jothy S, Dagnino L, Arbiser J, Klement G, Dumont DJ. (2005). A cyclosporine-sensitive psoriasis-like disease produced in Tie2 transgenic mice. *Am J Pathol* 166(3): 843-55.

Wang H, Zhang Y, Toratani S, Okamoto T. (2004). Transformation of vascular endothelial cells by a point mutation in the Tie2 gene from human intramuscular haemangioma. *Oncogene* 23(53): 8700-4.

Wang Y, Haider HK, Ahmad N, Xu M, Ge R, Ashraf M. (2006). Combining pharmacological mobilization with intramyocardial delivery of bone marrow cells over-expressing VEGF is more effective for cardiac repair. *J Mol Cell Cardiol* 40(5): 736-45.

Witzenbichler B, Maisonpierre PC, Jones P, Yancopoulos GD, Isner JM. (1998). Chemotactic properties of angiopoietin-1 and -2, ligands for the endothelial-specific receptor tyrosine kinase Tie2. *J Biol Chem* 273(29): 18514-21.

Yau TM, Kim C, Li G, Zhang Y, Fazel S, Weisel RD, Li RK. (2007). Enhanced angiogenesis with multimodal cell-based gene therapy. *Ann Thorac Surg* 83(3): 1110-9.

Ye L, Haider H, Jiang S, Tan RS, Ge R, Law PK, Sim EK. (2007). Improved angiogenic response in pig heart following ischaemic injury using human skeletal myoblast simultaneously expressing VEGF165 and angiopoietin-1. *Eur J Heart Fail* 9(1): 15-22.

Ye L, Haider H, Jiang S, Tan RS, Toh WC, Ge R, Sim EK. (2007). Angiopoietin-1 for myocardial angiogenesis: a comparison between delivery strategies. *Eur J Heart Fail* 9(5): 458-65.

Ye L, Haider H, Tan R, Toh W, Law PK, Tan W, Su L, Zhang W, Ge R, Zhang Y, Lim Y, Sim EK. (2007). Transplantation of nanoparticle transfected skeletal myoblasts overexpressing vascular endothelial growth factor-165 for cardiac repair. *Circulation* 116(11 Suppl): I113-20.

Yu Y, Varughese J, Brown LF, Mulliken JB, Bischoff J. (2001). Increased Tie2 expression, enhanced response to angiopoietin-1, and dysregulated angiopoietin-2 expression in hemangioma-derived endothelial cells. *Am J Pathol* 159(6): 2271-80.

Zhu WH, Han J, Nicosia RF. (2003). Requisite role of p38 MAPK in mural cell recruitment during angiogenesis in the rat aorta model. *J Vasc Res* 40(2): 140-8.

Zhu WH, MacIntyre A, Nicosia RF. (2002). Regulation of angiogenesis by vascular endothelial growth factor and angiopoietin-1 in the rat aorta model: distinct temporal patterns of intracellular signaling correlate with induction of angiogenic sprouting. *Am J Pathol* 161(3): 823-30.

Part 2

Pathogenesis of Myocarditis

10

The Key Players of Coxsackievirus-Induced Myocarditis

Pamela J. Lincez, Marine Walic and Marc S. Horwitz
Department of Microbiology and Immunology,
University of British Columbia
Canada

1. Introduction

Myocarditis is a devastating cardiac disease causing death in children and young adults worldwide (Esfandiarei et al. 2008). The disease is clinically characterized by inflammation of the myocardium and degeneration of myocytes. Clinical symptoms of viral myocarditis range from flu-like and/or gastrointestinal illness to ventricular dysfunction ending commonly in heart failure. Acute disease is accompanied by multi-organ abnormalities and presents mostly in neonates and young children. Chronic disease occurs in one third of patients and is likely a consequence of autoimmune-mediated myocardial injury and viral persistence. As cardiac myocytes are destroyed by virus and/or self-induced cytopathic immune effects, excessive repair or fibrosis of myocardial tissue impairs disease progression rather than protects the tissue from further damage. Fibrosis or scar tissue, can lead to abnormal ventricular architecture that inevitably leads to the disruption of its function. At this stage of disease, chronic myocarditis progresses to dilated cardiomyopathy and can eventually lead to congestive heart failure (Esfandiarei et al. 2008).

The exact cause for myocarditis is still unknown though pathogen infections, hypersensitivity reactions, and systemic and autoimmune diseases are all likely contributing factors. It is suggested that acute viral myocarditis that progresses to chronic disease mirrors the clinical pathology observed with dilated cardiomyopathy patients and is likely the result of an inappropriate immune response after virus infection that leads to chronic inflammation and virus persistence (Escher et al. 2011).

Tracking the incidence of myocarditis is challenging. It is difficult to determine the potential disease burden to populations since there is a range in clinical symptoms associated with disease and endomyocardial biopsy to diagnose disease is rarely practised (Blauwet et al. 2010). Though mounting evidence of viral genomes recovered from chronic dilated cardiomyopathy patients provides some insight in to the potential burden of this devastating cardiac disease (Kuhl et al. 2005). Viral-induced myocarditis and dilated cardiomyopathy leads to a worse prognosis than other possible myocarditis/dilated cardiomyopathy etiological agents. Isolation of enteroviral RNA from endocardial biopsies of myocarditis and dilated cardiomyopathy patients renders these patients six times more susceptible to death after two years from diagnosis compared to virus-negative patients (Why et al. 1994). Sex is another contributing factor to disease susceptibility. Initially, it was reported that men develop myocarditis twice as often as women and recent clinical work as supported this notion though the incidence is not quite as high as claimed in 1980 (Woodruff 1980; Mason et al. 1995; Kuhl et al. 2003; Cooper 2009).

Diagnosis and treatment of viral myocarditis is challenging due to the lack in specific clinical features and signature serological markers known for the acute phase of disease. The standard Dallas criteria that were typically used for diagnosis of myocarditis are not appropriate for determining viral or autoimmune myocarditis since they avoid the identification of inflammation or viral genome in the heart (Aretz 1987; Aretz et al. 1987). A more appropriate set of guidelines was established in 1995 by the WHO, with a classification of cardiomyopathies requiring endomyocardial biopsy, histological Dallas criteria, immunohistochemistry and viral PCR amongst the criteria for diagnosis (Richardson et al. 1996). Four stages of clinical disease in humans have been described since the implication of the 1995 WHO criteria: fulminant, subacute, chronic active and chronic persistent myocarditis. The first three stages involve mild to moderate dysfunction of the left ventricle, with the fourth, chronic persistent stage, characterized by normal ventricular function. Both chronic stages have ongoing inflammation with the development of scar tissue from myocardial damage. It is only during the chronic persistent stage that viral genome is detected from endomyocardial biopsy tissue (Lieberman et al. 1991; Olsen 1993). The incidence of viral infection, specifically coxsackievirus B infection, in human myocarditis, originates from seroepidemiologic and molecular studies between the 1950s and 1990s and from observations of viral genomes in cardiac tissue more prevalently in dilated cardiomyopathy patients compared to valvular or ischemic cardiomyopathies.

The true etiology and molecular pathogenesis responsible for viral myocarditis in humans remains unclear. Serological studies and endomyocardial biopsies from myocarditis patients have associated over 20 different viruses including coxsackieviruses, adenoviruses, cytomegaloviruses, parvoviruses, influenza viruses, and even human immunodeficiency viruses with the disease (Yajima et al. 2009; Blauwet et al. 2010). Of all the viruses implicated, it is the enteroviruses, specifically coxsackievirus B, which show the most likely contribution.

Coxsackievirus A and B are enteroviruses that are a part of the *Picornaviridae* family (Baboonian et al. 1997). They are human pathogens transmitted fecal-orally that cause enteric diseases (coxsackievirus A) as well as severe disease in the heart, pancreas, and central nervous system (coxsackievirus B) (Baboonian et al. 1997). Coxsackievirus A has 23 different serotypes, whereas coxsackievirus B has six. The six coxsackievirus B serotypes can instigate a variety of diseases including two very important autoimmune diseases: myocarditis and type I diabetes (Richer et al. 2009). It is also important to note that all coxsackievirus B serotypes are capable of triggering systemic disease in infants that can devastating lead to death (Esfandiarei et al. 2008). Relevant to myocarditis is the coxsackievirus B serotype 3 (coxsackievirus B3). Coxsackievirus B3 has been linked to approximately 30% of new dilated cardiomyopathy cases per anum though data establishing a direct link between coxsackievirus B3 pathogenesis and the onset of myocarditis in patients is lacking (Huber et al. 1998). The B3 serotype has a 7.4-kb single-stranded positive-sense RNA genome containing a VPg (3B) protein at the 5′ end. The 7-methyl guanosine-like cap influences replication and translation following virus entry (Flanegan et al. 1977). To gain entry in to a cell, coxsackieviruses interact with both coxsackievirus and adenovirus receptor (CAR) and decay accelerating factor (DAF) located both in the host cell membrane (Figure 1) (Pelletier et al. 1988).

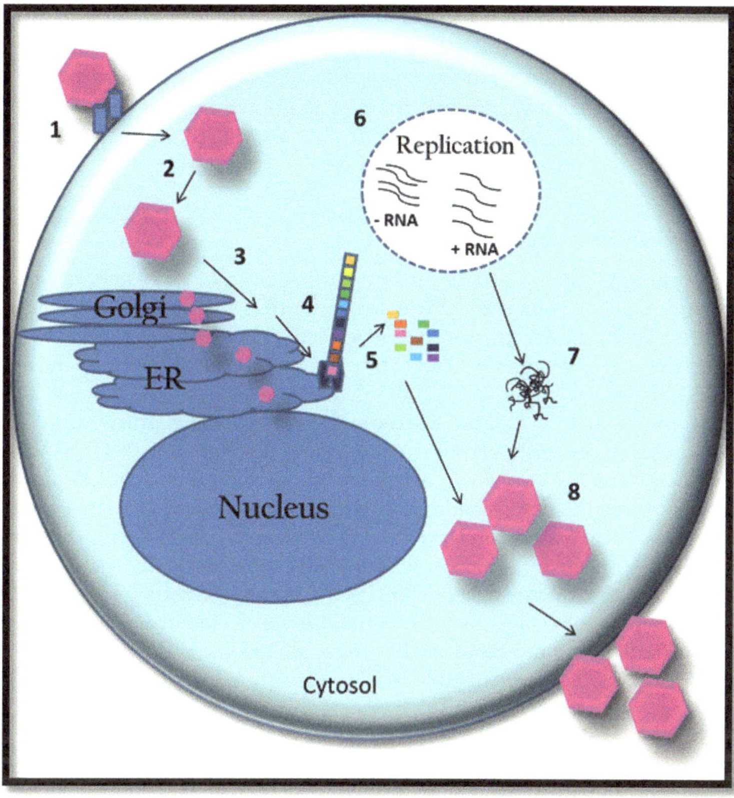

Fig. 1. Tentative coxsackievirus life cycle. The general host and virus components suggested to contribute to production of new coxksackievirus: 1) Viral entry through binding coxsackievirus and adenovirus receptor (CAR) and decay accelerating factor (DAF), 2) Internalization and transport of viral particles to the Golgi and endoplasmic reticulum (ER) 3) viral uncoating, 4) release of viral RNA, translation of RNA by ribosomes on the rough endoplasmic reticulum (ER) into viral polyprotein, 5) autocleavage of polyprotein into viral structural and functions proteins, 6) positive and negative strand RNA transcription to replicate viral genome, 7) release of viral genome in to the cytosol to encapsidate with structural proteins, 8) formation and release of viral progeny.

Once the virus enters the cytosol and uncoats, its positive-sense genome is released in the cytosol for translation and later, transcription. As a polyprotein comprised of the virus proteins VP4, VP3, VP2, VP, 2A, 2B, 2C, 3A, 3B, 3C, and 3D emerges from translation at the rough endoplasmic reticulum (ER), it is cleaved into its respective structural and functional proteins. The virally encoded $3D^{pol}$ is a RNA-dependent RNA polymerase that transcribes viral positive-sense RNA in to negative-sense RNA strands that serve as intermediates for the transcription of multiple positive-sense RNA strands needed for new progeny virions. After synthesis, the newly generated positive-RNA strands are packaged in new virus particles formed by the newly generated structural and functional virus proteins. The new progeny viruses are then released via plasma membrane by a mechanism likely mediated by viral protein 2B (van Kuppeveld et al. 1997; Esfandiarei et al. 2008). Though many groups have identified key virus and host interactions throughout the coxsackievirus B life cycle, there still remains many stages unsolved. Nevertheless, the role of coxsackievirus B in the onset of myocarditis has been extensively studied thus far in animal models and cell culture systems. Here, we will discuss clinical and mouse studies that have investigated coxsackievirus-induced myocarditis and the role of key immune players in disease pathogenesis.

2. *In vivo* experimental systems

Mice provide a model system to distinguish characteristics of disease between autoimmune myocarditis and viral myocarditis. Mice are advantageous models because they share similar genetics to humans, they are cost-effective in handling and breeding, many transgenic strains are available and they are responsive to cardiotropic viruses (Cunningham 2001; Fairweather et al. 2001; Esfandiarei et al. 2008). Coxsackievirus B3 has been detected in 30-50% of dilated cardiomyopathy patients, providing support for a coxsackievirus B3-induced myocarditis mouse model (Escher et al. 2011). Following a single dose of coxsackievirus B3, acute myocarditis, encephalomeningitis, hepatitis, and even pancreatitis can ensue. Severe systemic pathogenicity observed with coxsackievirus B3 infection has also been related to the presence of sarcoma (Src) family kinase Lck ($p56^{lck}$) (Liu et al. 2000). With coxsackievirus B3 infection, mice tend to either develop chronic dilated cardiomyopathy mirroring clinical disease after recovering from viral infection or mice die from severe cytopathic effects, thus making coxsackievirus B3-induced myocarditis an excellent yet challenging model to study (Liu et al. 2000).

Studies with mice have demonstrated the significant contribution of the Th1 immune response to disease severity even though coxsackievirus B3 directly targets and destroys the myocardium. The contribution of a Th1 response to viral myocarditis pathogenesis is supported by studies modulating and inhibiting immune components and improving cardiac damage and function (Jiang et al. 2008).

Interestingly and in parallel with human myocarditis, male mice infected with coxsackievirus B3 experience acute myocarditis with greater severity compared to females. Greater disease severity in males has been linked to enhanced cardiac and splenic mast cell and macrophage TLR-4 expression at 12 hours post-infection (Frisancho-Kiss et al. 2006; Frisancho-Kiss et al. 2007). In males virally infected, signalling through cardiac TLR-4 enhances the production of cardiac IL-1β and IL-18 and promotes a Th1 skewed immune response (Fairweather et al. 2003). Also, male mice infected with coxsackievirus B3 harbour macrophages of a different phenotype and have more severe disease compared to infected female mice though viral replication is at similar levels in the heart (Frisancho-Kiss et al. 2006; Frisancho-Kiss et al. 2007). Moreover, genes relating to cholesterol metabolism in macrophages and to androgen receptor, which are known predictors for myocarditis, dilated cardiomyopathy and heart failure in male mice and humans, are upregulated considerably in spleens of male mice (Onyimba et al. 2011). This not only affords support for a gender difference in the susceptibility to viral-myocarditis, but critically implicates the innate response in disease severity. Furthermore, to bring male mice to the same immunological plane as female mice during myocarditis, Frisancho-Kiss et al removed the gonads from BALB/c mice and observed an increase in IL-4 production, the activation of macrophages and induction of regulatory T cells in the heart (Frisancho-Kiss et al. 2009).

Myocarditis can be induced in female mice with TNF-α treatment on days 1 and 3 post coxsackievirus B3 infection (Huber 2010). The lack of disease susceptibility in females is attributed to low mRNA and protein levels of TNF-α and IL-Iβ as well as reduced CD1d expression on splenic lymphocytes. CD1d is an important non-classical major histocompatibility complex antigen that can be regulated by TNF-α to induce myocarditis susceptibility in female mice (Huber 2010).

Not only is susceptibility to developing myocarditis dictating by sex, but development of chronic disease depends on the mouse strain. A.BY/SnJ & SWR/J are susceptible mouse strains that can develop ongoing myocarditis, where viral RNA is detected within the myocardium. C57BL/6J & DBA/1J mice are resistant strains capable of eliminating virus just after the early acute phase of disease. Tomioka and colleagues investigated neutralizing antibodies and their role in virus-induced myocarditis and B-cell-mediated immunity using BALB/c mice (Esfandiarei et al. 2008). NK-deficient mice have been used to look at the role of natural killer (NK) cells in killing virus-infected cardiomyocytes (Godeny et al. 1986). Perforin knockout mice inoculated with coxsackievirus B3 have also been used to describe the interplay of virus infection and lymphocyte infiltration in the myocytes and their effect on disease outcome (Godeny et al. 1987). Interestingly, with coxsackievirus B3 infection in suckling, weaning and adolescent mice, coxsackievirus B3 replicates in the heart, pancreas, spleen, and brain and causes human disease-like symptoms. In fact, following IP injection, three distinct immunovirological phases of disease have been observed.

In mice, coxsackievirus B3 can induce two forms of inflammatory heart disease, acute only or acute and chronic (biphasic) autoimmune disease (Horwitz et al. 2000; Cunningham 2001; Fairweather et al. 2001). Interestingly, coxsackievirus B3 replication is mainly observed in the pancreas and to a lesser extent in the heart. In genetically susceptible mice, such as A/J2, Balb/c and NOD mice, chronic autoimmune myocarditis after coxsackievirus B3 infection is observed. Autoimmune myocarditis in mice presents as early as day 7 pi with inflammatory cell infiltration in the heart and the formation of multifocal inflammatory lesions. At this stage, autoantibodies (autoAbs) against heart antigens, like cardiac myosin (cardiac myosin), are seen. In NOD mice, isotype switching ensues after 2 to 3 weeks, with the autoAbs switching from IgM to IgG subclasses (Kaya et al. 2001; Kaya et al. 2002). It is particularly remarkable to note that the chronic autoimmune heart disease induced by coxsackievirus B3 in mice resembles inflammatory heart disease seen with myocarditis and dilated cardiomyopathy in humans. There are still many complications with the full characterization and study of chronic virus and/or autoimmune induced myocarditis in mice and humans. One such complication is the acute infection that precedes chronic disease.

3. Experimental autoimmune myocarditis

As described in the previous section, mouse models greatly aid the analysis of autoimmune diseases. To set apart the autoimmune phase of disease from acute infection an experimental induced autoimmune myocarditis model was developed (Blyszczuk et al. 2008). Experimental induced autoimmune myocarditis mimics the typical chronic phase of disease observed in genetically susceptible mice infected with coxsackievirus B and different stages of disease severity observed with experimental induced autoimmune myocarditis models are graded according to the extent of inflammatory infiltrates at the peak of inflammation. Autoimmune myocarditis can be induced by the injection of cardiac myosin with complete Freund's adjuvant and pertussis toxin. Mice injected with this combination of self- antigen and adjuvants are able to generate cardiac myosin-specific autoantibodies and present with heart pathology similar to coxsackievirus B3-induced disease 3 weeks post-injection (Figure 2) (Kodama et al. 1992).

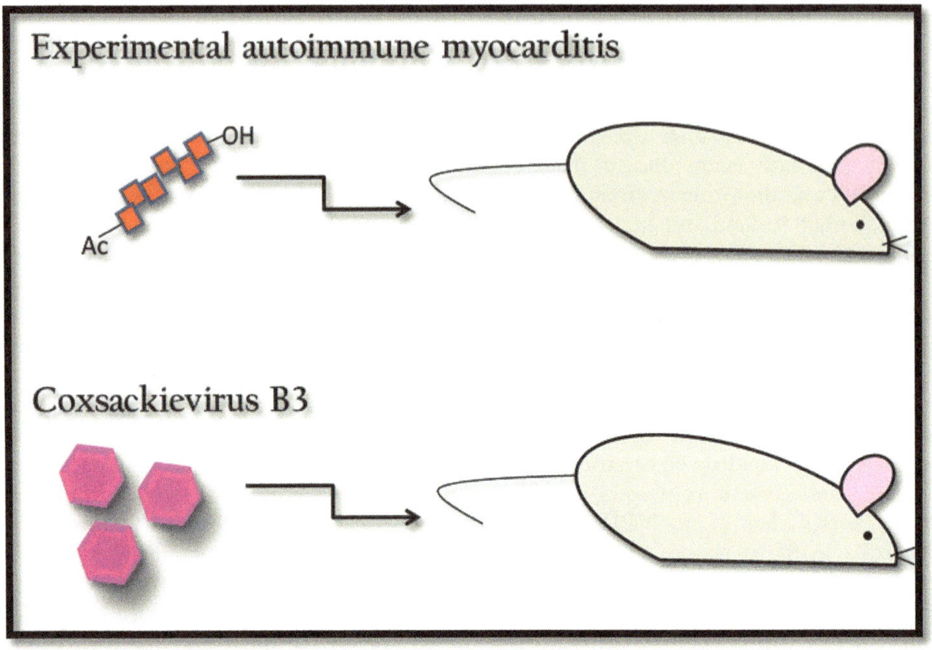

Fig. 2. Experimental autoimmune myocarditis versus coxsackievirus B3 induced myocarditis. Experimental autoimmune myocarditis involves the induction of autoimmunity by the injection of self-protein such as cardiac myosin or troponin I with adjuvants or without or injections of other cardiomyogenic peptides to induce chronic myocarditis as seen with coxsackievirus B3 infection in susceptible mice.

Neu et al suggest that autoimmune myocarditis is induced indirectly by viral infection and that one causative factor may be an autoimmune response to the cardiac myosin released or exposed after the virus-mediated myocyte damage (Neu et al. 1987). If this is the case, autoimmune disease should be induced by immunization with cardiac myosin alone and susceptibility to coxsackievirus B3-induced autoimmune myocarditis should be as likely as susceptibility to the myosin-induced autoimmune disease (Neu et al. 1987). Troponin I has also been used as an autoantigen for induced autoimmune myocarditis (Leuschner et al. 2009). Programmed cell death-1 receptor deficient mice develop cardiomyopathy with production of high-titered autoantibodies against cardiac troponin I (Okazaki et al. 2003). Cardiac troponin I induces a robust autoimmune response that encompasses both humoral and cellular responses that leads to severe inflammation and fibrosis in the myocardium of mice. Mice induced with cardiac troponin I have a genetic and sex biased susceptibility for myocardial inflammation compared to other autoimmune disease models (Leuschner et al. 2009). The key to reproducing ideal autoimmune disease conditions for studying myocarditis is to use a defined immunogen, ie cardiac myosin, troponin I etc. obtained from the same species as the study's model. Moreover, genetically defined inbred strains of susceptible and resistant mice allow results to be reproducible and facilitate detailed analysis of the autoimmune disease cellular and molecular components (Neu et al. 1987).

Other species such as rats and Guinea pigs have also greatly contributed to our understanding of myocarditis. Immunization of different animal models with heart homogenates derived from various species has not been, unfortunately, successful at inducing myocarditis, where the results were often controversial (Neu et al. 1987). In most of those models, mild lesions appeared in the heart. However, out of the differing species models, 2 reports: the guinea pig model by Hosenpud et al and the murine model by Neu et al, showed enlargement of the heart with autoimmune myocarditis (Hosenpud et al. 1985; Neu et al. 1987). The authors also noted discoloration of cardiac surfaces, pericardial effusion and lethal clinical course that were conditions not previously observed in experimental induced autoimmune myocarditis. Kodama et al were also able to produce such pathological and clinical conditions using the Lewis rat model (Kodama et al. 1992) though the cardiac myosin immunization murine model seems to have had the greatest impact on our understanding of autoimmune myocarditis.

There are many ways in which autoimmune myocarditis can been induced in animal models. Immunization of susceptible mice with cardiac myosin or with a myocardiogenic peptide derived from the alpha cardiac heavy chain emulsified in complete Freund's adjuvant induces myocarditis in mice with a peak of inflammation in the heart around day 21. This inflammation observed with induced autoimmune disease is similar to that seen in the coxsackievirus B3 induced autoimmune myocarditis model during the chronic phase, however in this case, does not include the earlier complication of a pathogen infection. The immunization with cardiac myosin is associated with production of cardiac myosin-specific autoantibodies and cardiac myosin-specific T cells (Kodama et al. 1992; Godsel et al. 2001; Leuschner et al. 2009; Rose 2010). It has been demonstrated that the induction of disease by immunization with cardiac myosin can only be successful in genetically susceptible mice (Neu et al. 1987). We suggest that the complex genetics of the host therefore determines whether an infection will resolve or proceed to an adverse autoimmune outcome (Poffenberger et al. 2010). Identifying particular traits that favour susceptibility or resistance to an autoimmune incidence helps us understand how infectious diseases culminate in autoimmune disease. Other methods used to induce autoimmune myocarditis include administration of 2 early, critical proinflammatory cytokines, IL1b and TNF-α and injection of mice with myosin in combination with CFA and additional lipopolysaccharide. Some groups have reported the induction of autoimmune myocarditis using immunization with porcine cardiac myosin (Wang et al. 1999). Interestingly, Wittner et al. produced myosin autoantibodies and myocarditis in rabbits using immunization with bovine heart myosin (Wittner et al. 1983). Daniels et al reported the development of a recombinant model of experimental induced autoimmune myocarditis, induced by immunization with a 68kDa fragment of cardiac myosin referred to as Myo4 (Daniels et al. 2008). Myo4 induces severe autoimmune myocarditis in A/J mice 21 days post immunization. The immune response to Myo4 immunization is characterized by Th1 and Th17 features. Myo4-experimental induced autoimmune myocarditis has advantages over other models in terms of immunogen production and the ability to measure antigen-specific functional immunity in *ex vivo* assays. Myo4 and other immunoantigen experimental induced autoimmune myocarditis provide a means to investigate epitope spreading and the effect on disease pathology as well as prophylactic and therapeutic treatment studies aimed at developing therapeutics to alleviate acute and chronic autoimmune myocarditis (Daniels et al. 2008).

Experimental induced autoimmune myocarditis is mediated by a CD4+ T cell immune response. Homing of cardiac myosin-specific CD4+ T cells into the myocardium is the first pathologic event observed with experimental induced autoimmune myocarditis. Subsequently, neurohumoral factors such as cytokines and chemokines are released in the myocardium. This then recruits various bystander inflammatory cells to cross vascular endothelial cell walls and enter the myocardium. In effect, blocking the recruitment of inflammatory mediators to the myocardium may present as a critical target for myocarditis therapy (Tanaka et al. 2011). Experimental induced autoimmune myocarditis development is also typically associated with elevated titers of heart-specific autoantibodies, though in rats and susceptible mouse strains the response depends on the induction and expansion of heart specific, autoreactive CD4+ T cells. In BALB/c mice, CD4+ T cells belong to a specific subset of IL-17 producing helper cells, i.e. Th17 cells (Chang et al. 2008). With experimental induced autoimmune myocarditis, heart-infiltrating alpha-myosin-specific CD4+ Th17 cells are pathogenic and cause ongoing inflammation in the myocardium (Blyszczuk et al. 2008). Notably, autoimmune myocarditis induced by myosin can be reiterated in mice adoptively transferred with pathogenic CD4+ T lymphocytes (Sukumaran et al. 2011). In addition to T cells, passive administration of antimyosin monoclonal antibodies induces myocarditis in DBA/2 but not in BALB/c mice. DBA/2 mice are susceptible to passively induced disease due to the presence of myosin or a myosin like protein in their extracellular matrix. In addition to antibodies and T cells contributing to the pathogenesis of inflammatory myocardial lesions (Leuschner et al. 2009), injection of activated bone marrow (BM)-derived dendritic cells loaded with heart-specific self peptide can instigate disease pathogenesis (Kania et al. 2009).

Autoimmune myocarditis can be induced experimentally by several means as is the case for protection from induced disease. Amelioration of disease has been demonstrated with oral administration of specific antigens in several autoimmune models (Gonnella et al. 2009). Protection from experimental induced autoimmune myocarditis has also been observed with many studies from Godsel et al (Godsel et al. 2001). They successfully administered syngeneic splenocytes covalently coupled with ethylene carbodiimide (ECDI) by intravenous injections to prevent and treat a number of autoimmune diseases in animal models. Initial application of this approach in humans has been fortunately successful. Godsel et al essentially demonstrate in animal models that coupled-cell tolerance is an effective approach for the prevention of myocarditis and may present as a useful antigen-specific immunotherapy for treating myocarditis in humans (Godsel et al. 2001). Antigen-specific peripheral tolerance induction also represents a powerful tool for dissecting the mechanisms involved in cardiac autoimmunity. Although myosin-specific tolerization is commonly used to prevent experimental induced autoimmune myocarditis, it is also important to note that tissue homogenates are equally useful. This approach has yet to be tested in other models of myocarditis including coxsackievirus myocarditis (Godsel et al. 2001). Horwitz et al's investigation in to cardiac myosin tolerance and protection from experimental induced autoimmune myocarditis conflicted with results presented in the Godsel et al studies (Horwitz et al. 2005). Since cardiac myosin is a major autoantigen in virus-induced myocarditis the question was asked whether inhibition of this autoantibody response to cardiac myosin could prevent destructive autoimmunity. In NOD mice, cardiac myosin-specific antibodies develop following both coxsackievirus B3 infection and experimental induced autoimmune myocarditis induction. To ask whether the induction of peripheral tolerance to a single self-antigen could be used to prevent coxsackieviral-induced autoimmune myocarditis, a disease likely directed at multiple self-antigens, NOD mice were tolerized to cardiac myosin using a covalently coupled antigen approach and subsequently challenged with coxsackievirus B3. Cardiac myosin tolerance to effectively prevent coxsackievirus B3-mediated autoimmune myocarditis was not observed, possibly reprimanding cardiac myosin as a single autoantigen player in viral-mediated disease (Horwitz et al. 2005).

Another possible player in viral-mediated disease as demonstrated with experimental induced autoimmune myocarditis may be multinucleated giant cells. Wang et al showed that the cardiac lesions in experimental induced autoimmune myocarditis are histologically similar to human myocarditis, with myocyte swelling, necrosis, and fibrosis that are accompanied by mononuclear cell infiltration consisting of granulocytes, macrophages, CD4+, CD8+ T cells, B cells and multinucleated giant cells (Wang et al. 1999; Blyszczuk et al. 2008; Daniels et al. 2008). Also, the histological features observed in myocarditis induced by cardiac myosin are very similar to the description of active giant-cell myocarditis in humans (Wang et al. 1999; Blyszczuk et al. 2008). Therefore, it has been inferred that macrophage-derived multinucleated giant cells, together with other inflammatory cells, are important mediators of myocyte destruction. The presence of a heterogeneous population of cellular components in the cardiac infiltrate also implies the existence of a complex, cytokine-rich microenvironment that may contribute to the pathogenesis of autoimmune myocarditis. TNF-α, IL-1β, IL-2, IFN-γ, IL-4 and IL-10 are cytokines that have been detected in culture supernatants of splenocytes derived from mice at the peak of myocardial disease. Their detected levels were higher in mice that developed myocarditis than mice immunized but not developing disease. Furthermore, it has been previously suggested that TNF-α contributes to myocarditis pathogenesis by either causing direct injury of cardiomyocytes or, together with IL1b, triggering the production of nitric oxide. The expression of E-selectin, VCAM-1 and ICAM-1 has also been found to be markedly increased in inflamed hearts during induced disease. The increased expression of these adhesion molecules on the vascular endothelium may contribute to the extravasation and accumulation of inflammatory cells observed in the myocardium (Wang et al. 1999; Blyszczuk et al. 2008).

There are limitations of using experimental induced autoimmune myocarditis as a model to separate the mechanisms of biphasic (acute infection and chronic) viral disease, where the model relies too heavily on the inoculation of a single antigen. There are undoubtedly other key immune players that contribute to the onset of autoimmune disease following virus infection with the innate immune system being one of the major contributors having a dual role: controlling and perpetuating disease. Despite the fact that the experimental induced autoimmune myocarditis models are rather artificial, they offer the advantage of studying disease pathogenesis and autoimmune mechanisms *in vivo* in the absence of an infective agent. Immunization with myosin peptide-loaded activated dendritic cells offers a useful tool to dissect the role of antigen-presenting cells (APCs) and effector cells while studying disease mechanisms. From the experimental induced autoimmune myocarditis model we can not only learn about autoimmune mechanisms contributing to disease development, but we can study the pathophysiology of inflammatory heart disease and design novel immunomodulating treatment strategies. In addition, the experimental induced autoimmune myocarditis model might offer a potential tool to improve the diagnostic accuracy of currently available and future imaging technologies (Blyszczuk et al. 2008).

Work from our lab using the experimental induced autoimmune myocarditis model has helped focus our attention to the role of innate immunity in response to an infectious agent and as a driving force in the development of autoimmune disease. The innate immune system includes many key players like pathogen recognition receptors that recognize highly conserved pathogen-associated molecular patterns on microbial invaders. These receptors include the Toll-like receptors and expression of these receptors on antigen presenting cells such as macrophages and dendritic cells determine not only innate immunity but the subsequent adaptive immune response.

4. Key players in immunity

4.1 Pathogen recognition receptors

Cardiotropic viruses can be cytopathic, killing off host cells, yet their viral RNA is detected and tends to persist in cardiac muscle. Viral persistence in the myocardium can then lead to chronic inflammatory cardiomyopathy. Pathogens such as viruses are recognized by Toll-like receptors (TLRs) and other pattern recognition receptors of the innate immune response. The recognition of a pathogenic insult releases proinflammatory cytokines that serve as protectors from infection and perpetrators of chronic inflammatory disease (Lane et al. 1993; Kawai et al. 2006). Activation of Toll-like receptors by pathogen associated molecular patterns and the subsequent production of proinflammatory cytokines can lead to protection as well as the exacerbation of an autoimmune response.

Pathogen-associated molecular patterns from viruses like double-stranded RNA are sensed by Toll-like receptor 3 (TLR3) (Schnare et al. 2001; Pasare et al. 2003). Infections with coxsackievirus B in TLR3 knock out mice have demonstrated an important role for TLR3 in host defense. The innate antiviral response is mediated, at least in part, by nucleic acid-sensing receptors such as TLR3, retinoic acid inducible gene I (RIG-I), and melanoma differentiation-associated protein-5 (MDA-5). The activation of RIG-I/MDA5 receptor pathways is thought to evoke type I IFN responses. TLR3, which recognizes double stranded RNA, is critical in the antiviral immune response against coxsackievirus B3. TLR3-deficient mice are highly susceptible to coxsackievirus B3, where impaired antiviral responses and acute myocarditis ensue. Increased disease in TLR knock out mice is associated with decreased production of IL-12p40, IFNγ and IL-1β post infection. Mice deficient in the TLR3 adaptor protein, Trif, have a similar disease course as TLR3 knock out mice suggesting that the TLR3-Trif pathway is also important in the host response to coxsackievirus B3 infection. Research from Negishi et al reveals a critical cooperation between the RIG-I/MDA5-type I IFN and TLR3-type II IFN signaling axes for efficient innate antiviral immune responses (Negishi et al. 2008). Importantly, a rare TLR3 variant has been identified in patients diagnosed with enteroviral myocarditis (Gorbea et al. 2010). These patients also held a greatly increased incidence of a common polymorphism. Gorbea et al also demonstrated that induction of the TLR3 variant or the TLR3 possessing the common polymorphism with synthetic double stranded RNA hindered proper TLR3-mediated signaling. Also, with coxsackievirus B3 infected cell lines, mutated TLR3 impaired type I IFN signalling and production and failed to control viral replication (Gorbea et al. 2010). The Gorbea et al study thus suggests that individuals who possess these particular TLR3 variants may have an ineffective innate anti-enteroviral response that fails to clear the virus and in turn, elevates the associative risk for cardiac disease. Interestingly, human cardiac myosin pathogenic epitopes can directly stimulate other human Toll-like receptors such as Toll-like receptors 2 and 8 (TLR2, TLR8). Stimulation of these receptors allows for the production of proinflammatory cytokines from human monocytes. TLR8, found within endosomes, detects single stranded RNA, such as the coxsackievirus B3 genome and instigates inflammation (Triantafilou et al. 2005; Zhang et al. 2009).

Signalling through another critical receptor, Toll-like receptor 4 (TLR4) also leads to the expression of proinflammatory cytokines, but has been implicated as a cardiomyopathy etiological factor. Satoh et al have suggested that myocardial expression of TLR4 is linked to coxsackievirus B3 replication in human cardiomyopathy and that TLR4 may be directly involved in the pathogenesis of disease (Satoh et al. 2004). Viral proteins have actually been found to co-localize with TLR4 in infected cardiac tissue. In coxsackievirus B infected mice, TLR4 deficiency reduces viral pathogenesis and the production of several cytokines including IL-1β and IL-18 (Pasare et al. 2003; Pasare et al. 2004).

Another major player in host defense is the critical adaptor protein for TLR signaling myeloid differentiation primary response gene (MyD88). MyD88 signaling has been associated with several aspects of the pathogenesis of chronic autoimmune myocarditis. MyD88 activates self-antigen presenting cells and promotes autoreactive CD4+ T-cell expansion in experimental induced autoimmune myocarditis. To determine the role of MyD88 in the progression of acute myocarditis to an end-stage heart failure, Blyszczuk et al used alpha-myosin heavy chain peptide (MyHC-alpha)-loaded activated dendritic cells (Blyszczuk et al. 2008). They induced myocarditis in wild-type and MyD88 knock out mice and observed comparable heart-infiltrating cell subsets and CD4+ T-cell responses. Injection of complete Freund's adjuvant or MyHC-alpha/complete Freund's adjuvant into diseased mice caused cardiac fibrosis, ventricular dilation, and disrupted heart function in wild-type but not MyD88 knock out mice (Pasare et al. 2003; Marty et al. 2006; Blyszczuk et al. 2008). The protection of MyD88 knock out mice from the induction of experimental induced autoimmune myocarditis is likely from the impairment of other key players of autoimmunity such as antigen presenting cells. The role of MyD88 in cardiac fibrosis has been demonstrated with chimeric mice, where the origin of fibroblasts that replace inflammatory infiltrates was determined to be from the bone marrow. MyD88 has thus been suggested to be critical for the development of cardiac fibrosis during progression to heart failure (Pasare et al. 2003; Marty et al. 2006). Fuse et al observed elevated MyD88 cardiac protein levels in the hearts of wild-type mice after exposure to coxsackievirus B3 and MyD88 knock out mice have a greater survival rate (86%) compared to wild type mice (35%) after coxsackievirus B3 exposure (Fuse et al. 2005). MyD88 is implicated not only in cardiac inflammation and mediating cytokine production, but is also associated with skewing the Th1/Th2 cytokine balance, increasing the expression of coxsackie-adenoviral receptor important for virus entry and viral titers after coxsackievirus B3 incidence. In the absence of MyD88, protection from virus infection and disease is observed and is suggested to be associated with IRF-3 and IFN-β activation (Fuse et al. 2005). From the above mentioned MyD88 work, it is fair to infer that MyD88 could be a useful target for preventative heart-specific autoimmunity and cardiomyopathy treatments (Marty et al. 2006). TLR signalling may be a major contributor to the initiation and progression of autoimmune myocarditis though there are many additional players such as the cells that express viral and self antigen sensors (antigen presenting cells) that remain poorly understood.

4.2 Antigen presenting cells (APCs)

Following viral infection, a cellular immune response is needed to completely clear the virus. However these same cells can drive chronic inflammation and autoimmune responses. Antigen presenting cells and other cell types critical in activating the cellular response to viral infection such as CD4+ T cells, CD8+ T cells, γδ T cells, B cells, macrophages, mast cells, neutrophils, NK cells and DC cells are all detected in the hearts of mice post coxsackievirus B3 infection and with experimental induced autoimmune myocarditis induction (Afanasyeva et al. 2004; Cooper 2009; Kemball et al. 2010).

Antigen presenting cells play a pivotal role in the stimulation of acquired immunity and can be manipulated by cytokines and environmental factors. The manipulation of antigen presenting cells modulates the T cell response and results in changes in tolerance to specific antigens. Antigen presenting cells influence lymphocyte responses by 1) promoting helper T-cell 1 (Th1), Th2 or Th17 responses, 2) inducing peripheral tolerance, and 3) activating regulatory T cells (Chatenoud et al. 2005; Ait-Oufella et al. 2006; Blyszczuk et al. 2008). From autoimmunity studies it has been curiously determined that regulatory T cells and Th17 cells have opposing functions during autoimmunity (Langrish et al. 2005). Th17 cells are an important pro-inflammatory T cell lineage during heightened tissue inflammation and autoimmunity, whereas regulatory T cells cells function to suppress immune responses (Richer et al. 2008; Korn et al. 2009; Marchant et al. 2010; Wing et al. 2010; Zou et al. 2010). Antigen presenting cells trigger changes in regulatory T cells and other T cell populations, which alters disease outcome and may be a promising therapeutic avenue to further investigate in viral-induced autoimmune diseases such as viral myocarditis.

Damage to the myocardium and the onset of coxsackievirus B3-induced acute myocarditis in mice is attributable to many immune factors including activated antigen-specific T cell activity. Two signals are required for activating T cells: first through the T-cell receptor engaging with antigen loaded MHC on antigen presenting cells and next through costimulatory molecules on antigen presenting cells such as CD40 and B7. CD40L on T cells engages CD40 on antigen presenting cells activating them to secrete cytokines and express adhesion molecules. Signalling from both the T cell receptor and costimulatory molecules promotes the proliferation of the antigen-specific T cells and stimulates an anti-antigen immune response. Early work with CD40/CD40L revealed enhanced CD40 expression on cardiac myocytes of coxsackievirus B3-infected mice and reduced myocardial inflammation with anti-CD40L/B7-1 monoclonal antibody treatment (Seko et al. 1998). Increased expression of CD40 and the B7 family of costimulatory molecules has also been observed in myocardial tissue from patients with dilated cardiomyopathy and acute myocarditis (Seko et al. 1998). Recently, CD40-Ig treatment was used post-coxsackievirus B3 infection to block the interaction between CD40/CD40L in male Balb/c mice and notably, this treatment reduced inflammation and coxsackievirus B3 transcription. CD40-Ig treatment also skewed the Th1/Th2 response in favour of Th2 cytokines rather than Th1 (Bo et al. 2010). This work and studies with myocardial tissue from patients has important implications not only for the role of CD40, but also for potential therapeutic options that downregulate the inflammatory Th1 response in coxsackievirus B3-mediated acute myocarditis.

Dendritic cells are highly specialized antigen presenting cells that upon encountering a pathogen undergo maturation. This process involves antigen processing, upregulation of major histocompatibility class (MHC) class II molecules, induction of costimulatory activity and migration to lymph nodes, where they prime antigen-specific T cells. With their antigen processing capability, dendritic cells can trigger activation of autoreactive T cells (Eriksson et al. 2003). Dendritic cells may also be involved in both host defense and maintenance of peripheral tolerance. Dendritic cells may also play an important role in autoimmune myocarditis (Marty et al. 2006). Dendritic cells from infected susceptible mice produce lower levels of cytokines and chemokines, particularly IP-10, a chemokine with cardioprotective properties. In the hearts of healthy wild type mice, tissue-resident dendritic cells take up and present endogenous heart-specific peptides (Eriksson et al. 2003). Activated and self-antigen loaded dendritic cells induce myocarditis and heart failure in genetically susceptible mice. The mechanism by which dendritic cells instigate damage to the myocardium is likely a combined effect from tissue damage and innate immunity activation that causes dendritic cells to activate autoreactive T cells and target the myocardium (Marty et al. 2006). This proposed mechanism was supported by Eriksson et al who have shown that injection of dendritic cells loaded with cardiac myosin peptide induces CD4+ T-cell-mediated autoimmune myocarditis (Eriksson et al. 2003). Interestingly, the dendritic cell-induced autoimmunity observed by Eriksson et al resulted only with TLR and CD40 stimulation. They demonstrated how TLR signalling following the onset and resolution of acute myocarditis instigates the reoccurrence of inflammatory infiltrates in the heart and the onset of autoimmunity. TLR signalling activation was also important for myocarditis induction in mice injected with damaged, immune stimulating cardiomyocytes (Eriksson et al. 2003). These few studies provide an insight into the possible role of dendritic cells in the induction of myocarditis and they offer an alternative, complete Freund's adjuvant-free method of inducing experimental induced autoimmune myocarditis (Afanasyeva et al. 2004).

The work done by Eriksson et al suggests targetting TLR signalling pathways may be needed as a therapeutic avenue to protect from heart-specific autoimmunity. In a scenario where microbial infections are acting concurrently with myocardial damage, such as with coxsackievirus B3 infection and myocarditis onset, self peptide–loaded dendritic cells might respond to the various pathogen associated molecular patterns in the environment that stimulate different TLRs and induce tolerance rather than act in antigenic mimicry. The end result may not be antigenic mimicry to instigate autoimmunity, but downregulation of autoreactive T cells and induction of tolerance (Eriksson et al. 2003; Blyszczuk et al. 2008). With this in mind, innate activation pathways such as TLR signaling, may be attractive targets for autoimmune myocarditis therapy.

Macrophages, another type of antigen presenting cell, play a critical role in the immune response to coxsackievirus B3 infection and have been implicated in the pathogenesis of coxsackievirus B3-induced autoimmune myocarditis. There are two groups of macrophages, type I or type II that are defined by their activation markers and cytokine production. Type II macrophages have been linked to the cardiac repair stage following acute myocarditis (Nahrendorf et al. 2007). The significance of macrophages in coxsackievirus B3 myocarditis was demonstrated in previous work by Richer et al and Horwitz et al, where a transgenic TGF-β mouse model demonstrated a protective role for TGF-β against autoimmune disease. This protection coincided with a reduction in macrophage maturation suggesting the important involvement of macrophage inflammatory properties (Horwitz et al. 2006; Richer et al. 2006). It has been suggested therefore, that a balance between the inflammatory macrophages that are necessary for defense against viruses and the macrophages necessary for the resolution of an immune response and tissue healing is critical for an appropriate antiviral immune response that avoids autoimmunity (Heath et al. 2004). Interestingly, macrophage phenotype can differ between male and female mice with coxsackievirus B3-induced myocarditis. Since coxsackievirus B3 infection induces severe myocarditis only in male mice it is possible that myocardial infiltrating macrophages detected in female mice will have a distinct functional phenotype that contributes to their protection from coxsackievirus B3-induced myocarditis. Li et al observed myocardial infiltrating macrophages from coxsackievirus B3-infected male mice expressing high levels of classically activated macrophages (type I) markers, such as inducible nitric oxide synthase, IL-12, TNF-α, and CD16/32, whereas macrophages from females had increased expression of arginase 1, IL-10, macrophage mannose receptor and macrophage galactose type C-type lectin that are typically associated with alternatively activated macrophages (type II) (Li et al. 2009). Li et al also demonstrated a distinct myocardial-derived cytokine signature that is sex-biased and contributes to differential macrophage polarization after coxsackievirus B3 infection. With adoptive transfer experiments using *ex vivo* programmed M1 macrophages, Li et al observed significantly increased myocarditis in both male and female mice. However, the transfer of M2 macrophages into susceptible male mice protected mice from myocardial inflammation (Li et al. 2009). This protection was postulated to be the result of a modulated local cytokine profile that contributed to the promotion of peripheral regulatory T cells differentiation. This work has helped our understanding of a possible mechanism that underlies the gender bias in coxsackievirus B3 myocarditis susceptibility. Developing therapeutic strategies that manipulate macrophage polarization may be a promising avenue for the treatment of inflammatory heart diseases.

4.3 Cytokines and chemokines

Cytokines and chemokines also play critical roles in the detection of pathogens and the response by the innate immune system. Unfortunately, they are also actively involved in the pathogenesis and progression of viral myocarditis. Transgenic mouse models expressing cytokines have facilitated our understanding of interplay between cytokines at the sites of infection and the development of autoimmune disease.

During experimental induced autoimmune myocarditis, it has been thought that CD4+ Th cells differentiate into IL-2- and IFNγ-producing Th1 and IL-4-, IL-10- and IL-13-producing Th2 cell subsets and that the balance in T-helper cytokines can influence susceptibility and outcome of myocarditis (Horwitz et al. 2000). In recent research, it has been revealed that IL-1, IL-6, and IL-23 promote the differentiation of a distinct CD4+ T cell population that produces IL-17 and develops independently of Th1 and Th2 lineages (Blyszczuk et al. 2008). This new population denoted Th17, plays an important role for various models of immune-mediated tissue injury, including organ-specific autoimmunity diseases like myocarditis (Horwitz et al. 2000).

Work from our laboratory has established a critical link between IL-6 and disease severity. Work done by Poffenberger and colleagues has shown a significant increase in disease severity with the absence of IL-6 after coxsackievirus B3 infection in mice. An increase in inflammatory mediators associated with the progression of myocarditis such as TNF-α and MCP1 was observed in concordance with the increase in disease severity (Poffenberger et al. 2009). Without IL-6 to regulate the early immune response after infection, the early inflammatory response leads to increased chronic myocarditis severity as the disease progresses (Poffenberger et al. 2009).

An important factor affecting the immune response to the virus and viral clearance is the pro-inflammatory cytokine interferon-γ (IFNγ). Coxsackievirus B3 infection in mice deficient in IFNγ results in increased disease severity and increased viral replication in the heart (Eriksson et al. 2001; Fairweather et al. 2005). Expression of IFNγ in the pancreas can control viral replication as well as the virus-mediated damage in the heart and ensuing autoimmune disease (Horwitz et al. 2000). This cytokine also controls disease severity in an adjuvant induction disease model. In essence, IFNγ likely limits myocarditis pathology by decreasing viral replication and virus-mediated damage. Resolution of inflammation and progressive remodeling are associated with high levels of another cytokine transforming growth factor-β (TGF-β) in the myocardium.

TGF-β is a pleiotropic, immunomodulating cytokine that greatly contributes to myocardial repair and remodelling (Khan et al. 2006; Rubtsov et al. 2007). Cardiac fibroblasts are the predominant source of secreted TGF-β within the heart. Secretion of TGF-β drives differentiation of cardiac fibroblasts into their more active myofibroblast form (Lijnen et al. 2002). It is with this active connective tissue cell form and stimulation by TGF-β that copious amounts of collagen can be secreted (Petrov et al. 2002). Fibrillar collagen is a leading contributor to extensive fibrosis. With disproportionate amounts of secreted collagen, ventricles tighten, restricting proper diastolic function (Kania et al. 2009). TGF-β contributes to the secretion of collagen via the TGF-β-Smad pathway that promotes collagen gene activation and translation (Khan et al. 2006). TGF-β also enhances the production of adhesion molecules that in turn, promote the longevity of myofibroblasts (Vaughan et al. 2000). Macrophages also secrete TGF-β in the heart (Riemann et al. 1994). They colocalize with myofibroblasts in fibrotic heart tissue and act as either initiating or supplemental sources of TGF-β1 (Hinglais et al. 1994; Kuwahara et al. 2004).

Coxsackievirus B3 first targets and replicates in the pancreas before reaching the heart. To inhibit coxsackievirus B3 spread to the heart and initiation of chronic disease, Horwitz et al developed a transgenic TGF-β mouse model where TGF-β is overexpressed in the pancreas. The expression of TGF-β in the pancreatic beta cells recruited macrophages into the pancreas, reduced viral replication, and inhibited the onset of coxsackievirus B3-induced autoimmune myocarditis. This study also demonstrated that the protective effect was strictly attributed to TGF-β and not IL-4, which has been linked to both autoimmunity suppression and antigen-presenting cell activation (Horwitz et al. 2006). Later on, Richer et al demonstrated that LPS from *Salmonella minnesota* and signalling through TLR-4 was capable of bypassing the protective effect provided by TGF-β in coxsackievirus B3-mediated autoimmune myocarditis (Richer et al. 2006). The authors also showed that neither antibody isotype switching, the extent of viral replication, nor the expression of CD40 was modulated with LPS induced TLR-4 signalling, rather the circumventing effect was due to failed APC expression of CD40 and inherent TLR-4 signalling effects such as the production of pro-inflammatory cytokines (Richer et al. 2006).

Though over-expression of TGF-β in the pancreas can protect from coxsackievirus B3-induced autoimmune myocarditis, there is still evidence that increased levels of TGF-β1 in the heart enhance, rather than protect from chronic disease. Elevated levels of TGF-β have also been tied to dilated, ischemic and hypertrophic cardiomyopathies (Khan et al. 2006). As mentioned previously, TGF-β can enhance collagen secretion and thus promote extensive tissue fibrosis. A recent study examined the effect of astragaloside IV, a Chinese medical herb that has anti-myocardial injury and immunoregulatory properties, to inhibit myocardial fibrosis in Balb/c mice inoculated with coxsackievirus B3 (Chen et al. 2011). Interestingly, astragaloside IV exhibited a protective effect alike TGF-β against myocardial fibrosis and significantly ameliorated survival in coxsackievirus B3-infected mice that developed dilated cardiomyopathy. The authors also suggest that the protective role exerted by astragaloside IV is likely due to its ability to interfere with TGF-β-Smad signalling through the direct downregulation of Smad2/3 and Smad 4 (Chen et al. 2011).

Lipopolysaccharide injection at the time of coxsackievirus B3 infection helps overcome genetic resistance in susceptible mice. This investigation also identified interleukin (IL)-1 as the mediator responsible for causing the change in disease course. Injection of IL-1 alone overcomes the genetic resistance to induced myocarditis similarly to lipopolysaccharide treatment. The change in disease susceptibility is likely due to increased IL-1 production in the heart. Production of IL-1 begins during the acute stage of disease but persists into the chronic phase of disease. Interestingly, the levels of IL-1 in the heart correlate with the degree of fibrotic lesions during disease. Eriksson et al demonstrated that injection of an IL-1 receptor agonist prior to infection sufficiently decreases viral titres in the heart and reduced chances of mortality. They also showed that IL-1 receptor stimulation is required for efficient dendritic cell activation, the subsequent induction of autoreactive CD4+ T cells, and resulting autoimmune disease (Eriksson et al. 2003).

Another important immunomodulating cytokine that contributes to viral-induced myocarditis and controls macrophage activation is IL-10. IL-10 is produced in the myocardium during both the acute and chronic stages of virus-induced myocarditis. Chronic coxsackievirus B3-induced myocarditis features viral RNA persistence and chronic inflammation that is primarily mediated by macrophages and T cells therefore, cytokines like IL-10 that control these critical immune cells are important to investigate. IL-10 gene-deficient mice have been used to confirm the regulatory role of IL-10 in the outcome of coxsackievirus B3 myocarditis. Mice deficient in IL-10 have uncontrolled nitric oxide synthase production, which likely contributes to their ongoing myocardial injury (Szalay et al. 2006). IL-10 in experimental induced autoimmune myocarditis mice hearts is mainly detected in non-cardiomyocytic non-inflammatory cells (ie. fibroblasts, smooth muscle cells, and endothelial cells) and IL-10-targeting cells. The IL-10-targetting cells, which express both IL-10 receptors 1 and 2, are mainly T cells expressing αβT cell antigen receptors (αβT cells) and CD11b+ cells such as macrophages, dendritic cells, and granulocytes. Several studies have demonstrated a therapeutic effect for IL-10 in autoimmune and inflammatory diseases. In myocarditis models, IL-10 has been shown to inhibit the secretion of proinflammatory cytokines such as TNF-α, IFN-γ, iNOS, IL-2 and IL-12 and has displayed major effects on immune cells (Horwitz et al. 2000). These few studies suggest that the role of IL-10 in disease development could be predominantly protective.

IL-12, another key cytokine, is comprised of p40 and p35 subunits. IL-12 signals through a heterodimeric receptor composed of two units, IL-12Rβ1 and IL-12Rβ2. p40 and IL-12Rβ1 deficient mice show less or no myocardial disease with adjuvant-induction and treatment of wild type mice with IL-12, exacerbates disease suggesting IL-12 as a driving force in disease development similar to the actions of IL-1β and TNFα (Eriksson et al. 2001; Afanasyeva et al. 2004). However, Fairweather et al have found that IL-12 deficiency does not prevent myocarditis, rather viral replication significantly increases, causing more myocardial tissue damage. A decrease in inflammatory infiltrates was also observed and corresponded to with reduced TNF-α and IFN-γ levels in the heart. IL-12 and IFNg positively regulate each other and type I inflammatory responses. Type I inflammatory responses are believed to be responsible for tissue damage in autoimmune diseases. Eriksson et al further investigated the role of the IL-12/IFN-γ (Th1) axis in the development of autoimmune myocarditis. They observed resistance to disease in IL-12p40-deficient mice that were bred on a susceptible background. In the absence of IL-12, they suggested that autospecific CD4+ T cells proliferated poorly and exerted Th2 cytokine responses. IFN-γ-deficient mice developed fatal autoimmune disease. Interestingly, blocking IL-4R signalling did not confer susceptibility to myocarditis in IL-12p40-deficient mice. This suggests that IL-12 triggers autoimmunity in a manner independent of the cytokines IFN-γ and IL-4 (Eriksson et al. 2001).

IL-13 is another cytokine that can protect mice from both viral and adjuvant induced myocarditis. Cihakova et al demonstrated that IL-13 knock out BALB/c mice develop severe autoimmune myocarditis and their pathology is characterized by increased cardiac inflammation, increased total intracardiac CD45+ leukocytes, elevated anti-cardiac myosin autoantibodies, and increased cardiac fibrosis, with impaired cardiac function and heart failure. Hearts of IL-13 knock out mice showed elevated levels of the proinflammatory and profibrotic cytokines including IL-1β, IL-18, IFN-γ, TGF-β, and IL-4. CD4+ T cells were also highly increased in IL-13 knock out hearts. Splenic T cells from the knock out mice were greatly activated and with myosin stimulation, immensely proliferated. Regulatory T-cells harvested from spleens were also affected in knock out mice, where they showed a decrease in numbers compared to wild type mice. IL-13 knock out also reduced alternatively activated CD206(+) and CD204(+) macrophages and hightened levels of classically activated macrophages. Caspase-1 activation was increased, which then likely increased production of both IL-1β and IL-18. This study exemplified IL-13 as another important immunomodulating cytokine that protects against myocarditis by manipulating T cell and macrophage populations (Cihakova et al. 2008).

Examining T cells subsets is another avenue investigated to determine pathogenic or protective factors in myocarditis development. Mice deficient in T-bet, a T-box transcription factor required for Th1 cell differentiation and IFN-γ production, develop severe autoimmune heart disease. T-bet can also regulate autoimmunity by controlling nonspecific CD8+ T cell bystander functions in the inflamed target organ such as the heart. CD4+ Th1 cells producing INFγ are protective in experimental induced autoimmune myocarditis. This protection is likely attributed to regulation of IL-17 production by Th17 cells. Th17 cells produce IL-17, a proinflammatory cytokine that activates T cells and other immune cells to produce a variety of cytokines, chemokines and cell adhesion molecules. Rangachari et al have shown that Th17 cells are involved in acute viral myocarditis and enhance humoral responses (Rangachari et al. 2006). The relationship between Th17 cells and coxsackievirus B3 replication still remained unclear so they infected BALB/c mice with the virus and observed increased viral replication, expression of splenic Th17 cells, serum IL-17, and cardiac IL-17 mRNA that were all accompanied by progressive cardiac injury. Interestingly, Th1 and CD8+ T cell expression was elevated and the neutralization of IL-17 further upregulated splenic Th1 and CD8+ T cell numbers and levels of cardiac IFN-γ mRNA. Cardiac pathology was improved after IL-17 neutralization and correlated with reduced viral replication and decreases in cardiac inflammatory cytokines IL-17, TNF-α, and IL-1β. This study implicates Th17 cells in contributing coxsackeivirus B3 replication in viral myocarditis, and implicates IL-17 as a target for regulating antiviral immune responses (Yuan et al. 2010). Th17 cells are activated by IL-23, a cytokine likely produced by activated macrophages and dendritic cells, through receptor interactions made of IL-12Rβ1 and IL-23 receptor (Langrish et al. 2005). IL-23 is a heterodimeric cytokine like IL-12 that is composed of a p19 and p40 subunit similar to IL-12. IL-23–mediated immune responses have a different gene expression pattern than IL-12–driven T cell responses and IL-23 does not promote the development of IFN-γ-producing Th1 cells as does IL-12. IL-23 is however, one of the many contributors to pathogenic CD4+ T cell expansion. With its anti-IFN-γ and Th1 cell activity, IL-23 helps establish and maintain organ-specific inflammatory autoimmune diseases such as myocarditis (Langrish et al. 2005). Understanding the molecular basis for the differential gene expression pattern observed with IL-23–dependent T cell populations and investigating IL-23's cellular mechanism of action in autoimmunity could provide additional therapeutic targets for the treatment of inflammatory autoimmune diseases.

Experimental and preliminary human studies have demonstrated that TNF-α plays a crucial role in viral-induced myocarditis. Calabrese et al investigated the expression of TNF-α and both its receptors (TNFRI and TNFRII) in both viral and non viral myocarditis. Expression of TNF-α was significantly enhanced in viral myocarditis compared to non viral myocarditis. Importantly, cardiac myocytes express TNFα receptors TNFR1 (TNFRp55) and TNFR2 (TNFRp75), implicating the possible importance of enhance TNF-α in the myocardium. Histological analysis revealed that myocardial necrosis and cellular infiltration are more prominent in TNF-α-positive cases further supporting the notion that the expression of TNF-α significantly contributes to the pathogenesis of viral myocarditis and including the severity of cardiac dysfunction (Calabrese et al. 2004).

Chemokines act as chemotactic mediators in leukocyte trafficking to sites of infection (Groom et al. 2011). In addition to their chemo-attractant activity, chemokines can influence disease severity by modifying immune response strength and polarity. This immune modulating capability thus makes them attractive targets for viral myocarditis therapeutics. Chemokines apart of the CC chemokine family such as CCL2, CCL4, and CCL19 have been shown to mediate mononuclear cell migration to the heart in coxsackievirus B3-induced myocarditis (Chen et al. 2009). In fact, a recent gene therapy approach using a CCL2 mutant that lacked chemo-attractant activity in a Balb/c coxsackievirus B3-infection model impaired appropriate Th1 immune responses and significantly controlled myocardial disease (Yue et al. 2011). Blocking CCL2 with expression of the mutant did not assist in viral clearance. The potential therapeutic effect of blocking CCL2 lies in the CCL2 mutant's ability to weaken the pro-inflammatory Th1 immune response (Yue et al. 2011).

The CDC family of chemokines also contribute to myocarditis pathogenesis. CDC chemokines act on monoculear CXCR3 expressing cells and include such members as IFN-inducible protein 10 (IP10/CXCL10), monokine induced by IFN-γ (Mig/CXCL9), and IFN-inducible T-cell a chemoattractant (I-TAC/CXCL11) (Groom et al. 2011). CXCL10 and its interaction with its receptor CXCR3 have been implicated in many virus disease models. CXCL10 is a key contributor in the innate immune response to viral infection. By interacting with its receptor CXCR3, CXCL10 manipulates natural killer cell trafficking and their production of IFN-γ. Yuan et al recently found CXCL10 levels in the heart to be inversely related to viral titers after coxsackievirus B3 infection and a massive infiltration of $CXCR3^+$, $CD4^+$, and $CD8^+$ cells (Yuan et al. 2009). The production of associated inflammatory cytokines followed with the infiltration of leukocytes though the anti-viral response was not effective in clearing the virus or ensuring survival in coxsackievirus B3-infected CXCL10 transgenic mice (Yuan et al. 2009). CXCL10 did assist viral clearance and protect myocytes from damage in the early stages of infection by robustly attracting NK cells and enhancing IFN-γ production to infection sites (Yuan et al. 2009). Though CXCL10 appears to improve cardiac pathology and reduce viral persistence during initial infection stages, the caveat with using this chemokine as a potential coxsackievirus B3-induced myocarditis therapy lies with its inherent actions as a Th1-type chemeokine. Th1 immune responses escalate detrimental cardiac fibrosis during the reclamation stage of disease so enhancing important contributors to this repair process may acceleration rather than prevent the development of chronic disease.

Determining the effect of CXCL10 on viral replication and recruitment of innate immune cells in other organs than the heart such as the liver and pancreas must still be pursued. As seen with another immunomodulatory factor, TGF-β, the immune responses in other organs than the heart can affect susceptibility to severe myocardial injury and the development of chronic disease.

Recent research has demonstrated that coxsackievirus B3-infected Balb/c mice have increased levels of cardiac CXCL10 and this level fluctuates in a time and dose-dependent manner (Yue et al. 2011). The same research group treated coxsackievirus B3-infected mice with a CXCL10 mutant that lacks the critical chemo-attractant part. This mutant effectively blocked endogenous CXCL10 activity and protected coxsackievirus B3-infected mice from developing myocarditis (Yue et al. 2011). The CXCL10 mutant expressing mice had greater survival, less changes in body weight, less inflammation and necrosis in the heart. Cardiac Th1 cytokines IFN-γ, IL-12, TNF-α, were also found to be significantly reduced with CXCL10/CXCR3 signalling inhibition. This suggests that dampening the Th1 response to coxsackievirus B3 infection through blocking CXCL10 activity may present as an effective strategy to suppress immune inflammation and myocardial damage in coxsackievirus B3-mediated myocarditis (Yue et al. 2011).

The production of immunomodulating mediators such as cytokines and chemokines affects not only antigen presenting cell and T cell populations acting at the site of injury, but greatly influences the outcome of disease. The expression of particular cytokines and chemokines after a pathogenic insult, such as coxsackievirus B3 infection, influences the balance of effector versus regulatory responses that ensue. Once the balance between effector versus regulatory responses tips in a particular direction, chronic autoimmune-type disease or the prevention of disease will materialize (Rouse et al. 2010; Wing et al. 2010) (Figure 3). It is therefore critical to bear in mind the possibility of tipping the immunity balance when manipulating key immune players in coxsackievirus-induced myocarditis.

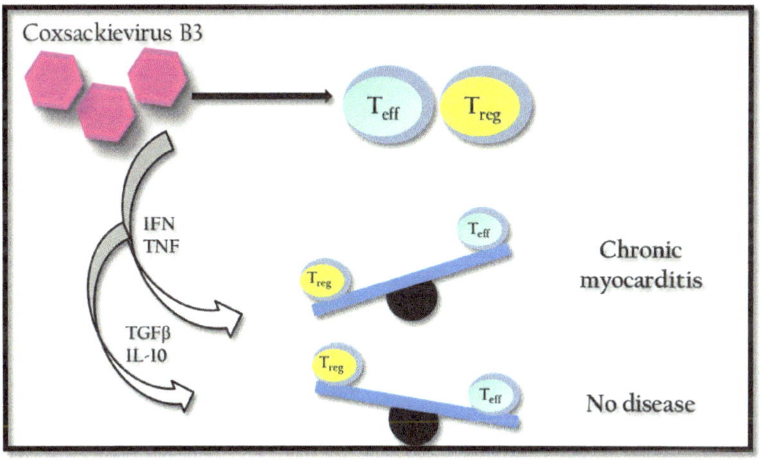

Fig. 3. Immunomodulation of the immune balance and the effects on disease outcome. With coxsackievirus B3 infection, populations of regulatory and effector cells are produced. It is with particular immunomodulating mediators such as cytokines interferon (IFN) and tumor necrosis factor (TNF) that enhanced production and proliferation of effector T cells (T_{eff}) is promoted and leads to the persistent destruction of the myocardium and chronic myocarditis disease. Pro-regulatory cytokines transforming growth factor-β (TGF-β) and interleukin-10 (IL-10) are examples of immune modulators that promote the enhanced production of regulatory T cells (regulatory T cells) and the prevention of autoimmune myocarditis disease.

5. Therapeutic challenges and future directions

Treatment for myocarditis mainly involves targeting the symptoms of heart dysfunction. If the disease progresses to dilated cardiomyopathy, heart transplantation is necessitated. Regrettably, for 50% of patients progressing to dilated cardiomyopathy, survival is limited to 5 years. Broad-spectrum antivirals tested in clinical trials with children and adults have been few and mildly successful. Specific therapies designed against viruses (enteroviruses) for prevention and/or management of viral myocarditis are still desperately needed. One challenge in designing specific antivirals or vaccines for viral myocarditis is the range of possible etiologies and immune mechanisms that may be responsible. Although enteroviral infection inducing or exacerbating an autoimmune response is a likely cause for viral myocarditis, supporting data defining a link between viral infection and the onset of acute and/or chronic myocarditis in humans must still be determined. The existence of many viral serotypes for promising etiological agents like coxsackievirus B also poses a problem in designing specific antiviral therapies.

Dampening the Th1 immune response in viral myocarditis is a therapeutic avenue consistently featured in past and recent studies. Many key innate immune players, such as cytokines and chemokines, are targets of potential Th1 skewing therapeutics. Cytokines presenting at the site of viral infection have a significant influence on whether a tolerant or autoimmune response is chosen. Targeting cytokines, chemokines and other immunomodulating factors for myocarditis therapy may depend on the timing and duration of the particular factor and the maintenance of immune balance to prevent the development of autoimmunity.

6. Conclusion

For quite some time scientists have investigated virus and host cellular and molecular events that underlie the pathogenesis of enteroviral-induced myocarditis. Our lab has demonstrated the significance of many key innate players that contribute to coxsackievirus-B3 induced myocarditis in mouse models. Horwitz et al first revealed the importance of IFN-γ expression in the pancreas for the protection from coxsackievirus B3 infection and the induction of myocarditis (Horwitz et al. 2000). Later on, Horwitz et al again demonstrated a protective role against coxsackievirus B3-induced myocarditis with cytokine expression in the pancreas, this time, with transgenic expression of TGF-β in the beta cells (Horwitz et al. 2006). This work was followed by Richer et al, who provided a role for TLR4 and stimulation by *Salmonella minnesota* lipopolysaccharide in bypassing the protective effect exerted by TGF-β in coxsackievirus B3-induced myocarditis (Richer et al. 2006). Our lab has also investigated the role of IL-6 in disease severity. Poffenberger et al demonstrated that in the absence of IL-6, a greater early immune response occurred, instigating a severe chronic disease pathology (Poffenberger et al. 2009). Recently, Poffenberger et al described susceptibility loci on chromosome 17 that implicate the highly suggested genetic component as a factor dictating viral myocarditis pathogenesis (Poffenberger et al. 2010). Though work from our lab has contributed a great deal to the understanding of coxsackievirus B3-induced myocarditis, there remains many unanswered questions with regards to the true key immune players that dictate disease pathogenesis. It is likely that an interplay of genetic and environmental factors influence the susceptibility and severity of virus-induced myocarditis however, we must not discount the significance of the innate immune response in shaping the outcome of virus-induced disease. It is possible that this early immune response may ultimately dictate whether an acute or chronic immune response ensues with enteroviral infection.

7. References

Afanasyeva, M., D. Georgakopoulos, et al. (2004). "Autoimmune myocarditis: cellular mediators of cardiac dysfunction." Autoimmun Rev 3(7-8): 476-486.

Ait-Oufella, H., B. L. Salomon, et al. (2006). "Natural regulatory T cells control the development of atherosclerosis in mice." Nat Med 12(2): 178-180.

Aretz, H. T. (1987). "Myocarditis: the Dallas criteria." Hum Pathol 18(6): 619-624.

Aretz, H. T., M. E. Billingham, et al. (1987). "Myocarditis. A histopathologic definition and classification." Am J Cardiovasc Pathol 1(1): 3-14.

Baboonian, C., M. J. Davies, et al. (1997). "Coxsackie B viruses and human heart disease." Curr Top Microbiol Immunol 223: 31-52.

Blauwet, L. A. and L. T. Cooper (2010). "Myocarditis." Prog Cardiovasc Dis 52(4): 274-288.

Blyszczuk, P., A. Valaperti, et al. (2008). "Future therapeutic strategies in inflammatory cardiomyopathy: insights from the experimental autoimmune myocarditis model." Cardiovasc Hematol Disord Drug Targets 8(4): 313-321.

Bo, H., L. Zhenhu, et al. (2010). "Blocking the CD40-CD40L interaction by CD40-Ig reduces disease progress in murine myocarditis induced by CVB3." Cardiovasc Pathol 19(6): 371-376.

Calabrese, F., E. Carturan, et al. (2004). "Overexpression of tumor necrosis factor (TNF)alpha and TNFalpha receptor I in human viral myocarditis: clinicopathologic correlations." Mod Pathol 17(9): 1108-1118.

Chang, H., H. Hanawa, et al. (2008). "Alteration of IL-17 related protein expressions in experimental autoimmune myocarditis and inhibition of IL-17 by IL-10-Ig fusion gene transfer." Circ J 72(5): 813-819.

Chatenoud, L. and J. F. Bach (2005). "Regulatory T cells in the control of autoimmune diabetes: the case of the NOD mouse." Int Rev Immunol 24(3-4): 247-267.

Chen, P., R. Chen, et al. (2009). "Coxsackievirus B3 infection promotes generation of myeloid dendritic cells from bone marrow and accumulation in the myocardium." Int Immunopharmacol 9(11): 1304-1312.

Chen, P., Y. Xie, et al. (2011). "Astragaloside IV attenuates myocardial fibrosis by inhibiting TGF-beta1 signaling in coxsackievirus B3-induced cardiomyopathy." Eur J Pharmacol 658(2-3): 168-174.

Cihakova, D., J. G. Barin, et al. (2008). "Interleukin-13 protects against experimental autoimmune myocarditis by regulating macrophage differentiation." Am J Pathol 172(5): 1195-1208.

Cooper, L. T., Jr. (2009). "Myocarditis." N Engl J Med 360(15): 1526-1538.

Cunningham, M. W. (2001). "Cardiac myosin and the TH1/TH2 paradigm in autoimmune myocarditis." Am J Pathol 159(1): 5-12.

Daniels, M. D., K. V. Hyland, et al. (2008). "Recombinant cardiac myosin fragment induces experimental autoimmune myocarditis via activation of Th1 and Th17 immunity." Autoimmunity 41(6): 490-499.

Eriksson, U., M. O. Kurrer, et al. (2001). "Dual role of the IL-12/IFN-gamma axis in the development of autoimmune myocarditis: induction by IL-12 and protection by IFN-gamma." J Immunol 167(9): 5464-5469.

Eriksson, U., M. O. Kurrer, et al. (2003). "Activation of dendritic cells through the interleukin 1 receptor 1 is critical for the induction of autoimmune myocarditis." J Exp Med 197(3): 323-331.
Eriksson, U., R. Ricci, et al. (2003). "Dendritic cell-induced autoimmune heart failure requires cooperation between adaptive and innate immunity." Nat Med 9(12): 1484-1490.
Escher, F., D. Westermann, et al. (2011). "Development of diastolic heart failure in a 6-year follow-up study in patients after acute myocarditis." Heart 97(9): 709-714.
Esfandiarei, M. and B. M. McManus (2008). "Molecular biology and pathogenesis of viral myocarditis." Annu Rev Pathol 3: 127-155.
Fairweather, D., S. Frisancho-Kiss, et al. (2005). "IL-12 protects against coxsackievirus B3-induced myocarditis by increasing IFN-gamma and macrophage and neutrophil populations in the heart." J Immunol 174(1): 261-269.
Fairweather, D., Z. Kaya, et al. (2001). "From infection to autoimmunity." J Autoimmun 16(3): 175-186.
Fairweather, D., S. Yusung, et al. (2003). "IL-12 receptor beta 1 and Toll-like receptor 4 increase IL-1 beta- and IL-18-associated myocarditis and coxsackievirus replication." J Immunol 170(9): 4731-4737.
Flanegan, J. B., R. F. Petterson, et al. (1977). "Covalent linkage of a protein to a defined nucleotide sequence at the 5'-terminus of virion and replicative intermediate RNAs of poliovirus." Proc Natl Acad Sci U S A 74(3): 961-965.
Frisancho-Kiss, S., M. J. Coronado, et al. (2009). "Gonadectomy of male BALB/c mice increases Tim-3(+) alternatively activated M2 macrophages, Tim-3(+) T cells, Th2 cells and Treg in the heart during acute coxsackievirus-induced myocarditis." Brain Behav Immun 23(5): 649-657.
Frisancho-Kiss, S., S. E. Davis, et al. (2007). "Cutting edge: cross-regulation by TLR4 and T cell Ig mucin-3 determines sex differences in inflammatory heart disease." J Immunol 178(11): 6710-6714.
Frisancho-Kiss, S., J. F. Nyland, et al. (2006). "Sex differences in coxsackievirus B3-induced myocarditis: IL-12Rbeta1 signaling and IFN-gamma increase inflammation in males independent from STAT4." Brain Res 1126(1): 139-147.
Fuse, K., G. Chan, et al. (2005). "Myeloid differentiation factor-88 plays a crucial role in the pathogenesis of Coxsackievirus B3-induced myocarditis and influences type I interferon production." Circulation 112(15): 2276-2285.
Godeny, E. K. and C. J. Gauntt (1986). "Involvement of natural killer cells in coxsackievirus B3-induced murine myocarditis." J Immunol 137(5): 1695-1702.
Godeny, E. K. and C. J. Gauntt (1987). "Murine natural killer cells limit coxsackievirus B3 replication." J Immunol 139(3): 913-918.
Godsel, L. M., K. Wang, et al. (2001). "Prevention of autoimmune myocarditis through the induction of antigen-specific peripheral immune tolerance." Circulation 103(12): 1709-1714.
Gonnella, P. A., P. J. Del Nido, et al. (2009). "Oral tolerization with cardiac myosin peptide (614-629) ameliorates experimental autoimmune myocarditis: role of STAT 6 genes in BALB/CJ mice." J Clin Immunol 29(4): 434-443.
Gorbea, C., K. A. Makar, et al. (2010). "A role for Toll-like receptor 3 variants in host susceptibility to enteroviral myocarditis and dilated cardiomyopathy." J Biol Chem 285(30): 23208-23223.
Groom, J. R. and A. D. Luster (2011). "CXCR3 ligands: redundant, collaborative and antagonistic functions." Immunol Cell Biol 89(2): 207-215.

Heath, W. R., G. T. Belz, et al. (2004). "Cross-presentation, dendritic cell subsets, and the generation of immunity to cellular antigens." Immunol Rev 199: 9-26.
Hinglais, N., D. Heudes, et al. (1994). "Colocalization of myocardial fibrosis and inflammatory cells in rats." Lab Invest 70(2): 286-294.
Horwitz, M. S., A. Ilic, et al. (2005). "Induction of antigen specific peripheral humoral tolerance to cardiac myosin does not prevent CB3-mediated autoimmune myocarditis." J Autoimmun 25(2): 102-111.
Horwitz, M. S., M. Knudsen, et al. (2006). "Transforming growth factor-beta inhibits coxsackievirus-mediated autoimmune myocarditis." Viral Immunol 19(4): 722-733.
Horwitz, M. S., A. La Cava, et al. (2000). "Pancreatic expression of interferon-gamma protects mice from lethal coxsackievirus B3 infection and subsequent myocarditis." Nat Med 6(6): 693-697.
Hosenpud, J. D., S. M. Campbell, et al. (1985). "Experimental autoimmune myocarditis in the guinea pig." Cardiovasc Res 19(10): 613-622.
Huber, S. (2010). "Tumor necrosis factor-alpha promotes myocarditis in female mice infected with coxsackievirus B3 through upregulation of CD1d on hematopoietic cells." Viral Immunol 23(1): 79-86.
Huber, S. A., C. J. Gauntt, et al. (1998). "Enteroviruses and myocarditis: viral pathogenesis through replication, cytokine induction, and immunopathogenicity." Adv Virus Res 51: 35-80.
Jiang, Z., W. Xu, et al. (2008). "Remission of CVB3-induced viral myocarditis by in vivo Th2 polarization via hydrodynamics-based interleukin-4 gene transfer." J Gene Med 10(8): 918-929.
Kania, G., P. Blyszczuk, et al. (2009). "Heart-infiltrating prominin-1+/CD133+ progenitor cells represent the cellular source of transforming growth factor beta-mediated cardiac fibrosis in experimental autoimmune myocarditis." Circ Res 105(5): 462-470.
Kawai, T. and S. Akira (2006). "Innate immune recognition of viral infection." Nat Immunol 7(2): 131-137.
Kaya, Z., M. Afanasyeva, et al. (2001). "Contribution of the innate immune system to autoimmune myocarditis: a role for complement." Nat Immunol 2(8): 739-745.
Kaya, Z., K. M. Dohmen, et al. (2002). "Cutting edge: a critical role for IL-10 in induction of nasal tolerance in experimental autoimmune myocarditis." J Immunol 168(4): 1552-1556.
Kemball, C. C., M. Alirezaei, et al. (2010). "Type B coxsackieviruses and their interactions with the innate and adaptive immune systems." Future Microbiol 5(9): 1329-1347.
Khan, R. and R. Sheppard (2006). "Fibrosis in heart disease: understanding the role of transforming growth factor-beta in cardiomyopathy, valvular disease and arrhythmia." Immunology 118(1): 10-24.
Kodama, M., Y. Matsumoto, et al. (1992). "In vivo lymphocyte-mediated myocardial injuries demonstrated by adoptive transfer of experimental autoimmune myocarditis." Circulation 85(5): 1918-1926.
Korn, T., E. Bettelli, et al. (2009). "IL-17 and Th17 Cells." Annu Rev Immunol 27: 485-517.
Kuhl, U., M. Pauschinger, et al. (2005). "High prevalence of viral genomes and multiple viral infections in the myocardium of adults with "idiopathic" left ventricular dysfunction." Circulation 111(7): 887-893.
Kuhl, U., M. Pauschinger, et al. (2003). "Interferon-beta treatment eliminates cardiotropic viruses and improves left ventricular function in patients with myocardial persistence of viral genomes and left ventricular dysfunction." Circulation 107(22): 2793-2798.

Kuwahara, F., H. Kai, et al. (2004). "Hypertensive myocardial fibrosis and diastolic dysfunction: another model of inflammation?" Hypertension 43(4): 739-745.

Lane, J. R., D. A. Neumann, et al. (1993). "Role of IL-1 and tumor necrosis factor in coxsackie virus-induced autoimmune myocarditis." J Immunol 151(3): 1682-1690.

Langrish, C. L., Y. Chen, et al. (2005). "IL-23 drives a pathogenic T cell population that induces autoimmune inflammation." J Exp Med 201(2): 233-240.

Leuschner, F., H. A. Katus, et al. (2009). "Autoimmune myocarditis: past, present and future." J Autoimmun 33(3-4): 282-289.

Li, K., W. Xu, et al. (2009). "Differential macrophage polarization in male and female BALB/c mice infected with coxsackievirus B3 defines susceptibility to viral myocarditis." Circ Res 105(4): 353-364.

Lieberman, E. B., G. M. Hutchins, et al. (1991). "Clinicopathologic description of myocarditis." J Am Coll Cardiol 18(7): 1617-1626.

Lijnen, P. and V. Petrov (2002). "Transforming growth factor-beta 1-induced collagen production in cultures of cardiac fibroblasts is the result of the appearance of myofibroblasts." Methods Find Exp Clin Pharmacol 24(6): 333-344.

Liu, P., K. Aitken, et al. (2000). "The tyrosine kinase p56lck is essential in coxsackievirus B3-mediated heart disease." Nat Med 6(4): 429-434.

Marchant, D. J. and B. M. McManus (2010). "Regulating viral myocarditis: allografted regulatory T cells decrease immune infiltration and viral load." Circulation 121(24): 2609-2611.

Marty, R. R., S. Dirnhofer, et al. (2006). "MyD88 signaling controls autoimmune myocarditis induction." Circulation 113(2): 258-265.

Marty, R. R. and U. Eriksson (2006). "Dendritic cells and autoimmune heart failure." Int J Cardiol 112(1): 34-39.

Mason, J. W., J. B. O'Connell, et al. (1995). "A clinical trial of immunosuppressive therapy for myocarditis. The Myocarditis Treatment Trial Investigators." N Engl J Med 333(5): 269-275.

Nahrendorf, M., F. K. Swirski, et al. (2007). "The healing myocardium sequentially mobilizes two monocyte subsets with divergent and complementary functions." J Exp Med 204(12): 3037-3047.

Negishi, H., T. Osawa, et al. (2008). "A critical link between Toll-like receptor 3 and type II interferon signaling pathways in antiviral innate immunity." Proc Natl Acad Sci U S A 105(51): 20446-20451.

Neu, N., K. W. Beisel, et al. (1987). "Autoantibodies specific for the cardiac myosin isoform are found in mice susceptible to Coxsackievirus B3-induced myocarditis." J Immunol 138(8): 2488-2492.

Neu, N., N. R. Rose, et al. (1987). "Cardiac myosin induces myocarditis in genetically predisposed mice." J Immunol 139(11): 3630-3636.

Okazaki, T., Y. Tanaka, et al. (2003). "Autoantibodies against cardiac troponin I are responsible for dilated cardiomyopathy in PD-1-deficient mice." Nat Med 9(12): 1477-1483.

Olsen, E. G. (1993). "Morphological recognition of viral heart disease." Scand J Infect Dis Suppl 88: 45-47.

Onyimba, J. A., M. J. Coronado, et al. (2011). "The innate immune response to coxsackievirus B3 predicts progression to cardiovascular disease and heart failure in male mice." Biol Sex Differ 2: 2.

Pasare, C. and R. Medzhitov (2003). "Toll pathway-dependent blockade of CD4+CD25+ T cell-mediated suppression by dendritic cells." Science 299(5609): 1033-1036.

Pasare, C. and R. Medzhitov (2004). "Toll-dependent control mechanisms of CD4 T cell activation." Immunity 21(5): 733-741.
Pelletier, J., G. Kaplan, et al. (1988). "Cap-independent translation of poliovirus mRNA is conferred by sequence elements within the 5' noncoding region." Mol Cell Biol 8(3): 1103-1112.
Petrov, V. V., R. H. Fagard, et al. (2002). "Stimulation of collagen production by transforming growth factor-beta1 during differentiation of cardiac fibroblasts to myofibroblasts." Hypertension 39(2): 258-263.
Poffenberger, M. C., I. Shanina, et al. (2010). "Novel nonmajor histocompatibility complex-linked loci from mouse chromosome 17 confer susceptibility to viral-mediated chronic autoimmune myocarditis." Circ Cardiovasc Genet 3(5): 399-408.
Poffenberger, M. C., N. Straka, et al. (2009). "Lack of IL-6 during coxsackievirus infection heightens the early immune response resulting in increased severity of chronic autoimmune myocarditis." PLoS ONE 4(7): e6207.
Rangachari, M., N. Mauermann, et al. (2006). "T-bet negatively regulates autoimmune myocarditis by suppressing local production of interleukin 17." J Exp Med 203(8): 2009-2019.
Richardson, P., W. McKenna, et al. (1996). "Report of the 1995 World Health Organization/International Society and Federation of Cardiology Task Force on the Definition and Classification of cardiomyopathies." Circulation 93(5): 841-842.
Richer, M. J., D. Fang, et al. (2006). "Toll-like receptor 4-induced cytokine production circumvents protection conferred by TGF-beta in coxsackievirus-mediated autoimmune myocarditis." Clin Immunol 121(3): 339-349.
Richer, M. J. and M. S. Horwitz (2009). "The innate immune response: an important partner in shaping coxsackievirus-mediated autoimmunity." J Innate Immun 1(5): 421-434.
Richer, M. J., N. Straka, et al. (2008). "Regulatory T-cells protect from type 1 diabetes after induction by coxsackievirus infection in the context of transforming growth factor-beta." Diabetes 57(5): 1302-1311.
Riemann, D., H. G. Wollert, et al. (1994). "Immunophenotype of lymphocytes in pericardial fluid from patients with different forms of heart disease." Int Arch Allergy Immunol 104(1): 48-56.
Rose, N. R. (2010). "Autoimmunity, infection and adjuvants." Lupus 19(4): 354-358.
Rouse, B. T. and S. Sehrawat (2010). "Immunity and immunopathology to viruses: what decides the outcome?" Nat Rev Immunol 10(7): 514-526.
Rubtsov, Y. P. and A. Y. Rudensky (2007). "TGFbeta signalling in control of T-cell-mediated self-reactivity." Nat Rev Immunol 7(6): 443-453.
Satoh, M., M. Nakamura, et al. (2004). "Toll-like receptor 4 is expressed with enteroviral replication in myocardium from patients with dilated cardiomyopathy." Lab Invest 84(2): 173-181.
Schnare, M., G. M. Barton, et al. (2001). "Toll-like receptors control activation of adaptive immune responses." Nat Immunol 2(10): 947-950.
Seko, Y., N. Takahashi, et al. (1998). "Expression of costimulatory molecule CD40 in murine heart with acute myocarditis and reduction of inflammation by treatment with anti-CD40L/B7-1 monoclonal antibodies." Circ Res 83(4): 463-469.
Seko, Y., N. Takahashi, et al. (1998). "Expression of costimulatory molecules B7-1, B7-2, and CD40 in the heart of patients with acute myocarditis and dilated cardiomyopathy." Circulation 97(7): 637-639.

Sukumaran, V., K. Watanabe, et al. (2011). "Telmisartan ameliorates experimental autoimmune myocarditis associated with inhibition of inflammation and oxidative stress." Eur J Pharmacol 652(1-3): 126-135.

Szalay, G., M. Sauter, et al. (2006). "Sustained nitric oxide synthesis contributes to immunopathology in ongoing myocarditis attributable to interleukin-10 disorders." Am J Pathol 169(6): 2085-2093.

Tanaka, K., M. Ito, et al. (2011). "Sulfated polysaccharide fucoidan ameliorates experimental autoimmune myocarditis in rats." J Cardiovasc Pharmacol Ther 16(1): 79-86.

Triantafilou, K., G. Orthopoulos, et al. (2005). "Human cardiac inflammatory responses triggered by Coxsackie B viruses are mainly Toll-like receptor (TLR) 8-dependent." Cell Microbiol 7(8): 1117-1126.

van Kuppeveld, F. J., J. G. Hoenderop, et al. (1997). "Coxsackievirus protein 2B modifies endoplasmic reticulum membrane and plasma membrane permeability and facilitates virus release." EMBO J 16(12): 3519-3532.

Vaughan, M. B., E. W. Howard, et al. (2000). "Transforming growth factor-beta1 promotes the morphological and functional differentiation of the myofibroblast." Exp Cell Res 257(1): 180-189.

Wang, Y., M. Afanasyeva, et al. (1999). "Characterization of murine autoimmune myocarditis induced by self and foreign cardiac myosin." Autoimmunity 31(3): 151-162.

Why, H. J., B. T. Meany, et al. (1994). "Clinical and prognostic significance of detection of enteroviral RNA in the myocardium of patients with myocarditis or dilated cardiomyopathy." Circulation 89(6): 2582-2589.

Wing, K. and S. Sakaguchi (2010). "Regulatory T cells exert checks and balances on self tolerance and autoimmunity." Nat Immunol 11(1): 7-13.

Wittner, B., B. Maisch, et al. (1983). "Quantification of antimyosin antibodies in experimental myocarditis by a new solid phase fluorometric assay." J Immunol Methods 64(1-2): 239-247.

Woodruff, J. F. (1980). "Viral myocarditis. A review." Am J Pathol 101(2): 425-484.

Yajima, T. and K. U. Knowlton (2009). "Viral Myocarditis: From the Perspective of the Virus." Circulation 119(19): 2615-2624.

Yuan, J., Z. Liu, et al. (2009). "CXCL10 inhibits viral replication through recruitment of natural killer cells in coxsackievirus B3-induced myocarditis." Circ Res 104(5): 628-638.

Yuan, J., M. Yu, et al. (2010). "Th17 cells contribute to viral replication in coxsackievirus B3-induced acute viral myocarditis." J Immunol 185(7): 4004-4010.

Yue, Y., J. Gui, et al. (2011). "Direct Gene Transfer with IP-10 Mutant Ameliorates Mouse CVB3-Induced Myocarditis by Blunting Th1 Immune Responses." PLoS ONE 6(3): e18186.

Yue, Y., J. Gui, et al. (2011). "Gene therapy with CCL2 (MCP-1) mutant protects CVB3-induced myocarditis by compromising Th1 polarization." Mol Immunol 48(4): 706-713.

Zhang, P., C. J. Cox, et al. (2009). "Cutting edge: cardiac myosin activates innate immune responses through TLRs." J Immunol 183(1): 27-31.

Zou, W. and N. P. Restifo (2010). "T(H)17 cells in tumour immunity and immunotherapy." Nat Rev Immunol 10(4): 248-256.

11

Pattern-Recognition Receptors Sensing Viral Infection in Myocarditis and Inflammatory Heart Disease

Volker Ruppert[1] and Thomas Meyer[2]
[1]*Klinik für Kardiologie, Philipps-Universität Marburg and*
[2]*Klinik für Psychosomatische Medizin und Psychotherapie, Georg-August-Universität Göttingen, Germany*

1. Introduction

Myocarditis is a potentially life-threatening heart disease affecting both children and adults which presents with a broad spectrum of clinical manifestations. Symptoms range from asymptomatic infection to a fulminant course that rapidly progresses to dilated cardiomyopathy (DCM) and heart failure. Viral infection of the heart is a major cause of acute myocarditis, leading to myocardial inflammation and tissue damage. Cellular infiltration in acute viral myocarditis may be caused by direct cytopathic effects of the virus, pathologic responses to persistent viral replication as well as autoimmunity triggered by the virus (Liu and Mason, 2001; Bowles and Vallejo, 2003; Linde et al., 2007; Rose et al., 2009; Rutschow et al., 2010). The cardiovirulence of the viral agent, together with the host´s genetic susceptibility and the variability in the innate and acquired immune system, appear to determine the extent of the inflammatory reaction, thereby predicting clinical outcome (Kindermann et al., 2008).

Recently, meaningful advances have been made in our understanding of cellular mechanisms that are aimed to suppress viral propagation in inflammatory heart disease. In the first line of defense against viral replication, the host´s innate immune system is activated by unspecific, albeit effective interactions of cellular receptors with distinct pathogen-derived ligands. A variety of pattern-recognition receptors have been shown to be implicated in the detection of invading microbial agents (Kawai and Akira, 2010; Takeuchi and Akira, 2010). Upon viral infection of the heart, different signal pathways initiate an inflammatory response and orchestrate the concerted anti-viral defense machinery in a complex manner. Toll-like and RIG-I-like receptors are essential for the recognition of pathogen-associated molecular patterns and their activation induces intracellular signalling pathways which lead to the production of pro-inflammatory cytokines, chemokines, and interferons (Bowles and Vallejo, 2003; Fairweather et al., 2005; Triantafilou et al., 2005; Frantz et al., 2007; Linde et al., 2007; Yajima and Knowlton, 2009; Kawai and Akira, 2010; Takeuchi and Akira, 2010; Yamamoto and Takeda, 2010; Zhu and Mohan, 2010). Vice verse, interferons appear to induce the expression of a subset of toll-like receptors (Khoo et al., 2011). Type I interferons execute anti-viral responses by modulating cell growth, establishing an anti-viral state and influencing the activation of various immune cells. These potent anti-viral cytokines are best known for their role as innate immune mediators (Yajima and Knowlton, 2009). In the course of viral myocarditis, apoptotic signalling pathways are activated and modulate disease pathogenesis. However, cardiotropic viruses have evolved a battery of highly specific strategies to circumvent this innate protective response of the host and successfully replicate in cardiomyocytes (Versteeg and García-Sastre, 2010). Viral factors with or without homology to host proteins specifically target key components of the anti-viral defense machinery, some of which are transcription factors involved in establishing an anti-viral state.

In the present review we focus on the contribution of pattern-recognition receptors engaged in the early response cascade against cardiotropic viruses. In particular, we report on different signal transduction pathways emerging from membrane-associated and cytosolic receptors that inhibit viral dissemination and, furthermore, give a brief overview of the various adaptor molecules involved in these pathways. Not covered in this review are the diverse viral mechanisms for antagonizing the innate immune response and the precise cellular actions of cytokines in executing this anti-viral defense. Understanding the exact mechanisms by which viral components activate pattern-recognition receptors in the heart and modify gene expression profiles may help to improve novel therapeutic regimes for the treatment of viral myocarditis (Topkara et al., 2010).

2. Clinical course of myocarditis

Myocarditis is defined as a heterogeneous common disease pathway for myocardial inflammation resulting from a variety of infectious, immune and non-immune insults. The histopathologic hallmark of the disease is characterized by inflammatory infiltrates of the myocardium with concomitant necrosis or degeneration of adjacent cardiomyocytes in the absence of predominant ischemia. Despite this clear definition, the classification and diagnosis of myocarditis continue to present clinical problems. In recent years our understanding of the pathophysiology and natural clinical course of the disease has improved, probably because histological findings obtained from endomyocardial biopsies have routinely been combined with modern molecular biological and immunological tools in the detection of viral genomes persisting in the heart (Heidecker et al., 2011).

From epidemiological studies, it is known that viruses are the most frequent cause of myocarditis in Europe and North America although in rare cases bacteria, protozoa, and even fungi have also been implicated as infectious agents (Ellis and Di Salvo, 2007). Among the more common cardiotropic viruses are enteroviruses including Coxsackie virus, adenoviruses, parvovirus B19, hepatitis C virus, and human immunodeficiency virus (Kühl et al., 2005; Magnani and Dec, 2006; Mahrholdt et al., 2006; Noutsias et al., 2009; Rose, 2009; Pankuweit and Maisch, 2010). Other non-infectious etiologies of myocardial inflammation include hypersensitivity reactions against drugs, unexplained toxic reactions, and immunological syndromes including Churg-Strauss syndrome, giant cell myocarditis, systemic lupus erythematosus, sarcoidosis, Wegener´s granulomatosis, and others (Magnani and Dec, 2006; Ellis and Di Salvo, 2007; Rose, 2009). Although infections with cardiotropic viruses are believed to be the most common cause of acute lymphocytic myocarditis, a large number of patients have no identifiable source of the illness (Liu and Mason, 2001; Rose, 2009). Particularly, when the inflammatory process in the myocardium is moderate, the diagnosis frequently remains a challenge for clinicians. The diagnostic sensitivity for viral myocarditis is comparably low, even when applying modern molecular biological techniques, probably because, due to sampling error, the diagnostic accuracy of endomyocardial biopsy remains a significant limitation (Magnani and Dec, 2006; Ellis and Di Salvo, 2007). The Dallas criteria, originally proposed in an effort to standardize the histopathologic diagnosis of myocarditis, have been shown to be of limited use for epidemiological investigations (Magnani and Dec, 2006; Ellis and Di Salvo, 2007). Thus, despite recent advances in the recognition of myocardial inflammation, the true incidence and prevalence of acute viral myocarditis is still unknown.

The spectrum of clinical manifestations of viral myocarditis is extensive, ranging from asymptomatic infection to fever, myalgias, palpitations, exertional dyspnea, and hemodynamic collapse. Fulminant myocarditis may lead to systolic failure, malignant ventricular arrhythmias and sudden cardiac death (Baughman, 2005; Magnani and Dec, 2006; Rose, 2009, Blauwet and Cooper, 2010). The cardiac symptoms may also be present in more chronic forms of DCM, therefore contributing much to the difficulties in establishing the correct diagnosis. The main reason for the clinical variability appears to lie in the characteristics of the viral agent, together with the host´s innate immune system and genetic susceptibility to infection. Given the diversity and insidious onset of clinical manifestations, endomyocardial biopsy in combination with other techniques such as immuno-histochemistry, serological analyses, PCR and *in situ* hydridization remains the gold standard for the detection of virus-induced myocardial inflammation (Magnani and Dec, 2006; Rose, 2009).

Although, in severely affected individuals, fulminant viral myocarditis can lead to rapid progressive heart failure, the disease usually resolves spontaneously without persisting ventricular dysfunction (Baughman, 2005; Magnani and Dec, 2006; Rose, 2009, Blauwet and Cooper, 2010). Continuing cardiovascular symptoms in the absence of ventricular compromise may indicate that chronic persistent myocarditis has developed, which is characterized by the maintenance of lymphocytic infiltrates combined with foci of myocyte necrosis. Whereas it has been well-established that chronic active myocarditis can induce heart failure, there is still a controversy with respect to the causal relationship of asymptomatic viral infections for the pathogenesis of idiopathic DCM (Yajima and Knowlton, 2009). Several studies have suggested an association between viral persistence in the myocardium and the development of DCM. However, the etiologic significance of viral genomes detected in endomyocardial biopsies from DCM patients is currently unknown (Bock et al., 2010).

3. Toll-like receptors in the inflamed heart

Despite a wealth of information regarding the symptomatology and clinical course of the disease, the complex pathophysiological mechanisms underlying inflammatory heart disease are only partially understood. Lessons learned from transgenic mouse models have shed some light on the essential role of endogenous receptors and transcriptional regulators engaged in early anti-viral response. From clinical and animal studies we know that the host´s innate immune system acts as the first line of defense against viral replication in a wide array of pathogenic viruses. The innate immune system, which senses pathogen invasion and primes antigen-specific adaptive immunity, has long been considered to be only non-specific and somewhat simpler than that of the adaptive system. However, recent findings on pattern-recognition receptors and their downstream signalling pathways have led to a reconsideration of the role of innate immunity now seen as a highly potent defense apparatus against microbial pathogens which works in close cooperation with adaptive immunity.

Initial sensing of invading microorganisms by the innate immune system is mediated by pattern-recognition receptors (PRRs), which include toll-like receptors (TLRs), RIG-I-like-receptors, NOD-like receptors, and C-type lectin receptors (Akira et al., 2006; Bauer et al., 2009; Yajima and Knowlton, 2009; Kawai and Akira, 2010; Takeuchi and Akira, 2010). These four classes of germline-encoded PRR families are responsible for recognizing exogenous structures conserved among microbial species, which are called pathogen-associated molecular patterns (PAMPs). Currently, the paradigm of PRRs has changed, since it has been shown that PRRs also recognize endogenous molecules released from damaged cells, collectively termed damage-associated molecular patterns (DAMPs) (Piccinini and Midwood, 2010; Lamkanfi, 2011).

Among the PRRs, toll-like receptors and C-type lectin receptors are transmembrane glycoproteins, whereas retinoic acid-inducible gene (RIG)-I-like receptors and NOD-like receptors function as cytosolic PRRs (Figure 1). Toll-like receptors were first discovered in Drosophila as evolutionary ancient molecules that function as receptors for endogenous ligands such as proteolytically cleaved Spätzle protein, but later were found to be present also in the mammalian system where they respond to microbial components as well as endogenous ligands including heat shock proteins HSP60, HSP70, and gp96 (Medzhitov et al., 1997; Ohashi et al., 2000; Vabulas et al., 2002; Vabulas et al., 2002b; Kim et al., 2009; Arnot et al., 2010). Toll-like receptors are expressed on macrophages, dendritic cells, endothelial cells, and interestingly also on cardiac myocytes (Boyd et al., 2006). Structurally, they are characterized by a highly variable amino-terminal region containing a leucine-rich repeat (LRR) ectodomain, followed by a hydrophobic transmembrane region and a cytoplasmic toll/interleukin 1 receptor (TIR) homology domain, which mediates interaction between TLRs and downstream signalling molecules (Choe et al., 2005; Bell et al., 2006; Jin et al., 2007; Kang et al., 2009; Park et al., 2009). Ligand binding is mediated by the extracellular LRR ectodomain, which is composed of 19-25 tandem copies of the "xLxxLxLxx" motif (Jin and Lee, 2008). In humans, 10 members of the germline-encoded TLR family have been identified so far, TLR1-TLR9 being conserved in humans and mice. Due to a retroviral insertion, TLR10 is not functional in mice and the murine TLRs 11-13 are not present in humans (O'Neill, 2008; Kawai and Akira, 2010).

Ligand binding of PAMPs by TLRs occurs at the plasma membrane (TLR1, TLR2, TLR4-6) as well as in endolysosomal compartments and the endoplasmic reticulum (TLR3, TLR7-9) (Frantz et al., 2007. Kawai and Akira, 2010; Takeuchi and Akira, 2010; Yamamoto and Takeda, 2010). The difference in the downstream signalling cascades activated can be partly explained by the individual TLR molecule, which recognizes a specific subset of PAMPs and recruits different TIR domain-containing adaptors to the receptor. Ligands for TLRs include a broad range of various microbial components, such as bacterial lipoprotein moieties (TLR1-2, TLR6), lipopolysaccharide (TLR4), and flagellin protein (TLR5). Toll-like receptor 3, the first TLR family member to be implicated in the recognition of viral nucleic acids, binds to double-stranded RNA (dsRNA) molecules, which are produced as intermediates during the replication cycle of many viruses (Alexopoulou et al., 2001). TLR7 and TLR8 receptors recognize single-stranded RNA (ssRNA) and are expressed in a variety of immune cells, including dendritic cells, lymphocytes, monocytes, and NK cells (Bauer et al., 2008). Triantafilou and co-workers reported that inflammatory responses in human myocarditis

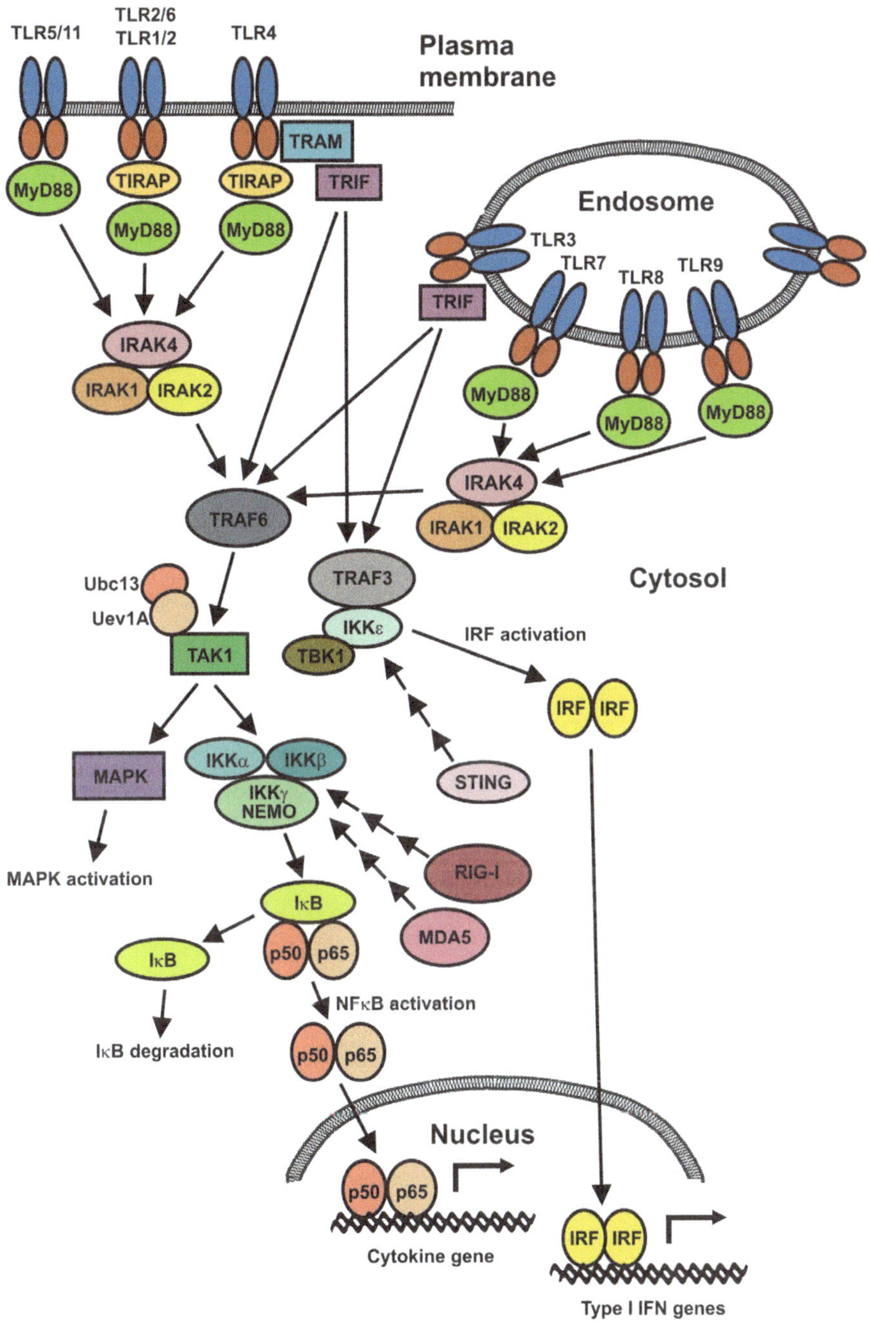

Fig. 1. Signalling pathways engaged in the detection of highly conserved, relatively invariant structural motifs of pathogens. Depicted are different pathways for the recognition

of microbial infection including toll-like receptor (TLR)-mediated MyD88-dependent and TRIF-dependent pathways as well as cytosolic sensors for foreign nucleic acid sequences (STING, RIG-I, and MDA5). For details on key receptors, their signalling adaptors and downstream mediators see text. **Abbreviations:** IKK; IκB kinase, IRAK; IL1-receptor-associated kinase, IRF; interferon-regulatory factor, MDA5; melanoma differentiation-associated gene 5, MyD88; myeloid differentiation primary response gene 88, NEMO; NF-κB essential modulator, NF-κB; nuclear factor-κB, RIG-I; retinoic acid-inducible gene-I, STING; stimulator of interferon genes, TAK1; transforming growth factor-β-activated kinase 1, TBK1; TANK-binding kinase 1, TIRAP; toll-interleukin 1 receptor (TIR) domain-containing adaptor protein, TLR; toll-like receptor, TRAF; tumour necrosis factor receptor-associated factor, TRIF; TIR-domain-containing adaptor protein inducing interferon-β (also known as TICAM), TRAM; TRIF-related adaptor molecule.

induced by Coxsackie virus B3 (CVB3) are mediated through TLR8 and to a lesser extent through TLR7 (Triantafilou et al., 2005). Elevated expression levels of TLR8 have been associated with heart failure and adverse clinical outcome in patients with enterovirus-associated dilated cardiomyopathy (Satoh et al., 2007). Toll-like receptor 9 functions as a sensor for unmethylated cytosine-phosphate-guanine (CpG) sequences in bacterial and viral DNA, which are rarely found in vertebrates (Barton et al., 2006; Guggemoos et al., 2008). Riad and colleagues demonstrated that, in the acute phase of CVB3-induced myocarditis, TLR9 knockout mice displayed improved LV function associated with reduced cardiac inflammation as compared to CVB3-infected wild-type mice. The cardioprotective effects due to TLR9 deficiency were associated with suppression of the TLR9 downstream pathway as indexed by reduced cardiac levels of the adapter protein MyD88 and the proinflammatory cytokine TNF-α (Riad et al., 2010).

In non-infected cells, TLR3 and TLR7-9 reside in the endoplasmic reticulum, whereas after uncoating and exposure to viral nucleic acids they traffic to the endosomal compartments, where they finally trigger a signal cascade resulting in the activation of the transcription factor NF-κB. The subcellular localization of the various TLR family members appears to be tightly regulated, probably because this avoids unbalanced activation to self-DNA in the absence of viral encounter. The diverse distributions of individual TLRs allow for the surveillance of different intracellular compartments, as viral entry usually occurs by receptor-mediated endocytosis and endosomal fusion or by direct fusion with the plasma membrane (Barton et al., 2006; Barton and Kagan, 2009).

Structural studies have revealed that the hydrophobic ligands of TLR1, TLR2, and TLR4 interact with internal protein pockets on the ectodomain, while hydrophilic dsRNA binds to the solvent-exposed surface of TLR3. Binding to cognate ligands induces homodimerization of the TLR ectodomains, whereas TLR2 forms heterodimers with TLR1 or TLR6 which interact with triacyl- and diacyl lipoproteins, respectively (Jin et al., 2007; Kang et al., 2009; Kawai and Akira, 2010). The membrane-adjacent carboxy-termini of the extracellular domains then converge and probably facilitate dimer formation of the cytoplasmic TIR domains to activate intracellular signalling.

Upon stimulation, the dimeric TLR molecules, except for TLR3, recruit a cytoplasmic adaptor called MyD88 (myeloid differentiation primary response gene 88), which is composed of a death domain (DD) in addition to a TIR domain (Muzio et al., 1997; Frantz et al., 2007; Kawai and Akira, 2010). CpG-DNA activates the TLR signaling pathway via MyD88 and TRAF6 (tumour necrosis factor receptor-associated factor 6), leading to activation of kinases of the IκB kinase complex (Häcker et al., 2000). When infected with the spirochete *Borrelia burgdorferi*, mice deficient in MyD88 expression develop myocarditis and arthritis similar to the disease in wild-type mice (Liu et al., 2004). However, the pathogen burden was much higher in MyD88$^{-/-}$ mice than in wild-type mice, probably because degradation of the bacteria was critically impaired.

In response to stimulation with dsRNA, TLR3 recruits another adaptor molecule referred to as TRIF (TIR domain-containing adaptor protein inducing interferon-β, also known as TICAM), which associates with TRAF6 and RIP1 (receptor interacting protein 1) (Yamamoto et al., 2003). TRIF plays a critical role in MyD88-independent TLR3 signalling via TRAF6 and TANK-binding kinase (TBK)-1, leading to the activation of two distinct transcription factors, NF-κB and interferon-regulatory factor 3 (Sato et al., 2003). Hardarson and colleagues reported that TLR3 is an essential component of the innate stress response in encephalomyocarditis virus (EMCV)-induced cardiac injury (Hardarson et al., 2007). Mice lacking TLR3 expression were more susceptible to EMCV infection and had a significantly higher viral load in the heart, but lesser inflammatory changes of the myocardium as compared to control mice. TLR3-deficient mice had impaired proinflammatory cytokine and chemokine production in the heart, while expression of interferon-β was not impaired (Hardarson et al., 2007).

Satoh and colleagues reported that in 44 patients with myocarditis increased expression of TLR4 was associated with replication of enteroviral RNA and that these RNA levels were related to cardiac dysfunction (Satoh et al., 2003). In TLR4 signalling, the ligand-bound receptor utilizes MyD88 and TIRAP (toll-interleukin 1 receptor (TIR) domain-containing adaptor protein) for MyD88-dependent as well as TRIF and TRAM (TRIF-related adaptor molecule) for MyD88-independent pathways (Yamamoto et al., 2003b; Fitzgerald et al., 2003). The adaptor protein TRAM is required for activation of TRIF and recently a splice variant of TRAM called TAG (TRAM adaptor with GOLD domain) has been identified that acts as a negative regulator of TRIF-dependent signalling (Palsson-McDermott et al., 2009). TLR1, TLR2, TLR4, and TLR6 signalling requires, in addition, TIRAP which is important for bridging between the cytoplasmic TLR tail and MyD88 (Fitzgerald et al., 2001). Recently, it was shown that infection with Coxsackie virus group B serotype 3 (CVB3) resulted in cardiac remodelling, severe heart failure, and high mortality in TRIF-deficient mice, while wild-type mice showed only mild myocarditis and normal survival postinfection (Riad et al., 2011). Furthermore, virus control was markedly reduced in mice lacking TRIF expression and, interestingly, TRIF-deficient myocytes displayed a TLR4-dependent suppression of interferon-β. These findings suggest that TRIF confers cardioprotection against CVB3 infection.

The recruitment of these adaptors triggers a cascade of signalling events, which leads to the activation of the transcription factors NF-κB and interferon-regulatory factors (IRFs). These transcription factors ultimately induce the expression of various inflammatory cytokines, which execute important functions in anti-viral defence. The first step in the synthesis of cytokines leads to the activation of interleukin 1 receptor-associated kinase 4 (IRAK4), which functions as a serine/threonine kinase with an aminoterminal death domain (DD) (Suzuki et al., 2002; Suzuki et al., 2002b). Subsequently, IRAK1 and IRAK2 are phosphorylated by IRAK4 and, after dissociation of MyD88, a complex with TRAF3 and TRAF6 is formed (Kawagoe et al., 2007; Kawagoe et al., 2008; Lin et al., 2010). TRAF6 acts as an E3 ligase in conjugation with the E2 ubiquitin-conjugating enzymes Ubc13 and Uev1A and catalyzes the formation of a lysine63-linked polyubiquitin chain on target proteins, including TRAF6 itself, IRAK, and the NF-κB essential modulator (NEMO) (Deng et al., 2000). Transforming growth factor-β-activated kinase 1 (TAK1) is recruited and ubiquitinylated by TRAF6 (Wang et al., 2001). Subsequently, the IKK complex composed of IKKα, IKKβ and NEMO is formed which phosphorylates inhibitor of NF-κB (IκB) kinase-ß (IKKβ). The activated IKK complex then induces phosphorylation and subsequent degradation of IκB by the proteasome. Upon degradation of IκB, the freed NF-κB is no longer sequestered in the cytosol, but translocates into the nucleus, where it drives the expression of cytokine genes. Simultaneously, TAK1 activates the mitogen-activated protein kinase (MAPK) cascade leading to the activation of the transcription factor AP-1, which also targets gene expression of cytokine genes (Wang et al., 2001).

4. Cytosolic sensors for recognizing foreign nucleic acids

Members of the cytosolic RIG-I-like receptor (RLR) family act as cytosolic sensors for genomic RNA of dsRNA viruses and dsRNA intermediates that are generated during replication of ssRNA viruses (Yoneyama et al., 2004; Kato et al., 2005; Bowzard et al., 2009; Ranjan et al., 2009). Retinoic acid-induced protein I is composed of two amino-terminal caspase activation and recruitment domains (CARDs), a central DEAD box helicase/ATPase domain, and a carboxy-terminal regulatory domain (Yoneyama et al., 2004). The latter domain plays a critical role in the specific recognition of dsRNA and 5'-triphosphorylated ssRNA. Other members of the RIG-I family include MDA5 (melanoma differentiation-associated gene 5) and LGP2 (laboratory of genetics and physiology 2). RIG-I and MDA5 distinguish between different RNA viruses and contribute to the host´s anti-viral response through recognition of either 5'-triphosphorylated and uncapped ssRNA or dsRNA, species not found among endogenous self-RNA (Kato et al., 2006). Transgenic mice, deficient in RIG-I or MDA5 expression, are highly susceptible to infection with RNA viruses compared to control mice (Kato et al., 2006). The RIG-I homolog LGP2, which lacks the amino-terminal CARDs, potentiates viral RNA recognition by RIG-I and MDA5 through its ATPase domain and has been found to be essential for type I interferon production in response to picornaviridae infection (Satoh et al., 2010). Recently, it has been shown that also DNA-dependent RNA polymerase III is pivotal in sensing viral DNA in the cytoplasm (Ablasser et al., 2009; Chiu et al, 2009). AT-rich dsDNA can serve as a template for RNA polymerase III, which is transcribed enzymatically into dsRNA containing a 5'-triphosphorylated moiety. Activation of RIG-I by dsRNA ultimately induces production of type I interferon and activation of the transcription factor NF-κB.

Recently, it was reported that overexpression of STING (stimulator of interferon genes), a transmembrane protein found in the endoplasmic reticulum of numerous cells such as macrophages, dendritic, endothelial and epithelial cells, induces activation of NF-κB and IRF3 to stimulate type I interferon synthesis (Ishikawa et al., 2009; Barber, 2011). STING-knockout mice were susceptible to lethal infection after exposure to herpes simplex virus 1, suggesting that STING plays an important role in detecting foreign DNA.

Another cytosolic sensor for both bacterial and viral pathogens is AIM2 (absent in melanoma 2), which is essential for inflammasome activation in response to *Fransicella tularensis*, vaccinia virus, and mouse cytomegalovirus (Rathinam et al., 2010). AIM2 regulates caspase-1-dependent maturation of IL-1β and IL-18 and plays a role in natural killer cell-dependent production of interferon-γ, as has been shown for AIM2-deficient mice. However, the role of AIM2 in the pathogenesis of myocarditis has not been investigated so far.

PRRs	Ligand	Localization	Origin of the ligand	Selected references
TLR2	Lipoprotein	Plasma membrane	Bacteria, viruses	Following coronary artery ligation, *tlr*2-/- mice show reduced mortality and preserved left ventricular function as compared to wild-type mice (Shishido et al., 2003; Riad et al., 2008). Ischemia-reperfusion results in smaller infarct size (Favre et al., 2007). *Tlr*2-/- mice are protected from doxorubicin-induced cardiomyopathy (Nozaki et al., 2004).
TLR3	dsRNA	Endolysosome	Viruses	*Tlr*3-/- mice are more susceptible to EMCV infection and have a higher viral load, but lesser myocardial inflammation (Hardarson et al., 2007).
TLR4	Lipopoly-saccharide (LPS)	Plasma membrane	Bacteria, viruses	*Tlr*4-/- mice are protected from ischemia-reperfusion injury (Chong et al, 2004; Oyama et al., 2004; Kim et al., 2007) and LPS-induced mortality and cardiac dysfunction (Tavener et al., 2004; Nemoto et al, 2009). *Tlr*4-/- mice develop less-severe cardiac hypertrophy following pressure overload by aortic banding than wild-type mice (Ha et al., 2005).
TLR5	Flagellin	Plasma membrane	Bacteria	Exposure to the TLR5 ligand flagellin triggers cardiac innate immune responses that result in acute contractile dysfunction (Rolli et al., 2010).
TLR6	Diacyl lipoprotein	Plasma membrane	Bacteria, viruses	TLR6 Ser249Pro polymorphism has been associated with lower left ventricular thickness in hypertensive women (Sales et al., 2010).
TLR7 (TLR8)	ssRNA	Endolysosome	Bacteria, viruses	*Tlr*7-/- mice show markedly reduced myocardial cellular infiltration in experimental autoimmune myocarditis (Pagni et al., 2010). TLR8 expression is higher in DCM patients than in controls (Satoh et al., 2007).
TLR9	CpG-DNA	Endolysosome	Bacteria, viruses	Upon murine cytomegalovirus-induced myocarditis, *tlr*9-/- mice show higher severity of myocardial infiltration compared to wild-type (Pagni et al., 2010). Myocardial TLR9 expression is reduced in DCM patients (Ruppert et al., 2008).
RIG-I	Short dsRNA	Cytoplasm	Viruses	RIG-I mRNA is expressed at high levels in normal heart tissue (Ellis et al., 2002). Interferon-γ upregulates RIG-I in pericardial mesothelial cells, suggesting that RIG-I may be involved in the pathogenesis of pericarditis (Hatakeyama et al., 2007)

Table 1. Pattern recognition receptors (PRR) and their ligands engaged in myocarditis and inflammatory heart disease.

5. Concluding remarks

Beside direct effects of replicating viruses, unbalanced autoimmune responses associated with the production of auto-antibodies against cardiac tissue may also contribute to the progression of myocardial injury in inflammatory heart disease (Eriksson et al., 2003). The detection of auto-reactive antibodies directed against a number of different cardiac antigens is a prominent feature of all forms of persistent myocarditis and inflammatory cardiomyopathy, and there are reports demonstrating that the presence of anti-myosin autoantibodies is associated with deterioration of left ventricular function (Liu and Mason, 2001; Shishido et al., 2003; Dörner et al., 2005; Rose, 2009). In addition to the critical role of TLRs in mediating cardiac dysfunction in infectious conditions, emerging evidence suggests that the TLRs are also involved in modulating cardiomyocyte survival and ischemic myocardial injury (Chao, 2009; Riad et al., 2008). Despite significant progress in the identification of receptors triggering innate immune responses, further research is necessary to unravel the cooperative interactions between the innate and acquired immune system active in the protection of the heart against viral or autoimmune damage.

6. Acknowledgements

This work was supported by grants from the Deutsche Forschungsgemeinschaft und Deutsche Krebshilfe to T.M. Disclose of conflict of interest: none.

7. References

Ablasser A, Bauernfeind F, Hartmann G, Latz E, Fitzgerald KA, Hornung V. RIG-I-dependent sensing of poly(dA:dT) through the induction of an RNA polymerase III-transcribed RNA intermediate. Nat Immunol. 2009;10:1065-1072.

Akira S, Uematsu S, Takeuchi O. Pathogen recognition and innate immunity. Cell. 2006;124:783-801.

Alexopoulou L, Holt AC, Medzhitov R, Flavell RA. Recognition of double-stranded RNA and activation of NF-kappaB by Toll-like receptor 3. Nature. 2001;413:732-738.

Arnot CJ, Gay NJ, Gangloff M. Molecular mechanism that induces activation of Spätzle, the ligand for the Drosophila Toll receptor. J Biol Chem. 2010;285:19502-19519.

Barber GN. Innate immune DNA sensing pathways: STING, AIMII and the regulation of interferon production and inflammatory responses. Curr Opin Immunol. 2011;23:10-20.

Barton GM, Kagan JC. A cell biological view of Toll-like receptor function: regulation through compartmentalization. Nat Rev Immunol. 2009;9:535-542.

Barton GM, Kagan JC, Medzhitov R. Intracellular localization of Toll-like receptor 9 prevents recognition of self DNA but facilitates access to viral DNA. Nat Immunol. 2006;7:49-56.

Bauer S, Müller T, Hamm S. Pattern recognition by Toll-like receptors. Adv Exp Med Biol. 2009;653:15-34.

Bauer S, Pigisch S, Hangel D, Kaufmann A, Hamm S. Recognition of nucleic acid and nucleic acid analogs by Toll-like receptors 7, 8 and 9. Immunobiology. 2008;213:315-328.

Baughman KL. Clinical presentations of myocarditis. Heart Fail Clin. 2005;1:363-376.

Bell JK, Askins J, Hall PR, Davies DR, Segal DM. Crystal structure of human toll-like receptor 3 (TLR3) ectodomain. Proc Natl Acad Sci U S A. 2006;103:8792-8797.

Bock CT, Klingel K, Kandolf R. Human parvovirus B19-associated myocarditis. N Engl J Med. 2010;362:1248-1249.

Bowles NE, Vallejo J. Viral causes of cardiac inflammation. Curr Opin Cardiol. 2003;18:182-188.

Blauwet LA, Cooper LT. Myocarditis. Prog Cardiovasc Dis. 2010;52:274-288.

Bowzard JB, Ranjan P, Sambhara S, Fujita T. Antiviral defense: RIG-Ing the immune system to STING. Cytokine Growth Factor Rev. 2009;20:1-5

Boyd JH, Mathur S, Wang Y, Bateman RM, Walley KR. Toll-like receptor stimulation in cardiomyocytes decreases contractility and initiates an NF-kappaB dependent inflammatory response. Cardiovasc Res. 2006;72:384-393.

Chao W. Toll-like receptor signaling: a critical modulator of cell survival and ischemic injury in the heart. Am J Physiol Heart Circ Physiol. 2009;296:H1-12.

Chiu YH, Macmillan JB, Chen ZJ. RNA polymerase III detects cytosolic DNA and induces type I interferons through the RIG-I pathway.Cell. 2009;138:576-591.

Choe J, Kelker MS, Wilson IA. Crystal structure of human toll-like receptor 3 (TLR3) ectodomain. Science. 2005;309:581-585.

Chong AJ, Shimamoto A, Hampton CR, Takayama H, Spring DJ, Rothnie CL, Yada M, Pohlman TH, Verrier ED. Toll-like receptor 4 mediates ischemia/reperfusion injury of the heart. J Thorac Cardiovasc Surg. 2004;128:170-179.

Deng L, Wang C, Spencer E, Yang L, Braun A, You J, Slaughter C, Pickart C, Chen ZJ. Activation of the IkappaB kinase complex by TRAF6 requires a dimeric ubiquitin-conjugating enzyme complex and a unique polyubiquitin chain. Cell. 2000;103:351-361.

Dörner A, Kallwellis-Opara A, Pauschinger M, Kühl U, Schultheiss HP. Cardiac autoantibodies in viral myocarditis. Heart Fail Clin. 2005;1:333-343.

Ellis CR, Di Salvo T. Myocarditis: basic and clinical aspects. Cardiol Rev. 2007;15:170-177.

Ellis CA, Vos MD, Howell H, Vallecorsa T, Fults DW, Clark GJ. Rig is a novel Ras-related protein and potential neural tumor suppressor. Proc Natl Acad Sci USA. 2002;99:9876-9881.

Eriksson U, Ricci R, Hunziker L, Kurrer MO, Oudit GY, Watts TH, Sonderegger I, Bachmaier K, Kopf M, Penninger JM. Dendritic cell-induced autoimmune heart failure requires cooperation between adaptive and innate immunity. Nat Med. 2003;9:1484-1490.

Fairweather D, Frisancho-Kiss S, Rose NR. Viruses as adjuvants for autoimmunity: evidence from Coxsackievirus-induced myocarditis. Rev Med Virol. 2005;15:17-27.

Favre J, Musette P, Douin-Echinard V, Laude K, Henry JP, Arnal JF, Thuillez C, Richard V. Toll-like receptors 2-deficient mice are protected against postischemic coronary endothelial dysfunction. Arterioscler Thromb Vasc Biol. 2007;27:1064-1071.

Fitzgerald KA, Palsson-McDermott EM, Bowie AG, Jefferies CA, Mansell AS, Brady G, Brint E, Dunne A, Gray P, Harte MT, McMurray D, Smith DE, Sims JE, Bird TA, O'Neill LA. Mal (MyD88-adapter-like) is required for Toll-like receptor-4 signal transduction. Nature. 2001;413:78-83.

Fitzgerald KA, Rowe DC, Barnes BJ, Caffrey DR, Visintin A, Latz E, Monks B, Pitha PM, Golenbock DT. LPS-TLR4 signaling to IRF-3/7 and NF-kappaB involves the toll adapters TRAM and TRIF. J Exp Med. 2003;198:1043-1055.

Frantz S, Ertl G, Bauersachs J. Mechanisms of disease: Toll-like receptors in cardiovascular disease. Nat Clin Pract Cardiovasc Med. 2007;4:444-454.

Guggemoos S, Hangel D, Hamm S, Heit A, Bauer S, Adler H. TLR9 contributes to antiviral immunity during gammaherpesvirus infection. J Immunol. 2008;180:438-443.

Ha T, Li Y, Hua F, Ma J, Gao X, Kelley J, Zhao A, Haddad GE, Williams DL, William Browder I, Kao RL, Li C. Reduced cardiac hypertrophy in toll-like receptor 4-deficient mice following pressure overload. Cardiovasc Res. 2005;68:224-234.

Häcker H, Vabulas RM, Takeuchi O, Hoshino K, Akira S, Wagner H. Immune cell activation by bacterial CpG-DNA through myeloid differentiation marker 88 and tumor necrosis factor receptor-associated factor (TRAF)6. J Exp Med. 2000;192:595-600.

Hardarson HS, Baker JS, Yang Z, Purevjav E, Huang CH, Alexopoulou L, Li N, Flavell RA, Bowles NE, Vallejo JG. Toll-like receptor 3 is an essential component of the innate stress response in virus-induced cardiac injury. Am J Physiol Heart Circ Physiol. 2007;292:H251-258.

Hatakeyama M, Imaizumi T, Terasaki F, Mori F, Tanji K, Sato F, Kijima H, Suma H, Wakabayashi K, Yoshida H, Fukuda I, Satoh K. Interferon-gamma upregulates retinoic acid-inducible gene-I in human pericardial mesothelial cells. Acta Cardiol. 2007;62:553-557.

Heidecker B, Kittleson MM, Kasper EK, Wittstein IS, Champion HC, Russell SD, Hruban RH, Rodriguez ER, Baughman KL, Hare JM. Transcriptomic biomarkers for the accurate diagnosis of myocarditis. Circulation 2011;123:1174-1184.

Ishikawa H, Ma Z, Barber GN. STING regulates intracellular DNA-mediated, type I interferon-dependent innate immunity. Nature. 2009;461:788-792.

Jin MS, Kim SE, Heo JY, Lee ME, Kim HM, Paik SG, Lee H, Lee JO. Crystal structure of the TLR1-TLR2 heterodimer induced by binding of a tri-acylated lipopeptide. Cell. 2007;130:1071-1082.

Jin MS, Lee JO. Structures of the toll-like receptor family and its ligand complexes. Immunity. 2008;29:182-191.

Kang JY, Nan X, Jin MS, Youn SJ, Rvu YH, Mah S, Han SH, Lee H, Paik SG, Lee JO. Recognition of lipopeptide patterns by Toll-like receptor 2-Toll-like receptor 6 heterodimer. Immunity 2009;31:873-884.

Kato H, Sato S, Yoneyama M, Yamamoto M, Uematsu S, Matsui K, Tsujimura T, Takeda K, Fujita T, Takeuchi O, Akira S. Cell type-specific involvement of RIG-I in antiviral response. Immunity. 2005;23:19-28.

Kato H, Takeuchi O, Sato S, Yoneyama M, Yamamoto M, Matsui K, Uematsu S, Jung A, Kawai T, Ishii KJ, Yamaguchi O, Otsu K, Tsujimura T, Koh CS, Reis e Sousa C, Matsuura Y, Fujita T, Akira S. Differential roles of MDA5 and RIG-I helicases in the recognition of RNA viruses. Nature. 2006;441:101-105.

Kawagoe T, Sato S, Jung A, Yamamoto M, Matsui K, Kato H, Uematsu S, Takeuchi O, Akira S. Essential role of IRAK-4 protein and its kinase activity in Toll-like receptor-mediated immune responses but not in TCR signaling. J Exp Med. 2007 14;204:1013-1024.

Kawagoe T, Sato S, Matsushita K, Kato H, Matsui K, Kumagai Y, Saitoh T, Kawai T, Takeuchi O, Akira S. Sequential control of Toll-like receptor-dependent responses by IRAK1 and IRAK2. Nat Immunol. 2008;9:684-691.

Kawai T, Akira S. The role of pattern-recognition receptors in innate immunity: update on Toll-like receptors. Nat Immunol. 2010;11:373-384.

Khoo JJ, Forster S, Mansell A. Toll-like receptors as interferon-regulated genes and their role in disease. J Interferon Cytokine Res. 2011;31:13-25.

Kim SC, Ghanem A, Stapel H, Tiemann K, Knuefermann P, Hoeft A, Meyer R, Grohé C, Knowlton AA, Baumgarten G. Toll-like receptor 4 deficiency: smaller infarcts, but no gain in function. BMC Physiol. 2007;7:5.

Kim SC, Stice JP, Chen L, Jung JS, Gupta S, Wang Y, Baumgarten G, Trial J, Knowlton AA. Extracellular heat shock protein 60, cardiac myocytes, and apoptosis. Circ Res. 2009;105:1186-1195.

Kindermann I, Kindermann M, Kandolf R, Klingel K, Bültmann B, Müller T, Lindinger A, Böhm M. Predictors of outcome in patients with suspected myocarditis. Circulation. 2008;118:639-648.

Kühl U, Pauschinger M, Noutsias M, Seeberg B, Bock T, Lassner D, Poller W, Kandolf R, Schultheiss HP. High prevalence of viral genomes and multiple viral infections in the myocardium of adults with "idiopathic" left ventricular dysfunction. Circulation. 2005;111:887-893.

Lamkanfi M. Emerging inflammasome effector mechanisms. Nat Rev Immunol. 2011;11:213-220.

Lin SC, Lo YC, Wu H. Helical assembly in the MyD88-IRAK4-IRAK2 complex in TLR/IL-1R signalling. Nature. 2010;465:885-890.

Linde A, Mosier D, Blecha F, Melgarejo T. Innate immunity and inflammation. New frontiers in comparative cardiovascular pathology. Cardiovasc Res. 2007;73:26-36

Liu N, Montgomery RR, Barthold SW, Bockenstedt LK. Myeloid differentiation antigen 88 deficiency impairs pathogen clearance but does not alter inflammation in *Borrelia burgdorferi*-infected mice. Infect Immun. 2004;72:3195-3203.

Liu PP, Mason JW. Advances in the understanding of myocarditis. Circulation. 2001;104:1076-1082.

Magnani JW, Dec GW. Myocarditis: current trends in diagnosis and treatment. Circulation. 2006;113:876-890.

Mahrholdt H, Wagner A, Deluigi CC, Kispert E, Hager S, Meinhardt G, Vogelsberg H, Fritz P, Dippon J, Bock CT, Klingel K, Kandolf R, Sechtem U. Presentation, patterns of myocardial damage, and clinical course of viral myocarditis. Circulation. 2006;114:1581-1590.

Medzhitov R, Preston-Hurlburt P, Janeway CA Jr. A human homologue of the Drosophila Toll protein signals activation of adaptive immunity. Nature. 1997;388:394-397.

Muzio M, Ni J, Feng P, Dixit VM. IRAK (Pelle) family member IRAK-2 and MyD88 as proximal mediators of IL-1 signaling. Science. 1997;278:1612-1615.

Nemoto S, Vallejo JG, Knuefermann P, Misra A, Defreitas G, Carabello BA, Mann DL. *Escherichia coli* LPS-induced LV dysfunction: role of toll-like receptor-4 in the adult heart. Am J Physiol Heart Circ Physiol. 2002;282:H2316-2323.

Noutsias M, Pankuweit S, Maisch B. Pathophysiological mechanisms of parvovirus B19 infection. J Clin Microbiol. 2009;47:2358-2359.

Nozaki N, Shishido T, Takeishi Y, Kubota I. Modulation of doxorubicin-induced cardiac dysfunction in toll-like receptor-2-knockout mice. Circulation. 2004;110:2869-2874.

Ohashi K, Burkart V, Flohé, Kolb H. Cutting edge: heat shock protein 60 is a putative endogenous ligand of the toll-like receptor-4 complex. J Immunol 2000;164:558-561.

Oyama J, Blais C Jr, Liu X, Pu M, Kobzik L, Kelly RA, Bourcier T. Reduced myocardial ischemia-reperfusion injury in toll-like receptor 4-deficient mice. Circulation. 2004;109:784-789.

O'Neill LA. The interleukin-1 receptor/Toll-like receptor superfamily: 10 years of progress. Immunol Rev. 2008;226:10-18.

Pagni PP, Traub S, Demaria O, Chasson L, Alexopoulou L. Contribution of TLR7 and TLR9 signaling to the susceptibility of MyD88-deficient mice to myocarditis. Autoimmunity. 2010; 43:275-287.

Palsson-McDermott EM, Doyle SL, McGettrick AF, Hardy M, Husebye H, Banahan K, Gong M, Golenbock D, Espevik T, O'Neill LA. TAG, a splice variant of the adaptor TRAM, negatively regulates the adaptor MyD88-independent TLR4 pathway. Nat Immunol. 2009;10:579-586.

Pankuweit S, Maisch B. The heart in viral infections. Internist (Berl). 2010;51:836-843.

Park BS, Song DH, Kim HM, Choi BS, Lee H, Lee JO. The structural basis of lipopolysaccharide recognition by the TLR4-MD-2 complex. Nature. 2009;458:1191-1195.

Piccinini AM, Midwood KS. DAMPening inflammation by modulating TLR signalling. Mediators Inflamm. 2010;e672395:1-21.

Ranjan P, Bowzard JB, Schwerzmann JW, Jeisy-Scott V, Fujita T, Sambhara S. Cytoplasmic nucleic acid sensors in antiviral immunity. Trends Mol Med. 2009;15:359-368.

Rathinam VA, Jiang Z, Waggoner SN, Sharma S, Cole LE, Waggoner L, Vanaja SK, Monks BG, Ganesan S, Latz E, Hornung V, Vogel SN, Szomolanyi-Tsuda E, Fitzgerald KA. The AIM2 inflammasome is essential for host defense against cytosolic bacteria and DNA viruses. Nat Immunol. 2010;11:395-402.

Riad A, Jäger S, Sobirey M, Escher F, Yaulema-Riss A, Westermann D, Karatas A, Heimesaat MM, Bereswill S, Dragun D, Pauschinger M, Schultheiss HP, Tschöpe C. Toll-like receptor-4 modulates survival by induction of left ventricular remodeling after myocardial infarction in mice. J Immunol. 2008;180:6954-6961.

Riad A, Westermann D, Escher F, Becher PM, Savvatis K, Lettau O, Heimesaat MM, Bereswill S, Volk HD, Schultheiss HP, Tschöpe C. Myeloid differentiation factor-88 contributes to TLR9-mediated modulation of acute coxsackievirus B3-induced myocarditis in vivo. Am J Physiol Heart Circ Physiol. 2010;298:H2024-2031.

Riad A, Westermann D, Zietsch C, Savvatis K, Becher PM, Bereswill S, Heimesaat MM, Lettau O, Lassner D, Dörner A, Poller W, Busch M, Felix SB, Schultheiss HP, Tschöpe C. TRIF is a critical survival factor in viral cardiomyopathy. J Immunol. 2011;186:2561-2570.

Rolli J, Rosenblatt-Velin N, Li J, Loukili N, Levrand S, Pacher P, Waeber B, Feihl F, Ruchat P, Liaudet L. Bacterial flagellin triggers cardiac innate immune responses and acute contractile dysfunction. PLoS One. 2010;5:e12687.

Rose NR. Myocarditis: infection versus autoimmunity. J Clin Immunol. 2009;29:730-737.

Ruppert V, Meyer T, Pankuweit S, Möller E, Funck RC, Grimm W, Maisch B; German Heart Failure Network. Gene expression profiling from endomyocardial biopsy tissue allows distinction between subentities of dilated cardiomyopathy. J Thorac Cardiovasc Surg. 2008;136:360-369.

Rutschow S, Leschka S, Westermann D, Puhl K, Weitz A, Ladyszenskij L, Jaeger S, Zeichhardt H, Noutsias M, Schultheiss HP, Tschope C, Pauschinger M. Left ventricular enlargement in coxsackievirus-B3 induced chronic myocarditis--ongoing inflammation and an imbalance of the matrix degrading system. Eur J Pharmacol. 2010;630:145-151.

Sales ML, Schreiber R, Ferreira-Sae MC, Fernandes MN, Piveta CS, Cipolli JA, Cardoso CC, Matos-Souza JR, Geloneze B, Franchini KG, Nadruz W Jr. Toll-like receptor 6 Ser249Pro polymorphism is associated with lower left ventricular wall thickness and inflammatory response in hypertensive women. Am J Hypertens. 2010;23:649-654.

Sato S, Sugiyama M, Yamamoto M, Watanabe Y, Kawai T, Takeda K, Akira S. Toll/IL-1 receptor domain-containing adaptor inducing IFN-beta (TRIF) associates with TNF receptor-associated factor 6 and TANK-binding kinase 1, and activates two distinct transcription factors, NF-kappa B and IFN-regulatory factor-3, in the Toll-like receptor signaling. J Immunol. 2003;171:4304-4310.

Satoh M, Akatsu T, Ishikawa Y, Minami Y, Takahashi Y, Nakamura M. Association between toll-like receptor 8 expression and adverse clinical outcomes in patients with enterovirus-associated dilated cardiomyopathy. Am Heart J. 2007;154:581-588.

Satoh T, Kato H, Kumagai Y, Yoneyama M, Sato S, Matsushita K, Tsujimura T, Fujita T, Akira S, Takeuchi O. LGP2 is a positive regulator of RIG-I- and MDA5-mediated antiviral responses. Proc Natl Acad Sci U S A. 2010;107:1512-1517.

Satoh M, Nakamura M, Akatsu T, Iwasaka J, Shimoda Y, Segawa I, Hiramori K. Expression of Toll-like receptor 4 is associated with enteroviral replication in human myocarditis. Clin Sci (Lond). 2003;104:577-584.

Shishido T, Nozaki N, Yamaguchi S, Shibata Y, Nitobe J, Miyamoto T, Takahashi H, Arimoto T, Maeda K, Yamakawa M, Takeuchi O, Akira S, Takeishi Y, Kubota I. Toll-like receptor-2 modulates ventricular remodeling after myocardial infarction. Circulation. 2003;108:2905-2910.

Suzuki N, Suzuki S, Duncan GS, Millar DG, Wada T, Mirtsos C, Takada H, Wakeham A, Itie A, Li S, Penninger JM, Wesche H, Ohashi PS, Mak TW, Yeh WC. Severe impairment of interleukin-1 and Toll-like receptor signalling in mice lacking IRAK-4. Nature. 2002;416:750-756.

Suzuki N, Suzuki S, Yeh WC. IRAK-4 as the central TIR signaling mediator in innate immunity. Trends Immunol. 2002b;23:503-506.

Takeuchi O, Akira S. Pattern recognition receptors and inflammation. Cell. 2010:140:805-820.

Tavener SA, Long EM, Robbins SM, McRae KM, Van Remmen H, Kubes P. Immune cell Toll-like receptor 4 is required for cardiac myocyte impairment during endotoxemia. Circ Res. 2004;95:700-707.

Topkara VK, Evans S, Zhang W, Epelman S, Staloch L, Barger PM, Mann DL. Therapeutic targeting of innate immunity in the failing heart. J Mol Cell Cardiol. 2010 [Epub ahead of print]

Triantafilou K, Orthopoulos G, Vakakis E, Ahmed MA, Golenbock DT, Lepper PM, Triantafilou M. Human cardiac inflammatory responses triggered by Coxsackie B viruses are mainly Toll-like receptor (TLR) 8-dependent. Cell Microbiol. 2005;7:1117-1126.

Vabulas RM, Ahmad-Nejad P, Ghose S, Kirschning CJ, Issels RD, Wagner H. HSP70 as endogenous stimulus of the Toll/interleukin-1 receptor signal pathway. J Biol Chem. 2002;277:15107-15112.

Vabulas RM, Braedel S, Hilf N, Singh-Jasuja H, Herter S, Ahmad-Nejad P, Kirschning CJ, Da Costa C, Rammensee HG, Wagner H, Schild H. The endoplasmic reticulum-resident heat shock protein Gp96 activates dendritic cells via the Toll-like receptor 2/4 pathway. J Biol Chem. 2002b;277:20847-20853.

Versteeg GA, García-Sastre A. Viral tricks to grid-lock the type I interferon system. Curr Opin Microbiol. 2010;13:508-516.

Wang C, Deng L, Hong M, Akkaraju GR, Inoue J, Chen ZJ. TAK1 is a ubiquitin-dependent kinase of MKK and IKK. Nature. 2001;6844:346-351.

Yajima T, Knowlton KU. Viral myocarditis: from the perspective of the virus. Circulation. 2009;119:2615-2624.

Yamamoto M, Sato S, Hemmi H, Hoshino K, Kaisho T, Sanjo H, Takeuchi O, Sugiyama M, Okabe M, Takeda K, Akira S. Role of adaptor TRIF in the MyD88-independent toll-like receptor signaling pathway. Science. 2003;301:640-643.

Yamamoto M, Sato S, Hemmi H, Uematsu S, Hoshino K, Kaisho T, Takeuchi O, Takeda K, Akira S. TRAM is specifically involved in the Toll-like receptor 4-mediated MyD88-independent signaling pathway. Nat Immunol. 2003b;4:1144-1150.

Yamamoto M, Takeda K. Current views of toll-like receptor signaling pathways. Gastroenterol Res Pract. 2010;e240365:1-8.

Yoneyama M, Kikuchi M, Natsukawa T, Shinobu N, Imaizumi T, Miyagishi M, Taira K, Akira S, Fujita T. The RNA helicase RIG-I has an essential function in double-stranded RNA-induced innate antiviral responses. Nat Immunol. 2004;5:730-737.

Zhu J, Mohan C. Toll-like receptor signaling pathways. Therapeutic opportunities. Mediators Inflamm. 2010;e781235:1-7.

12

Innate Lymphocyte Effectors (Natural Killer, Natural Killer T and γδ T Cells) in Infection and Myocarditis

S.A. Huber
Department of Pathology, University of Vermont
Colchester, Vermont
U.S.A.

1. Introduction

Myocarditis is defined as an inflammation of myocardium where the infiltrating leukocytes are intimately associated with cardiomyocyte necrosis or drop-out (Liu, 2005; Woodruff, 1980). Cardiac damage may be minimal and self-limiting or may result in chronic fibrosis and cardiac dysfunction leading to death in children and young adults (Eckart et al., 2004; Fabre, 2006; Solberg et al., 2010). As discussed in other chapters of this book, infections with a highly diverse group of viruses, bacteria, fungi, and worms have been implicated in infectious myocarditis (Friman et al., 1995). Enteroviruses and adenoviruses are usually considered as the predominant viral etiological agents, and are associated with approximately 80% of clinical myocarditis where a viral infection is documented. However, virtually any virus infection may initiate myocarditis (Bowles et al., 2003; Woodruff, 1980). While seasonal influenza virus is only a minor etiological agent in myocarditis, evidence from the most recent influenza H1N1 pandemic (Vila de Muga et al., 2010; Wiegand et al., 2010; Zheng et al., 2010) suggests a higher incidence of both mortality and morbidity, and accounts for 5% of complications in infected children (Zheng et al., 2010).
Myocardial injury results either directly from replication and induction of death or dysfunction in infected cardiocytes, or from host responses to infection (Huber, 2010). Although anti-viral host responses (innate or adaptive) are intended to control and eliminate the infection, cytokines and by-products such as nitric oxide or oxygen free radicals may also damage adjacent uninfected cells (Szalay et al., 2006). Innate immunity is the initial host response to infection and usually occurs within hours or days of virus introduction. The major characteristic of the innate response, besides its rapidity, is that it is broadly reactive to multiple infectious agents. While it is highly unlikely that innate immunity can completely eliminate the infection, it can suppress microbial replication until the far more potent and highly specific adaptive immune response kicks in. The reason for this is quite simple, viruses replicate rapidly with, for example, one picornavirus infected cell in tissue culture producing up to a million progeny virions within 18-24 hrs. In vivo, such rapid and uncontrolled growth could result in extensive tissue injury or death of the organism prior to a useful adaptive immune response being established since during a primary immune response, production of meaningful numbers of virus-specific T cells could

take 7-10 days after virus inoculation. The best known innate immunity results from microbial products binding to and activating Toll-Like Receptors (TLR) or RNA helicases (RIG-I and MDA-5) which activate transcription factors (NFkB) leading to expression of cytokines (TNFα, IL-1β and IL-6) and nitric oxide (Hosoi et al., 2004; Michelsen et al., 2004); or interferon response factors (IRF3/7) leading to expression of type 1 interferons (IFNα/β) RANTES and IP-10 (O'Neill, 2004; Vogel et al., 2003). These roles for TLR are discussed elsewhere. This review will concentrate on lymphocytes belonging to the innate immune response and discuss their role in myocarditis. These lymphocytes include natural killer (NK), natural killer T (NKT) and γδ T cells.

2. Natural killer cells

Natural killer (NK) cells are capable of distinguishing between infected/transformed cells and uninfected/non-transformed cells and are able to kill the former using perforin or granzyme dependent mechanism (Topham & Hewitt, 2009). The best recognized mechanism for NK cell activation is through Type 1 interferons (IFNα/β). Type 1 interferons upregulate multiple interferon response factors (IRFs) and two of these IRFs are strongly implicated in NK cell proliferation and activation (Taniguchi et al., 2001). NK cell numbers are dramatically reduced in IRF2-/- mice (Lohoff et al., 2000). NK cell numbers are also reduced in IRF1-/- mice but in this case, the defect is not inherent in the NK cell progenitor since adoptive transfer of IRF1-/- bone marrow into wild-type mice results in NK cell proliferation (Ogasawara et al., 1998). Rather, IRF-1 appears to control IL-15 expression in bone marrow stromal cells and IL-15 promotes NK cell generation. Similarly, other cytokines including IL-2, IL-12 and IL-18 promote NK cell responses (Agaugue et al., 2008). In contrast to IRF1, IRF2 is inherently important in the NK cell progenitor since adoptive transfer of IRF2-/- bone marrow into wild-type recipients fails to generate NK cells. How NK cells recognize aberrant cells has received substantial study since these effectors are non-T cells, lack the T cell receptor and CD3, and do not undergo genetic recombination of recognition receptors (Biron et al., 1999; Orange et al., 2002). NK cells express substantial numbers of both activating and inhibiting receptors (reviewed in (Lanier, 2008)), and despite lacking classical T cell receptors, NK cells can recognize microbial molecules. Examples include NKp46 recognition of the influenza hemagglutinin protein (Mandelboim et al., 2001), Ly49H recognition of m157 (mCMV) (Arase et al., 2002), NKp44/NKp46 recognition of NDV hemagglutinin-neuraminidase (Jarahian et al., 2009), and Ly49P recognition of m04 (mCMV) (Kielczewska et al., 2009). NK activation receptors pair with ITAM-bearing DAP12, FcεRI-γ and CD3-ζ signaling molecules. Stimulation of the NK activating receptors leads to phosphorylation of the ITAM components and recruitment of Syk and ZAP-70. This results in actin cytoskeletal reorganization, which promotes secretion of preformed cytokines. The cytokines primarily produced by NK cells are IFNγ/TNFα, or perforin/granzyme. Activation also increases transcription of cytokine genes. In contrast, inhibitory NK receptors are either monomeric type 1 glycoproteins of the immunoglobulin superfamily [examples include: killer cell immunoglobulin-like receptors (KIRs) and leukocyte immunoglobulin-like receptors (LILRs)] or type II glycoproteins containing a C-type lectin–like scaffold [examples include: Ly49 and CD94-NKG2A]. Both types of receptor contain immunoreceptor tyrosine-based inhibitory motifs (ITIMs) in their intracellular domains which, when activated, recruit tyrosine phosphatases that block the phosphorylation steps initiated by the NK activating receptors and thus inhibit NK cell functions (Lanier, 2008).

NK inhibitory receptors recognize major histocompatibility complex class I (MHC I) molecules which represents one mechanism by which NK cells distinguish between infected and normal cells, as many viruses attempt to evade the immune system through down-regulation of MHC molecules (Hewitt, 2003).

Evidence for a major role of NK cells in clinical myocarditis is rather weak. NK cells were not observed in heart tissue from 18 cases of biopsy proven myocarditis (Chow et al., 1989). Other studies have found either increased numbers of NK like cells in peripheral blood of dilated cardiomyopathy patients (Yokoyama, 1988) or diminution of NK cell activity in such patients (Maisch et al., 1985). Studies in patients with Chagas' disease find no alteration in NK cells early in the disease but an increase in these innate effectors occurs at later stages (Sathler-Avelar et al., 2003). One potential problem with clinical studies is that diagnosis of myocarditis or dilated cardiomyopathy is a relatively late event in the disease process and may be quite removed from the initiating acute infection (Woodruff, 1980). In fact, while viral genomic sequences can be detected in clinical heart biopsies for months and possibly for years, it is rare for infectious virus to be isolated from the hearts of myocarditis patients. Any role for NK cells may be over by the time human tissue is studied. The best evidence that NK cells might participate in viral myocarditis comes from mouse models. These studies indicate that NK cells are important in controlling coxsackievirus B infections in vivo (Gauntt et al., 1988; Gauntt et al., 1989; Vella & Festenstein, 1992) as depletion of these cells substantially increases virus titers in the heart or pancreas. The ability of NK cells to suppress virus infection may relate to their cytolytic activity to infected cardiocytes. Rapid elimination of infected cells before virus replication is complete would restrict the number of progeny virions produced and therefore limit the next cycle of infection. The second mechanism by which NK cells may help control virus infection is through either augmenting or accelerating the adaptive immune response to the virus. NK cells directly interact with both dendritic cells and activated T cells causing maturation of the dendritic cells and increased activation of the T cells (Zingoni et al., 2005). Interactions occur through up-regulation of OX40L on the NK cells and OX40 on activate CD4+ lymphocytes. Also, NK cells contain high concentration of pre-formed cytokines which can be rapidly released upon NK receptor engagement and these cytokines provide the environment necessary for optimal adaptive immunity development. As with the mouse model of CVB3 myocarditis, NK cells also control spread of Trypanosoma cruzi in the mouse model of Chagas' disease (Brener & Gazzinelli, 1997).

3. Natural killer T and γδ T cells

The other two major innate lymphocyte populations are natural killer T (NKT) and γδ T cells. NKT cells primarily recognize lipid antigens presented by CD1d molecules. The γδ T cells represent a more diverse population and in many cases, the antigen specificity of these cells is not known. However, as discussed below, the γδ T cells known to be involved in experimental viral myocarditis are also CD1d restricted. For this reason, description of the CD1 family of molecules is provided followed by discussion of the NKT and γδ T cells in innate immunity.

3.1 CD1 molecules and regulation of their expression

There are five distinct CD1 molecules, CD1a, CD1b, CD1c, CD1d and CD1e (Figure 1). Although these different molecules most likely arose from a single common ancestral gene and are located as a cluster of genes on the same chromosome (De Libero & Mori, 2003), they share only approximately 30% homology and have distinct expression patterns and functional characteristics (Blumberg et al., 1995; Calabi et al., 1989; Kasmar et al., 2009). These proteins belong to a family of non-polymorphic, class I-like major histocompatibility complex (MHC) molecules (Boes et al., 2009). Humans express CD1a, CD1b, CD1c, CD1e (Group 1 CD1 molecules) and CD1d (Group 2 CD1 molecule). Mice express two isoforms of CD1d but lack any of the Group 1 CD1 molecules (Bradbury et al., 1990; Sugita et al., 1999). Other mammals express varying combinations of the different CD1 isoforms. For example, ruminants, such as cattle, express CD1a, three isoforms of CD1b and CD1e but lack either homologues of CD1c or CD1d (Van Rhijn et al., 2006). To date, all mammals have at least one CD1 molecule and a similar CD1-like molecule has been recently found in birds (Dvir et al., 2010). The wide distribution of CD1 expression among species underlines the importance of these molecules in immunity. A major difference between the non-classical CD1 molecules and the classical MHC I and MHC II molecules is that the latter molecules primarily present peptide antigens while CD1 molecules present amphipathic glycolipid (Kasmar et al., 2009; Kulkarni, 2010) and possibly hydrophobic peptide (Van Rhijn et al., 2009) antigens to T cells which provides a more comprehensive sampling of microbial products than the classical MHC molecules alone could provide. There are few CD1 genes (maximum of 12 but not all are present in all species) compared to the classical MHC molecules (>200), and CD1 proteins are highly conserved with few if any allelic variations. However, crystal structure analysis suggests that CD1 proteins have substantial flexibility and can conformationally change to present diverse microbial and self glycolipids (Zajonc et al., 2008).

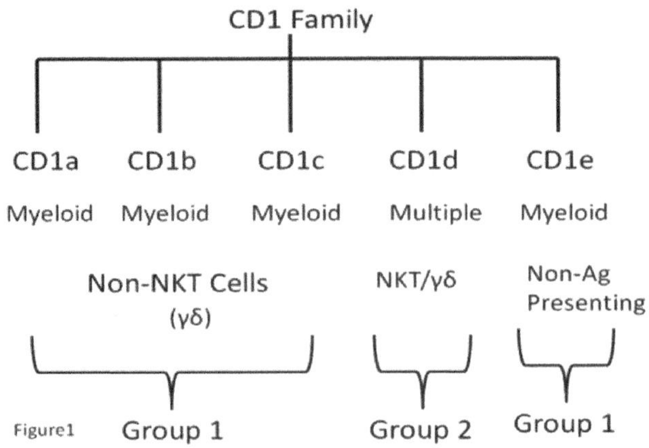

Fig. 1. CD1 family of non-classical MHC class I-like molecules.

There are five known members of the CD1 family divided into Group 1 and Group 2 molecules. All CD1 molecules present lipid antigens, unlike classical MHC molecules which primarily present peptide antigens. All CD1 genes derive from a common ancestral gene.
Unlike the other four members of the CD1 family, CD1e is only found as a soluble form in endosomes where it aids in trimming phosphatidylinositol for presentation by CD1b (de la Salle et al., 2005). CD1a, b, and c molecules are expressed on myeloid cells while CD1d is

expressed on these cells and additionally on non-hemopoietic cells including cardiac myocytes and endothelial cells (Blumberg et al., 1995; Exley et al., 2001; Huber et al., 2003) . CD1 molecules structurally resemble class I MHC molecules since they consist of a single polypeptide chain coded by the CD1 gene and are associated with β2 microglobulin. However, antigen presentation more closely resembles class II MHC molecules since antigen loading occurs in the endosome pathway and is TAP independent (Boes et al. , 2009; Brutkiewicz et al., 1995; Odyniec et al., 2004). The CD1 extracellular domain has a deep antigen binding groove containing two to four hydrophobic pockets into which the alkyl lipid tails of antigens are inserted leaving the glycosylated portion available for T cell recognition (Cheng et al., 2006; Zajonc et al., 2003; Zajonc et al., 2008). The cytoplasmic tails of CD1b, CD1c and CD1d contain a tyrosine motif which directs these molecules to the late endosome while the CD1a cytoplasmic tail lacks this motif and directs this molecule to the early endosome. The difference in trafficking of the CD1 molecules may reflect an evolutionary process since bacteria localize to different cellular organelles and expression of CD1 isoforms to distinct endosome compartments should promote maximal capture and presentation of microbial antigens to host immunity (De Libero & Mori, 2003). CD1b presents bacterial lipids including mycobacterial mycolic acids (Beckman et al., 1994), lipoarabinomannan (Sieling et al., 1995), glucose monomycolate (Moody, 2001), and self-glycosphingolipids such as GM1 ganglioside (Shamshiev et al., 2000). CD1a and CD1c present bacterial phospholipids (Beckman et al., 1996). CD1d presents a bacterial sphingolipid from *Sphingomonas* (Kinjo et al., 2005), alphaproteobacterium from *N. aromaticivorans* (Mattner et al., 2008), glycolipids from *B. burgdorferi* (Kinjo et al., 2006), and a self-sphingolipid isogloboside (Mattner et al., 2005). The sphingolipid α-galactosylceramide (αGalCer) isolated from marine sponges, is the classical CD1d ligand (Kawano et al., 1997), but CD1d has also been shown to present an α-galactosyl-diacylglycerol of *B. burgdorferi* (BbGL-II) (Kinjo et al., 2008; Kinjo et al., 2006). Evidence for CD1 presentation of viral antigens is sparse despite the fact that CD1-restricted T cells have been shown to respond in various viral infections including HIV, HSV, influenza and picornavirus (De Santo et al., 2008; Exley et al., 2001; Li & Xu, 2008; Yuan et al., 2006). Indeed, it would be highly unlikely that CD1 could directly present picornavirus molecules since these are non-enveloped viruses and should therefore lack any potential for glycolipid or lipopeptide antigens. Possible explanations for CD1-restricted immune responses to viruses exist. For example, infection may promote cellular lipidation of virus proteins (Van Rhijn et al., 2005) or infection may cause increased expression of endogenous glycolipid antigens (De Libero et al., 2005; Paget et al., 2007). Lysosomal α-galactosidase A is an enzyme which degrades endogenous lipid antigens (Darmoise et al., 2010). However, subsequent to many infections, α-galactosidase A activity can be severely curtailed leading to endogenous lipid accumulation. This means that CD1d dependent innate immunity may be directed to both exogenous and endogenous antigens during infections.

Endogenous glycosphingolipids binding to CD1 include GM1 ganglioside, sulfatide, galactosylceramide, and sphingomyelin (Darmoise et al., 2010; De Libero & Mori, 2003; Franchini et al., 2007; Hegde et al., 2010; Roy et al., 2008). The self-glycosphingolipids are not only important as self-antigens for T cell activation, but their presence may stabilize and promote CD1 expression on the cell surface (De Libero & Mori, 2003). Unlike microbial glycolipids which require processing in the endosomes, glycosphingolipids can directly bind to CD1 molecules expressed on the cell surface and can displace glycolipids already in these surface CD1 molecules (De Libero & Mori, 2003). Although endogenous glycosphingolipids have been primarily viewed as the probable self antigen in CD1-dependent immunity, recent studies by Pei et al (Pei et al., 2010) demonstrated that cell lines incapable of glycosphingolipid biosynthesis were nonetheless capable of activating CD1-restricted cells. Thus, the types of self antigen capable of activating the CD1-dependent innate immune response are likely to be broader than originally thought.

Group 1 CD1 molecules are not expressed on monocytes in the blood and recent studies have shown that serum immunoglobulin and lipids suppress expression of these molecules (Leslie et al., 2008; Smed-Sorensen et al., 2008). However, once monocytes leave the circulation, Group 1 CD1 molecules can be induced by signaling through TLR2 (Roura-Mir et al., 2005), TLR2/TLR5 agonists, or cytokines (GM-CSF and IL-4) (Moody, 2006). CD1d is not up-regulated by GM-CSF and IL-4 (Exley et al., 2001; Sallusto & Lanzavecchia, 1994). CD1d is constitutively expressed in dendritic cells, monocytes and macrophage, but levels can be further increased subsequent to infection (Dougan et al. , 2007; Durante-Mangoni et al., 2004; Huber et al., 2003; Skold & Behar, 2003). Such up-regulation depends upon signaling through TLR and cytokines (IFNγ, IFNβ, TNFα) (Raghuraman et al., 2006; Skold et al., 2005). While microbial infections can up-regulate CD1 expression, they can also result in CD1 down-regulation (Donovan et al., 2007; Raftery et al., 2006). Viruses are well-known for their ability to evade immunity through multiple different mechanisms (Alcami & Koszinowski, 2000; Antoniou & Powis, 2008; Vossen et al., 2002). While most investigations of immune evasion by viruses center on the adaptive immune response, viruses also interfere with innate immunity. The HIV Nef protein binds to CD1d decreasing CD1d transport to the cell surface (Hage et al., 2005). Similarly, HSV, suppresses CD1 expression by interrupting the CD1 recycling pathway (Yuan et al., 2006). Karposi sarcoma-associated herpesvirus (KSHV) uses its modulator of immune recognition (MIR) proteins to ubiquitinize the cytoplastic tail of the CD1d molecule leading to its endocytosis (Sanchez et al., 2005). Activation of TLR7/8 blocks CD1 expression at the protein and mRNA levels (Assier et al., 2007). Finally, infection can change the endosomal processing of glycolipids which could restrict antigen availability to CD1 molecules.

Unlike Group 1 CD1 molecules, CD1d can be expressed on non-hemopoeitic cells (Huber et al., 2003; Monzon-Casanova et al. ; Sikder et al., 2009) CVB3 infection augments CD1d expression on macrophage, dendritic cells and T cells (Huber, 2006). The virus also causes de novo CD1d expression on non-hemopoietic cells (cardiac endothelial cells and myocytes), but only in non-hemopoietic cells actively replicating virus. Uninfected myocytes/endothelial cells immediately adjacent to infected cells remain CD1d negative (Huber et al., 2003). The requirement for active virus replication strongly suggests that TLR signal pathways such as TLR3 (recognizing single stranded RNA) or TLR7/8 (recognizing double stranded RNA) are necessary. However, virus replication alone is insufficient. Mice or cells infected with a non-pathogenic variant of CVB3, H310A1 (Knowlton et al., 1996), fail to up-regulate CD1d either on hemopoeitic or non-hemopoeitic cells (Huber et al., 2003; Huber & Sartini, 2005b). A major difference between the non-pathogenic and pathogenic (H3) variants of CVB3 is that the pathogenic virus is a potent inducer of TNFα. Further studies showed that TNFα and H310A1 infection up-regulated CD1d expression whereas either TNFα or H310A1 infection alone did not. In the mouse model of CVB3 induced myocarditis, CD1d is required for cardiac inflammation and injury. Mice lacking CD1d fail to develop myocarditis despite high levels of virus replication in the heart (Huber et al., 2003). Since CD1d is up-regulated on both hemopoeitic and non-hemopoeitic cells subsequent to CVB3 infection, a major question is where expression of this molecule is most important in pathogenesis. CD1d-restricted effectors are cytolytic to CVB3 infected cardiocytes in vitro and expression of CD1d on infected cardiocytes in vivo may contribute directly to their death through cytolytic T lymphocyte activity. To address this question, bone marrow transplantation was performed between wild-type (CD1d+/+) and CD1d-/- mice where either the hemopoeitic cells were CD1d+ and the non-hemopoeitic cells (heart) was CD1d- or the opposite (Huber, 2006). These studies showed that CD1d expression on both hemopoeitic and non-hemopoeitic cells contributed to heart disease, although CD1d expression on hemopoeitic cells was of primary importance. There are no published studies showing the importance of CD1in clinical myocarditis. It is therefore not possible to evaluate the significance of CD1-dependent innate immunity in the human disease. However, based on the tight control of CD1 for pathogenesis in the experimental disease, the strong association between various microbial infections and clinical myocarditis, and the importance of CD1-restricted immunity in many different microbial infections; future investigation into a role for CD1 in this disease would be warranted.

3.2 Natural killer T cells and CD1-restricted γδ T cells

Many T cells respond to CD1 molecules (Barral & Brenner, 2007; Kaufmann, 1996) and express either T cell receptors (TCR) consisting of α/β or γ/δ polypeptide chains. Group 1 CD1-restricted αβ T cells are clonally diverse with fine antigen specificity, recognition of both self and foreign lipid antigens and either double negative (CD4-CD8-) or single positive (CD4+ or CD8+) (Barral & Brenner, 2007; Kaufmann, 1996; Vincent et al., 2005). The αβ T cell response is slow, similar to classical MHC αβ T cell responses indicating that these CD1-restricted effectors probably do not belong to the innate immune system. There are two major populations of γδ T cells in humans (Vδ1 and Vδ2) with Vδ2 cells primarily present in the circulation and Vδ1 cells primarily found in tissues and intestine (Das et al., 2004). Subsets of both γδ populations recognize antigens in context of non-classical MHC class I-like molecules including group 1 CD1(Rincon-Orozco et al., 2005; Russano et al., 2007). Activation of the group 1 CD1 restricted effectors requires IL-12, NKG2D activation on the effector and adhesion molecule interactions (LFA3/CD2, LFA1/ICAM1) in addition to TCR engagement. Since mice lack Group 1 CD1 molecules, this species does not have Group 1 CD1-restricted immunity. However, these effectors may function in humans.

T cells reacting to CD1d (Group 2 CD1) are also diverse. CD1d-restricted natural killer T (NKT) cells are designated as either invariant NKT (iNKT, also known as Type 1) or diverse NKT (also known as Type 2) cells (Barral & Brenner, 2007; Kronenberg, 2005; Ronchi & Falcone, 2008; Taniguchi et al., 2010). Type 1 iNKT cells have a TCR comprised of a single type of TCRα chain (Vα14Jα18 for mice and Vα24Jα18 for humans) and one of a limited number of distinct TCRβ chains resulting in limited clonal diversity. In contrast, Type 2 NKT cells use TCR comprised of diverse α and β chains. iNKT cells comprise between 2-40% of CD3+ cells in various tissues (Bendelac et al., 2007; Terabe & Berzofsky, 2008), have a constitutively activated phenotype, and rapidly secret large amounts of cytokines (IFN-γ, IL-4, IL-17, IL-5, and IL-13) upon activation due to the presence of pre-formed cytokine mRNA in the cells (Kronenberg, 2005; Michel, 2007; Olson et al., 2009; Stetson et al., 2003). Three mechanisms of iNKT cell activation have been described (Figure 2). Direct activation involves recognition of microbial antigens presented by CD1d on antigen presenting cells (TCR-mediated). In contrast, indirect activation either involves microbial stimulation of antigen presenting cells to release cytokines (IL-12 and Type 1 IFN) and presentation of self/altered self lipid antigens on CD1d; or cytokines (IL-12 and IL-18) in the absence of CD1d antigen presentation (Brigl et al., 2003). Both inflammation and TLR activation can affect expression of enzymes involved in lipid metabolism (Khovidhunkit et al., 2004; Salio et al., 2007) and this may either increase total self lipid in endosomes or alter self lipids making them appear more foreign to the immune system. The mechanism of iNKT cell activation can impact the types of cytokines released with direct CD1d activation resulting in both Th1 (IFNγ) and Th2 (IL-4/IL-13) release while indirect activation causes predominantly Th1 (IFNγ) expression (Brigl et al., 2003). iNKT cells producing Th2 cytokines modulate NK cells to express TGFβ and TGFβ promotes T regulatory cell activation(Chen et al., 2009; Monteiro et al., 2010). Thus, depending upon the mode of iNKT cell activation, these effectors can be either pro- or anti-inflammatory. Type 2 NKT cells also can have a Th1 or Th2 phenotype with corresponding cytokine profiles, and therefore may have either potentiating or protective roles in infections and autoimmune diseases (Arrenberg et al., 2009). A number of reports indicate that Type 1 and Type 2 NKT cells are antagonistic to each other and form a regulatory network to control adaptive immunity. Most reports suggest an anti-inflammatory role for Type 2 NKT cells which can be protective in autoimmune diabetes in NOD mice (Duarte et al., 2004), experimental allergic encephalomyelitis (Jahng et al., 2004) and Con-A induced hepatitis (Halder et al., 2007). Furthermore, while type 1 NKT cells may increase tumor immunosurveillance, Type 2 NKT cells may suppress anti-tumor immunity (Ambrosino et al., 2007; Terabe & Berzofsky, 2008). Activation pathways for γδ T cells can also be diverse with both direct antigen presentation in MHC or MHC-like molecules or indirect with minimal or no antigen presentation (Kaufmann, 1996). Unlike NKT cells, γδ T cells may either react to CD1 itself in the absence of any antigen or to antigen without presentation by MHC/MHC-like molecule involvement. Although both human and mouse γδ T cells have been found to recognize antigens presented by Group 1 CD1 and other non-classical MHC antigens (Chien & Konigshofer, 2007; Cui et al., 2009; Spada et al., 2000; Van Kaer et al., 1991), only this laboratory has reported a subpopulations of γδ cells (Vγ4 TCR) recognizing CD1d (Huber et al., 2003).

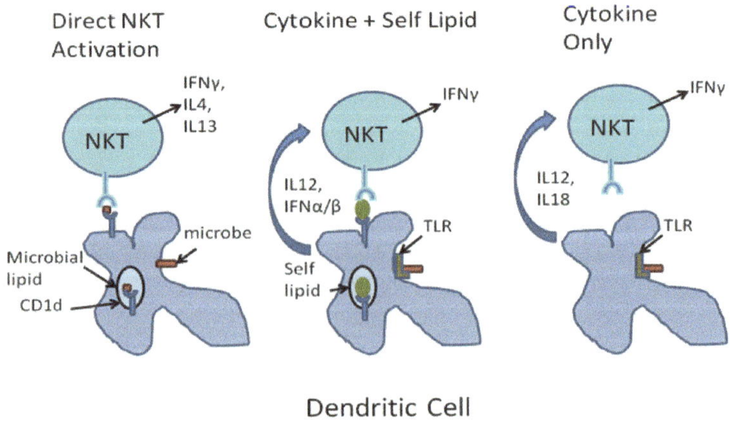

Fig. 2. Mechanisms for NKT cell activation.

There are three major mechanisms for activating NKT cells. Direct activation involves phagocytosis of microbes and binding of microbial lipids into the CD1d groove in the late endosome with transport of the CD1d-lipid complex to the antigen presenting cell surface. NKT cells activated through this pathway produce a broader range of Th1 and Th2 cytokines. A second pathway involves microbial stimulation of TLR on the antigen presenting cell which can both affect self-lipid expression/availability and stimulate cytokine expression from the antigen presenting cells. NKT cells stimulated by the recognition of self-lipid/CD1d and the cytokine milieu secrete primarily Th1 cytokines. The third mechanism is either not or substantial less dependent upon CD1d recognition by the NKT cells but NKT cell activation is primarily induced through cytokines alone.

3.3 NKT and γδ T Cells in myocarditis

Several cases of clinical cardiomyopathy have been reported where substantial numbers of γδ cells are in the inflammatory infiltrate (Eck et al., 1997; Takeda et al., 2008; Takeda et al., 2005). However, there is little direct evidence for a pathogenic role for these innate effectors in humans. As indicated above for NK cells, the lack of direct evidence for innate effectors in clinical myocarditis may simply reflect the fact that innate immunity should function early after infection and may disappear from the heart by the time that clinical symptoms are evident. In contrast to myocarditis in humans, substantial evidence implicates innate lymphocyte effectors in mouse models of coxsackievirus B3 (CVB3) and Borrelia burgdorferi (Lyme disease) myocarditis (Figure 3). As described above, mice lacking CD1d fail to develop myocarditis subsequent to CVB3-H3 (highly myocarditic variant of CVB3 (Knowlton et al., 1996)) infection despite high levels of virus replication in the heart (Huber et al., 2003). Infecting iNKT deficient mice with CVB3-H3 had no effect indicating that iNKT cells do not contribute to pathogenesis with this CVB3 variant. Surprisingly, CD1d deficient mice had significantly reduced numbers of activated γδ T cells belonging to the Vγ4 subset, and further analysis demonstrated that these Vγ4 cells are CD1d restricted as they killed CVB3-H3 infected CD1d+ but not infected CD1d- cardiac myocytes and cytotoxicity of the CD1d+ myocytes was blocked by anti-CD1d antibodies but not by antibodies to the classical MHC I and MHC II antigens (Huber, 2000; Huber et al., 2003). More importantly, activation of Vγ4 cells correlated to induction of CD4+IFNγ+ (Th1) virus-specific cells, which indicates that γδ cells might impact myocarditis through their effects on the antigen-specific, adaptive immune response (Huber & Sartini, 2005a; Huber et al., 2002). Previous studies had shown that heart-specific, autoimmune CD8+ cytolytic T lymphocytes are the primary immunopathogenic effector in CVB3 induced myocarditis (Guthrie et al., 1984; Henke et al., 1995; Huber & Lodge, 1984; Huber et al., 1988; Huber et al., 2002). These autoimmune CD8 cells kill uninfected cardiocytes through recognition of cardiac myosin epitopes (Huber & Gauntt, 2000) and can adoptively transfer myocarditis into uninfected recipients (Huber et al., 1987). However, the autoimmune CD8 T cell response is absolutely dependent on CD4+IFNγ+ cells (Huber et al., 2002). This is not surprising as many studies have shown that CD4+ Th1 cells promote CD8 T cell activation (Krawczyk et al., 2007; Serre et al., 2006). Although Vγ4 cells are required for generation of CD4+IFNγ+ cells, once the CD4+IFNγ+ cells exist, Vγ4+ cells are no longer necessary for autoimmune CD8 cell induction or myocarditis (Huber et al., 2002). The CVB3 model is not the only one showing that γδ T cells are required for immunopathogenic CD4 and CD8 T cell responses. Trypanosoma cruzi, the etiological agent in Chagas' disease, causes myocarditis with cardiac injury at least partially mediated by T cells and IFNγ (dos Santos et al., 2001; Marin-Neto et al., 2007; Ribeiro-Dos-

Santos et al., 2001; Soares et al., 2001). As with the CVB3 model, γδ cells are required for the pathogenic CD4 and CD8 responses in T. cruzi infections (Nomizo et al., 2006). However, unlike the CVB3 myocarditis model, the relevant γδ cell in T. cruzi infection expresses the Vγ1 T cell receptor. Why Vγ4 cells are operational in CVB3 disease while Vγ1 cells function in T. cruzi infection, is not currently known, but might reflect the difference between a virus and protozoa as the etiological agent. Nonetheless, the principle is the same: innate effectors control the activation of pathogenic antigen-specific adaptive immunity which subsequently causes cardiac damage.

The next question is how γδ cells control induction of adaptive immunity. Regulatory T cells (Tregs) are important negative immune modulators, constitute up to 10% of peripheral CD4+ T cells in naive mice and humans, and express CD25 (IL-2 receptor α chain) (Sakaguchi, 2005; Sakaguchi et al., 2008; Torgerson, 2006). There are several types of T regulatory cells which can basically be divided into natural (nTreg) and inducible (iTreg) populations. nTreg cells are generated in the thymus, and presumably arise from T cells with high affinity TCR for self antigens. nTreg cells are functionally mature when leaving the thymus and do not require antigen exposure peripherally to generate immunosuppressive activity. In contrast to nTreg cells, iTreg can be converted from effector T cell populations in the periphery subsequent to antigen challenge. The transcription factor, FoxP3, is usually associated with Treg cell development and transduction of exogenous FoxP3 into CD4+CD25- cells converts these cells into CD4+CD25+ Treg cells (Sakaguchi et al., 2008). Induction of FoxP3 expression and therefore, Treg cell activation depends upon the presence of TGFβ (Mantel & Schmidt-Weber, 2010). While FoxP3 is necessary for conversion of CD4+ cells to Treg cells, IL-2 is required for Treg cell maintenance/survival. Animals lacking either CD25 (IL-2R) or IL-2 develop lymphoproliferative and autoimmune diseases (Malek & Bayer, 2004) associated with a decrease in Treg cells. Three mechanisms have been proposed for Treg cell function (Sakaguchi et al., 2008). The first mechanism hypothesizes that Treg cells out-compete effector T cells for MHC-antigen complexes on antigen presenting cells which effectively blocks effector T cell activation. In the second mechanism, Treg cells directly interact with dendritic cells through CTLA4 which down-regulates required accessory molecule expression needed for successful antigen stimulation of effector T cells. Finally, Treg cell secretion of TGFβ or IL-10 may inhibit T cell differentiation (Ozdemir et al. , 2009; Ray et al., 2010).

CVB3 infection up-regulates CD1d on infected cardiac myocytes and myeloid cells. CD1d activates NKT and Vγ4 T cells which can either recognize CD1d on myocytes leading to myocyte death or interact with dendritic cells (DC) through CD1d to alter antigen presentation function of the dendritic cells or to produce cytokines. NKT cells may also activate NK cells. NK and NKT cells promote activation of Treg cells by promoting myeloid derived suppressor cell differentiation, while Vγ4 T cells have the opposite effect and either directly kill Treg cells through CD1d expressed on the Treg cell population or induce dendritic cell maturation and enhanced antigen presentation to adaptive immune (CD4, CD8) effectors. Treg cells inhibit activation of CD4+IFNγ+ (Th1) cells which are required for generation of cytolytic, autoimmune CD8 effector cells. The CD8 effector cells are the primary immunopathogenic mediator to cardiac injury in CVB3 induced myocarditis.

Treg cells prevent autoimmunity in myocarditis (Frisancho-Kiss et al., 2006; Huber et al., 2006; Wang, 2010). Distinct populations of innate effector T cells can have dramatically different effects on Treg cell responses. iNKT cells can promote Treg cell activation (Nowak et al., 2006; Roelofs-Haarhuis et al., 2004; Roelofs-Haarhuis et al., 2003). Under appropriate stimulation (see Figure 2), iNKT cells produce IL-13, a Th2 cytokine, which can induce TGFβ production from CD11b+Gr-1+ myeloid derived suppressor cells. TGFβ promotes FoxP3 expression and Treg cell differentiation (Mantel & Schmidt-Weber, 2010). Indirectly, NKT cells activate NK cells (Carnaud et al., 1999) and subpopulations of NK cells suppress adaptive immunity either through their effects on dendritic cells or T cells (Flodstrom-Tullberg et al., 2009; Lunemann et al., 2009). CD1d and NKT cells are crucial to Treg cell development (Sonoda et al., 1999), and treating mice with αGalCer increases Treg cell activation (La Cava et al. , 2006) and suppresses autoimmune diabetes in NOD mice (Cardell, 2006; Ly et al., 2006). NKT cells secret high levels of TGFβ and IL-10 (Sonoda et al., 2001; Stein-Streilein et al., 2000) which alter dendritic cell (DC) cytokine (IL-10) and accessory molecule (CD40, CD80 and/or CD86) expression (Kumanogoh et al., 2001; McGuirk & Mills, 2002; Salomon et al., 2000) that favors T regulatory cell responses. (Bach et al., 2004; Chen et al., 2009). NKT cells are protective in Chagas' disease (Duthie & Kahn, 2006; Olson et al., 2009) and IFNγ expression by the NKT cells appears to be crucial to their protective effect. Similarly, treating CVB3 infected mice with αGalCer is protective, again indicating a role for NKT cells in preventing myocarditis (Wu et al., 2010). However, whether these NKT cells also suppress immunopathogenicity by enhancing Treg cell responses is not clear. γδ T cells appear to have the opposite effect on Treg cell responses. IL-23 activated γδ cells prevent conversion of effector T cells to iTreg cells (Petermann et al., 2010). Similarly γδ cells reduce IL-10 producing Treg cells in the lung in an asthma model γδ cells (Hahn et al., 2008). Vγ2Vδ2 cells prevent IL-2 induced expansion of CD4+CD25+FoxP3+ T (Gong et al., 2009). γδ T cells promote dendritic cell maturation and enhance antigen presentation. Also, these innate effectors suppress IL-2 expression which is needed for Treg cell maintenance. Recently, it has been shown that CVB3-H3 infection of mice deficient in γδ cells results in significant increases in Treg cells and accumulation of a population of CD1d+ Treg cells (Huber, 2009, 2010). These CD1d+ Treg cells are substantially more immunosuppressive to myocarditis than the CD1d- Treg cells on a per cell basis. These CD1d+ Treg cells are absent in mice containing γδ cells, and adoptive transfer of activated γδ cells into CVB3-H3 infected γδKO mice both restores myocarditis susceptibility and eliminates the CD1d+ Treg cell population. Direct co-culture of the activated γδ cells on CD1d+ and CD1d- Treg cell populations shows that the γδ effector cells are lytic to the CD1d+ Treg in a CD1d- and caspase-dependent manner. (Huber, 2010).

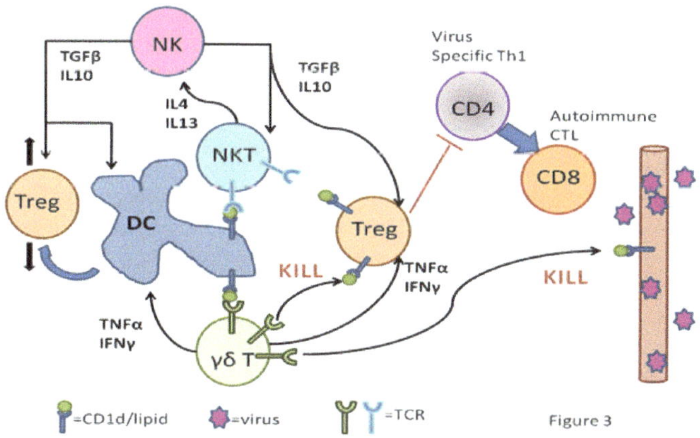

Fig. 3. Cross-talk between innate effectors in control of adaptive immunity.

4. Conclusions

Innate immunity is the rapid host response and occurs within hours of microbial infections. Although a major role for innate immunity is to help dampen microbe replication until the adaptive immune response is adequately developed for final microbial elimination, another major role for innate immunity is to control and direct the developing adaptive immune response. There is substantial cross-talk between innate lymphocyte effectors during myocarditis. Both NKT and a population of γδ cells recognize CD1d, a non-classical MHC class I-like molecule. However, evidence implies that while NKT cells are protective in myocarditis, γδ cells are pro-inflammatory and pathogenic. Interesting similarities have been found in the role of NKT and γδ cells in two different myocarditis mouse models: CVB3 and Trypanosoma cruzi induced myocarditis. The fact that similar immune processes of pathogenicity and protection appear to function in these two models provides circumstantial evidence that these innate effectors may have identical roles in other forms of myocarditis and also in clinical disease. To date, little evidence actually exists for innate effectors in clinical disease. However, the strong association between microbial infections and myocarditis in humans means that innate immunity should be important.

5. Acknowledgements

This work was supported by HL108371 from the National Institutes of Health.

6. References

Agaugue, S., Marcenaro, E., Ferranti, B., Moretta, L., and Moretta, A. (2008). Human natural killer cells exposed to IL-2, IL-12, IL-18, or IL-4 differently modulate priming of naive T cells by monocyte-derived dendritic cells. *Blood,* Vol. 112 (September 2008), No. 5, pp. 1776-83, ISSN 0006-4971.

Alcami, A., and Koszinowski, U. (2000). Viral mechanisms of immune evasion. *Immunology Today,* Vol. 21 (September 2000), No. 9, pp. 447-455, ISSN 0167-5699.

Ambrosino, E., Terabe, M., Halder, R. C., Peng, J., Takaku, S., Miyake, S., Yamamura, T., Kumar, V., and Berzofsky, J. A. (2007). Cross-regulation between type I and type II NKT cells in regulating tumor immunity: a new immunoregulatory axis. *Journal of Immunology,* Vol. 179 (October 2007), No. 8, pp. 5126-36, ISSN 0022-1767.

Antoniou, A. N., and Powis, S. J. (2008). Pathogen evasion strategies for the major histocompatibility complex class I assembly pathway. *Immunology,* Vol. 124 (May, 2008), No. 1, pp. 1-12, ISSN 0019-2805.

Arase, H., Mocarski, E. S., Campbell, A. E., Hill, A. B., and Lanier, L. L. (2002). Direct recognition of cytomegalovirus by activating and inhibitory NK cell receptors. *Science,* Vol. 296(May 2007), No. 5571, pp. 1323-6, ISSN 0193-4511.

Arrenberg, P., Halder, R., and Kumar, V. (2009). Cross-regulation between distinct natural killer T cell subsets influences immune response to self and foreign antigens. *Journal of Cellular Physiology,* Vol. 218 (February 2009), No. 2, pp. 246-50, ISSN 0021-9541.

Assier, E., Marin-Esteban, V., Haziot, A., Maggi, E., Charron, D., and Mooney, N. (2007). TLR7/8 agonists impair monocyte-derived dendritic cell differentiation and maturation. *Journal of Leukocyte Biology,* Vol. 81(January 2007), No. 1, pp. 221-8, ISSN 0741-5400.

Bach, J. F., Bendelac, A., Brenner, M. B., Cantor, H., De Libero, G., Kronenberg, M., Lanier, L. L., Raulet, D. H., Shlomchik, M. J., and von Herrath, M. G. (2004). The role of innate immunity in autoimmunity. The *Journal of Experimental Medicine,* Vol. 200 (December 2004), No.12, pp. 1527-31, ISSN 0022-1007.

Barral, D. C., and Brenner, M. B. (2007). CD1 antigen presentation: how it works. *Nature Reviews Immunology,* Vol. 7 (December 2007), No. 12, pp. 929-41, ISSN 1474-1733.

Beckman, E. M., Melian, A., Behar, S. M., Sieling, P. A., Chatterjee, D., Furlong, S. T., Matsumoto, R., Rosat, J. P., Modlin, R. L., and Porcelli, S. A. (1996). CD1c restricts responses of mycobacteria-specific T cells. Evidence for antigen presentation by a second member of the human CD1 family. *Journal of Immunology,* Vol. 157 (October 1996), No. 7, pp. 2795-803, ISSN 0022-1767.

Beckman, E. M., Porcelli, S. A., Morita, C. T., Behar, S. M., Furlong, S. T., and Brenner, M. B. (1994). Recognition of a lipid antigen by CD1-restricted alpha beta+ T cells. *Nature,* Vol. 372 (December 1994), No. 6507, pp. 691-4, ISSN 0028-0836.

Bendelac, A., Savage, P. B., and Teyton, L. (2007). The biology of NKT cells. *Annual Review of Immunology,* Vol. 25 (April 2007), pp.297-336, ISSN 0732-0582.

Biron, C. A., Nguyen, K. B., Pien, G. C., Cousens, L. P., and Salazar-Mather, T. P. (1999). Natural killer cells in antiviral defense: function and regulation by innate cytokines. *Annual Review of Immunology,* Vol. 17 (April 199), pp. 189-220, ISSN 0732-0582.

Blumberg, R. S., Gerdes, D., Chott, A., Porcelli, S. A., and Balk, S. P. (1995). Structure and function of the CD1 family of MHC-like cell surface proteins. *Immunological Reviews,* Vol. 147 (October 1995), pp. 5-29, ISSN 0105-2896.

Boes, M., Stoppelenburg, A. J., and Sille, F. C. (2009). Endosomal processing for antigen presentation mediated by CD1 and Class I major histocompatibility complex: roads to display or destruction. *Immunology,* Vol. 127 (June 2009), No. 2, pp. 163-70, ISSN 0019-2805.

Bowles, N. E., Ni, J., Kearney, D. L., Pauschinger, M., Schultheiss, H. P., McCarthy, R., Hare, J., Bricker, J. T., Bowles, K. R., and Towbin, J. A. (2003). Detection of viruses in myocardial tissues by polymerase chain reaction. evidence of adenovirus as a common cause of myocarditis in children and adults. *Journal of American College of Cardiology,* Vol. 42 (August 2003), No. 3, pp. 466-72, ISSN 0735-1097.

Bradbury, A., Calabi, F., and Milstein, C. (1990). Expression of CD1 in the mouse thymus. *European Journal of Immunology,* Vol. 20 (August 1990), No. 8, pp. 1831-6, ISSN 0014-2980.

Brener, Z., and Gazzinelli, R. T. (1997). Immunological control of Trypanosoma cruzi infection and pathogenesis of Chagas' disease. *International Archices of Allergy and Immunology,* Vol. 114 (October 1997), No. 2, pp. 103-10, ISSN 1018-2438.

Brigl, M., Bry, L., Kent, S. C., Gumperz, J. E., and Brenner, M. B. (2003). Mechanism of CD1d-restricted natural killer T cell activation during microbial infection. *Nature Immunology,* Vol. 4 (December 2003), No. 12, pp. 1230-7, ISSN 1529-2908.

Brutkiewicz, R. R., Bennink, J. R., Yewdell, J. W., and Bendelac, A. (1995). TAP-independent, beta 2-microglobulin-dependent surface expression of functional mouse CD1.1. *The Journal of Experimental Medicine,* Vol. 182 (December 1995), No. 6, pp. 1913-9, ISSN 0022-1007.

Calabi, F., Jarvis, J. M., Martin, L., and Milstein, C. (1989). Two classes of CD1 genes. *European Journal of Immunology,* Vol. 19 (February 1989), No. 2, pp. 285-92, ISSN 0014-2980.

Cardell, S. L. (2006). The natural killer T lymphocyte: a player in the complex regulation of autoimmune diabetes in non-obese diabetic mice. *Clinical and Experimental Immunology,* Vol. 143 (February 2006), No. 2, pp. 194-202, ISSN 0009-9104.

Carnaud, C., Lee, D., Donnars, O., Park, S. H., Beavis, A., Koezuka, Y., and Bendelac, A. (1999). Cutting edge: Cross-talk between cells of the innate immune system: NKT cells rapidly activate NK cells. *Journal of Immunology,* Vol. 163 (November 1999), No. 9, pp. 4647-50, ISSN 0022-1767.

Chen, G., Han, G., Wang, J., Wang, R., Xu, R., Shen, B., Qian, J., and Li, Y. (2009). Natural killer cells modulate overt autoimmunity to homeostasis in nonobese diabetic mice after anti-CD3 F(ab')2 antibody treatment through secreting transforming growth factor-beta. *The American Journal of Pathology,* Vol. 175 (September 2009), No. 3, pp. 1086-94, ISSN 0002-9440.

Cheng, T. Y., Relloso, M., Van Rhijn, I., Young, D. C., Besra, G. S., Briken, V., Zajonc, D. M., Wilson, I. A., Porcelli, S., and Moody, D. B. (2006). Role of lipid trimming and CD1 groove size in cellular antigen presentation. *The EMBO Journal,* Vol. 25 (July 2006), No. 13, pp. 2989-99, ISSN 0261-4189.

Chien, Y. H., and Konigshofer, Y. (2007). Antigen recognition by gammadelta T cells. *Immunological Reviews,* Vol. 215 (February 2007), pp. 46-58, ISSN 0105-2896.

Chow, L. H., Ye, Y., Linder, J., and McManus, B. M. (1989). Phenotypic analysis of infiltrating cells in human myocarditis. An immunohistochemical study in paraffin-embedded tissue. *Archives of Pathology & Laboratory Medicine,* Vol. 113 (December 1989), No. 12, pp. 1357-62, ISSN 0003-9985.

Cui, Y., Kang, L., Cui, L., and He, W. (2009). Human gammadelta T cell recognition of lipid A is predominately presented by CD1b or CD1c on dendritic cells. *Biology Direct,* Vol. 4 (December 2009), pp. 47, ISSN 1745-6150.

Darmoise, A., Teneberg, S., Bouzonville, L., Brady, R. O., Beck, M., Kaufmann, S. H., and Winau, F. (2010). Lysosomal alpha-galactosidase controls the generation of self lipid antigens for natural killer T cells. *Immunity,* Vol. 33 (August 2010), No. 2, pp. 216-28, ISSN 1074-7613.

Das, H., Sugita, M., and Brenner, M. B. (2004). Mechanisms of Vdelta1 gammadelta T cell activation by microbial components. *Journal of Immunology,* Vol. 172 (June 2004), No. 11, pp. 6578-86, ISSN 0022-1767.

de la Salle, H., Mariotti, S., Angenieux, C., Gilleron, M., Garcia-Alles, L. F., Malm, D., Berg, T., Paoletti, S., Maitre, B., Mourey, L., Salamero, J., Cazenave, J. P., Hanau, D., Mori, L., Puzo, G., and De Libero, G. (2005). Assistance of microbial glycolipid antigen processing by CD1e. *Science,* Vol. 310 (November 2005), No. 5752, pp. 1321-4, ISSN 0193-4511.

De Libero, G., Moran, A. P., Gober, H. J., Rossy, E., Shamshiev, A., Chelnokova, O., Mazorra, Z., Vendetti, S., Sacchi, A., Prendergast, M. M., Sansano, S., Tonevitsky, A., Landmann, R., and Mori, L. (2005). Bacterial infections promote T cell recognition of self-glycolipids. *Immunity,* Vol. 22 (June 2005), No. 6, pp. 763-72, ISSN 1074-7613.

De Libero, G., and Mori, L. (2003). Self glycosphingolipids: new antigens recognized by autoreactive T lymphocytes. *News in Physiological Sciences,* Vol. 18 (April 2003), pp. 71-6, ISSN 0886-1714.

De Santo, C., Salio, M., Masri, S. H., Lee, L. Y., Dong, T., Speak, A. O., Porubsky, S., Booth, S., Veerapen, N., Besra, G. S., Grone, H. J., Platt, F. M., Zambon, M., and Cerundolo, V. (2008). Invariant NKT cells reduce the immunosuppressive activity of influenza A virus-induced myeloid-derived suppressor cells in mice and humans. *The Journal of Clinical Investigation,* Vol 118 (December 2008), No. 12, pp. 4036-48, ISSN 0021-9738.

Donovan, M. J., Jayakumar, A., and McDowell, M. A. (2007). Inhibition of groups 1 and 2 CD1 molecules on human dendritic cells by Leishmania species. *Parasite Immunology,* Vol. 29 (October 2007), No. 10, pp. 515-24, ISSN 0141-9838.

dos Santos, P. V., Roffe, E., Santiago, H. C., Torres, R. A., Marino, A. P., Paiva, C. N., Silva, A. A., Gazzinelli, R. T., and Lannes-Vieira, J. (2001). Prevalence of CD8(+)alpha beta T cells in Trypanosoma cruzi-elicited myocarditis is associated with acquisition of CD62L(Low)LFA-1(High)VLA-4(High) activation phenotype and expression of IFN-gamma-inducible adhesion and chemoattractant molecules. *Microbes and Infection,* Vol. 3 (October 2001), No. 12, pp. 971-84, ISSN 1286-4579.

Dougan, S. K., Kaser, A., and Blumberg, R. S. (2007). CD1 expression on antigen-presenting cells. *Current Topics in Microbiology and Immunology,* Vol. 314, pp. 113-41, ISSN 0070-217X.

Duarte, N., Stenstrom, M., Campino, S., Bergman, M. L., Lundholm, M., Holmberg, D., and Cardell, S. L. (2004). Prevention of diabetes in nonobese diabetic mice mediated by CD1d-restricted nonclassical NKT cells. *Journal of Immunology,* Vol. 173 (September 2004), No. 5, pp. 3112-8, ISSN 0022-1767.

Durante-Mangoni, E., Wang, R., Shaulov, A., He, Q., Nasser, I., Afdhal, N., Koziel, M. J., and Exley, M. A. (2004). Hepatic CD1d expression in hepatitis C virus infection and recognition by resident proinflammatory CD1d-reactive T cells. *Journal of Immunology,* Vol. 173 (August 2004), No. 3, pp. 2159-66, ISSN 0022-1767.

Duthie, M. S., and Kahn, S. J. (2006). During acute Trypanosoma cruzi infection highly susceptible mice deficient in natural killer cells are protected by a single alpha-galactosylceramide treatment. *Immunology,* Vol. 119 (November 2006), No. 3, pp. 355-61, ISSN 0019-2805.

Dvir, H., Wang, J., Ly, N., Dascher, C. C., and Zajonc, D. M. (2010). Structural basis for lipid-antigen recognition in avian immunity. *Journal of Immunology,* Vol. 184 (March 2010), No. 5, pp. 2504-11, ISSN 0022-1767.

Eck, M., Greiner, A., Kandolf, R., Schmausser, B., Marx, A., and Muller-Hermelink, H. K. (1997). Active fulminant myocarditis characterized by T-lymphocytes expressing the gamma-delta T-cell receptor: a new disease entity? The *American Journal of Surgical Pathology,* Vol. 21 (September 1997), No. 9, pp. 1109-12, ISSN 0147-5185.

Eckart, R. E., Scoville, S. L., Campbell, C. L., Shry, E. A., Stajduhar, K. C., Potter, R. N., Pearse, L. A., and Virmani, R. (2004). Sudden death in young adults: a 25-year review of autopsies in military recruits. *Annals of Internal Medicine,* Vol. 141 (December 2004), No. 11, pp. 829-34, ISSN 0003-4819.

Exley, M., Bigley, N., Cheng, O., Tahir, S., Smiley, S., Carter, Q., Stills, H., Grusby, M., Koezuka, Y., Taniguchi, M., and Balk, S. (2001). CD1d-reactive T-cell activation leads to amelioration of disease caused by diabetogenic encephalomyocarditis virus. *Journal of Leukocyte Biology,* Vol. 69 (May 2001), No. 5, pp. 713-718, ISSN 0741-5400.

Fabre A, S. M. (2006). Sudden adult death syndrome and other non-ischaemic causes of sudden cardiac death: a UK experience. *Heart,* Vol. 92 (March 2006), No. 3, pp. 316-320, ISSN 1355-6037.

Flodstrom-Tullberg, M., Bryceson, Y. T., Shi, F. D., Hoglund, P., and Ljunggren, H. G. (2009). Natural killer cells in human autoimmunity. *Current Opinion in Immunology,* Vol. 21 (December 2009), No. 6, pp. 634-40, ISSN 0952-7915.

Franchini, L., Matto, P., Ronchetti, F., Panza, L., Barbieri, L., Costantino, V., Mangoni, A., Cavallari, M., Mori, L., and De Libero, G. (2007). Synthesis and evaluation of human T cell stimulating activity of an alpha-sulfatide analogue. *Bioorganic & Medicinal Chemistry* Vol. 15 (August 2007), No. 16, pp. 5529-36, ISSN 0968-0896.

Friman, G., Wesslen, L., Fohlman, J., Karjalainen, J., and Rolf, C. (1995). The epidemiology of infectious myocarditis, lymphocytic and dilated cardiomyopathy. *European Heart Journal,* Vol. 16 (December 1995), No. Suppl o, pp. 36-41, ISSN 0195-668X.

Frisancho-Kiss, S., Nyland, J. F., Davis, S. E., Barrett, M. A., Gatewood, S. J., Njoku, D. B., Cihakova, D., Silbergeld, E. K., Rose, N. R., and Fairweather, D. (2006). Cutting edge: T cell Ig mucin-3 reduces inflammatory heart disease by increasing CTLA-4 during innate immunity. *Journal of Immunology,* Vol. 176 (June 2006), No. 11, pp. 6411-5, ISSN 0022-1767.

Gauntt, C., Godney, E., and Lutton, C. (1988). Host factors regulating viral clearance. *Pathology and Immunopathology Research,* Vol. 7, pp. 251-265, ISSN 0257-2761.

Gauntt, C., Godney, E., Lutton, C., and Fernandes, G. (1989). Role of natural killer cells in experimental murine myocarditis. *Springer Seminars in Immunopathology,* Vol. 11, pp. 51-59, ISSN 0344-4325.

Gong, G., Shao, L., Wang, Y., Chen, C. Y., Huang, D., Yao, S., Zhan, X., Sicard, H., Wang, R., and Chen, Z. W. (2009). Phosphoantigen-activated V gamma 2V delta 2 T cells antagonize IL-2-induced CD4+CD25+Foxp3+ T regulatory cells in mycobacterial infection. *Blood,* Vol. 113 (January 2009), No. 4, pp. 837-45, ISSN 0006-4971.

Guthrie, M., Lodge, P. A., and Huber, S. A. (1984). Cardiac injury in myocarditis induced by Coxsackievirus group B, type 3 in Balb/c mice is mediated by Lyt 2 + cytolytic lymphocytes. *Cellular Immunology,* Vol. 88 (October 1984), No. 2, pp. 558-67, ISSN 0008-8749.

Hage, C. A., Kohli, L. L., Cho, S., Brutkiewicz, R. R., Twigg, H. L., 3rd, and Knox, K. S. (2005). Human immunodeficiency virus gp120 downregulates CD1d cell surface expression. *Immunology Letters,* Vol. 98 (April 2005), No. 1, pp. 131-5, ISSN 0165-2478.

Hahn, Y. S., Ji, X. Y., Woo, S. I., Choi, Y. K., Song, M. S., Shin, K. S., Jin, N., O'Brien, R. L., and Born, W. K. (2008). Vgamma1+ gammadelta T cells reduce IL-10-producing CD4+CD25+ T cells in the lung of ovalbumin-sensitized and challenged mice. *Immunology Letters,* Vol. 121 (December 2008), No. 2, pp. 87-92, ISSN 0165-2478.

Halder, R. C., Aguilera, C., Maricic, I., and Kumar, V. (2007). Type II NKT cell-mediated anergy induction in type I NKT cells prevents inflammatory liver disease. *The Journal of Clinical Investigation,* Vol. 117 (August 2007), No. 8, pp. 2302-12, ISSN 0021-9738.

Hegde, S., Fox, L., Wang, X., and Gumperz, J. E. (2010). Autoreactive natural killer T cells: promoting immune protection and immune tolerance through varied interactions with myeloid antigen-presenting cells. *Immunology,* Vol. 130 (August 2010), No. 4, pp. 471-83, ISSN 0019-2805.

Henke, A., Huber, S., Stelzner, A., and Whitton, J. (1995). The role of CD8+ T lymphocytes in coxsackievirus B3-induced myocarditis. *Journal of Virology,* Vol. 69 (November 1995), No. 11, pp. 6720-6728, ISSN 0022-538X.

Hewitt, E. W. (2003). The MHC class I antigen presentation pathway: strategies for viral immune evasion. *Immunology,* Vol. 110 (October 2003), No. 2, pp.163-9, ISSN 1365-2567.

Hosoi, T., Suzuki, S., Nomura, J., Ono, A., Okuma, Y., Akira, S., and Nomura, Y. (2004). Bacterial DNA induced iNOS expression through MyD88-p38 MAP kinase in mouse primary cultured glial cells. *Brain Research Molecular Brain Research,* Vol. 124 (May 2004), No. 2, pp. 159-64, ISSN 0169-328X.

Huber, S. (2000). T cells expressing the gamma-delta T cell receptor induce apoptosis in cardiac myocytes. *Cardiovascular Research,* Vol. 45 (February 2000), No. 3, pp. 579-587, ISSN 0008-6363.

Huber, S. (2010). γδ T lymphocytes kill T regulatory cells through CD1d. *Immunology,* Vol. 131 (October 2010), No. 2, pp. 202-209, ISSN 0019-2805.

Huber, S., and Gauntt, C. (2000). Antigenic mimicry between self and coxsackievirus protein leads to both humoral and cellular autoimmunity to heart proteins, In: *Molecular Mimicry in Disease,* M. Cunningham and R. Fijinami, pp. 51, ASM Press, ISBN 1555811949, Washington DC.

Huber, S., and Lodge, P. (1984). Coxsackievirus B3 myocarditis in Balb/c mice: evidence for autoimmunity to myocyte antigens. *The American Journal of Pathology,* Vol. 116 (July 1984), No. 1, pp. 21-9, ISSN 0002-9440.

Huber, S., Lodge, P., Herzum, M., Estrin, M., and Olszewski, J. (1987). The role of T lymphocytes in the pathogenesis of coxsackievirus B3 myocarditis, In: *Cardiomyopathy Update 1: Pathogenesis of Myocarditis and Cardiomyopathy,* C. Kawai, W. Abelmann and A. Matsumori, pp. 9-21. University of Tokyo Press, ISBN 0860084191, Tokyo Japan.

Huber, S., and Sartini, D. (2005a). T cells expressing the Vgamma1 T-cell receptor enhance virus-neutralizing antibody response during coxsackievirus B3 infection of BALB/c mice: differences in male and female mice. *Viral Immunology,* Vol. 18, No. 4, pp. 730-9, ISSN 0882-8245.

Huber, S., Sartini, D., and Exley, M. (2003). Role of CD1d in coxsackievirus B3-induced myocarditis. *Journal of Immunology,* Vol. 170 (March 2003), No. 6, pp. 3147-53 (ISSN 0022-1767).

Huber, S., Shi, C., and Budd, R. C. (2002). Gammadelta T cells promote a Th1 response during coxsackievirus B3 infection in vivo: role of Fas and Fas ligand. *Journal of Virology,* Vol. 76 (July 2002), No. 13, pp. 6487-94, ISSN 0022-538X.

Huber, S., Weller, A., Herzum, M., Lodge, P., Estrin, M., Simpson, K., and Guthrie, M. (1988). Immunopathogenic mechanisms in experimental picornavirus-induced autoimmunity. *Pathology and Immunopathology Research,* Vol. 7, No. 4, pp. 279-91, ISSN 0257-2761.

Huber, S. A. (2006). CD1d expression on hemopoietic cells promotes CD4+ Th1 response in coxsackievirus B3 induced myocarditis. *Virology,* Vol. 352 (August 2006), No. 1, pp. 226-36, ISSN 0042-6822.

Huber, S. A. (2009). Depletion of gammadelta+ T cells increases CD4+ FoxP3 (T regulatory) cell response in coxsackievirus B3-induced myocarditis. *Immunology,* Vol. 127 (August 2009), No. 4, pp. 567-76, ISSN 0019-2805.

Huber, S. A., Feldman, A. M., and Sartini, D. (2006). Coxsackievirus B3 induces T regulatory cells, which inhibit cardiomyopathy in tumor necrosis factor-alpha transgenic mice. *Circulation Research,* Vol. 99 (November 2006), No. 10, pp. 1109-16, ISSN 0009-7330.

Huber, S. A., and Sartini, D. (2005b). Roles of tumor necrosis factor alpha (TNF-alpha) and the p55 TNF receptor in CD1d induction and coxsackievirus B3-induced myocarditis. *Journal of Virology,* Vol. 79 (March 2005), No. 5, pp. 2659-65, ISSN 0022-538X.

Huber, S. A., Sartini, D., and Exley, M. (2002). Vgamma4(+) T cells promote autoimmune CD8(+) cytolytic T-lymphocyte activation in coxsackievirus B3-induced myocarditis in mice: role for CD4(+) Th1 cells. *Journal of Virology,* Vol. 76 (November 2002), No. 21, pp. 10785-90, ISSN 0022-538X.

Jahng, A., Maricic, I., Aguilera, C., Cardell, S., Halder, R. C., and Kumar, V. (2004). Prevention of autoimmunity by targeting a distinct, noninvariant CD1d-reactive T cell population reactive to sulfatide. *The Journal of Experimental Medicine,* Vol. 199 (April 2004), No. 7, pp. 947-57, ISSN 0022-1007.

Jarahian, M., Watzl, C., Fournier, P., Arnold, A., Djandji, D., Zahedi, S., Cerwenka, A., Paschen, A., Schirrmacher, V., and Momburg, F. (2009). Activation of natural killer cells by newcastle disease virus hemagglutinin-neuraminidase. *Journal of Virology,* Vol. 83 (August 2009), No. 16, pp. 8108-21.

Kasmar, A., Van Rhijn, I., and Moody, D. B. (2009). The evolved functions of CD1 during infection. *Current Opinion in Immunology,* Vol. 21 (August 2009), No. 4, pp. 397-403, ISSN 0952-7915.

Kaufmann, S. H. (1996). gamma/delta and other unconventional T lymphocytes: what do they see and what do they do? *Proceedings of the National Academy of Sciences of the United States of America,* Vol. 93 (March 1996), No. 6, pp. 2272-9, ISSN 0027-8424.

Kawano, T., Cui, J., Koezuka, Y., Toura, I., Kaneko, Y., Motoki, K., Ueno, H., Nakagawa, R., Sato, H., Kondo, E., Koseki, H., and Taniguchi, M. (1997). CD1d-restricted and TCR-mediated activation of valpha14 NKT cells by glycosylceramides. *Science,* Vol. 278 (November 1997), No. 5343, pp. 1626-9, ISSN 0193-4511.

Khovidhunkit, W., Kim, M. S., Memon, R. A., Shigenaga, J. K., Moser, A. H., Feingold, K. R., and Grunfeld, C. (2004). Effects of infection and inflammation on lipid and lipoprotein metabolism: mechanisms and consequences to the host. *Journal of Lipid Research,* Vol. 45 (July 2004), No. 7, pp. 1169-96, ISSN 0022-2275.

Kielczewska, A., Pyzik, M., Sun, T., Krmpotic, A., Lodoen, M. B., Munks, M. W., Babic, M., Hill, A. B., Koszinowski, U. H., Jonjic, S., Lanier, L. L., and Vidal, S. M. (2009). Ly49P recognition of cytomegalovirus-infected cells expressing H2-Dk and CMV-encoded m04 correlates with the NK cell antiviral response. *The Journal of Experimental Medicine,* Vol. 206 (March 2009), No. 3, pp. 515-23, ISSN 0022-1007.

Kinjo, Y., Pei, B., Bufali, S., Raju, R., Richardson, S. K., Imamura, M., Fujio, M., Wu, D., Khurana, A., Kawahara, K., Wong, C. H., Howell, A. R., Seeberger, P. H., and Kronenberg, M. (2008). Natural Sphingomonas glycolipids vary greatly in their ability to activate natural killer T cells. *Chemistry & Biology,* Vol. 15 (July 2008), No. 7, pp. 654-64, ISSN 1074-5521.

Kinjo, Y., Tupin, E., Wu, D., Fujio, M., Garcia-Navarro, R., Benhnia, M. R., Zajonc, D. M., Ben-Menachem, G., Ainge, G. D., Painter, G. F., Khurana, A., Hoebe, K., Behar, S. M., Beutler, B., Wilson, I. A., Tsuji, M., Sellati, T. J., Wong, C. H., and Kronenberg, M. (2006). Natural killer T cells recognize diacylglycerol antigens from pathogenic bacteria. *Nature Immunology,* Vol. 7 (September 2006), No. 9, pp. 978-86, ISSN 1529-2908.

Kinjo, Y., Wu, D., Kim, G., Xing, G. W., Poles, M. A., Ho, D. D., Tsuji, M., Kawahara, K., Wong, C. H., and Kronenberg, M. (2005). Recognition of bacterial glycosphingolipids by natural killer T cells. *Nature,* Vol. 434 (March 2005), No. 7032, pp. 520-5, ISSN 0028-0836.

Knowlton, K. U., Jeon, E. S., Berkley, N., Wessely, R., and Huber, S. (1996). A mutation in the puff region of VP2 attenuates the myocarditic phenotype of an infectious cDNA of the Woodruff variant of coxsackievirus B3. *Journal of Virology,* Vol. 70 (November 1996), No. 11, pp. 7811-8, ISSN 0022-538X.

Krawczyk, C. M., Shen, H., and Pearce, E. J. (2007). Memory CD4 T cells enhance primary CD8 T-cell responses. *Infection and Immunity,* Vol. 75 (July 2007), No. 7, pp. 3556-60, ISSN 0019-9567.

Kronenberg, M. (2005). Toward an understanding of NKT cell biology: progress and paradoxes. *Annual Review of Immunology,* Vol. 23 (January 2005), pp. 877-900, ISSN 0732-0582.

Kulkarni RR, H. S., Sharif S. (2010). The invariant NKT cell subset in anti-viral defenses: a dark horse in anti-influenza immunity? *Journal of Leukocyte Biology, Vol.* 88 (October 2010), No. 4, pp. 635-43, ISSN 0741-5400.

Kumanogoh, A., Wang, X., Lee, I., Watanabe, C., Kamanaka, M., Shi, W., Yoshida, K., Sato, T., Habu, S., Itoh, M., Sakaguchi, N., Sakaguchi, S., and Kikutani, H. (2001). Increased T cell autoreactivity in the absence of CD40-CD40 ligand interactions: a role of CD40 in regulatory T cell development. *Journal of Immunology.* Vol. 166 (January 2001), No. 1, pp. 353-60, ISSN 0022-1767.

La Cava, A., Van Kaer, L., and Fu Dong, S. (2006). CD4+CD25+ Tregs and NKT cells: regulators regulating regulators. *Trends in Immunology,* Vol. 27 (July 2006), No. 7, pp. 322-7, ISSN 1471-4906.

Lanier, L. L. (2008). Up on the tightrope: natural killer cell activation and inhibition. *Nature Immunology,* Vol. 9 (May 2008), No. 5, pp. 495-502, ISSN 1529-2908.

Leslie, D. S., Dascher, C. C., Cembrola, K., Townes, M. A., Hava, D. L., Hugendubler, L. C., Mueller, E., Fox, L., Roura-Mir, C., Moody, D. B., Vincent, M. S., Gumperz, J. E., Illarionov, P. A., Besra, G. S., Reynolds, C. G., and Brenner, M. B. (2008). Serum lipids regulate dendritic cell CD1 expression and function. *Immunology,* Vol. 125 (November 2008), No. 3, pp. 289-301, ISSN 0019-2805.

Li, D., and Xu, X. N. (2008). NKT cells in HIV-1 infection. *Cell Research,* Vol. 18 (August 2008), No. 8, pp. 817-22, ISSN 1001-0602.

Liu W, L. W., Gao C, Sun NL (2005). Effects of atorvastatin on the Th1/Th2 polarization of ongoing experimental autoimmune myocarditis in Lewis rats. . *Journal of Autoimmunity,* Vol. 25 (December 2005), No. 4, pp. 258-263, ISSN 0896-8411.

Lohoff, M., Duncan, G. S., Ferrick, D., Mittrucker, H. W., Bischof, S., Prechtl, S., Rollinghoff, M., Schmitt, E., Pahl, A., and Mak, T. W. (2000). Deficiency in the transcription factor interferon regulatory factor (IRF)-2 leads to severely compromised development of natural killer and T helper type 1 cells. *The Journal of Experimental Medicine,* Vol. 192 (August 2000), No. 3, pp. 325-36, ISSN 0022-1007.

Lunemann, A., Lunemann, J. D., and Munz, C. (2009). Regulatory NK-cell functions in inflammation and autoimmunity. *Molecular Medicine,* Vol. 15 (September-October 2009), No. 9-10, pp. 352-8, ISSN 1076-1551.

Ly, D., Mi, Q. S., Hussain, S., and Delovitch, T. L. (2006). Protection from type 1 diabetes by invariant NK T cells requires the activity of CD4+CD25+ regulatory T cells. *Journal of Immunology,* Vol. 177 (September 2006), No. 6, pp. 3695-704, ISSN 0022-1767.

Maisch, B., Bulowius, U., Schmier, K., Klopf , D., Koper, D., Sivelis, T., and Kochsiek, K. (1985). Immunological cellular regulator and effector mechanisms in myocarditis. *Herz,* Vol. 10 (February 1985), No. 1, pp. 8-14, ISSN 0340-9937.

Malek, T. R., and Bayer, A. L. (2004). Tolerance, not immunity, crucially depends on IL-2. *Nature Reviews Immunology, Vol.* 4 (September 2004), No. 9, pp. 665-74, ISSN 1474-1733.

Mandelboim, O., Lieberman, N., Lev, M., Paul, L., Arnon, T. I., Bushkin, Y., Davis, D. M., Strominger, J. L., Yewdell, J. W., and Porgador, A. (2001). Recognition of haemagglutinins on virus-infected cells by NKp46 activates lysis by human NK cells. *Nature,* Vol. 409 (February 2001), No. 6823, pp.1055-60, ISSN 0028-0836.

Mantel, P. Y., and Schmidt-Weber, C. B. (2010). Transforming growth factor-beta: recent advances on its role in immune tolerance. *Methods in Molecular Biology,* Vol. 677, pp. 303-38, ISSN 1064-3745.

Marin-Neto, J. A., Cunha-Neto, E., Maciel, B. C., and Simoes, M. V. (2007). Pathogenesis of chronic Chagas heart disease. *Circulation,* Vol. 115 (March 2007), No. 9, pp. 1109-23, ISSN 0009-7322.

Mattner, J., Debord, K. L., Ismail, N., Goff, R. D., Cantu, C., 3rd, Zhou, D., Saint-Mezard, P., Wang, V., Gao, Y., Yin, N., Hoebe, K., Schneewind, O., Walker, D., Beutler, B., Teyton, L., Savage, P. B., and Bendelac, A. (2005). Exogenous and endogenous glycolipid antigens activate NKT cells during microbial infections. *Nature,* Vol. 434 (March 2005), No. 7032, pp. 525-9, ISSN 0028-0836.

Mattner, J., Savage, P. B., Leung, P., Oertelt, S. S., Wang, V., Trivedi, O., Scanlon, S. T., Pendem, K., Teyton, L., Hart, J., Ridgway, W. M., Wicker, L. S., Gershwin, M. E., and Bendelac, A. (2008). Liver autoimmunity triggered by microbial activation of natural killer T cells. *Cell Host & Microbe,* Vol. 3 (May 2008), No. 5, pp. 304-15, ISSN 1931-3128.

McGuirk, P., and Mills, K. H. (2002). Pathogen-specific regulatory T cells provoke a shift in the Th1/Th2 paradigm in immunity to infectious diseases. *Trends in Immunology,* Vol. 23 (September 2002), No. 9, pp. 450-5, ISSN 1471-4906.

Michel ML, K. A., Paget C, Fujio M, Trottein F, Savage PB, Wong CH, Schneider E, Dy M, Leite-de-Moraes MC. (2007). Identification of an IL-17-producing NK1.1(neg) iNKT cell population involved in airway neutrophilia. *The Journal of Experimental Medicine.,* Vol. 204 (May 2007), No. 5, pp. 995-1001, ISSN 0022-1007.

Michelsen, K. S., Doherty, T. M., Shah, P. K., and Arditi, M. (2004). TLR signaling: an emerging bridge from innate immunity to atherogenesis. *Journal of Immunology,* Vol. 173 (November 2004), No. 10, pp. 5901-7, ISSN 0022-1767.

Monteiro, M., Almeida, C. F., Caridade, M., Ribot, J. C., Duarte, J., Agua-Doce, A., Wollenberg, I., Silva-Santos, B., and Graca, L. (2010). Identification of regulatory Foxp3+ invariant NKT cells induced by TGF-beta. *Journal of Immunology,* Vol. 185 (August 2010), No. 4, pp. 2157-63, ISSN 0022-1767.

Monzon-Casanova, E., Steiniger, B., Schweigle, S., Clemen, H., Zdzieblo, D., Starick, L., Muller, I., Wang, C. R., Rhost, S., Cardell, S., Pyz, E., and Herrmann, T. (2010). CD1d expression in paneth cells and rat exocrine pancreas revealed by novel

monoclonal antibodies which differentially affect NKT cell activation. *PLoS One*, Vol. 5 (September 2010), No. 9, ISSN 1932-6203.
Moody, D. B. (2001). Polyisoprenyl glycolipids as targets of CD1-mediated T cell responses. *Cellular and Molecular Life Sciences*, Vol. 58 (September 2001), No. 10, pp. 1461-74, ISSN 1420-682X.
Moody, D. B. (2006). The surprising diversity of lipid antigens for CD1-restricted T cells. *Advances in Immunology*, Vol. 89, pp. 87-139, ISSN 0065-2776.
Nomizo, A., Cardillo, F., Postol, E., de Carvalho, L. P., and Mengel, J. (2006). V gamma 1 gammadelta T cells regulate type-1/type-2 immune responses and participate in the resistance to infection and development of heart inflammation in Trypanosoma cruzi-infected BALB/c mice. *Microbes & Infection*, Vol. 8 (March 2006), No. 3, pp. 880-8, ISSN 1286-4579.
Nowak, M., Kopp, F., Roelofs-Haarhuis, K., Wu, X., and Gleichmann, E. (2006). Oral nickel tolerance: Fas ligand-expressing invariant NK T cells promote tolerance induction by eliciting apoptotic death of antigen-carrying, effete B cells. *Journal of Immunology*, Vol. 176 (April 2006), No. 8, pp. 4581-9, ISSN 0022-1767.
O'Neill, L. A. (2004). TLRs: Professor Mechnikov, sit on your hat. *Trends in Immunology*, Vol. 25 (December 2004), No. 12, pp. 687-93, ISSN 1471-4906.
Odyniec, A., Szczepanik, M., Mycko, M. P., Stasiolek, M., Raine, C. S., and Selmaj, K. W. (2004). Gammadelta T cells enhance the expression of experimental autoimmune encephalomyelitis by promoting antigen presentation and IL-12 production. *Journal of Immunology*, Vol. 173 (July 2004), No. 1, pp. 682-94, ISSN 1754-1441.
Ogasawara, K., Hida, S., Azimi, N., Tagaya, Y., Sato, T., Yokochi-Fukuda, T., Waldmann, T. A., Taniguchi, T., and Taki, S. (1998). Requirement for IRF-1 in the microenvironment supporting development of natural killer cells. *Nature*, Vol. 391 (February 1998), No. 6668, pp. 700-3, ISSN 0028-0836.
Olson, C. M., Jr., Bates, T. C., Izadi, H., Radolf, J. D., Huber, S. A., Boyson, J. E., and Anguita, J. (2009). Local production of IFN-gamma by invariant NKT cells modulates acute Lyme carditis. *Journal of Immunology*, Vol. 182 (March 2009), No. 6, pp. 3728-34, ISSN 0022-1767.
Orange, J. S., Fassett, M. S., Koopman, L. A., Boyson, J. E., and Strominger, J. L. (2002). Viral evasion of natural killer cells. *Nature Immunology*, Vol. 3 (November 2002), No. 11, pp. 1006-12, ISSN 1529-2908.
Ozdemir, C., Akdis, M., and Akdis, C. A. (2009). T regulatory cells and their counterparts: masters of immune regulation. *Clinical and Experimental Allergy*, Vol. 39 (May 2009), No. 5, pp. 626-39, ISSN 0954-7894.
Paget, C., Mallevaey, T., Speak, A. O., Torres, D., Fontaine, J., Sheehan, K. C., Capron, M., Ryffel, B., Faveeuw, C., Leite de Moraes, M., Platt, F., and Trottein, F. (2007). Activation of invariant NKT cells by toll-like receptor 9-stimulated dendritic cells requires type I interferon and charged glycosphingolipids. *Immunity*, Vol. 27 (October 2007), No. 4, pp. 597-609, ISSN 1074-7613.
Pei, B., Speak, A. O., Shepherd, D., Butters, T., Cerundolo, V., Platt, F. M., and Kronenberg, M. (2010). Diverse endogenous antigens for mouse NKT cells: self-antigens that are not glycosphingolipids. *Journal of Immunology*, Vol. 186 (February 2011), No. 3, pp. 1348-60, ISSN 0022-1767.
Petermann, F., Rothhammer, V., Claussen, M. C., Haas, J. D., Blanco, L. R., Heink, S., Prinz, I., Hemmer, B., Kuchroo, V. K., Oukka, M., and Korn, T. (2010). gammadelta T cells

enhance autoimmunity by restraining regulatory T cell responses via an interleukin-23-dependent mechanism. *Immunity,* Vol. 33 (September 2010), No. 3, pp. 351-63, ISSN 1074-7613.

Raftery, M. J., Winau, F., Kaufmann, S. H., Schaible, U. E., and Schonrich, G. (2006). CD1 antigen presentation by human dendritic cells as a target for herpes simplex virus immune evasion. *Journal of Immunology,* Vol. 177 (November 2006), No. 9, pp. 6207-14, ISSN 0022-1767.

Raghuraman, G., Geng, Y., and Wang, C. R. (2006). IFN-beta-mediated up-regulation of CD1d in bacteria-infected APCs. *Journal of Immunology,* Vol. 177 (December 2006), No. 11, pp. 7841-8, ISSN 0022-1767.

Ray, A., Khare, A., Krishnamoorthy, N., Qi, Z., and Ray, P. (2010). Regulatory T cells in many flavors control asthma. *Society for Mucosal Immunology,* Vol. 3 (May 2010), No. 3, pp. 216-29, ISSN 1933-0219.

Ribeiro-Dos-Santos, R., Mengel, J. O., Postol, E., Soares, R. A., Ferreira-Fernandez, E., Soares, M. B., and Pontes-De-Carvalho, L. C. (2001). A heart-specific CD4+ T-cell line obtained from a chronic chagasic mouse induces carditis in heart-immunized mice and rejection of normal heart transplants in the absence of Trypanosoma cruzi. *Parasite Immunology,* Vol. 23 (February 2001), No. 2, pp. 93-101, ISSN 0141-9838.

Rincon-Orozco, B., Kunzmann, V., Wrobel, P., Kabelitz, D., Steinle, A., and Herrmann, T. (2005). Activation of V gamma 9V delta 2 T cells by NKG2D. *Journal of Immunology,* Vol. 175 (August 2005), No. 4, pp. 2144-51, ISSN 0022-1767.

Roelofs-Haarhuis, K., Wu, X., and Gleichmann, E. (2004). Oral tolerance to nickel requires CD4+ invariant NKT cells for the infectious spread of tolerance and the induction of specific regulatory T cells. *Journal of Immunology,* Vol. 173 (July 2004), No. 2, pp.1043-50, ISSN 0022-1767.

Roelofs-Haarhuis, K., Wu, X., Nowak, M., Fang, M., Artik, S., and Gleichmann, E. (2003). Infectious nickel tolerance: a reciprocal interplay of tolerogenic APCs and T suppressor cells that is driven by immunization. *Journal of Immunology,* Vol. 171 (September 2003), No. 6, pp. 2863-72, ISSN 0022-1767.

Ronchi, F., and Falcone, M. (2008). Immune regulation by invariant NKT cells in autoimmunity. *Frontiers in Bioscience,* Vol. 13 (May 2008), pp. 4827-37, ISSN 1945-0494.

Roura-Mir, C., Wang, L., Cheng, T. Y., Matsunaga, I., Dascher, C. C., Peng, S. L., Fenton, M. J., Kirschning, C., and Moody, D. B. (2005). Mycobacterium tuberculosis regulates CD1 antigen presentation pathways through TLR-2. *Journal of Immunology,* Vol. 175 (August 2005), No. 3, pp. 1758-66, ISSN 0022-1767.

Roy, K. C., Maricic, I., Khurana, A., Smith, T. R., Halder, R. C., and Kumar, V. (2008). Involvement of secretory and endosomal compartments in presentation of an exogenous self-glycolipid to type II NKT cells. *Journal of Immunology,* Vol. 180 (March 2008), No. 5, pp. 2942-50, ISSN 0022-1767.

Russano, A. M., Bassotti, G., Agea, E., Bistoni, O., Mazzocchi, A., Morelli, A., Porcelli, S. A., and Spinozzi, F. (2007). CD1-restricted recognition of exogenous and self-lipid antigens by duodenal gammadelta+ T lymphocytes. *Journal of Immunology,* Vol. 178 (March 2007), No. 6, pp. 3620-6, ISSN 0022-1767.

Sakaguchi, S. (2005). Naturally arising Foxp3-expressing CD25+CD4+ regulatory T cells in immunological tolerance to self and non-self. *Nature Immunology,* Vol. 6 (April 2005), No. 4, pp. 345-52, ISSN 1529-2908.

Sakaguchi, S., Yamaguchi, T., Nomura, T., and Ono, M. (2008). Regulatory T cells and immune tolerance. *Cell,* Vol. 133 (May 2008), No. 5, pp. 775-87.

Salio, M., Speak, A. O., Shepherd, D., Polzella, P., Illarionov, P. A., Veerapen, N., Besra, G. S., Platt, F. M., and Cerundolo, V. (2007). Modulation of human natural killer T cell ligands on TLR-mediated antigen-presenting cell activation. *Proceedings of the National Academy of Sciences of the United States of America,* Vol. 104 (December 2007), No. 51, pp. 20490-5, ISSN 0027-8424.

Sallusto, F., and Lanzavecchia, A. (1994). Efficient presentation of soluble antigen by cultured human dendritic cells is maintained by granulocyte/macrophage colony-stimulating factor plus interleukin 4 and downregulated by tumor necrosis factor alpha. *The Journal of Experimental Medicine,* Vol. 179 (April 1994), No. 4, pp. 1109-18, ISSN 0022-1007.

Salomon, B., Lenschow, D. J., Rhee, L., Ashourian, N., Singh, B., Sharpe, A., and Bluestone, J. A. (2000). B7/CD28 costimulation is essential for the homeostasis of the CD4+CD25+ immunoregulatory T cells that control autoimmune diabetes. *Immunity,* Vol. 12 (April 2000), No. 4, pp. 431-40, ISSN 1074-7613.

Sanchez, D. J., Gumperz, J. E., and Ganem, D. (2005). Regulation of CD1d expression and function by a herpesvirus infection. *The Journal of Clinical Investigation,* Vol. 115 (May 2005), No. 5, pp. 1369-78, ISSN 0021-9738.

Sathler-Avelar, R., Lemos, E. M., Reis, D. D., Medrano-Mercado, N., Araujo-Jorge, T. C., Antas, P. R., Correa-Oliveira, R., Teixeira-Carvalho, A., Eloi-Santos, S. M., Favato, D., and Martins-Filho, O. A. (2003). Phenotypic features of peripheral blood leucocytes during early stages of human infection with Trypanosoma cruzi. *Scandinavian Journal of Immunology,* Vol. 58 (December 2003), No. 6, pp. 655-63, ISSN 0300-9475.

Serre, K., Giraudo, L., Siret, C., Leserman, L., and Machy, P. (2006). CD4 T cell help is required for primary CD8 T cell responses to vesicular antigen delivered to dendritic cells in vivo. *European Journal of Immunology,* Vol. 36 (June 2006), No. 6, pp. 1386-97, ISSN 0014-2980.

Shamshiev, A., Donda, A., Prigozy, T. I., Mori, L., Chigorno, V., Benedict, C. A., Kappos, L., Sonnino, S., Kronenberg, M., and De Libero, G. (2000). The alphabeta T cell response to self-glycolipids shows a novel mechanism of CD1b loading and a requirement for complex oligosaccharides. *Immunity,* Vol. 13 (August 2000), No. 2, pp. 255-64, ISSN 1074-7613.

Sieling, P. A., Chatterjee, D., Porcelli, S. A., Prigozy, T. I., Mazzaccaro, R. J., Soriano, T., Bloom, B. R., Brenner, M. B., Kronenberg, M., Brennan, P. J., and et al. (1995). CD1-restricted T cell recognition of microbial lipoglycan antigens. *Science,* Vol. 269 (July 1995), No. 5221, pp. 227-30, ISSN 0193-4511.

Sikder, H., Zhao, Y., Balato, A., Chapoval, A., Fishelevich, R., Gade, P., Singh, I. S., Kalvakolanu, D. V., Johnson, P. F., and Gaspari, A. A. (2009). A central role for transcription factor C/EBP-beta in regulating CD1d gene expression in human keratinocytes. *Journal of Immunology,* Vol. 183 (August 2009), No. 3, pp. 1657-66, ISSN 0022-1767.

Skold, M., and Behar, S. M. (2003). Role of CD1d-restricted NKT cells in microbial immunity. *Infection and Immunity.* Vol. 71 (October 2003), No. 10, pp. 5447-55, ISSN 0019-9567.

Skold, M., Xiong, X., Illarionov, P. A., Besra, G. S., and Behar, S. M. (2005). Interplay of cytokines and microbial signals in regulation of CD1d expression and NKT cell activation. *Journal of Immunology,* Vol. 175 (July 2005), No. 6, pp. 3584-93, ISSN 0022-1767.

Smed-Sorensen, A., Moll, M., Cheng, T. Y., Lore, K., Norlin, A. C., Perbeck, L., Moody, D. B., Spetz, A. L., and Sandberg, J. K. (2008). IgG regulates the CD1 expression profile and lipid antigen-presenting function in human dendritic cells via FcgammaRIIa. *Blood,* Vol. 111 (May 2008), No. 10, pp. 5037-46, ISSN 0006-4971.

Soares, M. B., Silva-Mota, K. N., Lima, R. S., Bellintani, M. C., Pontes-de-Carvalho, L., and Ribeiro-dos-Santos, R. (2001). Modulation of chagasic cardiomyopathy by interleukin-4: dissociation between inflammation and tissue parasitism. *The American Journal of Pathology,* Vol. 159 (August 2001), No. 2, pp. 703-9, ISSN 0002-9440.

Solberg, E. E., Gjertsen, F., Haugstad, E., and Kolsrud, L. (2010). Sudden death in sports among young adults in Norway. *European Journal of Cardiovascular Prevention and Rehabilitation,* Vol. 17 (June 2010), No. 3, pp. 337-41, ISSN 1741-8267.

Sonoda, K. H., Exley, M., Snapper, S., Balk, S. P., and Stein-Streilein, J. (1999). CD1-reactive natural killer T cells are required for development of systemic tolerance through an immune-privileged site. *The Journal of Experimental Medicine,* Vol. 190 (November 1999), No. 9, pp. 1215-26, ISSN 0022-1007.

Sonoda, K. H., Faunce, D. E., Taniguchi, M., Exley, M., Balk, S., and Stein-Streilein, J. (2001). NK T cell-derived IL-10 is essential for the differentiation of antigen-specific T regulatory cells in systemic tolerance. *Journal of Immunology,* Vol. 166 (January 2001), No. 1, pp. 42-50, ISSN 0022-1767.

Spada, F. M., Grant, E. P., Peters, P. J., Sugita, M., Melian, A., Leslie, D. S., Lee, H. K., van Donselaar, E., Hanson, D. A., Krensky, A. M., Majdic, O., Porcelli, S. A., Morita, C. T., and Brenner, M. B. (2000). Self-recognition of CD1 by gamma/delta T cells: implications for innate immunity. *The Journal of Experimental Medicine,* Vol. 191 (March 2000), No. 6, pp. 937-48, ISSN 0022-1007.

Stein-Streilein, J., Sonoda, K. H., Faunce, D., and Zhang-Hoover, J. (2000). Regulation of adaptive immune responses by innate cells expressing NK markers and antigen-transporting macrophages. *Journal of Leukocyte Biology,* Vol. 67 (April 2000), No. 4, pp. 488-94, ISSN 0741-5400.

Stetson, D. B., Mohrs, M., Reinhardt, R. L., Baron, J. L., Wang, Z. E., Gapin, L., Kronenberg, M., and Locksley, R. M. (2003). Constitutive cytokine mRNAs mark natural killer (NK) and NK T cells poised for rapid effector function. *The Journal of Experimental Medicine,* Vol. 198 (October 2003), No. 7, pp. 1069-76, ISSN 0022-1007

Sugita, M., Grant, E. P., van Donselaar, E., Hsu, V. W., Rogers, R. A., Peters, P. J., and Brenner, M. B. (1999). Separate pathways for antigen presentation by CD1 molecules. *Immunity,* Vol. 11 (December 1999), No. 6, pp. 743-52, ISSN 1074-7613.

Szalay, G., Sauter, M., Hald, J., Weinzierl, A., Kandolf, R., and Klingel, K. (2006). Sustained nitric oxide synthesis contributes to immunopathology in ongoing myocarditis attributable to interleukin-10 disorders. The *American Journal of Pathology,* Vol. 169 (December 2006), No. 6, pp. 2085-93, ISSN 0002-9440.

Takeda, N., Seko, Y., Oriuchi, N., and Nagai, R. (2008). Gamma-delta T-cell-mediated dilated cardiomyopathy. *International Journal of Cardiology,* Vol. 125 (March 2008), No. 1, pp. 130-2, ISSN 0167-5273.

Takeda, N., Takahashi, T., Seko, Y., Maemura, K., Nakasone, H., Sakamoto, K., Hirata, Y., and Nagai, R. (2005). Takayasu myocarditis mediated by cytotoxic T lymphocytes. *Internal Medicine,* Vol. 44 (March 2005), No. 3, pp. 256-60, ISSN 0918-2918.

Taniguchi, M., Tashiro, T., Dashtsoodol, N., Hongo, N., and Watarai, H. (2010). The specialized iNKT cell system recognizes glycolipid antigens and bridges the innate and acquired immune systems with potential applications for cancer therapy. *International Immunology,* Vol. 22 (January 2010), No. 1, pp. 1-6, ISSN 0953-8178.

Taniguchi, T., Ogasawara, K., Takaoka, A., and Tanaka, N. (2001). IRF family of transcription factors as regulators of host defense. *Annual Review of Immunology,* Vol. 19 (April 2001), pp. 623-55, ISSN 0732-0582.

Terabe, M., and Berzofsky, J. A. (2008). The role of NKT cells in tumor immunity. *Advances in Cancer Research,* Vol. 101(December 2008), pp. 277-348, ISSN 0065-230X.

Topham, N. J., and Hewitt, E. W. (2009). Natural killer cell cytotoxicity: how do they pull the trigger? *Immunology,* Vol. 128 (September 2009), No. 1, pp. 7-15, ISSN 0019-2805.

Torgerson, T. R. (2006). Regulatory T cells in human autoimmune diseases. *Springer Seminars in Immunopathology,* Vol. 28 (August 2006), No. 1, pp. 63-76, ISSN 0344-4325.

Van Kaer, L., Wu, M., Ichikawa, Y., Ito, K., Bonneville, M., Ostrand-Rosenberg, S., Murphy, D. B., and Tonegawa, S. (1991). Recognition of MHC TL gene products by gamma delta T cells. *Immunological Reviews,* Vol. 120 (April 1991), pp. 89-115, ISSN 0105-2896.

Van Rhijn, I., Koets, A. P., Im, J. S., Piebes, D., Reddington, F., Besra, G. S., Porcelli, S. A., van Eden, W., and Rutten, V. P. (2006). The bovine CD1 family contains group 1 CD1 proteins, but no functional CD1d. *Journal of Immunology,* Vol. 176 (April 2006), No. 8, pp. 4888-93, ISSN 0022-1767.

Van Rhijn, I., Young, D. C., De Jong, A., Vazquez, J., Cheng, T. Y., Talekar, R., Barral, D. C., Leon, L., Brenner, M. B., Katz, J. T., Riese, R., Ruprecht, R. M., O'Connor, P. B., Costello, C. E., Porcelli, S. A., Briken, V., and Moody, D. B. (2009). CD1c bypasses lysosomes to present a lipopeptide antigen with 12 amino acids. *The Journal of Experimental Medicine,* Vol. 206 (June 2009), No. 6, pp. 1409-22, ISSN 0022-1007.

Van Rhijn, I., Zajonc, D. M., Wilson, I. A., and Moody, D. B. (2005). T-cell activation by lipopeptide antigens. *Current Opinions in Immunology,* Vol. 17 (June 2005), No. 3, pp. 222-9, ISSN 0952-7915.

Vella, C., and Festenstein, H. (1992). Coxsackievirus B4 infection of the mouse pancreas: the role of natural killer cells in the control of virus replication and resistance to infection. *The Journal of General Virology,* Vol. 73 (June 1992), No. Pt 6, pp. 1379-86, ISSN 0022-1317.

Vila de Muga, M., Torre Monmany, N., Asensio Carretero, S., Traveria Casanovas, F. J., Martinez Mejias, A., Coll Sibina, M. T., and Luaces Cubells, C. (2010). [Clinical features of influenza A H1N1 2009: a multicentre study.]. *Anales de Pediatria (Barc), (March 2011), ISSN 1695-4033.*

Vincent, M. S., Xiong, X., Grant, E. P., Peng, W., and Brenner, M. B. (2005). CD1a-, b-, and c-restricted TCRs recognize both self and foreign antigens. *Journal of Immunology,* Vol. 175 (November 2005), No. 10, pp. 6344-51, ISSN 0022-1767.

Vogel, S. N., Fitzgerald, K. A., and Fenton, M. J. (2003). TLRs: differential adapter utilization by toll-like receptors mediates TLR-specific patterns of gene expression. *Molecular Interventions,* Vol. 3 (December 2003), No. 8, pp. 466-77, ISSN 1534-0384.

Vossen, M. T., Westerhout, E. M., Soderberg-Naucler, C., and Wiertz, E. J. (2002). Viral immune evasion: a masterpiece of evolution. *Immunogenetics,* Vol. 54 (November 2002), No. 8, pp. 527-42, ISSN 0093-7711.

Wang S, L. J., Wang M, Zhang J, Wang Z. (2010). Treatment and prevention of experimental autoimmune myocarditis with CD28 superagonists. *Cardiology,* Vol. 115 (January 2010), No. 2, pp. 107-113, ISSN 0008-6312.

Wiegand, J. A., Torgersen, C., Bloechlinger, S., Takala, J., and Dunser, M. W. (2010). Influenza A(H1N1) infection and severe cardiac dysfunction in adults: A case series. *Wiener Klinische Wochenschrift,* Vol. 123(February 2011), No. 3-4, pp. 120-123, ISSN 0043-5325.

Woodruff, J. (1980). Viral myocarditis. *The American Journal of Pathology,* Vol. 101 (November 1980), No 2, pp. 425-483, ISSN 0002-9440.

Wu, C. Y., Feng, Y., Qian, G. C., Wu, J. H., Luo, J., Wang, Y., Chen, G. J., Guo, X. K., and Wang, Z. J. (2010). alpha-Galactosylceramide protects mice from lethal Coxsackievirus B3 infection and subsequent myocarditis. *Clinical and Experimental Immunology,* Vol. 162 (October 2010), No. 1, pp. 178-87, ISSN 0009-9104.

Yokoyama, A. (1988). Natural killer cells in dilated cardiomyopathy. *The Tohoku Journal of Experimental Medicine.* Vol. 154 (April 1988), No. 4, pp. 335-44, ISSN 0040-8727.

Yuan, W., Dasgupta, A., and Cresswell, P. (2006). Herpes simplex virus evades natural killer T cell recognition by suppressing CD1d recycling. *Nature Immunology,* Vol. 7(August 2006), No. 8, pp. 835-42, ISSN 1529-2908.

Zajonc, D. M., Elsliger, M. A., Teyton, L., and Wilson, I. A. (2003). Crystal structure of CD1a in complex with a sulfatide self antigen at a resolution of 2.15 A. *Nature Immunology,* Vol. 4 (August 2003), No. 8, pp. 808-15, ISSN 1529-2908.

Zajonc, D. M., Savage, P. B., Bendelac, A., Wilson, I. A., and Teyton, L. (2008). Crystal structures of mouse CD1d-iGb3 complex and its cognate Valpha14 T cell receptor suggest a model for dual recognition of foreign and self glycolipids. *Journal of Molecular Biology,* Vol. 377 (April 2008), No. 4, pp. 1104-16, ISSN 0022-2836.

Zheng, Y., He, Y., Deng, J., Lu, Z., Wei, J., Yang, W., Tang, Z., Li, B., Zhang, J., Wang, L., Zhao, H., Li, X., Yu, Z., Song, P., Ma, Y., Li, Y., and Li, C. (2010). Hospitalized children with 2009 influenza a (H1N1) infection in Shenzhen, China, november-december 2009. *Pediatric Pulmonology.* Vol. 46 (March 2011), No. 3, pp. 246-252, ISSN 8755-6863.

Zingoni, A., Sornasse, T., Cocks, B. G., Tanaka, Y., Santoni, A., and Lanier, L. L. (2005). NK cell regulation of T cell-mediated responses. *Molecular Immunology,* Vol. 42 (February 2005), No. 4, pp. 451-4, ISSN 0161-5890.

13

Cellular and Immunological Regulation of Viral Myocarditis

David Marchant, Farshid S. Garmaroudi and Bruce M. McManus
UBC James Hogg Research Centre, Institute for Heart + Lung Health,
St. Paul's Hospital, University of British Columbia
Canada

1. Introduction

Since the discovery of coxsackievirus type B3 (CVB3) more than 50 years ago there has been considerable progress in the understanding of viral heart disease. Coxsackievirus was first discovered as a filterable agent associated with a paralytic syndrome, so named for its identification in Coxsackie, New York (coxsackievirus type A) (Dalldorf and Sickles, 1948). Coxsackievirus type B (CVB) was isolated the following year from patients with aseptic meningitis and by the mid-1950s an association with acute myocarditis in humans was apparent (Melnick et al., 1949). Many other viruses have since been shown to cause myocarditis and its long term sequelae, arrhythmias, dilated cardiomyopathy (DCM) and heart failure. By example, adenovirus, herpes viruses, and influenza can cause myocarditis in humans and models of heart failure. The viral agent most often reported as being the cause of viral myocarditis is CVB3. For example, CVB3 RNA can be detected in the heart muscle of 10 - 35 % of DCM patients (Feldman and McNamara, 2000; Hosenpud et al., 2001), depending on the study cohort.

1.1 Myocarditis etiologies

Inflammation of the heart muscle can have many causes, not least of which is viral infection. Cocaine [(Jentzen, 1989) reviewed in (Maraj et al., 2010)], virus induced, autoimmune (possibly due to resolved microbial infection), and even vaccine induced myocarditis (Cassimatis et al., 2004) have all been reported with a wide degree of occurrence. Though very rare, the vaccine induced aetiology is classified as idiopathic due to the poorly understood mechanism of inflammation. This manifestation of myocarditis is so rare it is probably very complex in cause and mechanism, requiring both environmental and genetic susceptibility factors of the host to trigger myocardial immune invasion. The subject of this chapter is one of the most common forms of myocarditis, and perhaps the most studied: myocarditis due to viral infection. In such cases, myocyte dropout and provisional matrix fibrosis, focal lesions of immune cell invasion are marked and key observations in the diagnosis of these cases.

1.2 Clinical presentation

With an experimental understanding of CVB3 induced myocarditis comes a better understanding of the breadth of symptoms presented by the admitted patient, before, during and after a hospital visit. The patient is most often admitted to hospital with general chest pain or discomfort, combined with other symptoms of an infection, which are often suspected as other ailments (Brady et al., 2004). These symptoms of infection can be so apparent that they divert the attention of the clinician away from cardiac dysfunction. Further work-up of the case reveals elevated creatinine phosphokinase and troponin with rhythmic disturbances and reduced cardiac output, often presented by shortness of breath with minimal exertion (Brady et al., 2004). Most cases resolve with little or no supportive therapy, but a minor percentage of cases progress to dilated cardiomyopathy and congestive heart failure, for which there is no cure other than heart transplantation.

1.3 Diagnosis: the Dallas criteria

The Dallas criteria for myocarditis are a set of histology based criteria proposed by a publication in 1987 by Aretz et al. (Aretz et al., 1987). These criteria rely upon histological observations made of left ventricular biopsies, obtained by either the Cordis or Scholten bioptomes. Several biopsies of the ventricle are required for a definitive diagnosis and there is a high possibility of false negatives using this method. Though not necessarily a problem inherent in the method itself but the need for a large number of samples due to the often localised and focal nature of the disease. The chances of false negatives combined with procedural discomfort are driving forward a need to develop new and less invasive procedures like blood-based biomarker-detection.

The Dallas criteria for diagnosis of myocarditis require an inflammatory infiltrate with associated myocyte necrosis, or otherwise damage that is not characteristic of ischemia. Less intense immune infiltration with little or no evidence of myocyte destruction is classified as borderline myocarditis (Aretz et al., 1987).

Understanding the etiology of myocarditis will improve the success rate of diagnosis, which in turn, improves management of the disease and prognosis (Baughman, 2006; Felker et al., 2000). The Dallas criteria were a good stepping stone toward a standardised diagnostic method, however there remain significant drawbacks to this biopsy based histological criteria. It has been demonstrated that myocarditis could only be accurately diagnosed in 25 % of single biopsies obtained from patients who had died of myocarditis (Chow et al., 1989; Hauck et al., 1989), and more than 5 biopsies are required to diagnose myocarditis in two thirds of patients (Hauck et al., 1989), and 17 biopsies are required for an 80 % level of confidence in diagnosis (Hauck et al., 1989; Schultz et al., 2009). Therefore only positive samples obtained by endomyocardial biopsy should be considered diagnostic. These poor rates of definitive diagnosis are a product of the small size of the bioptome sample from a relatively large area afflicted with a disease that is often focal and of relatively narrow localisation.

The Dallas criteria were a good start for a disease that had no diagnostic criteria at the time of publication (1987). To this day, the Dallas criteria are used to diagnose myocarditis from endomyocardial biopsies, though the existence of sensitive methods for disease detection, particularly in the blood, biomarker discovery should make this methodology supplementary or even obsolete. Therefore, there is a need for the development of sensitive methods for the differential and definitive diagnosis of non-ischemic cardiomyopathies like myocarditis. This chapter will not cover diagnosis or new detection strategies any further as these topics are covered in greater detail, elsewhere in this book.

2. Viral replication as the central regulator of viral myocarditis

The advent of virus replication in the heart of an individual is thought to occur secondarily to a more general and systemic virus infection (Carthy et al., 1997; Mena et al., 2000; Vuorinen et al., 1994), the spleen, gut, pancreas and lymph nodes are often infected; patients often report malaise, fatigue and more general 'flu-like' symptoms about 1- 2 weeks prior to chest pains and cardiac rhythm disturbances. Immune infiltration in the heart has taken hold by the time the patient has been seen by a physician and any evidence of direct virus-induced damage has been superseded by T cell invasion at the foci of infection. It is not surprising that there have been many reports that claim the predominant source of damage is immune infiltration of the myocardium, as inflammation is what defines this disease. Autoimmune etiologies due to an antiviral response gone awry have been proposed as one of the major causes of pathology (Lv et al., 2011). Regardless, there are numerous publications that suggest a large amount of damage is inflicted by the virus itself, in the murine model, early post-infection, that is correlated with the number of myocarditic lesions spatially coincident with positivity by *in situ* hybridization for CVB3 genome (Cheung et al., 2008; Chow et al., 1992; Marchant et al., 2009a; McManus et al., 1993). These observations are supported by findings in autopsy cases, particularly in infants (Iwasaki et al., 1985a; Iwasaki et al., 1985b).

2.1 The cytotoxic nature of enterovirus replication

Coxsackievirus B3 is a member of the *Enteroviridae* of the *Picornaviridae* family, which are fast replicating and exquisitely cytotoxic viruses. Another member of this family is poliovirus, which is also highly cytotoxic, producing a paralytic syndrome reminiscent of the aseptic meningitis and encephalitis sometimes caused by CVB3. The very nature of enterovirus replication makes these viruses very cytotoxic because the infected cell must burst to permit the release of progeny virus virions for infection of bystander cells and further replication cycles. This aspect of CVB3 replication means that every virus infected cell will die within 8 - 24 hrs of infection, releasing numerous rounds of progeny virus into the heart before the innate immune system has had a chance to control infection. The degree of immune infiltration and damage inflicted on the heart muscle is therefore a function of the amount of virus inoculum that takes hold in the heart, dictating the degree of damage done to the myocardium.

The virus polarises the protein expression machinery entirely to the benefit of the virus by a number of mechanisms and so in combination with the inability of the cell to perform its natural housekeeping functions inevitably leads to cell destruction. The viral proteases act to cleave capped cellular mRNAs thereby skewing protein translation in the cell from cap-dependent translation initiation to internal ribosome entry site (IRES) translation. Coxsackievirus B3 translates it's RNA genome via IRES translation initiation so destruction of the cell's own capped mRNAs removes any competition of the virus' own IRES RNAs for the cell's ribosomes. This usurping of control of the cell's protein expression machinery effectively brings the normal housekeeping function of the cell to a halt.

The massive amount of protein produced by the virus, devolution of the endoplasmic reticulum (ER) and other membranous structures combined with the oxidative stress placed upon the cell by virus replication, all destabilise the homeostasis of the infected cell. The large protein-nucleic acid aggregates that make up progeny virion are not normal to the cell and induce numerous UPR responses; due to their toxic nature, protein aggregates are normally sequestered to vimentin-cytoskeleton encased aggrosomes (Garcia-Mata et al., 1999; Johnston et al., 1998). For example, the irregular folding of viral proteins can lead to sequestering of virus protein products into cellular aggresomes (Spiropoulou et al., 2003). These combined facets of CVB3 replication contribute to the inherently toxic nature of virus replication, even in the absence of the onset of programmed cell death.

2.2 Virus entry into the host cell

The replication cycle of CVB3 in the cell begins in a very similar manner to poliovirus infection via receptor mediated endocytosis into the target host cell. Coxsackievirus B3 binds its cellular receptor(s), the coxsackie-adenovirus receptor (CAR) and ,sometimes, decay acceleration factor (DAF), to achieve entry via endocytosis into the host cell. Once the virus has achieved delivery inside the cell there is massive rearrangement of internal membrane structures and then complete usurping of the host cell protein translation machinery for the purposes of virus replication and virion assembly. The RNA polarity (positive-polarity RNA) of the CVB3 genome means that viral polypeptide can be translated directly after delivery into the host cell. All of the proteins encoded by the CVB3 genome are expressed as 1 poly-protein that is then cleaved by virus proteases, 2A and 3C, into the individual viral proteins VP4, VP2, VP3, VP1, 2A, 2B, 2C, 3A, 3B, 3C, and 3D.

2.3 Death and lysis of virus infected cells

Direct virus-induced damage inflicted by CVB3 upon the infected cell is through simultaneous activation of multiple cell death pathways, by direct and indirect mechanisms. For example, all of the known caspase cell death activation pathways are activated during CVB3 infection: the FAS/FADD receptor-mediated caspase- 8 pathway and the mitochondrial cytochrome c -caspase- 9 pathway are activated to ultimately trigger the death effector, caspase-3 (Carthy et al., 1998; Carthy et al., 2003). Normally, the activation of caspases during apoptosis leads to programmed cell death: cleavage of cellular DNA by endonucleases and shrinking of the cell's contents into a cytoskeleton-vimentin cage, for engulfment by phagocytes at some later time. This process is programmed, and most importantly, 'neat,' preventing the dissemination of the dead cell's contents throughout the tissue. The debris released from cells are hydrolytic and oxidative, some are apoptotic, which would lead to bystander necrosis of surrounding cells and tissue if not disposed of 'neatly' through programmed cell death. However, CVB3 infected cells do not die in a programmed and neat manner. The act of virus replication; viral proteases and activation of numerous cell death pathways all at once cause infected cells to rapidly lyse and release cellular contents, along with virus progeny virions, for further rounds of replication in surrounding bystander cells.

Necrotic cell death during CVB3 infection is most likely caused by a myriad of pathways that act in concert to result in the uncontrolled lysis of the cell for the purpose of virus progeny release. Evolution of the virus has favoured a more chaotic lysis/necrosis type death as opposed to a programmed and controlled method of killing the host cell. We will summarise the pathways of CVB3 induced cell death below:

2.3.1 Caspase-induced cell death during CVB3 infection

The caspase pathways of apoptosis were the first mechanisms of programmed cell death that were discovered [(Lazebnik et al., 1994; Miura et al., 1993; Yuan et al., 1993; Yuan and

Horvitz, 1990) reviewed in (Yuan and Horvitz, 2004)]. The first cellular pathways implicated in cell death due to CVB3 infection were also caspase mediated (Carthy et al., 1998; Colston et al., 1998), since these were the predominant mechanisms of cell death being studied at the time (Andrade et al., 1998; Atkinson et al., 1998; Barry et al., 2000). As new mechanisms of cell death were discovered, such as GSK-3β, some were attributed to virus induced cell death.

Comprehensive studies of caspase cleavage and activation during infection have demonstrated a pan-caspase activation profile during viral infection (Carthy et al., 1998; Carthy et al., 2003), from activation of the tumour necrosis factor (TNF) receptor activated caspase-8 to the mitochondrial cytochrome *c* release that results in the activation of caspase-9. All of the above mentioned pathways converge upon the activation of the effector caspase, caspase-3. The most notable caspase-8 activated pathway is triggered by Fas ligand binding and activation of Fas receptor, a member of the TNF superfamily of receptors. Various oxidative states, toxins and aberrant protein expression can lead to a permeable mitochondrial membrane that releases cytochrome *c* into the cytoplasm which leads to caspase-9 activation. Though the caspase-8 and -9 pathways are quite different in that they are extrinsic and intrinsic pathways of cell death, respectively, they both lead to cleavage and activation of caspase-3, a death effector caspase. In cells destined to die by either of these routes of apoptosis there is cleavage of poly ADP-ribose polymerase (PARP) and DNA fragmentation factor (DFF) by caspase-3. Cleavage of DFF by this caspase reveals an endonuclease that enters the nucleus and cleaves DNA, resulting in DNA fragmentation (Figure 1A).

Two of the experimental hallmarks of apoptotic cell death are PARP fragmentation, as observed on a Western blot, and fragmented genomic DNA as viewed by agarose gel electrophoresis. It was demonstrated that inhibition of caspase-3 PARP and DFF cleavage did not inhibit virus induced cell death completely (Carthy et al., 1998), however some alleviation of cytopathic effect was notable. The broad spectrum zVAD.fmk caspase inhibitor is not 100 % effective at inhibiting all caspases, and there is the possibility that in the absence of caspase activation that a redundant mechanism of cell death becomes dominant in mediating cytotoxicity. In this scenario we would expect zVAD.fmk to appear ineffectual at inhibiting cell death. It was apparent that the caspases were activated though this was clearly not the mechanism that was entirely responsible for CVB3 induced cytopathic effect. Below we will outline more mechanisms responsible for cell death and that may run parallel to caspase mediated cytotoxicity. Later in this chapter we will also cover new systems biology approaches that could be applied toward the understanding of the dominant/ pertinent pathways of CVB3 induced cell lysis and the networks employed by the virus to drive cell death.

2.3.2 Glycogen synthase kinase-3β

In addition to the roles of caspases during cell death, the actions of glycogen synthase kinase-3 β (GSK-3β) have also been implicated in the induction of cytopathic effect by CVB3 replication (Yuan et al., 2005; Zhang et al., 2003). Phosphorylation of transcription factors by GSK-3β can lead to either the activation or down-regulation of transcription, and activation of GSK-3β has been observed relatively early in the CVB3 replication cycle (Yuan et al. 2005). The catenins are poly-phosphorylated by activated GSK-3β, leading to degradation in the proteasome (Doble and Woodgett, 2003; Harwood, 2001). During CVB3 infection, the activation of GSK-3β has been proposed to lead to instability of cell viability due to degradation of a protein called β-catenin (Figure 1C). The catenins interact with the actin cytoskeleton and act to maintain morphological integrity by connecting the actin cytoskeleton with the cell membrane. The loss of these connections through enhanced GSK-3β activation and β-catenin degradation is consistent with the profound cell rounding that occurs during intermediate to late phases of CVB3 replication. The accumulation of β-catenin in the cytoplasm leads to translocation into the nucleus where it transactivates survival signalling via T-cell factor (TCF)/lymphocyte enhancer factor (LEF) family members (Doble and Woodgett, 2003; Hardt and Sadoshima, 2002; Harwood, 2001). Consistent with these findings, the inhibition of GSK-3β or the over-expression of β-catenin resulted in the suppression of viral progeny release, but not viral protein production (Yuan et al., 2005). Therefore GSK-3β is pivotal in regulating the rupture of infected cells for progeny release.

2.3.3 The endoplasmic reticulum unfolded protein response

CVB3 induces the unfolded protein response (UPR), which is an acute stress response that leads to ER stress (Zhang et al., 2010). Poliovirus, CVB3 and other viruses have been shown to replicate their genomes and translate protein on the surfaces of double membrane vesicles derived from the ER and autophagosomes (Suhy et al., 2000; Wong et al., 2008; Zhang et al., 2011). This activity in combination with interruption of regular protein translation and a massive upregulation of protein production by the virus probably leads to activation of the UPR. This process involves 3 different pathways of independent activation, initiated by 3 respective stress sensors in the proximal ER: ATF6a, IRE1-XBP-1, (X box binding protein 1), and PERK (PKR-like ER protein kinase). It has been shown that infection with CVB3 invokes activation of ATF6a and XBP-1, possibly through replication of the virus on the surface of double membrane vesicles derived from the ER and autophagosome (Wong et al., 2008). Other viruses that replicate in the cytosol, such as West Nile Virus, have been shown to activate this pathway to promote virus replication and cell death ((Medigeshi et al., 2007) review). The UPR response to massive viral protein synthesis and usurped cellular pathways most likely acts to initiate or augment the onset of death in the infected host cell. However if these pathways are activated too early in the virus replication cycle the cell will die before virus protein production and virus progeny can be completed and released, respectively. This would surely result in the termination of virus replication. Zhang et al. showed that expression of the UPR response protein, XBP-1 acts to delay the onset of cell lysis and release of progeny virion (Figure 1B). Therefore, pathways like XBP-1 are used by the virus to counter early destruction of the cell; so CVB3 has evolved mechanisms to prevent premature death of the infected cell. Major cellular survival pathways, like Akt, are also invoked to counter the death reflex, which we will discuss later in the chapter.

2.3.4 Cell death and lysis through activation of many simultaneous pathways

The overwhelming and rapid activation of many different pathways simultaneously leads to cell death and lysis (Figure 1), liberating progeny virion. It is possible, that cell death pathways may even be synergistic, additively driving the cell toward more rapid and thus uncontrolled death, leading to lysis. The cytochrome c- caspase-9 pathway requires a minimum of 15 hours to kill a cell that has been chemically induced, almost twice as long as it takes CVB3 to lyse an infected cell (Qu and Qing, 2004). The plant toxin abrin requires upwards of 15 - 36 hours to kill a culture of HeLa cells (Qu and Qing, 2004), the E2 protein of human papillomavirus requires 20 - 24 hrs to induce apoptosis (Desaintes et al., 1999), whereas CVB3 will have induced apoptosis and destroyed a similar culture of HeLa cells in just 8 - 10 hours. The rapid nature of CVB3 induced cell lysis suggests the synergy between numerous death pathways 'criss-cross' and interact to enhance their collective cell-death effect.

The loss of checked and contained cell death results in necrosis and lysis of the CVB3 infected host cell. Even though the pathways of cell death are clearly defined in this arena, the precise mechanisms of initiation are still unclear, and potential pathway interactions are unknown. Many reports have indicated that a particular pathway may be involved in CVB3 induced cell death although there hasn't been 100 % recovery of cell viability demonstrated from experiments that inhibit just one pathway. However, zVAD, a pan caspase inhibitor does not completely inhibit virus induced death and lysis just as GSK3β inhibition doesn't completely inhibit cell-rounding and death. Therefore there is still much to be learned about the initiation and interaction of cell death pathways during CVB3 infection, but we may never be able to completely inhibit CVB3 induced cell death because once virus replication is initiated the cell may already be past the threshold of viability.

2.3.5 Necroptosis?

Necroptosis (necrotic apoptosis) is a tumour necrosis factor receptor activated form of programmed cell death that is activated by the same class of receptors that activate caspase-8 mediated apoptosis (Declercq et al., 2009; Hitomi et al., 2008; Yuan and Kroemer, 2010). This is a more recently discovered pathway of cell death that has not been reported in the context of CVB3 infection. However, instead of caspase-8 activation that normally results from TNF receptor ligation there is activation of a receptor interacting protein (RIP)-1/RIP-3 pathway that results in rupture of the cell through loss of membrane integrity; a mode of cell death reminiscent of CVB3 induced cell lysis. Transgenic caspase-8 null animals undergo RIP-3 necroptosis instead of apoptosis, leading to embryonic lethality and non-viability of the line. However caspase-8 -/-, RIP-3 -/- double transgenic mice are viable, suggesting that caspase- 8 holds RIP-3 'in check', preventing initiation of programmed necrosis (Kaiser et al., 2011). The necroptosis pathway has not yet been described with respect to CVB3 infection but given the similarities between CVB3 induced cell lysis and necroptosis this pathway of cell death and the RIP-1/RIP-3 proteins may provide some insight.

2.4 Virus induced cell death and lysis – 'Timing is everything'

There have been reports showing that cell death activated early in the virus life cycle significantly inhibits viral replication (Zhang et al., 2010). Release of the cell contents prior to progeny virion production and more programmed processes of cell death will halt virus replication by killing the cell prior to assembly of progeny virus virion or confinement of progeny virion into vimentin cages, respectively.

Virus replication is cytotoxic and can cause cell death before production of progeny virion, terminating the life-cycle of the virus. For example, reactive oxygen species are a byproduct of CVB3 replication very early in the life-cycle of the virus, placing stress on the cell such that the mitochondrial cytochrome *c* pathway of caspase-9 mediated cell death might be activated prior to virion assembly. To prevent premature death of the host cell coxsackievirus triggers the activation of pro-survival proteins and their associated cascades to suppress cell lysis until progeny virion can be assembled. Perhaps the most studied pro-survival protein, Akt, is activated during the CVB3 replication cycle (Esfandiarei et al., 2007; Esfandiarei et al., 2004; Liu et al., 2008). It may appear counter-intuitive for a cytolytic virus to evolve to activate pro-survival pathways, particularly if the virus requires the cell to lyse at the end of the cycle. However, as we discussed in section 2.1 CVB3 replication is cytotoxic from the onset so pro-survival pathways may be selected evolutionarily to support the survival of the cell while viral protein synthesis and viral progeny assembly are taking place. These mechanisms of cell survival during virus infection act in favour of viral replication because they allow maximum amounts of virus progeny to be assembled prior to cell lysis and release of viral progeny. Subsequently, these same survival pathways must be inhibited to then permit cell death and lysis for release of assembled viral progeny virions.

2.5 Coxsackievirus induced cell death: many dimensions of complexity

It is now apparent that several cell death pathways and perhaps dozens of proteins are activated in a web of molecular interaction in order to short circuit normal death mechanisms, to cause rapid and aberrant rupture of the infected cell (Figure 1). New pathways of cell death, such as necroptosis, may as yet be shown to mediate death of the CVB3 infected cell. Nevertheless, there already exists a large web of seemingly disparate pathways of CVB3 induced cellular lysis. As we discussed earlier, it is difficult to determine the foundation pathway that is responsible for virally induced cell lysis of infected cardiomyocytes, and which ones are triggered, merely as a matter of coincident activation. New methods of data organisation and analysis are clearly needed as more pathways and mechanisms of CVB3 induced cell death are revealed. Knowledge of the truly pertinent and central pathways of cell death could lead to the most robust antivirals. Toward the end of this chapter we will discuss the use of systems biology to organise the myriad of pathways activated during CVB3 infection (proteolytic and kinase) and how it could be applied to elucidate the dominant pathways of virus induced cell death.

3. Inflammatory regulation of myocarditis by the host: regulatory T cells and healthy vs pathological signalling

3.1 Mouse genetic determinants of immune infiltration

Once virus infection has taken hold in the heart there is infiltration and onset of immune responses to clear infection and lay down provisional matrix in place of damaged tissue. As we discussed earlier in the chapter, the severity of the immune response varies broadly from patient to patient, from mild to massive immune infiltration that can lead to DCM and congestive heart failure. We know from the mouse models of CVB3 induced myocarditis that immune infiltration is correlated with the amount of virus inoculum, and therefore with the degree of damage that has been mediated by virus. However experiments comparing the susceptibility of various inbred strains of mice to CVB3 induced myocarditis showed that there could be a genetic predisposition to myocarditis severity (McManus et al., 1993). These data suggest that a genetic predisposition of the individual patient to mild or severe myocarditis, combined with viremia and cardiac viral load could act in concert to determine severity and number of myocarditic foci. The studies conducted with inbred mouse strains have implicated the MHC class II (H2) locus (Wolfgram et al., 1986), in addition to other genetic loci (Traystman et al., 1991) associated with the severity and susceptibility to CVB3 myocarditis, both acute, chronic and autoimmune. Not surprisingly, the H2 locus of the MHC II complex has been implicated in clearance of acute coxsackievirus infection

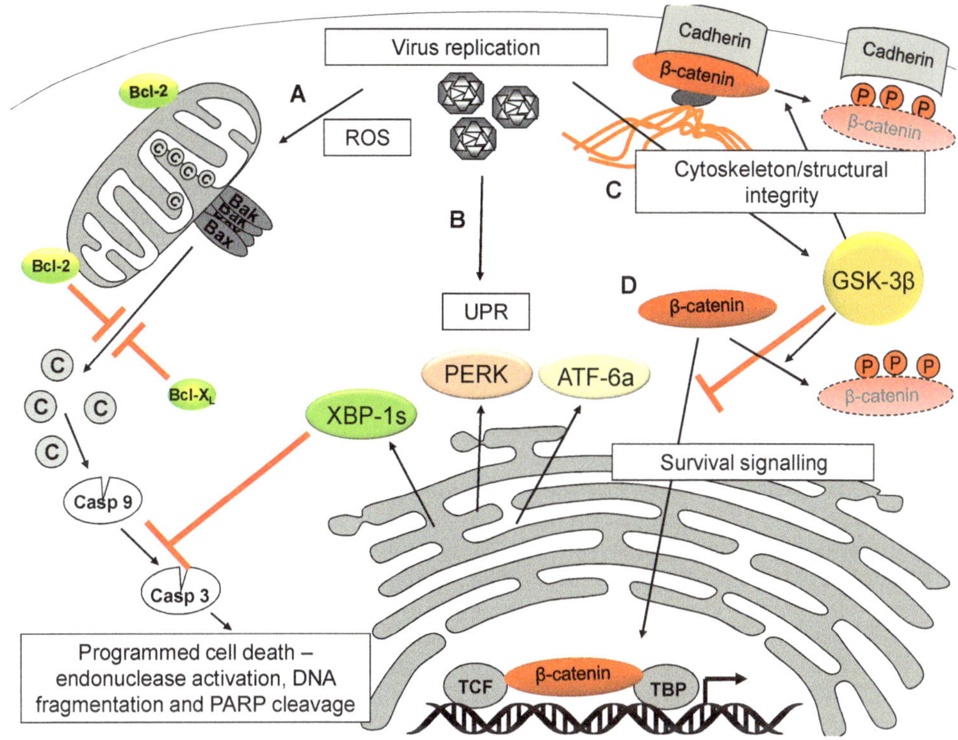

Fig. 1. Pathways of cell death in CVB3 infected cardiomyocytes. A. Coxsackievirus replication results in production of reactive oxygen species which promote the release of cytochrome c from mitochondria. The formation of Bak and Bax at the membrane surface mediate passage of cytochrome c into the cytosol. Overexpression of the anti-apoptotic proteins BCl 2 and BCl-XL during CVB3 infection significantly reduce cytochrome *c* release and activation of the caspase-9 pathway of apoptosis, which leads to caspase-3 death effector caspase activation. ROS – reactive oxygen species. B. The unfolded protein response (UPR) of the endoplasmic reticulum (ER) is activated during CVB3 infection of cardiomyocytes leading to activation of all 3 known pathways of the UPR: spliced XBP-1s, PERK and ATF6a ER stress sensors are all activated during CVB3 infection. Virus replication occurs on the surface of double membrane vesicles and membrane derived from the ER, activating the ER stress sensors. The result of XBP-1s activation is to slow the onset of cell death to prevent the cell from rupturing prior to the assembly of progeny virus virions. UPR = unfolded protein response. C and D. Glycogen synthase kinase -3β (GSK-3β) is activated during CVB3 infection resulting in phosphorylation and subsequent proteosomal degradation of its target, β -catenin, in the cytosol. C. Loss of β -catenin in the cytosol results in loss of connections between the actin cytoskeleton and cadherin receptors, via connections to α and β -catenins. D. Less β -catenin in the cytosol means that there will be less available to translocate across the nucleus to activate survival gene expression via TCF and TBP transcription factors.

(Wolfgram et al., 1986). The presence of a strong adaptive response that includes robust neutralising antibodies is required to control CVB3 infection in mice (Wolfgram et al., 1986) and patients (McKinney et al., 1987; Misbah et al., 1992), as well as other picornaviruses, like polio (MacLennan et al., 2004). Therefore, the host's own genetic makeup will determine how quickly and how completely virus infection is cleared from the body. An inability to mount a broad immune response will lead to more virus replication, more immune infiltraton of the myocardium, more matrix deposition and longer recovery times. In addition to these host dependent factors there may also be environmental factors that play roles during infection and inflammation: extrinsic source stress, pollution/allergens and population density could also contribute to susceptibility and severity of viral myocarditis.

3.2 Chronic infection and the cycle of virus-immune mediated damage

Over the last 3 decades it has become apparent that viral load is a primary determinant of viral myocarditis severity (Cheung et al., 2008; Chow et al., 1992; Lim et al., 2005; Marchant et al., 2009a; McManus et al., 1993), the virus causes extensive, early direct injury to the myocardium through its replication. The studies cited above all indicate significant injury to the myocardium prior to cardiac immune infiltration, supporting the view that considerable damage to the heart is directly mediated by the virus alone. An argument has been made previously for the importance of chronic virus replication in myocarditis and as a basis of dilated cardiomyopathy (Szalay et al., 2006) and chronic heart failure. Enhanced immunoproteasome expression in chronically CVB3 infected cardiomyocytes (Szalay et al., 2006) may increase the expression and presentation of auto-antigens, leading to more severe myocarditis through autoimmune avenues. Chronic virus replication will lead to consistent damage which will, in turn, result in provisional matrix turnover. This type of damage-repair loop will propagate the fibrosis that is evident during chronic myocarditis and DCM. As we covered in the apoptosis/death pathway sections of this chapter the release of cell constituents and debris, and progeny virus and proinflammatory cytokines, from an infected cell will lead to inflammation at the site of virus insult. Therefore, the damage inflicted by the virus itself will be exacerbated by the onset of cytolytic immune infiltration and fibrosis.

3.3 Regulatory T cells

Not all T cell infiltration and immunity are harmful as there are moderating arms of the immune response that solely act to moderate the strength of a response, preventing autoimmunity. Li et al recently reported that allografted M2 (anti-inflammatory) macrophages led to improvement of virus-induced myocarditis (Li et al., 2009) which was associated with enhanced levels of regulatory T cells (Treg). Huber et al have also reported decreased viral load and immune infiltration after adoptive transfer of a CD4+ CD25+ regulatory-like T cell population into a mouse model of CVB3 infection (Huber et al., 2006). Regulatory T cells are CD4 + cells that express the α-subunit of the IL2 receptor CD25, and are negative for CD127. The hallmark protein expressed in these cells is the transcription factor FoxP3 and they circulate as a functionally distinct T cell subpopulation, preventing autoimmune and other aberrant responses to innocuous environmental antigens (Wing and Sakaguchi). The T-reg population prevents the proliferation of self-reactive effector T cell populations and were aptly named suppressor T cells when first discovered for their ability to secrete IL10 and moderate Th1 immunity (Wing and Sakaguchi). Thus, it would be reasonable to postulate that adoptive transfer of T-regs into a mouse model of viral myocarditis would suppress the immune response and allow virus replication to proceed unchecked.

In a study by Shi et al (Shi et al., 2010) T-reg cells were adoptively transferred into CVB3 infected mice and the effect of the transferred cells upon viral load and signalling within the heart were investigated. Included in the study were PBS injection controls, but also naïve T cells. Decreased immune infiltration and enhanced Akt activation, as compared to the naïve CD4 T cell and PBS grafted controls, were notable in the T-reg adopted mice (Figure 2). Perhaps the most surprising of the results was the decreased viral load, not only in the heart but also in the pancreas and spleen, associated with lower expression of the Coxsackie-Adenovirus Receptor (CAR). The authors adoptively transferred, not only T-reg cells, but CD25 (-) CD4 T cells (naïve) as well (Figure 2A), into a separate group of mice. In fact, the naïve CD4 T cell treated control group fared worse than either the PBS or T-reg treated groups, related to less Akt activation and higher CAR receptor expression. As a result, the naive T cell population brought on a more severe myocarditis phenotype due to higher viral loads. Taken altogether, Shi *et al.* describe the protective role that T-reg cells play in immune infiltration of the heart during viral myocarditis, suggesting that there is a balance to be struck between clearance of infection and immune-associated damage to the myocardium. In fact, in this study there was observed decreased viral loads consonant with a decrease in immune infiltration due to reduced TNF-α release and lower CAR expression (Figure 2B). The authors found that though TNF-α could enhance CAR expression in mouse cardiomyocytes the co-addition of TGF-β eliminated TNF-α-induced CAR expression. To conclude, these findings suggest a more intimate link between inflammation and virus replication than previously posited. Thus, moderating the immune response may be critical for prevention of chronic virus replication.

Although the dominant factor in virus suppression during T-reg treatment was most likely down-regulation of CAR expression, we propose that the alteration in signaling evoked by T-regs is also playing a significant role in modulating virus replication. The basis of our argument is that CAR expression was suppressed 3-fold *in vivo* and 5-fold in a dividing cardiomyocyte cell line *in vitro*, but the suppression of viral load in the Treg group was almost 2-logarithms reduced as compared to the control group. Although the correlation between cell receptor expression and virus infection may not be linear, the decreased levels of CAR receptor may not explain the entire antiviral effect of T-regs in the myocardium during virus infection. It is entirely possible that the signalling environment altered by the adoptive transfer of T regs may have also contributed to a less favorable environment for virus replication. The authors reported activation of Akt in the myocardium of the T-reg treated groups, which suggests that the activation of other signalling proteins may have been altered by T-reg transfer. We have reported that Akt activation is required for successful CVB3 replication (Esfandiarei et al., 2007; Esfandiarei et al., 2004; Esfandiarei et al., 2006), a pro-survival protein required by the virus to optimize the longevity of the infected cell to promote optimal progeny virus production. On the other hand, the Akt activation reported by Shi *et al.* may merely be a reflection of a healthier environment created by allografted T-reg cells in the myocardium. It is quite clear that an unbraked immunologically active environment supports enhanced cellular signalling driven by viruses for successful replication (Esfandiarei et al., 2006; Marchant et al., 2009a; Marchant et al., 2008). For example, we have previously reported that the powerful immune-stimulating protein p38 is required for effective virus replication in a CVB3 myocarditis mouse model (Marchant et al., 2009a). The activation of p38 MAP kinase was not investigated by Shi *et al.*, but we would predict less net activation of p38 in the presence of T-regs, and thus an environment that is less conducive to virus replication. Although p38 MAP kinase activation is required for suppressor (T-reg) T cell activity and function (Adler et al., 2007), we propose that adoptive transfer of T-regs may have decreased the immune infiltrate in the myocardium with less activation of p38 MAP kinase.

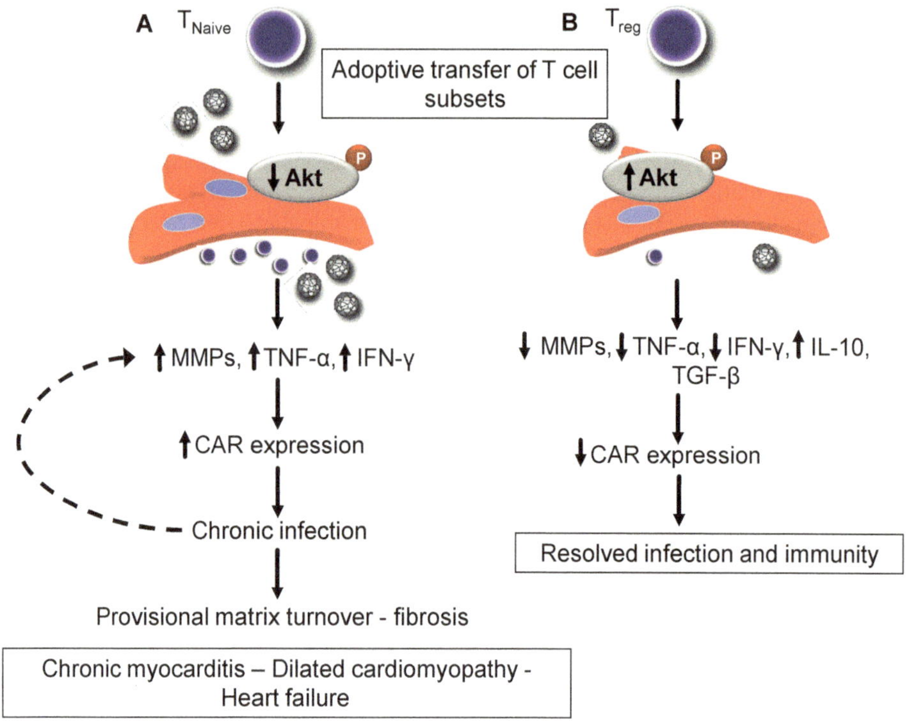

Fig. 2. Adoptive transfer of T cells into CVB3 infected mice has assisted in the elucidation of the beneficial arms of the immune response that aid in clearance of virus from the heart. A. Transfer of naïve T cells or control treatment with PBS, followed by infection with CVB3 results in high viral load in the heart followed by a large influx of T cells. An indication of myocarditis in the mouse model is the detection of decreased Akt activation, and MMP, TNF-α, and IFN-γ expression. Shi et al demonstrated that TNF- α induces coxsackie-adenovirus receptor (CAR) expression in myocardium during CVB3 replication which may promote chronic virus replication which could lead to dilated cardiomyopathy and heart failure through successive rounds of provisional matrix deposition and degradation. B. Adoptive transfer of syngeneic regulatory T cells reduces the immunologically reactive environment which results in less MMP, TNF-α, and IFN-γ expression. The result is lower CAR expression, lower viral loads and enhanced Akt activation, leading to a healthier, less immunologically reactive environment.

3.4 ERK and p38 MAP kinases

Activation of p38 MAP kinase is required for virus replication to take place, such that inhibition of p38 MAP kinase is an effective antiviral strategy *in vitro* (Si et al., 2005) and *in vivo* (Marchant et al., 2009a). The activation of ERK MAP kinase was first reported in the context of CVB3 infection both *in vitro* (Luo et al., 2002) and *in vivo* (Opavsky et al., 2002). The activation of this molecule by virus binding the CAR receptor may be involved in triggering endocytosis uptake of CVB3 during entry (Marchant et al., 2009b). The activation of p38 MAP kinase was later shown to be required for cell lysis and release of progeny virion. Si et al reported that inhibition of p38 MAP kinase could block progeny virus production but not virus protein expression (Si et al., 2005). Underlining the importance of p38 during virus replication was a relatively recent study that investigated the role of p38 during the life cycle of several different viruses. The activation of p38 MAP kinase was demonstrated as a common and dominant signalling molecule during the replication of many different types of viruses (Marchant et al., 2010). This molecule's intimate link to the immune response is perhaps not surprising; one might expect that Akt activation, p38 inhibition and T-reg immune control lead to improved outcome and result in lower viral load and immune infiltration.

With regard to new treatment strategies, this does not necessarily mean that we should be injecting T-reg cells into afflicted patients, but methods should be pursued that mediate the immune response to swing the pendulum in favor of viral clearance and reparation, and away from immune infiltration of the myocardium that favors higher viral loads. The work of several recent studies [(Li et al., 2009; Shi et al., 2010) reviewed in (Yajima and Knowlton, 2009)] have demonstrated the virus' evolved ability to bias immune activation and associated signaling queues for the benefit of virus replication. Given the results presented by Shi *et al.*, one might initially conclude that immune suppression would be a sound therapeutic strategy. However the Myocarditis Treatment Trial, wherein patients were treated with immunosuppressive agents (Mason et al., 1995), showed that such administration had no significant benefit for outcome of human myocarditis. As such, pan-immune suppression is not the way forward and better targeted methods of immune modulation are needed. Shi *et al.* demonstrated that TGF-β secreted by T-reg cells may have been responsible for the decreased CAR expression and enhanced Akt activation (Figure 1). Such suggests that we need not inhibit the immune response entirely, but rather target, modulate and encourage the arm of the immune system that promotes virus clearance. The way forward may not be adoptive transfer of T-regs, but administration of a drug that can promote T-reg differentiation and function.

3.5 The matrix metalloproteinases

The Matrix MetalloProteinases (MMPs) have been implicated in the immune response to CVB3 infection in addition to delaying matrix remodelling that takes place after acute infection.

The MMPs are collectively termed 'matrixins' and were first discovered for their ability to degrade the tails of tadpoles during frog morphogenesis (Visse and Nagase, 2003). These enzymes are zinc endoproteinases and there have since been 24 vertebrate MMP genes discovered that play a large number of roles during immune and developmental processes. There are several gene knock-out strains of MMPs that have been used to elucidate the roles of these enzymes during development and immunity. For example, MMP-8$^{-/-}$ mice are more prone to skin cancers due to delayed neutrophil infiltration and an aberrant immune response (Balbin et al., 2003). Matrix MetalloProteinase-12$^{-/-}$ mice are more susceptible to bacterial infection due to an innate antimicrobial property of MMP-12 in intracellular compartments (Houghton et al., 2009). This MMP was shown to bind to bacterial membranes within the endosomes of macrophages and destabilise bacteria, thus acting as an antimicrobial.

3.5.1 MMPs as modulators of the antiviral immune response

MMP-9 was one of the first MMPs to be implicated in the mechanism of myocarditis and cardiac dilatation. Heymans et al first showed that inhibition of MMP action through suppression of urokinase-type plasminogen activator, a potent activator of MMPs, and exogenous expression of tissue inhibitor of metalloproteinase-1 (TIMP-1) decreased cardiac inflammation and reduced myocardial necrosis at 7 days, decreasing cardiac fibrosis at 35 days after CVB3 infection (Heymans et al., 2006). When the activity of MMP-2 and -9 were decreased there was a concomitant recovery of cardiac function with decreased immune infiltration. However, shortly after the publication of this paper Cheung et al demonstrated that MMP-9 was in fact a necessary constituent of the antiviral immune response (Cheung et al., 2008). They demonstrated no difference in viral load between MMP-8$^{-/-}$ mice and their WT counterparts. However, MMP-9$^{-/-}$ mice had higher viral loads and virus mediated myocardial damage, during CVB3 infection. Though the antiviral mechanism of MMP-9 action was not explicitly reported, there were significantly elevated levels of interferon-β (IFN-β) in the MMP-9$^{-/-}$ mice. This MMP has been shown previously to cleave and inactivate IFN-β (Nelissen et al., 2003), and IFN-β is known to have a negative feedback effect upon IFN-γ expression (Hanada and Yoshimura, 2002; Yoshimura et al., 2003). The viral loads were similar at early time points (3 – 5 days) post-infection between the genetic MMP-9 knock-outs and WT mice, suggesting that the innate-early immune response was intact, but there were higher viral loads seen in the MMP-9$^{-/-}$ mice 9 days post-infection. These results suggest that there was a deficiency in adaptive immunity in the MMP-9$^{-/-}$ mice, consistent with IFN-β negative feedback inhibition on IFN-γ regulated adaptive immunity in the MMP-9$^{-/-}$ mice.

4. Virus induced cell signalling and global aspects of cellular signalling responses

Thus far we have discussed a large number of parallel signalling molecules and pathways that are simultaneously activated during CVB3 infection, from proteolytic death pathways to phospho-signalling kinase cascades that activate a myriad of functions. Systems biology approaches now exist whereby one may survey a large number of pathways and molecules at the same time, query these results using complex statistical methods and elucidate the pathways that are truly required for a particular pathogenic function, and determine which of those that are merely coincident to viral infection.

4.1 Defining cell signalling network models in virus-host interactions

Host cells have evolved complex systems to detect and eradicate viruses; on the other hand, viruses have evolved mechanisms to compromise essential cellular processes and suppress the host cell defence. In these complex systems, protein phosphorylation events control most aspects of cellular function and homeostasis, and the failure of control mechanisms causes disease (Cohen and Tcherpakov, 2010). Most notably, protein phosphorylation events mediated by kinases and phosphatases are used by viruses as they are crucial for pathogen replication, propagation, and evasion from host immune responses (Ribet and Cossart, 2010). Several studies have showed that multiple phosphorylated-proteins individually regulate the events that constitute virus replication [reviewed in (Esfandiarei and McManus, 2008)], yet the phospho-proteins are part of an intracellular signal-transduction network, composed of several pathways. Thus, systems perspective studies have enabled us to address network mechanisms active during host-virus interactions, with specific emphasis on elucidating key determinants of disease severity and the effective translation of these concepts into new systems-oriented therapeutic targets.

Virus infection is equivalent to a network perturbation, in that viruses have evolved effective strategies to manipulate multiple signalling pathways and induce crosstalk and feedback loops among pathways to form a network (Garmaroudi et al., 2010). In fact, viruses activate signal-transduction networks through multiple independent events, which include viral docking to receptors, viral protein synthesis, viral progeny release and virus-induced inflammatory responses (Tam, 2006). Thus, to properly understand how signal-transduction networks are disrupted by viruses, a global multivariate approach is required (Ideker et al., 2001; Kleppe et al., 2006).

One of the major challenges of defining a signal-transduction network model in the context of a disease is to study a holistic picture of molecular structures, coming together to make complex and dynamic networks. New tools are required to systematically perturb and monitor signalling processes and functions within cells. Indeed, the emergence of high-throughput, extremely parallel technologies enable biologists to monitor multiple cellular components all together (Albeck et al., 2008). These tools have provided researchers the opportunity to collect comprehensive and large datasets. Nowadays, in the era of "new biology" researchers are 'drowning' in data, in that one emerging challenge is how to organize, interpret and extract pertinent information. The complex web of death pathways discussed in section 2.3 or the complex nature of the immune response discussed in section 3.0, all argue a need for higher level analysis through machine learning. Though this analysis requires skilled computational biologists, using mathematical, statistical and computational techniques to put together the biological components into functional molecular and cellular network models in a systematic fashion (Janes and Yaffe, 2006).

One work that has emerged from recent studies of networked systems in the virus-infected host cell revealed ~260 host cellular factors, affecting virus infection (Brass et al., 2008), however only a small subset of these proteins played a role in the early stage of virus infection. Interestingly, a complementary study showed how a multi-parameter approach could unravel host-virus protein interactions that likely act as a network to facilitate the early steps of HIV-1 infection (König et al., 2008). Recently, small-molecule inhibitor pairs were used to perturb pairs of phospho-proteins to reveal causal mechanisms within the signal-transduction network response of cardiomyocytes to coxsackievirus B3 (CVB3) infection. Hierarchical cluster analysis of the resulting dataset showed that paired-inhibitor data was required for accurate predictions of the network. In this study we also depicted a high-confidence network based on partial correlations, which identified phospho-IκBα as a central "hub" in a measured phosphorylation signature (Garmaroudi et al., 2010). Now, biologists are poised to understand the network mechanisms in virus infection, in that these networks might be used to improve patient diagnosis, monitoring, and treatment.

4.2 Proposing novel therapeutic targets for viral myocarditis through systems biology analysis of host cell signal-transduction networks

As we have already discussed, cardio-tropic viruses like CVB3 can directly and indirectly further the progression of viral myocarditis to heart failure [(McManus et al., 1993) reviewed in (Marchant et al., 2008)]. To date, there is no curative treatment beyond heart transplantation for viral myocarditis-associated heart failure. Therapies that have been used in patients with myocarditis are immune serum globulin and pleconaril (Pevear et al., 1986; Rotbart, 1999). The anti-picornaviral agent, pleconaril perturbs viral uncoating and in turn blocks viral attachment to host cell receptors. Although, directly targeting viruses has been successful in controlling viral diseases, it suffers from some serious weaknesses, including failure to eliminate chronic viral myocarditis, narrow spectrum of action, and the inherent capacity to force outgrowth of drug resistance mutations (Tan et al., 2007). Thus, the discovery of novel antiviral targets, host cell-based antiviral agents is a more promising approach and deserves more attention (Saladino et al., 2010).

At the cellular level, studies have shown that host cell phospho-proteins essential for viral replication, are potentially targetable [(Marchant 2009) reviewed in (Marchant et al., 2008)]. It is known, however, that phospho-protein networks embrace a system that contains redundant, convergent and even distinct signaling pathways (Borisy et al., 2003). Such combinative properties of signaling networks may counteract the therapeutic efficacy of highly selective drugs due to signalling pathway redundancy. Thus, combination therapy may be necessary to achieve efficacy due to less treatment resistance (Fitzgerald et al., 2006). However, motivation for this initiative, therapeutic synergy of a combination is tempered by concerns about introducing synergistic side effects. Nevertheless, an *in vivo* study that has emerged from recent studies of the healing process in a rat asthma model showed that combining drugs performed better than single ones (Lehar et al., 2009).

Together, to propose novel and promising drugs and therapies requires us to understand network mechanisms at the cellular, tissue and organism level. Using high-throughput technologies in genomics, proteomics, phosphoproteomics, metabolomics and lipidomics, we can develop interactome network models, in that these models ultimately translate to network analysis and data-driven questions in a specific disease context, that can be used to analyse a broad range of different states and disease contexts. There have been recent reports that used systems biology analysis tools in an attempt to untangle the web of kinase signalling pathways that are activated during CVB3 infection of cardiomyocytes (Garmaroudi et al., 2010). There is a current unclaimed niche of research that exists to use similar systems biology tools to analyse the pathways of cell death in order to better understand not only the dominant pathways of virus induced cell death but to also characterise the type of cell death that causes necrotic rupture of infected cells. To perturb specific molecules or biological processes in a combination as directed by network models can be a capable strategy to treat complex diseases.

5. Conclusion

In every facet of CVB3 replication there are a large number of pathways and proteins involved, forming a large network of pathways and complexity too large to analyse by conventional means. The large number of death pathways activated by CVB3 may not all be required to mediate lysis of the infected host cell. The question still remains as to whether there are pathways activated as a matter of coincidence or whether death pathways are all consequential. There are also a large number of immune constituents involved in the clearance but also the pathogenesis of myocarditis, from naive T cells to regulatory T cell subsets and a large number of MMPs. Systems biology should prove useful in the near future to elucidate the interactions of proteins and pathways and show the truly pertinent proteins and pathways responsible for cell death, virus replication or MMP mediated tissue remodelling. New questions regarding pathway coincidence and consequence can be investigated. New methods of analysis should assist in the understanding of beneficial vs pathological arms of the immune system. With this knowledge we should be able to design highly useful and robust biomarkers, antivirals and drugs to help direct appropriate repair and remodelling.

6. References

Adler, H.S., Kubsch, S., Graulich, E., Ludwig, S., Knop, J., and Steinbrink, K. (2007). Activation of MAP kinase p38 is critical for the cell-cycle-controlled suppressor function of regulatory T cells. Blood *109*, 4351-4359.

Albeck, J.G., Burke, J.M., Aldridge, B.B., Zhang, M., Lauffenburger, D.A., and Sorger, P.K. (2008). Quantitative analysis of pathways controlling extrinsic apoptosis in single cells. Mol Cell *30*, 11-25.

Andrade, F., Roy, S., Nicholson, D., Thornberry, N., Rosen, A., and Casciola-Rosen, L. (1998). Granzyme B directly and efficiently cleaves several downstream caspase substrates: implications for CTL-induced apoptosis. Immunity *8*, 451-460.

Aretz, H.T., Billingham, M.E., Edwards, W.D., Factor, S.M., Fallon, J.T., Fenoglio, J.J., Jr., Olsen, E.G., and Schoen, F.J. (1987). Myocarditis. A histopathologic definition and classification. Am J Cardiovasc Pathol *1*, 3-14.

Atkinson, E.A., Barry, M., Darmon, A.J., Shostak, I., Turner, P.C., Moyer, R.W., and Bleackley, R.C. (1998). Cytotoxic T lymphocyte-assisted suicide. Caspase 3 activation is primarily the result of the direct action of granzyme B. J Biol Chem *273*, 21261-21266.

Balbin, M., Fueyo, A., Tester, A.M., Pendas, A.M., Pitiot, A.S., Astudillo, A., Overall, C.M., Shapiro, S.D., and Lopez-Otin, C. (2003). Loss of collagenase-2 confers increased skin tumor susceptibility to male mice. Nat Genet *35*, 252-257.

Barry, M., Heibein, J.A., Pinkoski, M.J., Lee, S.F., Moyer, R.W., Green, D.R., and Bleackley, R.C. (2000). Granzyme B short-circuits the need for caspase 8 activity during granule-mediated cytotoxic T-lymphocyte killing by directly cleaving Bid. Mol Cell Biol *20*, 3781-3794.

Baughman, K.L. (2006). Diagnosis of myocarditis: death of Dallas criteria. Circulation *113*, 593-595.

Borisy, A.A., Elliott, P.J., Hurst, N.W., Lee, M.S., Lehar, J., Price, E.R., Serbedzija, G., Zimmermann, G.R., Foley, M.A., Stockwell, B.R., *et al.* (2003). Systematic discovery of multicomponent therapeutics. Proc Natl Acad Sci U S A *100*, 7977-7982.

Brady, W.J., Ferguson, J.D., Ullman, E.A., and Perron, A.D. (2004). Myocarditis: emergency department recognition and management. Emerg Med Clin North Am *22*, 865-885.

Brass, A.L., Dykxhoorn, D.M., Benita, Y., Yan, N., Engelman, A., Xavier, R.J., Lieberman, J., and Elledge, S.J. (2008). Identification of host proteins required for HIV infection through a functional genomic screen. Science *319*, 921-926.

Carthy, C.M., Granville, D.J., Watson, K.A., Anderson, D.R., Wilson, J.E., Yang, D., Hunt, D.W., and McManus, B.M. (1998). Caspase activation and specific cleavage of substrates after coxsackievirus B3-induced cytopathic effect in HeLa cells. J Virol *72*, 7669-7675.

Carthy, C.M., Yanagawa, B., Luo, H., Granville, D.J., Yang, D., Cheung, P., Cheung, C., Esfandiarei, M., Rudin, C.M., Thompson, C.B., *et al.* (2003). Bcl-2 and Bcl-xL overexpression inhibits cytochrome c release, activation of multiple caspases, and virus release following coxsackievirus B3 infection. Virology *313*, 147-157.

Carthy, C.M., Yang, D., Anderson, D.R., Wilson, J.E., and McManus, B.M. (1997). Myocarditis as systemic disease: new perspectives on pathogenesis. Clin Exp Pharmacol Physiol *24*, 997-1003.

Cassimatis, D.C., Atwood, J.E., Engler, R.M., Linz, P.E., Grabenstein, J.D., and Vernalis, M.N. (2004). Smallpox vaccination and myopericarditis: a clinical review. J Am Coll Cardiol *43*, 1503-1510.

Cheung, C., Marchant, D., Walker, E.K., Luo, Z., Zhang, J., Yanagawa, B., Rahmani, M., Cox, J., Overall, C., Senior, R.M., *et al.* (2008). Ablation of matrix metalloproteinase-9 increases severity of viral myocarditis in mice. Circulation *117*, 1574-1582.

Chow, L.H., Beisel, K.W., and McManus, B.M. (1992). Enteroviral infection of mice with severe combined immunodeficiency. Evidence for direct viral pathogenesis of myocardial injury. Lab Invest *66*, 24-31.

Chow, L.H., Radio, S.J., Sears, T.D., and McManus, B.M. (1989). Insensitivity of right ventricular endomyocardial biopsy in the diagnosis of myocarditis. J Am Coll Cardiol *14*, 915-920.

Cohen, P., and Tcherpakov, M. (2010). Will the ubiquitin system furnish as many drug targets as protein kinases? Cell *143*, 686-693.

Colston, J.T., Chandrasekar, B., and Freeman, G.L. (1998). Expression of apoptosis-related proteins in experimental coxsackievirus myocarditis. Cardiovasc Res *38*, 158-168.

Dalldorf, G., and Sickles, G.M. (1948). An Unidentified, Filtrable Agent Isolated From the Feces of Children With Paralysis. Science *108*, 61-62.

Declercq, W., Vanden Berghe, T., and Vandenabeele, P. (2009). RIP kinases at the crossroads of cell death and survival. Cell *138*, 229-232.

Desaintes, C., Goyat, S., Garbay, S., Yaniv, M., and Thierry, F. (1999). Papillomavirus E2 induces p53-independent apoptosis in HeLa cells. Oncogene *18*, 4538-4545.

Doble, B.W., and Woodgett, J.R. (2003). GSK-3: tricks of the trade for a multi-tasking kinase. J Cell Sci *116*, 1175-1186.

Esfandiarei, M., Boroomand, S., Suarez, A., Si, X., Rahmani, M., and McManus, B. (2007). Coxsackievirus B3 activates nuclear factor kappa B transcription factor via a phosphatidylinositol-3 kinase/protein kinase B-dependent pathway to improve host cell viability. Cell Microbiol *9*, 2358-2371.

Esfandiarei, M., Luo, H., Yanagawa, B., Suarez, A., Dabiri, D., Zhang, J., and McManus, B.M. (2004). Protein kinase B/Akt regulates coxsackievirus B3 replication through a mechanism which is not caspase dependent. J Virol *78*, 4289-4298.

Esfandiarei, M., and McManus, B.M. (2008). Molecular biology and pathogenesis of viral myocarditis. Annu Rev Pathol *3*, 127-155.

Esfandiarei, M., Suarez, A., Amaral, A., Si, X., Rahmani, M., Dedhar, S., and McManus, B.M. (2006). Novel role for integrin-linked kinase in modulation of coxsackievirus B3 replication and virus-induced cardiomyocyte injury. Circ Res *99*, 354-361.

Feldman, A.M., and McNamara, D. (2000). Myocarditis. N Engl J Med *343*, 1388-1398.

Felker, G.M., Thompson, R.E., Hare, J.M., Hruban, R.H., Clemetson, D.E., Howard, D.L., Baughman, K.L., and Kasper, E.K. (2000). Underlying causes and long-term survival in patients with initially unexplained cardiomyopathy. N Engl J Med *342*, 1077-1084.

Fitzgerald, J.B., Schoeberl, B., Nielsen, U.B., and Sorger, P.K. (2006). Systems biology and combination therapy in the quest for clinical efficacy. Nat Chem Biol *2*, 458-466.

Garcia-Mata, R., Bebok, Z., Sorscher, E.J., and Sztul, E.S. (1999). Characterization and dynamics of aggresome formation by a cytosolic GFP-chimera. J Cell Biol *146*, 1239-1254.

Garmaroudi, F.S., Marchant, D., Si, X., Khalili, A., Bashashati, A., Wong, B.W., Tabet, A., Ng, R.T., Murphy, K., Luo, H., *et al.* (2010). Pairwise network mechanisms in the host signaling response to coxsackievirus B3 infection. Proc Natl Acad Sci U S A *107*, 17053-17058.

Hanada, T., and Yoshimura, A. (2002). Regulation of cytokine signaling and inflammation. Cytokine Growth Factor Rev *13*, 413-421.

Hardt, S.E., and Sadoshima, J. (2002). Glycogen synthase kinase-3beta: a novel regulator of cardiac hypertrophy and development. Circ Res *90*, 1055-1063.

Harwood, A.J. (2001). Regulation of GSK-3: a cellular multiprocessor. Cell *105*, 821-824.

Hauck, A.J., Kearney, D.L., and Edwards, W.D. (1989). Evaluation of postmortem endomyocardial biopsy specimens from 38 patients with lymphocytic myocarditis: implications for role of sampling error. Mayo Clin Proc *64*, 1235-1245.

Heymans, S., Pauschinger, M., De Palma, A., Kallwellis-Opara, A., Rutschow, S., Swinnen, M., Vanhoutte, D., Gao, F., Torpai, R., Baker, A.H., *et al.* (2006). Inhibition of urokinase-type plasminogen activator or matrix metalloproteinases prevents cardiac injury and dysfunction during viral myocarditis. Circulation *114*, 565-573.

Hitomi, J., Christofferson, D.E., Ng, A., Yao, J., Degterev, A., Xavier, R.J., and Yuan, J. (2008). Identification of a molecular signaling network that regulates a cellular necrotic cell death pathway. Cell *135*, 1311-1323.

Hosenpud, J.D., Bennett, L.E., Keck, B.M., Boucek, M.M., and Novick, R.J. (2001). The Registry of the International Society for Heart and Lung Transplantation: eighteenth Official Report-2001. J Heart Lung Transplant *20*, 805-815.

Houghton, A.M., Hartzell, W.O., Robbins, C.S., Gomis-Ruth, F.X., and Shapiro, S.D. (2009). Macrophage elastase kills bacteria within murine macrophages. Nature *460*, 637-641.

Huber, S.A., Feldman, A.M., and Sartini, D. (2006). Coxsackievirus B3 induces T regulatory cells, which inhibit cardiomyopathy in tumor necrosis factor-alpha transgenic mice. Circ Res *99*, 1109-1116.

Ideker, T., Galitski, T., and Hood, L. (2001). A new approach to decoding life: systems biology. Annu Rev Genomics Hum Genet *2*, 343-372.

Iwasaki, T., Monma, N., Satodate, R., Kawana, R., and Kurata, T. (1985a). An immunofluorescent study of generalized Coxsackie virus B3 infection in a newborn infant. Acta Pathol Jpn *35*, 741-748.

Iwasaki, T., Monma, N., Satodate, R., Segawa, I., Oyama, K., Kawana, R., and Kurata, T. (1985b). Myocardial lesions by Coxsackie virus B3 and cytomegalovirus infection in infants. Heart Vessels Suppl *1*, 167-172.

Janes, K.A. (2010). Paring down signaling complexity. Nat Biotechnol *28*, 681-682.

Janes, K.A., and Yaffe, M.B. (2006). Data-driven modelling of signal-transduction networks. Nat Rev Mol Cell Biol *7*, 820-828.

Jentzen, J.M. (1989). Cocaine-induced myocarditis. Am Heart J *117*, 1398-1399.

Johnston, J.A., Ward, C.L., and Kopito, R.R. (1998). Aggresomes: a cellular response to misfolded proteins. J Cell Biol *143*, 1883-1898.

Kaiser, W.J., Upton, J.W., Long, A.B., Livingston-Rosanoff, D., Daley-Bauer, L.P., Hakem, R., Caspary, T., and Mocarski, E.S. (2011). RIP3 mediates the embryonic lethality of caspase-8-deficient mice. Nature *471*, 368-372.

Kleppe, R., Kjarland, E., and Selheim, F. (2006). Proteomic and computational methods in systems modeling of cellular signaling. Curr Pharm Biotechnol *7*, 135-145.

Konig, R., Zhou, Y., Elleder, D., Diamond, T.L., Bonamy, G.M., Irelan, J.T., Chiang, C.Y., Tu, B.P., De Jesus, P.D., Lilley, C.E., *et al.* (2008). Global analysis of host-pathogen interactions that regulate early-stage HIV-1 replication. Cell *135*, 49-60.

Lazebnik, Y.A., Kaufmann, S.H., Desnoyers, S., Poirier, G.G., and Earnshaw, W.C. (1994). Cleavage of poly(ADP-ribose) polymerase by a proteinase with properties like ICE. Nature *371*, 346-347.

Lehar, J., Krueger, A.S., Avery, W., Heilbut, A.M., Johansen, L.M., Price, E.R., Rickles, R.J., Short, G.F., 3rd, Staunton, J.E., Jin, X., *et al.* (2009). Synergistic drug combinations tend to improve therapeutically relevant selectivity. Nat Biotechnol *27*, 659-666.

Li, K., Xu, W., Guo, Q., Jiang, Z., Wang, P., Yue, Y., and Xiong, S. (2009). Differential macrophage polarization in male and female BALB/c mice infected with coxsackievirus B3 defines susceptibility to viral myocarditis. Circ Res *105*, 353-364.

Lim, B.K., Shin, J.O., Choe, S.C., Choi, S.W., Jeong, J.O., Seong, I.W., Kim, D.K., and Jeon, E.S. (2005). Myocardial injury occurs earlier than myocardial inflammation in acute experimental viral myocarditis. Exp Mol Med *37*, 51-57.

Liu, Z., Zhang, H.M., Yuan, J., Lim, T., Sall, A., Taylor, G.A., and Yang, D. (2008). Focal adhesion kinase mediates the interferon-gamma-inducible GTPase-induced phosphatidylinositol 3-kinase/Akt survival pathway and further initiates a positive feedback loop of NF-kappaB activation. Cell Microbiol *10*, 1787-1800.

Luo, H., Yanagawa, B., Zhang, J., Luo, Z., Zhang, M., Esfandiarei, M., Carthy, C., Wilson, J.E., Yang, D., and McManus, B.M. (2002). Coxsackievirus B3 replication is reduced by inhibition of the extracellular signal-regulated kinase (ERK) signaling pathway. J Virol *76*, 3365-3373.

Lv, H., Havari, E., Pinto, S., Gottumukkala, R.V., Cornivelli, L., Raddassi, K., Matsui, T., Rosenzweig, A., Bronson, R.T., Smith, R., *et al.* (2011). Impaired thymic tolerance to alpha-myosin directs autoimmunity to the heart in mice and humans. J Clin Invest.

MacLennan, C., Dunn, G., Huissoon, A.P., Kumararatne, D.S., Martin, J., O'Leary, P., Thompson, R.A., Osman, H., Wood, P., Minor, P., *et al.* (2004). Failure to clear persistent vaccine-derived neurovirulent poliovirus infection in an immunodeficient man. Lancet *363*, 1509-1513.

Maraj, S., Figueredo, V.M., and Lynn Morris, D. (2010). Cocaine and the heart. Clin Cardiol *33*, 264-269.

Marchant, D., Dou, Y., Luo, H., Garmaroudi, F.S., McDonough, J.E., Si, X., Walker, E., Luo, Z., Arner, A., Hegele, R.G., *et al.* (2009a). Bosentan enhances viral load via endothelin-1 receptor type-A-mediated p38 mitogen-activated protein kinase activation while improving cardiac function during coxsackievirus-induced myocarditis. Circ Res *104*, 813-821.

Marchant, D., Sall, A., Si, X., Abraham, T., Wu, W., Luo, Z., Petersen, T., Hegele, R.G., and McManus, B.M. (2009b). ERK MAP kinase-activated Arf6 trafficking directs coxsackievirus type B3 into an unproductive compartment during virus host-cell entry. J Gen Virol *90*, 854-862.

Marchant, D., Si, X., Luo, H., McManus, B., and Yang, D. (2008). The impact of CVB3 infection on host cell biology. Curr Top Microbiol Immunol *323*, 177-198.

Mason, J.W., O'Connell, J.B., Herskowitz, A., Rose, N.R., McManus, B.M., Billingham, M.E., and Moon, T.E. (1995). A clinical trial of immunosuppressive therapy for myocarditis. The Myocarditis Treatment Trial Investigators. N Engl J Med *333*, 269-275.

McKinney, R.E., Jr., Katz, S.L., and Wilfert, C.M. (1987). Chronic enteroviral meningoencephalitis in agammaglobulinemic patients. Rev Infect Dis *9*, 334-356.

McManus, B.M., Chow, L.H., Wilson, J.E., Anderson, D.R., Gulizia, J.M., Gauntt, C.J., Klingel, K.E., Beisel, K.W., and Kandolf, R. (1993). Direct myocardial injury by enterovirus: a central role in the evolution of murine myocarditis. Clin Immunol Immunopathol *68*, 159-169.

Medigeshi, G.R., Lancaster, A.M., Hirsch, A.J., Briese, T., Lipkin, W.I., Defilippis, V., Fruh, K., Mason, P.W., Nikolich-Zugich, J., and Nelson, J.A. (2007). West Nile virus infection activates the unfolded protein response, leading to CHOP induction and apoptosis. J Virol *81*, 10849-10860.

Melnick, J.L., Shaw, E.W., and Curnen, E.C. (1949). A virus isolated from patients diagnosed as non-paralytic poliomyelitis or aseptic meningitis. Proc Soc Exp Biol Med *71*, 344-349.

Mena, I., Fischer, C., Gebhard, J.R., Perry, C.M., Harkins, S., and Whitton, J.L. (2000). Coxsackievirus infection of the pancreas: evaluation of receptor expression, pathogenesis, and immunopathology. Virology *271*, 276-288.

Misbah, S.A., Spickett, G.P., Ryba, P.C., Hockaday, J.M., Kroll, J.S., Sherwood, C., Kurtz, J.B., Moxon, E.R., and Chapel, H.M. (1992). Chronic enteroviral meningoencephalitis in agammaglobulinemia: case report and literature review. J Clin Immunol *12*, 266-270.

Miura, M., Zhu, H., Rotello, R., Hartwieg, E.A., and Yuan, J. (1993). Induction of apoptosis in fibroblasts by IL-1 beta-converting enzyme, a mammalian homolog of the C. elegans cell death gene ced-3. Cell *75*, 653-660.

Natarajan, M., Lin, K.M., Hsueh, R.C., Sternweis, P.C., and Ranganathan, R. (2006). A global analysis of cross-talk in a mammalian cellular signalling network. Nat Cell Biol *8*, 571-580.

Nelissen, I., Martens, E., Van den Steen, P.E., Proost, P., Ronsse, I., and Opdenakker, G. (2003). Gelatinase B/matrix metalloproteinase-9 cleaves interferon-beta and is a target for immunotherapy. Brain *126*, 1371-1381.

Opavsky, M.A., Martino, T., Rabinovitch, M., Penninger, J., Richardson, C., Petric, M., Trinidad, C., Butcher, L., Chan, J., and Liu, P.P. (2002). Enhanced ERK-1/2 activation in mice susceptible to coxsackievirus-induced myocarditis. J Clin Invest *109*, 1561-1569.

Pevear, D.C., Melio, F., and Pfau, C.J. (1986). Lymphocytic choriomeningitis virus-induced disease of the central nervous system and the "antigen-sink" hypothesis. Med Microbiol Immunol *175*, 205-208.

Qu, X., and Qing, L. (2004). Abrin induces HeLa cell apoptosis by cytochrome c release and caspase activation. J Biochem Mol Biol *37*, 445-453.

Ribet, D., and Cossart, P. (2010). Pathogen-mediated posttranslational modifications: A re-emerging field. Cell *143*, 694-702.

Rotbart, H.A. (1999). Antiviral therapy for enteroviral infections. Pediatr Infect Dis J *18*, 632-633.

Saladino, R., Barontini, M., Crucianelli, M., Nencioni, L., Sgarbanti, R., and Palamara, A.T. (2010). Current advances in anti-influenza therapy. Curr Med Chem *17*, 2101-2140.

Schultz, J.C., Hilliard, A.A., Cooper, L.T., Jr., and Rihal, C.S. (2009). Diagnosis and treatment of viral myocarditis. Mayo Clin Proc *84*, 1001-1009.

Shi, Y., Fukuoka, M., Li, G., Liu, Y., Chen, M., Konviser, M., Chen, X., Opavsky, A., and Liu, P.P. (2010). Regulatory T cells Protect against Coxsackievirus-Induced Myocarditis through the TGFbeta-CAR Pathway. Circulation.

Si, X., Luo, H., Morgan, A., Zhang, J., Wong, J., Yuan, J., Esfandiarei, M., Gao, G., Cheung, C., and McManus, B.M. (2005). Stress-activated protein kinases are involved in coxsackievirus B3 viral progeny release. J Virol *79*, 13875-13881.

Spiropoulou, C.F., Goldsmith, C.S., Shoemaker, T.R., Peters, C.J., and Compans, R.W. (2003). Sin Nombre virus glycoprotein trafficking. Virology *308*, 48-63.

Suhy, D.A., Giddings, T.H., Jr., and Kirkegaard, K. (2000). Remodeling the endoplasmic reticulum by poliovirus infection and by individual viral proteins: an autophagy-like origin for virus-induced vesicles. J Virol *74*, 8953-8965.

Szalay, G., Meiners, S., Voigt, A., Lauber, J., Spieth, C., Speer, N., Sauter, M., Kuckelkorn, U., Zell, A., Klingel, K., *et al.* (2006). Ongoing coxsackievirus myocarditis is associated with increased formation and activity of myocardial immunoproteasomes. Am J Pathol *168*, 1542-1552.

Tam, P.E. (2006). Coxsackievirus myocarditis: interplay between virus and host in the pathogenesis of heart disease. Viral Immunol *19*, 133-146.

Tan, S.L., Ganji, G., Paeper, B., Proll, S., and Katze, M.G. (2007). Systems biology and the host response to viral infection. Nat Biotechnol *25*, 1383-1389.

Traystman, M.D., Chow, L.H., McManus, B.M., Herskowitz, A., Nesbitt, M.N., and Beisel, K.W. (1991). Susceptibility to Coxsackievirus B3-induced chronic myocarditis maps near the murine Tcr alpha and Myhc alpha loci on chromosome 14. Am J Pathol *138*, 721-726.

Visse, R., and Nagase, H. (2003). Matrix metalloproteinases and tissue inhibitors of metalloproteinases: structure, function, and biochemistry. Circ Res *92*, 827-839.

Vuorinen, T., Vainionpaa, R., Kettinen, H., and Hyypia, T. (1994). Coxsackievirus B3 infection in human leukocytes and lymphoid cell lines. Blood *84*, 823-829.

Wing, K., and Sakaguchi, S. Regulatory T cells exert checks and balances on self tolerance and autoimmunity. Nat Immunol *11*, 7-13.

Wolfgram, L.J., Beisel, K.W., Herskowitz, A., and Rose, N.R. (1986). Variations in the susceptibility to Coxsackievirus B3-induced myocarditis among different strains of mice. J Immunol *136*, 1846-1852.

Wong, J., Zhang, J., Si, X., Gao, G., Mao, I., McManus, B.M., and Luo, H. (2008). Autophagosome supports coxsackievirus B3 replication in host cells. J Virol *82*, 9143-9153.

Yajima, T., and Knowlton, K.U. (2009). Viral myocarditis: from the perspective of the virus. Circulation *119*, 2615-2624.

Yoshimura, A., Mori, H., Ohishi, M., Aki, D., and Hanada, T. (2003). Negative regulation of cytokine signaling influences inflammation. Curr Opin Immunol *15*, 704-708.

Yuan, J., and Horvitz, H.R. (2004). A first insight into the molecular mechanisms of apoptosis. Cell *116*, S53-56, 51 p following S59.

Yuan, J., and Kroemer, G. (2010). Alternative cell death mechanisms in development and beyond. Genes Dev *24*, 2592-2602.

Yuan, J., Shaham, S., Ledoux, S., Ellis, H.M., and Horvitz, H.R. (1993). The C. elegans cell death gene ced-3 encodes a protein similar to mammalian interleukin-1 beta-converting enzyme. Cell *75*, 641-652.

Yuan, J., Zhang, J., Wong, B.W., Si, X., Wong, J., Yang, D., and Luo, H. (2005). Inhibition of glycogen synthase kinase 3beta suppresses coxsackievirus-induced cytopathic effect and apoptosis via stabilization of beta-catenin. Cell Death Differ *12*, 1097-1106.

Yuan, J.Y., and Horvitz, H.R. (1990). The Caenorhabditis elegans genes ced-3 and ced-4 act cell autonomously to cause programmed cell death. Dev Biol *138*, 33-41.

Zhang, H.M., Ye, X., Su, Y., Yuan, J., Liu, Z., Stein, D.A., and Yang, D. (2010). Coxsackievirus B3 infection activates the unfolded protein response and induces apoptosis through downregulation of p58IPK and activation of CHOP and SREBP1. J Virol *84*, 8446-8459.

Zhang, H.M., Yuan, J., Cheung, P., Luo, H., Yanagawa, B., Chau, D., Stephan-Tozy, N., Wong, B.W., Zhang, J., Wilson, J.E., *et al.* (2003). Overexpression of interferon-gamma-inducible GTPase inhibits coxsackievirus B3-induced apoptosis through the activation of the phosphatidylinositol 3-kinase/Akt pathway and inhibition of viral replication. J Biol Chem *278*, 33011-33019.

Zhang, Y., Li, Z., Xinna, G., Xin, G., and Yang, H. (2011). Autophagy promotes the replication of encephalomyocarditis virus in host cells. Autophagy *7*.

14

Experimental Autoimmune Myocarditis: Role of Renin Angiotensin System

Kenichi Watanabe[1], Somasundaram Arumugam[1], Rajarajan A. Thandavarayan[1,2] and Makoto Kodama[3]

[1]*Department of Clinical Pharmacology, Faculty of Pharmaceutical Sciences, Niigata University of Pharmacy and Applied Life Sciences, Niigata,*
[2]*Department of Functional and Analytical Food Sciences, Niigata University of Pharmacy and Applied Life Sciences, Niigata,*
[3]*First Department of Medicine, Niigata University Graduate School of Medical and Dental Sciences, Niigata,*
Japan

1. Introduction

Myocarditis is defined as myocardial inflammation allied with edema, cellular infiltration, apoptosis and necrosis of cardiomyocytes (Rosenstein et al., 2000). It is likely to be a complex disease and its etiology has been associated with various infections, systemic diseases, drugs, and toxins. Among them, a wide array of organisms, including viral, bacterial, rickettsial, fungal, and parasitic organisms have been implicated as causative agents (Feldman & McNamara, 2000). There are two types of myocarditis viz, lymphocytic and giant cell myocarditis.

Acute myocarditis must be considered in patients who present with recent onset of cardiac failure or arrhythmia, though the onset of clinical cardiac symptoms may be vague in many patients. Fulminant myocarditis is a distinct entity characterized by the sudden onset of severe congestive heart failure or cardiogenic shock, usually following a flu-like illness. Giant cell myocarditis is a rare, frequently fatal disorder of unknown origin characterized by the presence of giant cell inflammatory infiltrate in the myocardium with widespread necrosis and degeneration of myocardial fibers (Batra & Lewis, 2001). It may be associated with various systemic autoimmune diseases (Kuhl & Schultheiss, 2010).

Heart reactive autoantibodies are found in a high percentage of patients with myocarditis. Identified autoantigens include the β1 adrenoreceptor adenine dinucleotide translocator, branched-chain keto acid dehydrogenase, cardiac myosin, sarcolemmal and myolemmal proteins, connective tissue, and extracellular matrix proteins including laminin. Antigenic mimicry between the dominant self molecules and the infectious agents also contributes to the disease process (Caforio et al., 1997; Neumann et al., 1990; Maisch, 1989).

2. Experimental autoimmune myocarditis (EAM)

The EAM model has been extensively used as a disease model of human myocarditis (Kodama et al., 1990). Experimental data revealed several similarities between this model

and the original disease in human. The current EAM model will provide the opportunity for further fundamental research into myocarditis.
EAM is similar to the giant cell myocardits and is more likely to progress into dilated cardiomayopathy (DCM) (Kodama et al., 1990). EAM can be induced by injection of cardiac myosin with Freund's adjuvant in to the footpads of Lewis rats. The immunized rats become ill and immobile at day 14 and then their activity gradually recovers beginning in the fourth week. The diseased rats show severe myocardial damage with inflammatory cell infiltration. Rats with EAM that survive the acute phase develop postmyocarditis DCM after 4 months or more (Watanabe et al., 2001).
Rat EAM is characterized by its high morbidity and mortality (Kamal et al., 2010). Pericardial effusions, cardiac enlargement and discoloration of the cardiac surface are the macroscopic findings of EAM (Kodama et al., 1992). These findings are common in the autopsy of the patients with myocarditis and EAM Lewis rats but rarely reported in other experimental animal models of myocarditis.

2.1 Pathogenesis of EAM

In the rat model of EAM, cardiac myosin is one of the major inflammation inducing agents used commonly. It is composed of two heavy chains of about 2000 amino acids and four light chains. This protein acts as antigen and stimulates the inflammatory reactions in the rat especially targeting the myocardium. In the rat immune system, T cells recognize 10-20 amino acid residues, and B cells recognize 5-10 amino acid peptides as antigens. Amino acid residues 1539-1555 of the rat cardiac myosin α-chain would be the myocarditogenic epitope of EAM (Pummerer et al., 1996). Direct sub fragment analysis revealed that actually several myocarditogenic epitopes existed on cardiac myosin. The most effective epitope is present on the residues 1070-1165 of the porcine cardiac myosin β-chain (Inomata et al., 1995). Antigen-specific breakdown of self-tolerance due to the molecular mimicry of myocarditogenic epitopes initiates the autoimmune reaction (Jones et al., 1997). This is followed by the stimulation and proliferation of myocarditogenic T cells. Activated T cells secrete many cytokines, chemokines and other mediators, which recruit and activate other inflammatory cells. The inflammatory mediators damage the myocardium and interfere with the cardiac function (Smith & Allen, 1992; Goren et al., 1998; Ishiyama et al., 1998).
Administration of porcine cardiac myosin with complete Freund's adjuvant, which comprises of inactivated and dried *Mycobacterium tuberculosis* leads to antigen presentation of cardiac myosin-specific T cells in the peripheral lymphatic organs. Freund's adjuvant, an immunopotentiator, plays an important role in the cell-mediated immunity leads to the breakdown of self-tolerance by activation of antigen presenting cells, enhancement of the expression of major histocompatibility molecules as well as increases in vascular permeability. T cells produced de novo in the bone marrow play a major role in the pathogenesis of the autoimmune myocarditis (Bergelson et al., 1997). Release of cardiac myosin from the damaged heart leads to further activation of specific T cells. Autoantibodies developed against the myosin bind to the injured heart and destroy them (Fedoseyeva et al., 2002).

2.2 Role of inflammation in myocarditis

Cytokines play important roles in the pathogenesis of myocarditis (Ding et al., 2010; Yuan et al., 2010; Huang et al., 2009; Ingkanisorn et al., 2006). Interleukin (IL) -2 mRNA appears in the EAM hearts at the onset of the disease (Okura et al., 1998). Subsequently, mRNA of IL-1β, interferon γ, and tumor necrosis factor (TNF) α increases (Maeda et al., 2005). In the recovery phase IL-10 appears in the heart. IL1, IL2, IL6 and TNFα are involved in the impairment of cardiac contractility, IL1 and IL6 may induce hypertrophy of myocytes whereas IL1 and TNFα may play a role in the development of myocardial fibrosis. Th2 cytokine IL-10 plays a protective role in the development of EAM (Watanabe et al., 2001). IL10 possesses immunomodulatory properties involving the inhibition of macrophage function and the production of proinflammatory cytokines (Nishio et al., 1999).

In rat EAM, infiltration of the inflammatory cells into the myocardium may be mediated by monocyte chemoattractant protein-1 (MCP-1) or other chemokines as MCP-1 mRNA is strongly expressed in the heart coincident with the onset of the disease and persists until the recovery phase (Goser et al., 2005). Nitric oxide may also play a role in the development of autoimmune myocarditis, by exacerbating inflammatory responses to cardiac infections (Kittleson et al., 2005).

Angiotensin (Ang) II, the principal effector peptide of the renin–angiotensin system (RAS), has been reported to induce immune and inflammatory response in various cardiac disease conditions, including atherosclerosis, hypertension, left ventricular hypertrophy, myocardial infarction, heart failure and myocarditis (Ferrario & Strawn, 2006; Schmieder et al., 2007).

3. Renin angiotensin system (RAS)

The RAS is a central element of the physiological and pathological responses of the cardiovascular system. Its primary effector hormone, Ang II, not only intercedes immediate physiological effects of vasoconstriction and blood pressure regulation, but is also implicated in inflammation, endothelial dysfunction, hypertension and heart failure (Opie & Sack, 2001). Many of the cellular effects of Ang II appear to be mediated by ROS generated by NAD(P)H oxidase (Koumallos et al., 2011). Two subtypes of Ang II receptors have been defined on the basis of their differential pharmacological and biochemical properties: Ang II type 1 receptors (AT1), which are involved in most of the well-known physiological effects of Ang II, and Ang II type 2 receptors (AT2), which have a less well-defined role but appear capable of counterbalancing some of the effects of AT1 stimulation. AT1 transactivates growth pathways and mediates major Ang II effects such as vasoconstriction, increased cardiac contractility, renal tubular sodium reabsorption, cell proliferation, vascular and cardiac hypertrophy, inflammatory responses, and oxidative stress. AT2 is believed to induce essentially opposite effects, including vasodilation, antigrowth and antihypertrophic effects, and to play a significant role in blood pressure (BP) regulation (Oudit & Penninger, 2011; Horiuchi et al., 1999; Matsubara, 1998; Siragy, 2000; Carey et al., 2001).

The discovery of Ang (1-7), an endogenous peptide which opposes the pressor, proliferative, profibrotic, and prothrombotic actions mediated by Ang II has contributed to the realization that the RAS is composed of two opposing arms: the pressor arm constituted by the enzyme angiotensin-converting enzyme (ACE), Ang II as the product, and the AT1 receptor as the main protein mediating the biological actions of Ang II; the second arm is composed of the monocarboxypeptidase ACE2, Ang (1-7) produced through hydrolysis of Ang II, and the Mas receptor as the protein conveying the vasodilator, antiproliferative, antifibrotic, and antithrombotic effects of Ang (1-7) (Petty et al., 2009; Ferrario, 2011).

Hypertrophy of cardiac myocytes is an adaptive response in the damaged heart. Initially, hypertrophy acts as a compensatory mechanism to preserve cardiac function, but when sustained, it becomes a major risk factor for congestive heart failure and sudden cardiac death. Until recently, most in vitro and in vivo studies of the roles of AT1 and AT2 indicated that AT1 mediates the growth promoting, fibrotic, and hypertrophic effects of Ang II on cardiovascular tissues and that AT2 exerts counterbalancing suppressant effects (Gao & Zucker, 2011). Evidence has been provided that the circulating and local RAS promote the development of myocardial fibrosis in hypertensive heart disease and chronic heart failure where both Ang II and aldosterone stimulate collagen synthesis in a dose-dependent manner while Ang II additionally suppresses the activity of matrix metalloproteinase 1, the key enzyme of interstitial collagen degradation, that synergistically leads to progressive collagen accumulation within the myocardial interstitium (Lijnen & Petrov, 2003). Therefore, the physiological role of RAS on the development of myocardial fibrosis could be established.

In addition to its role in the regulation of arterial pressure, Ang II is known to mediate effects on cell growth and apoptosis and to have pro-oxidative and proinflammatory effects. Apoptosis can be induced in cardiomyocytes by a variety of factors and pathways, a number of findings suggest that the effectors of the RAS can be critically involved in cardiomyocyte apoptosis (Fabris et al., 2011; Guleria et al., 2011; Yamada et al., 1996).

Peroxisome proliferator activated receptors (PPARs), members of the superfamily of ligand regulated transcription factors, are expressed in the cardiovascular system and control diverse vascular functions by mediating appropriate changes to gene expression. PPARα and PPARγ modulate the RAS by transcriptional control of renin, angiotensinogen, ACE and AT1 (Takeyama et al., 2000; Lansang et al., 2006).

4. Angiotensin receptor blockers (ARBs)

ARBs preferentially block AT1 and leave AT2 unopposed. Long-term administration of ARBs results in a several-fold increase in plasma Ang and thus a possible overstimulation of AT2. It is generally accepted that the effects of stimulation of AT2 on the cardiovascular system are beneficial and that no harm would result from increased activation of these receptors; indeed, activation of AT2 is believed to contribute to the benefits of blocking AT1 (Levy, 2004).

Various ARBs were screened for their role in the treatment of acute myocarditis and are found to have significant activity against acute myocarditis. ARBs prevent progression of systolic heart failure, thereby reducing cardiac morbidity and mortality (Lindholm et al., 2002; Cohn & Tognoni, 2001). They also reduce myocardial damage during myocarditis. The major cardiovascular actions of Ang II have been reported to be mediated by the AT1, and AT1 antagonists are therapeutically effective for the treatment of patients with heart failure by reducing cytokines and oxidative stress through their anti-inflammatory effects. Thus, the blockade of AT1 is an important way to interrupt the RAS (Sukumaran et al., 2010). Recently, an AT1 antagonist has been shown to ameliorate EAM by the suppression of myocardial damage and inflammatory events in the myocardium in addition to hemodynamic modifications, and it has been reported to inhibit nitric oxide (NO) production in macrophages and IL 1β production. ARB treatment decreased myocardial fibrosis and its marker molecules (i.e. RNA expression of TGF-β1 and collagen-III), and improved the survival rate and cardiac function in rats with DCM after myocarditis in a dose dependent manner. Treatment with oral ARB improved both systolic and diastolic functions, increased neurohormonal parameter, such as plasma Ang II, and ameliorated myocardial remodeling and its marker molecules (Sukumaran et al., 2010, 2011a, 2011b; Shirai et al., 2005).

4.1 ARB and oxidative stress

EAM rats also suffer from various stresses including reactive oxygen species (ROS) mediated oxidative stress. There are several evidences for the adverse cardiac effects triggered by redox cycling of ROS, generated in part by an NADPH oxidase dependent pathway. Reports also add the role of Ang II in triggering the oxidative stress in which increase in the levels of NADPH oxidase subunits like gp91phox, NOX4, p22phox, p40phox, p47phox, p67phox, rac1 and 3-Nitrotyrosine in rat EAM. ARBs can block the myocardial oxidative stress in EAM evidenced by the decreased levels of these markers (Sukumaran et al., 2011b; Seko, 2006; Singh et al., 2008).

4.2 ARB and hemodynamics

Central venous pressure (CVP) and left ventricular end diastolic pressure (LVEDP) were significantly higher and mean blood pressure (MBP), LVP and +dP/dt were significantly lower in EAM rats indicating systolic and diastolic dysfunction. CVP and LVEDP were significantly decreased in the ARB treated EAM rats. Myocardial contractility parameters including intraventricular pressure change were improved in EAM rats treated with ARB. Echocardiographic analysis also showed the improvement of cardiac remodeling with ARB treatment evidenced by decreased LVDd and LVDs and increased fractional shortening and ejection fraction (Sukumaran et al., 2010; 2011a; 2011b; Shirai et al., 2005; Tsutsui et al., 2007).

4.3 ARB and cardiomyocyte apoptosis

Inappropriate apoptosis contributes to the pathogenesis of a number of cardiac diseases and is recognized as an important factor in cardiovascular remodeling. AT1 mediated cardiomyocyte apoptosis is due to the pathologic involvement of RAS where ARB can block the actions of Ang II on AT1 thereby preventing the cellular apoptosis in the myocardium. There were several reports indicating the myocardial apoptosis in the EAM rats and ARBs can effectively prevent it due to their action on RAS. For instance, ARB can block the endoplamic reticulum stress and caspase12 activation in the EAM rats thus prevents cardiomyocyte apoptosis (Singh et al., 2008; Tsutsui et al., 2007; Ye et al., 2010; Matsusaka et al., 2006) (Figure 1).

4.4 ARB and inflammation in EAM

AT1 antagonists are reported to suppress cytokine production and the transcription of cytokine genes in vitro and in vivo (Matsubara, 1998; Siragy, 2000; Carey et al., 2001). ARBs can decrease the expression of IFN-gamma (interferon-gamma), FasL (Fas ligand), iNOS (inducible nitric oxide synthase) and PFP (pore-forming protein) in myocardial tissue, indicating suppression of the activation of infiltrating killer lymphocytes (Seko, 2006). ARB administration downregulates Th1 cytokines (IFN-gamma and IL-2) while upregulating Th2 cytokines (IL-4 and IL-10). Thus, studies of RAS antagonists in inflammatory diseases suggested that Ang II was involved in immune and inflammatory responses and ARBs are useful candidates in preventing the inflammation associated with those disorders. In our lab we have studied the action of ARB against EAM in rats. Out of 10 EAM rats used for treatment with ARB only 20% mortality was observed whereas control group showed 60% mortality. The disease severity was also decreased in the ARB treated group as shown by the less number of apoptotic cells, lesser fibrotic tissue replacement and also low level of inflammatory cellular infiltration when compared with the control group rats (Fig. 1).

5. Conclusion

ARBs, when added to conventional treatment for patients with heart failure, are associated with a reduction in morbidity and mortality as well as an improvement in quality of life. Clinical trials of ARB therapy indicate that these agents are generally well tolerated, both alone and in combination with other neurohormonal inhibitors (Patterson, 2003). Studies with ARB against EAM in rats provided several evidences for their protective role against the pathological alterations induced by Ang II (Figure 2). The treatment option with ARB against the cardiac complications involving Ang II has widened the area of cardiovascular research which will benefit the number of suffering population.

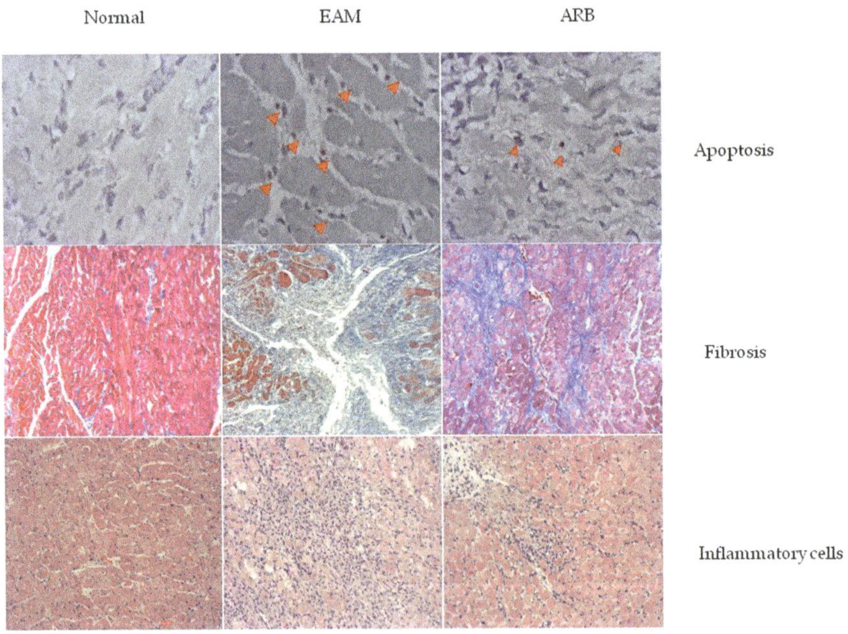

Fig. 1. Cross-sectional cardiac tissue slices with TUNEL staining depicting myocardial apoptosis, Azan-Mallory staining for fibrosis (blue area) and Hematoxylin and eosin staining depicting interstitial edema, vacuolization and degeneration of cardiac fibers respectively (X200). Normal, age-matched normal rats; EAM, Immunized rats without treatment; ARB, Immunized rats administered with ARB.

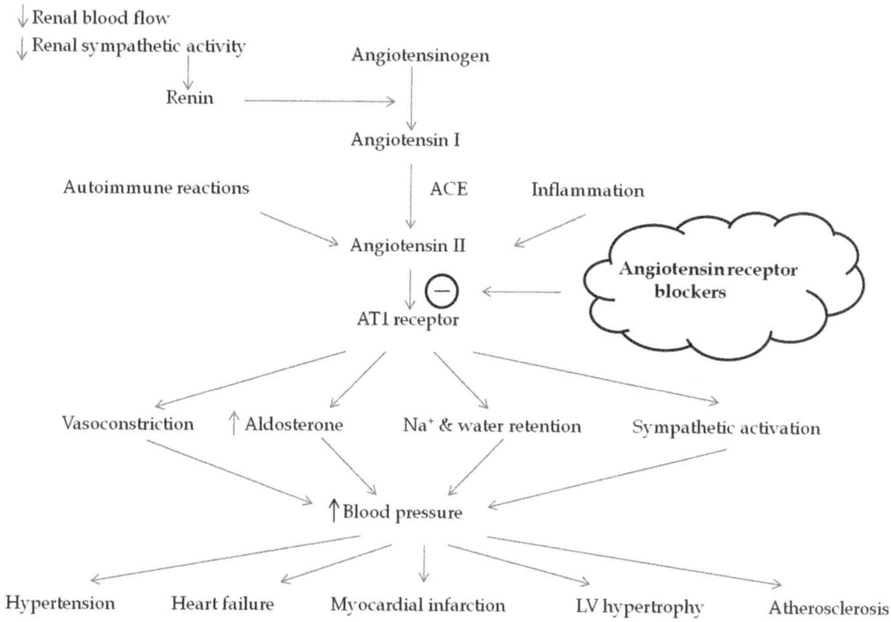

Fig. 2. Schematic representation of angiotensin pathway following angiotensin production. Angiotensin II binding to AT1 receptors leads to maintenance of homeostasis in normal physiology whereas pathological stimulation involves major cardiovascular complications. Treatment with ARB can potentially benefit the patients with these complications acting by blocking the actions of angiotensin II on AT1 receptors.

6. References

Batra, AS & Lewis, AB. (2001). Acute myocarditis. *Curr Opin Pediatr,* Vol. 13, No. 3, (June 2001), pp. 234-239.

Bergelson, JM, Cunningham, JA, Droguett, G, Kurt-Jones, EA, Krithivas, A, Hong, JS, Horwitz, MS, Crowell, RL & Finberg, RW. (1997). Isolation of common receptor for Coxsackie B viruses and adenoviruses 2 and 5. *Science,* Vol. 275, No. 5304, (Feb 1997), pp. 1320-1323.

Caforio, AL, Bauce, B, Boffa, GM, De Cian, F, Angelini, A, Melacini, P, Razzolini, R, Fasoli, G, Chioin, R, Schiaffino, S, Thiene, G, Dalla & Volta S. (1997). Autoimmunity in myocarditis and dilated cardiomyopathy: cardiac autoantibody frequency and clinical correlates in a patient series from Italy. *G Ital Cardiol,* Vol. 27, No. 2, (Feb 1997), pp. 106-112.

Carey, RM, Jin, XH & Siragy, HM. (2001). Role of the angiotensin AT2 in blood pressure regulation and therapeutic implications. *Am J Hypertens,* Vol. 14, No. 6, (June 2001), 98-102.

Cohn, JN & Tognoni, GA. (2001). A randomized trial of the angiotensin receptor blocker valsartan in chronic heart failure. *N Engl J Med,* Vol. 345, (Dec 2001), pp. 1667-1675.

Ding, L, Hanawa, H, Ota, Y, Hasegawa, G, Hao, K, Asami, F, Watanabe, R, Yoshida, T, Toba, K, Yoshida, K, Ogura, M, Kodama, M & Aizawa, Y. (2010). Lipocalin-2/neutrophil gelatinase-B associated lipocalin is strongly induced in hearts of rats with autoimmune myocarditis and in human myocarditis. *Circ J*, Vol 74, No. 3, (Mar 2010), pp. 523-530.

Ersoy, E, Kus, CN, Sener, U, Coker, I & Zorlu, Y. (2005). The effects of interferon-beta on interleukin-10 in multiple sclerosis patients. *Eur J Neurol*, Vol. 12, No. 3, (Mar 2005), pp. 208-211.

Fabris, B, Candido, R, Bortoletto, M, Toffoli, B, Bernardi, S, Stebel, M, Bardelli,M, Zentilin, L, Giacca, M & Carretta, R. (2011). Stimulation of cardiac apoptosis in ovariectomized hypertensive rats: potential role of the renin-angiotensin system. *J Hypertens*. Vol. 29, No. 2, (Feb 2011), pp. 273-281.

Fedoseyeva, EV, Kishimoto, K, Rolls, HK, Illigens, BM, Dong, VM, Valujskikh, A, Heeger, PS, Sayegh, MH & Benichou G. (2002). Modulation of tissue-specific immune response to cardiac myosin can prolong survival of allogeneic heart transplants. *J Immunol*, Vol. 169, No. 3, (Aug 2002), pp. 1168-1174.

Feldman, AM & McNamara, D. (2000). Myocarditis. *N Engl J Med*, Vol. 343, No. 19, (Nov 2000), pp. 1388–1398.

Ferrario, CM & Strawn, WB. (2006). Role of the renin-angiotensin-aldosterone system and proinflammatory mediators in cardiovascular disease. *Am J Cardiol*, Vol. 98, No. 1, (July 2006), pp. 121-128.

Ferrario, CM. (2011). ACE2: more of Ang-(1-7) or less Ang II? *Curr Opin Nephrol Hypertens*, Vol. 20, No. 1, (Jan 2011), pp. 1-6.

Gao, L & Zucker, IH. (2011). AT2 receptor signaling and sympathetic regulation. *Curr Opin Pharmacol*. Vol. 11, No. 2, (Apr 2011), pp. 124-130.

Goren, N, Leiros, CP, Sterin-Borda, L & Borda, E. (1998). Nitric oxide synthase in experimental autoimmune myocarditis dysfunction. *J Mol Cell Cardiol*, Vol. 30, No. 11, (Nov 1998), pp. 2467-2474.

Goser, S, Ottl, R, Brodner, A, Dengler, TJ, Torzewski, J, Egashira, K, Rose, NR, Katus, HA & Kaya, Z. (2005). Critical Role for Monocyte Chemoattractant Protein-1 and Macrophage Inflammatory Protein-1α in Induction of Experimental Autoimmune Myocarditis and Effective Anti–Monocyte Chemoattractant Protein-1 Gene Therapy. Circulation, Vol. 112, No. 22, (Nov 2005), pp. 3400-3407.

Guleria, RS, Choudhary, R, Tanaka, T, Baker, KM & Pan, J. (2011). Retinoic acid receptor-mediated signaling protects cardiomyocytes from hyperglycemia induced apoptosis: role of the renin-angiotensin system. *J Cell Physiol*. Vol. 226, No. 5, (May 2011), 1292-1307.

Horiuchi, M, Akishita, M & Dzau, VJ. (1999). Recent progress in angiotensin II type 2 receptor research in the cardiovascular system. *Hypertension,* Vol. 33, No. 2, (Feb 1999), pp. 613–621.

Huang, CH, Vallejo, JG, Kollias, G & Mann, DL. (2009). Role of the innate immune system in acute viral myocarditis. *Basic Res Cardiol*, Vol. 104, No. 3, (May 2009), pp. 228-237.

Ingkanisorn, WP, Paterson, DI, Calvo, KR, Rosing, DR, Schwartzentruber, DJ, Fuisz, AR & Arai AE. (2006). Cardiac magnetic resonance appearance of myocarditis caused by high dose IL-2: similarities to community-acquired myocarditis. *J Cardiovasc Magn Reson*, Vol. 8, No. 2, (2006), pp. 353-360.

Inomata, T, Hanawa, H, Miyanishi, T, Yajima, E, Nakayama, S, Maita, T, Kodama, M, Izumi, T, Shibata, A & Abo, T. (1995). Localization of porcine cardiac myosin epitopes that induce experimental autoimmune myocarditis. *Circ Res*, Vol. 76, No. 5, (May 1995), pp. 726-33.

Ishiyama, S, Hiroe, M, Nishikawa, T, Shimojo, T, Abe, S, Fujisaki, H, Ito, H, Yamakawa, K, Kobayashi, N, Kasajima, T & Marumo, F. (1998). The Fas/Fas ligand system is involved in the pathogenesis of autoimmune myocarditis in rats. *J. Immunol.*, Vol. 161, No. 9, (Nov 1998), pp. 4695-4701.

Jones, DE, Palmer, JM, Leon, MP, Yeaman, SJ, Bassendine, MF & Diamon, AG. (1997). T cell responses to tuberculin purified protein derivative in primary biliary cirrhosis: evidence for defective T cell function. Gut, Vol.40, No. 2, (Feb 1997), pp. 277-283.

Kamal, FA, Watanabe, K, Ma, M, Abe, Y, ElBarbary, R, Kodama, M & Aizawa, Y. (2010). A novel phenylpyridazinone, T-3999, reduces the progression of autoimmune myocarditis to dilated cardiomyopathy. *Heart and vessels*, Vol. 26, No. 1, (Jan 2010), pp. 81-90.

Kittleson, MM, Lowenstein, CJ, & Hare, JM. (2005). Novel Pathogenetic Mechanisms in Myocarditis: Nitric Oxide Signaling. Heart Failure Clinics, Vol. 1, No. 3, (Oct 2005), pp. 345-361.

Kodama, M, Matsumoto, Y & Fujiwara, M. (1992). In vivo lymphocyte-mediated myocardial injuries demonstrated by adoptive transfer of experimental autoimmune myocarditis. *Circulation*, Vol. 85, No. 5, (May 1992), pp. 1918-1926.

Kodama, M, Matsumoto, Y, Fujiwara, M, Masani, F, Izumi, T & Shibata, A. (1990). A novel experimental model of giant cell myocarditis induced in rats by immunization with cardiac myosin fraction. *Clin. Immunol. Immunopathol*, Vol. 57, No. 2, (Nov 1990), pp. 250–262.

Koumallos, N, Nteliopoulos, G, Paschalis, A, Dimarakis, I & Yonan, N. (2011). Therapeutic Interventions to Renin-Angiotensin-Aldosterone System, and Vascular Redox State. *Recent Pat Cardiovasc Drug Discov*. 2011 May 20.

Kuhl, U & Schultheiss, HP. (2010). Myocarditis in children. *Heart Fail Clin*, Vol. 6, No. 4, (Oct 2010) pp. 483-496.

Lansang, MC, Coletti, C, Ahmed, S, Gordon, MS & Hollenberg, NK. (2006). Effects of the PPAR-gamma agonist rosiglitazone on renal haemodynamics and the renin-angiotensin system in diabetes. *Journal of the Renin-Angiotensin-Aldosterone System*, Vol. 7, No. 3, (Sep 2006), pp. 175–180.

Levy, BI. (2004). Can Angiotensin II Type 2 Receptors Have Deleterious Effects in Cardiovascular Disease?: Implications for Therapeutic Blockade of the Renin-Angiotensin System. *Circulation*, Vol. 109, No. 1, (Jan 2004), pp. 8-13.

Lijnen, PJ & Petrov, VV. (2003). Role of intracardiac renin-angiotensin-aldosterone system in extracellular matrix remodeling. *Methods Find Exp Clin Pharmacol*. Vol. 25, No. 7, (Sep 2003), pp. 541-564.

Lindholm, LH, Ibsen, H, Dahlof, B, Devereux, RB, Beevers, G, de Faire, U, Fyhrquist, F, Julius, S, Kjeldsen, SE, Kristiansson, K, Lederballe-Pedersen, O, Nieminen, MS, Omvik, P, Oparil, S, Wedel, H, Aurup, P, Edelman, J & Snapinn, S. (2002). LIFE Study Group. Cardiovascular morbidity and mortality in patients with diabetes in the Losartan Intervention For Endpoint reduction in hypertension study (LIFE) a randomised trial against atenolol. *Lancet*, Vol. 359, No. 9311, (Mar 2002), pp. 1004–1010.

Maeda, K, Shioi, T, Kosugi, R, Yoshida, Y, Takahashi, K, Machida, Y & Izumi, T. (2005). Rapamycin ameliorates experimental autoimmune myocarditis. *Int Heart J*, Vol. 46, No. 3, (May 2005), pp. 513-530.

Maisch, B. (1989). Autoreactivity to the cardiac myocyte, connective tissue and the extracellular matrix in heart disease and postcardiac injury. *Springer seminars in Immunopathology*, Vol. 11, No. 4, (1989), pp. 369-395.

Matsubara, H. (1998). Pathophysiological role of angiotensin II type 2 receptor in cardiovascular and renal diseases. *Circ Res*, Vol. 83, No. 12, (Dec 1998), pp. 1182–1191.

Matsusaka, H, Kinugawa, S, Ide, T, Matsushima, S, Shiomi, T, Kubota, T, Sunagawa, K & Tsutsui, H. (2006). Angiotensin II type 1 receptor blocker attenuates exacerbated left ventricular remodeling and failure in diabetes-associated myocardial infarction. J *Cardiovasc Pharmacol*, Vol. 48, No. 3, (Sep 2006), pp. 95-102.

Neumann, DA, Burek, CL, Baughman, KL, Rose, NR & Herskowitz, A. (1990). Circulating heart-reactive antibodies in patients with myocarditis or cardiomyopathy. *J Am Coll Cardiol*, Vol. 16, No. 6, (Nov 1990), pp. 839-846.

Nishio, R, Matsumori, A, Shioi, T, Ishida, H & Sasayama, S. (1999). Treatment of Experimental Viral Myocarditis With Interleukin-10. Circulation, Vol. 100, No. 10, (Sep 1999), pp. 1102-1108.

Okura, Y, Yamamoto, T, Goto, S, Inomata, T, Hirono, S, Hanawa, H, Feng, L, Wilson, CB, Kihara, I, Izumi, T, Shibata, A, Aizawa, Y, Seki, S & Abo, T. (1997). Characterization of cytokine and iNOS mRNA expression in situ during the course of experimental autoimmune myocarditis in rats. *J Mol Cell Cardiol*, Vol. 29, No. 2, (Feb 1997), pp. 491-502.

Okura, Y, Takeda, Honda, S, Hanawa, H, Watanabe, H, Kodama, M, Izumi, T, Aizawa, Y, Seki & S, Abo, T. (1998). Recombinant Murine Interleukin-12 Facilitates Induction of Cardiac Myosin-Specific Type 1 Helper T Cells in Rats. *Circulation Research*, Vol. 82, No. 10, (Jun 1998), pp. 1035-1042.

Opie, LH & Sack, MN. (2001). Enhanced angiotensin II activity in heart failure: reevaluation of the counterregulatory hypothesis of receptor subtypes. *Circ Res*, Vol. 88, No. 7, (Apr 2001), pp. 654–658.

Oudit, GY & Penninger, JM. (2011). Recombinant Human Angiotensin-Converting Enzyme 2 as a New Renin-Angiotensin System Peptidase for Heart Failure Therapy. *Curr Heart Fail Rep*. 2011 May 26.

Patterson, JH. (2003). Angiotensin II receptor blockers in heart failure. *Pharmacotherapy*, Vol. 23, No. 2, (Feb 2003), pp. 173-182.

Petty, WJ, Miller, AA, McCoy, TP, Gallagher, PE, Tallant, EA & Torti, FM. (2009). Phase I and pharmacokinetic study of angiotensin-(1-7), an endogenous antiangiogenic hormone. *Clin Cancer Res*, Vol. 15, No. 23, (Dec 2009), pp. 7398-7404.

Pummerer, CL, Luze, K, Grässl, G, Bachmaier, K, Offner, F, Burrell, SK, Lenz, DM, Zamborelli, TJ, Penninger, JM & Neu, N. (1996). Identification of cardiac myosin peptides capable of inducing autoimmune myocarditis in BALB/c mice. *J Clin Invest*, Vol. 97, No. 9, (May 1996), pp. 2057–2062.

Rosenstein, ED, Zucker, MJ & Kramer, N. (2000). Giant cell myocarditis: most fatal of autoimmune diseases. *Semin Arthritis Rheum*,Vol. 30, No. 1, (Aug 2000), pp. 1–16.

Schmieder, RE, Hilgers, KF, Schlaich, MP & Schmidt, BM. (2007). Renin-angiotensin system and cardiovascular risk. *Lancet*, Vol. 369, No. 9568, (Apr 2007), pp. 1208-1219.

Seko, Y. (2006). Effect of the angiotensin II receptor blocker olmesartan on the development of murine acute myocarditis caused by coxsackievirus B3. *Clin Sci (Lond)*, Vol. 110, No. 3, (Mar 2006), pp. 379-386.

Shirai, K, Watanabe, K, Ma, M, Wahed, MI, Inoue, M, Saito, Y, Suresh, PS, Kashimura, T, Tachikawa, H, Kodama, M & Aizawa, Y. (2005). Effects of angiotensin-II receptor blocker candesartan cilexetil in rats with dilated cardiomyopathy. *Mol Cell Biochem*, Vol. 269, No. 1-2, (Jan 2005), pp. 137-142.

Singh, VP, Le, B, Khode, R, Baker, KM & Kumar, R. (2008). Intracellular angiotensin II production in diabetic rats is correlated with cardiomyocyte apoptosis, oxidative stress, and cardiac fibrosis. *Diabetes*, Vol. 57, No. 12, (Dec 2008), pp. 3297-306.

Siragy, HM. (2000). The role of the AT2 in hypertension. *Am J Hypertens*, Vol. 13, No. 5, (May 2000), 62–67.

Smith, SC & Allen, PM. (1992). Expression of myosin-class II major histocompatibility complexes in the normal myocardium occurs before induction of autoimmune myocarditis. *Proc. Natl. Acad. Sci. U. S. A.*, Vol. 89, No. 19, (Oct 1992), pp. 9131-9135.

Sukumaran, V, Watanabe, K, Veeraveedu, PT, Gurusamy, N, Ma, M, Thandavarayan, RA, Lakshmanan, AP, Yamaguchi, K, Suzuki, K & Kodama, M. (2011). Olmesartan, an AT(1) Antagonist, Attenuates Oxidative Stress, Endoplasmic Reticulum Stress and Cardiac Inflammatory Mediators in Rats with Heart Failure Induced by Experimental Autoimmune Myocarditis. *Int J Biol Sci*, Vol. 7, No. 2, (Feb 2011), pp. 154-167.

Sukumaran, V, Watanabe, K, Veeraveedu, PT, Ma, M, Gurusamy, N, Rajavel, V, Suzuki, K, Yamaguchi, K, Kodama, M & Aizawa, Y. (2011). Telmisartan ameliorates experimental autoimmune myocarditis associated with inhibition of inflammation and oxidative stress. *Eur J Pharmacol*, Vol. 652, No. 1-3, (Feb 2011), pp. 126-135.

Sukumaran, V, Watanabe, K, Veeraveedu, PT, Thandavarayan, RA, Gurusamy, N, Ma, M, Yamaguchi, K, Suzuki, K, Kodama, M & Aizawa, Y. (2010). Beneficial effects of olmesartan, an angiotensin II receptor type 1 antagonist, in rats with dilated cardiomyopathy. *Exp Biol Med (Maywood)*, Vol. 235, No. 11, (Nov 2010), pp. 1338-1346.

Takeyama, K, Kodera, Y, Suzawa, M & Kato, S. Peroxisome proliferator-activated receptor(PPAR)--structure, function, tissue distribution, gene expression. *Nippon Rinsho*, Vol. 58, No. 2, (Feb 2000), pp. 357-363.

Tsutsui, H, Matsushima, S, Kinugawa, S, Ide, T, Inoue, N, Ohta, Y, Yokota, T, Hamaguchi, S & Sunagawa, K. (2007). Angiotensin II type 1 receptor blocker attenuates myocardial remodeling and preserves diastolic function in diabetic heart. *Hypertens Res*, Vol. 30, No. 5, (May 2007), pp. 439-449.

Watanabe, K, Nakazawa, M, Fuse, K, Hanawa, H, Kodama, M, Aizawa, Y, Ohnuki, T, Gejyo, F, Maruyama, H, Miyazaki, J. (2001). Protection against autoimmune myocarditis by gene transfer of interleukin-10 by electroporation. Circulation, Vol 104, No. 10, (Sep 2001), pp. 1098 -1100.

Yamada, T, Horiuchi, M, Dzau, VJ. (1996). Angiotensin II type 2 receptor mediates programmed cell death. *Proc Nat Acad Sci U S A*, Vol. 93, No. 1, (Jan 1996), pp. 156–160.

Ye, Y, Keyes, KT, Zhang, CF, Perez-Polo, JR, Lin, Y & Birnbaum, Y. (2010). Additive effect of TAK-491, a new angiotensin receptor blocker, and pioglitazone, in reducing myocardial infarct size. *Cardiovasc Drugs Ther*, Vol. 24, No. 2, (Apr 2010), pp. 107-120.

Yuan, J, Cao, AL, Yu, M, Lin, QW, Yu, X, Zhang, JH, Wang, M, Guo, HP & Liao, YH. (2010). Th17 cells facilitate the humoral immune response in patients with acute viral myocarditis. *J Clin Immunol*, Vol. 30, No. 2, (Mar 2010), pp. 226-234.

15

Impaired Cardiac Function in Viral Myocarditis

Jerry Wong and Honglin Luo
James Hogg Research Center, Providence Heart and Lung Institute, St. Paul's Hospital and Department of Pathology and Laboratory Medicine, University of British Columbia, Vancouver, BC, Canada

1. Introduction

Viral myocarditis, the inflammation of the myocardium caused by viral infection, is an important cause of dilated cardiomyopathy (DCM) - a major cause of morbidity and mortality worldwide (Mason, 2003; Esfandiarei & McManus, 2008; Cooper, 2009). In North America, viral myocarditis and DCM together account for 20% of the sudden deaths and heart failure in children and adolescents (Okuni *et al.*, 1975; Drory *et al.*, 1991). To date, there is no effective therapeutic against these diseases. Patients diagnosed with late stage DCM are limited to supportive treatments such as ventricular assist device implantation and heart transplantation.

The clinical presentation of viral myocarditis comes in various severities. Most people have contracted and subsequently recovered from multiple viral infections of the heart without overt symptoms. Yet, retrospective studies revealed that ~20% of subclinical cases later develop congestive heart failure. In addition, some may experience acute fulminant viral myocarditis or persistent chronic myocarditis symptoms. About one-third of these patients with viral myocarditis subsequently develop DCM (Esfandiarei & McManus, 2008). A combination of new diagnostic technologies for viral myocarditis such as cardiovascular magnetic resonance techniques with conventional diagnostics including clinical presentation, histopathological examination, cardiac antibody assessment, and viral polymerase chain reaction (PCR), now helps better define disease stage and its respective management protocol (Baughman, 2006).

The presence of viral genome in the myocardium is associated with significantly worse outcome over two years (Why *et al.*, 1994). Analysis of human failing hearts by PCR unveiled trails of previous viral infection. The identified viruses include enterovirus, adenovirus, parvovirus B19, herpes simplex virus 6, cytomegalovirus, hepatitis C virus, and human immunodeficiency virus, which are clinically associated with viral myocarditis (Grist & Reid, 1997; Calabrese *et al.*, 2010). Among them, coxsackievirus B3 (CVB3), an enterovirus in the picornavirus family, is highly implicated in clinical cases of viral myocarditis, particularly in neonates and young children, and is the most thoroughly studied causative agent in experimental viral myocarditis models (Froeschle *et al.*, 1966; Abelmann, 1971; Reyes & Lerner, 1985; McManus *et al.*, 1988). CVB3 replicates rapidly in short infection cycles that begin with viral receptor engagement and subsequent internalization, followed by translation of viral RNA, amplification of viral genome, viral assembly, and complete with viral progeny release.

CVB3 infection of myocarditis susceptible mice results in severe heart failure. The disease progression of viral myocarditis in the experimental infection model can be classified into three phases: acute (viremia), subacute (inflammatory), and chronic (remodeling) phases. The acute (viremia) phase is signified by active viral replication and direct virus-induced cardiomyocyte damage. The subacute (inflammatory) phase is characterized by the infiltration of immune cells that helps viral clearance but nonetheless adds to myocardial damage. The chronic (remodeling) phase is featured by the continual efforts of the impaired heart to meet the hemodynamic demand by remodeling the myocardium. Cardiac hypertrophy is triggered during remodeling to compensate for reduced contractile function due to myocyte loss and interstitial fibrosis in the earlier phases. However, such an adaption is unsustainable in the longer term in face of increasingly hostile environments, i.e. reduced blood supply and increased reactive oxidative stress, thus leading to cardiomyocyte death and triggering further inflammation and fibrosis. The pathological remodeling process eventually leads to DCM and heart failure.

This book chapter focuses on the virus-host protein interactions in cardiomyocytes during viral myocarditis. We discuss the role of virus-induced protein cleavage and dysregulation of the host protein degradation systems in the pathogenesis of viral myocarditis and its subsequent progression to DCM.

2. Host protein cleavages by coxsackieviral proteases contributing to cardiac dysfunction

2.1 Viral proteases and dilated cardiomyopathy

CVB3 encodes two viral proteases, 2A and 3C, both of which are cysteine proteases that have chymotrypsin-like activity and play critical roles in successful viral replication (Chau *et al.*, 2007). First, the viral proteases are required to process the large viral polyprotein, a product of mono-cistronic translation of RNA genome, into the individual functional, structural and non-structural proteins. Second, the viral proteases facilitate viral replication by cleaving a number of host proteins that are involved in various cell functions such as transcription, translation, cell signaling, and cellular structure.

Viral myocarditis is originally thought to be an immune response driven disorder. The initial observation that established the importance of direct virus-mediated myocardial damage in the pathogenesis of viral myocarditis was made in severe combined immunodeficient (SCID) mice, which lack functional T and B lymphocytes and yet developed early and severe myocyte damage upon enterovirus challenge (McManus *et al.*, 1993). The significance of viral proteins in the development of viral myocarditis and DCM was further explored by Dr. Knowlton's research group. First, they showed that the cardiac-specific expression of a replication-restricted CVB3 mutant genome in transgenic mice, which only allows the expression of viral proteins without generating viral progenies and subsequent immune response, results in DCM phenotype (Wessely *et al.*, 1998). Then, they demonstrated that mice with cardiac-restricted expression of viral protease 2A display a severe DCM phenotype (Xiong *et al.*, 2007). These findings suggest that viral proteases play an important role in the development of viral-induced dilated cardiomyopathy.

2.2 Cleavage of dystrophin during CVB3 infection may contribute to dilated cardiomyopathy

The observation that mouse cardiac expression of viral protease 2A induces DCM has been explained based on the landmark finding that dystrophin, which links the cytoskeleton to the extracellular matrix (ECM) by forming the dystrophin glycoprotein complex (DGC), is cleaved during CVB3 infection by protease 2A (Badorff *et al.*, 1999; Badorff & Knowlton, 2004) (Fig. 1A). Dystrophin has three domains that serve different purposes. Its N-terminal domain anchors to the actin cytoskeleton and its rod domain provides the linkage to the C-terminal domain, which binds to β-dystroglycan that in turn connects to the sarcolemma and the extracellular matrix (Fig. 1A). Furthermore, dystrophin-deficient mice have been shown to have an increased susceptibility to viral myocarditis and develop severe cardiomyopathy (Xiong *et al.*, 2002). Human genetic mutations of the dystrophin gene cause Duchenne Muscular Dystrophy (DMD) (Nigro *et al.*, 1990). Approximately 20% of DMD patients suffer and die from a resultant cardiomyopathy. Other mutations of the dystrophin gene also cause X-linked DCM (Ferlini *et al.*, 1999). CVB3-induced dystrophin cleavage occurs at its 3′ hinge and therefore breaks its connection to the ECM. As a result, the sarcolemmal integrity is compromised and force transmission is reduced. This can further lead to cardiomyocyte necrosis due to the increased sarcolemmal permeability (Fig. 1A). Thereafter, dystrophin cleavage has been viewed as a major mechanism in enteroviral cardiomyopathy. However, dystrophin knockout mice (Mdx) display only mild cardiomyopathy phenotype, due to the compensatory upregulation of utrophin, a dystrophin homologue (Deconinck *et al.*, 1997; Grady *et al.*, 1997). Thus, other mechanisms may also contribute to the severe cardiomyopathy phenotype in viral protease 2A expressing mice.

2.3 Cleavage of serum response factor by viral protease 2A is associated with impaired cardiac function

Recent efforts have demonstrated for the first time that serum response factor (SRF) is cleaved in CVB3-infected mouse hearts and cultured murine cardiomyocytes (unpublished). SRF, which belongs to the MADS-box (MCM1, Agamous, Deficiens, and SRF) protein superfamily, is a muscle-enriched transcription factor that regulates the expression of contractile and regulatory genes, as well as microRNAs (miRNAs) (Miano, 2003; Niu *et al.*, 2007; Oka *et al.*, 2007) (Fig. 1B). SRF interacts with tissue specific cofactors such as myocardin, Nkx2.5, c-Fos, and binds to the serum response element (SRE) of its target genes. It contains two major domains: the N-terminal DNA binding and dimerization domain and the C-terminal transactivation domain (Fig. 1B). Genomic studies have identified over 1200 SRE containing genes and more than 250 of these have been verified (Sun *et al.*, 2006). Cardiac contractile genes under SRF regulation include cardiac α-actin, β-myosin heavy chain, myosin light chain, cardiac troponin I, etc. SRF is indispensable for mesoderm formation and plays a central role in cardiac development and function (Niu *et al.*, 2007). Therefore, SRF knockout results in embryonic lethality (Parlakian *et al.*, 2004). The construction of cardiac-specific inducible SRF knockout transgenic mice overcomes this problem and helps illustrate the importance of SRF in cardiac function (Parlakian *et al.*, 2005). It was shown that SRF knockout in the adult mouse heart results in damaged cardiac function, and subsequent progression to DCM. Genetic mutations of SRF in humans have not been described likely due to the associated lethality. However, the expression of alternatively spliced SRF isoforms, which was shown to have inhibitory effects on wild-type SRF, is increased in failing human and animal hearts (Davis *et al.*, 2002). Furthermore, a cleaved form of SRF lacking the transactivation domain was also found in human failing hearts as a result of caspase-3 activation during cardiomyocyte apoptosis (Chang *et al.*,

2003). This caspase-cleaved SRF fragment functions as a dominant-negative mutant that inhibits SRF-dependent activation of cardiac genes. On the other hand, SRF overexpression in transgenic mouse hearts leads to the development of cardiac hypertrophy and subsequent cardiomyopathy (Zhang *et al.*, 2001).

During CVB3 infection, SRF is cleaved into a ~47kD N-terminal fragment (SRF-N) and a ~20kD C-terminal fragment (SRF-C) by viral protease 2A (unpublished). As a result, the DNA-binding domain is detached from the transactivation domain, thus abolishing SRF function. In addition, the SRF-N fragment generated from the cleavage can compete with wild-type SRF for target gene binding, and thereby exhibits dominant-negative suppression of SRF target gene expression (Fig. 1B). This study suggests another important mechanism by which CVB3 damages cardiac function and leads to subsequent DCM. Further research using knock-in transgenic mice expressing non-cleavable SRF will help clarify the relative contribution of SRF cleavage in the pathogenesis of viral myocarditis.

2.4 Caspase activation by viral proteases

Both viral proteases 2A and 3C lead to late onset of host cell apoptosis through the direct cleavage of caspase-8 and the activation of caspase-3, as well as the cleavage of anti-apoptotic protein Bid that leads to mitochondrial cytochrome c release and subsequent initiation of the caspase cascade (Chau *et al.*, 2007). Cardiomyocyte apoptosis is a common phenomenon in various cardiac diseases. Apoptosis, also known as programmed cell death, is the self-destruction pathway activated when host cells decide to commit suicide. Apoptosis during viral myocarditis caused by viral protease-induced caspase activation, however, is "switched on" intentionally by viral mechanisms for the release of mature viral progenies. In cell culture, caspase activation results in cytoplasmic proteolysis and DNA fragmentation. However, despite ultrastructural evidence of cytochrome c release detected in many cardiomyocytes of heart failure patients, intact nuclei are seen in all of these myocytes (Narula *et al.*, 1998). This suggests that the terminally differentiated cardiomyocytes have evolved strategies to resist nuclear fragmentation despite ongoing cytoplasmic apoptosis. In fact, the number of apoptotic myocytes in a cardiomyopathic heart ranges only from 0.07% to 0.7% as compared to 0.003% in the normal myocardium (Narula *et al.*, 1998). Nevertheless, cytoplasmic apoptosis initiated during viral myocarditis may compromise mitochondrial ATP generation, as well as cause destruction to contractile proteins which add to systolic dysfunction in the disease pathogenesis.

2.5 Other mechanisms

Other mechanisms that viral proteases use to impair cardiomyocyte function include the interference of host gene transcription by the cleavage of cyclic AMP response element binding protein (CREB) (Yalamanchili *et al.*, 1997), the disruption of host protein translation through the cleavage of eukaryotic translation initiation factor 4γ (eIF4γ) (Chau *et al.*, 2007) and eIF5B (de Breyne *et al.*, 2008), the interception of cell signaling pathways via the cleavage of RasGAP (Huber *et al.*, 1999), and the weakening of the cytoskeletal network by the cleavage of cytokeratin-8 (Seipelt *et al.*, 2000). Although there are no known cardiac diseases associated with the aforementioned proteins, their cleavages exert additive effects to the final detriment of the infected cardiomyocytes.

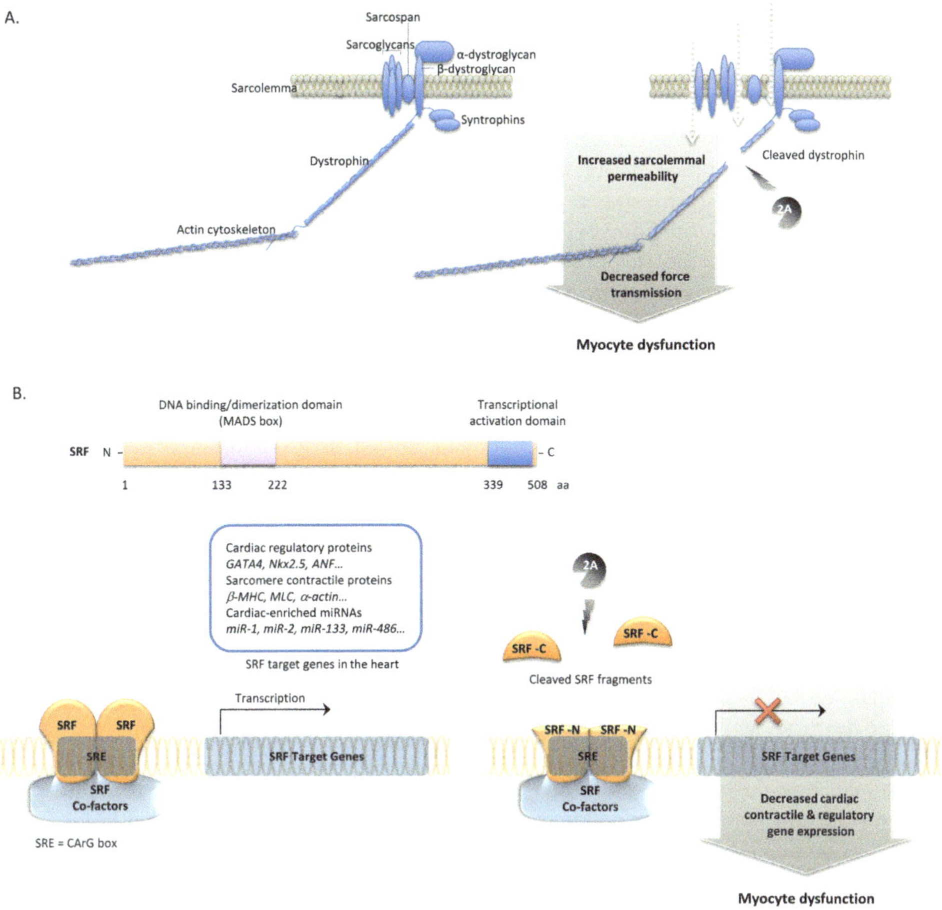

Fig. 1. Host protein cleavages by coxsackieviral proteases in viral myocarditis.
A. Coxsackieviral protease 2A cleaves dystrophin at its 3' hinge. Dystrophin is a component of the dystrophin-glycoprotein complex that links the cytoskeleton to the extracellular matrix. Dystrophin cleavage contributes to myocyte dysfunction by reducing contractile force transmission and increasing sarcolemmal permeability.
B. Viral protease 2A also cleaves serum response factor (SRF). SRF is a muscle-enriched transcription factor that regulates the expression of cardiac regulatory proteins, sarcomere contractile proteins, as well as cardiac-specific microRNAs (miRNAs). SRF associates with co-factors such as GATA4, Nkx2.5, MEF2, and myocardin and binds to serum response element (SRE) (also known as CArG box) to activate gene transcription. SRF cleavage results in myocyte dysfunction by the dissociation of the N-terminal DNA binding/dimerization domain from the C-terminal transcriptional activation domain, thus abolishing SRF-mediated gene expression. Furthermore, the N-terminal fragment (SRF-N) exhibits a dominant-negative effect on endogenous SRF function by competing for DNA binding.

3. Dysregulation of host protein degradation systems in viral cardiomyopathy

3.1 Protein degradation systems

Protein degradation is an integral part in the maintenance of cellular homeostasis. It allows for the selective removal of host proteins that are misfolded, damaged, and unnecessary, and balances the ongoing protein synthesis that is driven to provide the desirable cellular function in response to environmental changes. The dynamic interaction between protein synthesis and degradation is of particular importance to cardiomyocytes, the basic contractile units of the heart, due to the plasticity of the heart. It drives the hypertrophy or atrophy of individual cardiomyocytes, which contributes to sufficient contractile force generation that meets the hemodynamic demands. Consequently, the dysregulation of protein degradation jeopardizes cardiomyocyte vitality and function and plays an important role in the development of various cardiac diseases (Zheng & Wang, 2010).

Enteroviral infection leads to the dysregulation of host protein degradation pathways, which include the ubiquitin/proteasome system (UPS) and autophagy. Such viral-induced manipulation plays key roles not only in viral propagation, but also in the pathogenesis of viral myocarditis and the subsequent development of DCM. The following sections discuss the contributions of UPS and autophagy in viral propagation and the development of cardiomyopathy.

3.2 The ubiquitin/proteasome system

The ubiquitin/proteasome system is the major protein degradation pathway in eukaryotic cells that accounts for ~80% of host protein recycling (Zheng & Wang, 2010). By controlling the longevity/half-life of most proteins (predominantly short-lived but also some long-lived proteins), the UPS extends its role beyond protein recycling and regulates most aspects of cellular functions. UPS substrate selectivity is achieved by protein polyubiquitination, i.e. the attachment of ubiquitin (Ub) molecules onto the target protein. Ubiquitin is a small 76 amino acid protein modifier molecule that conjugates to target protein or to another Ub through one of its seven lysine residues. Ubiquitin linkage at different lysine residues serves different functions. For example, polyubiquitination via lysine 48 targets protein for UPS degradation, polyubiquitination via lysine 63 promotes signal transduction or targets degradation through the autophagy pathway, whereas monoubiquitination modulates protein intracellular localization and protein function.

Protein ubiquitination is regulated in a multi-step manner (Hershko & Ciechanover, 1998) (Fig. 2A). First, Ub is activated by the ubiquitin-activating enzyme (E1) using ATP. Then, it is transferred to ubiquitin-conjugating enzyme (E2). Finally, it is conjugated onto the target protein selectively brought in by the ubiquitin ligase (E3). A polyUb chain is formed by repeating the ubiquitination process. The expression of these important enzymes that regulate protein ubiquitination may change according to physiological stimuli. For instance, in cardiac atrophy mouse model, the E2 enzyme UbcH2 expression is upregulated in atrophic hearts to increase the capacity of protein degradation (Razeghi *et al.*, 2006).

The 26S proteasome is composed of the 20S proteolytic core and the 19S proteasome activator lid(s) (Luo *et al.*, 2010). The 20S proteolytic core is made up of two outer (α-subunits) and two inner (β-subunits) rings. It contains caspase-like, trypsin-like, and chymotrypsin-like protease activities conveyed by subunits β1, β2, and β5, respectively. The 19S lid(s), also known as proteasome activator 700 (PA700), helps the recognition and docking of polyubiquitinated target protein. 19S also serves to detach and hence recycle the Ub by its deubiquitinating enzyme (DUB) activity. Furthermore, 19S unfolds the target protein and feeds it to the 20S core for degradation.

The immunoproteasome is an alternative version of the proteasome expressed to accommodate inflammatory responses upon stimulation with interferon-γ (Rivett & Hearn, 2004). The immunoproteasome has a 20S core that substitutes the constitutive catalytic β-subunits with inducible β-counterparts (β1i, β2i, and β5i), which offer different proteolytic function and activity to generate small peptides suitable for antigen presentation by major histocompatibility complex (MHC) class I (Griffin *et al.*, 1998) (Fig. 2A). In addition to the 19S proteasome, the immunoproteasome can also have a different lid(s) - the 11S proteasome, also known as PA28 (proteasome activator 28). Different compositions of 11S exist: heteroheptamer of PA28α and PA28β that are induced by interferon-γ under intensified immune response (Murray *et al.*, 2000) and homoheptamer of PA28γ that resides in the nucleus and assists ATP- and ubiquitin-independent proteasomal activity (Mao *et al.*, 2008). Sometimes, hybrid proteasomes with both 11S and 19S lids are also observed. However, their functions remain to be explored.

3.2.1 The UPS and heart diseases

UPS dysregulation is a common phenomenon in heart diseases. It is accentuated with the accumulation of Ub-protein conjugates and is associated with markedly reduced proteasome proteolytic activity in failing human hearts as compared to non-failing hearts (Predmore *et al.*, 2010). This suggests that ubiquitinated proteins in hearts are not degraded due to impaired proteasomal function. While no changes were noted in protein expression of proteasome subunits (i.e. 20S, 19S, 11S), elevated levels of protein carbonyls and 4-hydroxynonenylated proteins were observed in failing hearts. Also, oxidative modification to the 19S ATPase subunit Rpt5 was found in these failing hearts. Together, these oxidative modifications to proteasome subunits and substrate proteins may lead to impaired proteasomal function. On the other hand, microarray studies demonstrate reduced transcript levels of some 20s α- and β-subunits in the failing hearts as compared to controls (Hwang *et al.*, 2002; Kaab *et al.*, 2004). The incongruence between protein and mRNA expression of proteasome subunits may be attributed to myocyte loss and fibrosis in the failing hearts.

Animal models of cardiac diseases also have an increased ubiquitinated protein expression, but are acommpanied with changes in their proteasome expression profile. Upregulation in protein expression of proteasome subunits was observed in a left ventricular hypertrophy mouse model (Depre *et al.*, 2006). Post-translational modifications of the proteasome subunits were also reported in these hypertrophic hearts (Depre *et al.*, 2006). Treatment with proteasome inhibitor effectively prevents cardiac hypertrophy development, suggesting that the upregulation of proteasome expression is central to this physiological adaptation. Similar beneficial effects of proteasome inhibition in the regression of cardiac hypertrophy were observed in other studies (Meiners *et al.*, 2008; Stansfield *et al.*, 2008). Besides hypertrophic cardiomyopathy, the accumulation of Ub-conjugated proteins was observed in hyperglycemia-induced cardiomyopathy mouse model (Powell *et al.*, 2008). A parallel drop in the basal ATP-dependent proteasomal activity was observed in these mice. However, an increased ATP-independent chymotryptic proteasomal activity was observed, which is accompanied by an increased expression of 11S lid subunits PA28α and PA28β, as well as the 20S subunits α3 and β5. Together, these data suggest a shift to immunoproteasomal activity is induced under hyperglycemic stress conditions to help the degradation of accumulated proteins.

The difference in cardiac proteasome expression profiles between human heart failure and various cardiomyopathy mouse models can be attributed to the limited time frame of animal studies. It is likely that stressed human hearts also induce the compensatory upregulation of proteasomal expression and activity at the earlier disease stages, but fail to maintain these changes over time.

3.2.2 The UPS and viral myocarditis

The UPS is also dysregulated in viral myocarditis (Fig. 2A). Accumulation of Ub-protein conjugates, as in other cardiomyopathies, was observed in CVB3-infected mouse hearts and cultured cells (Luo *et al.*, 2003; Gao *et al.*, 2008; Si *et al.*, 2008). The expression of several enzymes in the UPS pathway such as E1 enzyme E1A/E1B, E2 enzyme UbcH7, and DUB UCHL1 (ubiquitin carboxyl-terminal hydrolase L1) is upregulated in CVB3-infected mouse hearts, while ATP-dependent proteasomal activity is unaltered (Gao *et al.*, 2008). *In vitro* application of proteasome inhibitors such as MG132 (Luo *et al.*, 2003), lactacystin (Luo *et al.*, 2003), pyrrolidine dithiocarbamate (PDTC) (Si *et al.*, 2005), and curcumin (Si *et al.*, 2007) effectively attenuates viral RNA replication and protein synthesis. In addition, depletion of Ub by RNA interference also inhibits viral replication (Si *et al.*, 2008). Furthermore, it was shown that viral RNA-dependent polymerase 3D is ubiquitinated during viral replication, which may help its anchorage to intracellular membrane platforms required for the assembly of viral RNA replication machinery (Si *et al.*, 2008). *In vivo* administration of proteasome inhibitor to CVB3-infected mice also improves the outcome of viral myocarditis with reduced myocardial damage and inflammatory infiltration (Gao *et al.*, 2008). The viral titer, however, is not significantly reduced in the treated mice. This suggests that proteasome inhibitor treatment ameliorates viral myocarditis via multiple mechanisms: direct viral inhibition and immunomodulation. It was further demonstrated that the expression of 11S subunit PA28γ plays a role in CVB3 replication (Gao *et al.*, 2010). CVB3 infection leads to the redistribution of PA28γ from the nucleus to the cytosol, where it interacts with host proteins, such as tumor suppressor protein p53, and promotes their degradation via UPS. Overexpression of PA28γ enhances viral replication while its knockdown does the opposite.

Szalay et al. explored the involvement of the immunoproteasome in viral myocarditis. They found that the catalytic subunits of the immunoproteasome, LMP2 (β1i), LMP7 (β5i), and MECL-1 (β2i), are upregulated in CVB3-infected myocarditis-susceptible mouse hearts as compared to infected hearts from resistant mouse strains (Szalay *et al.*, 2006). Increased activity of the immunoproteasome in the susceptible myocardium helps generate the MHC class I-restricted peptide, boost antigen presentation and mount the subsequent adaptive immune response. A recent study demonstrates a differential immunoproteasome expression pattern between myocarditis-susceptible and -resistant mouse strains (Jakel *et al.*, 2009). In this study, immunoproteasome formation peaks early after CVB3 challenge in resistant mice, while it is postponed and expressed in greater extent in susceptible mice. The timing and magnitude of immunoproteasome activation determine in part the effectiveness of early viral clearance and the extent of direct viral-mediated damages, as well as the injury incurred during adaptive immune responses.

3.3 Autophagy

The other host protein degradation system is autophagy, i.e. "self-eating". It proceeds by the engulfing of a portion of the cytoplasm including long-lived and misfolded proteins and organelles by the autophagic membranes to form double-membraned vesicles called autophagosomes, followed by their delivery to lysosomes for degradation (Levine & Kroemer, 2008) (Fig. 2B). Autophagy is activated in two parallel cascades of enzymatic actions that are similar to the process of protein ubiquitination (Ravikumar *et al.*, 2010). First, Atg12 (autophagy-related gene 12) and Atg8 (also known as LC3, microtubule-associated protein light chain 3, in mammalian cells) are activated by the E1-like activating enzyme Atg7 using ATP. Then, Atg12 is conjugated to its E2 Atg10, while Atg8 is attached to another E2 Atg3. Atg12 is then transferred to its designated partner Atg5 forming the Atg12-Atg5 complex and further matures by the conjugation to Atg16. Finally, the Atg12-Ag5-Atg16 complex acts as an E3 to help Atg8 lipidation, forming the Atg8-PE (phosphatidylethanolamine) complex. Lipidation of Atg8 helps its incorporation onto the autophagic membrane. Atg8-PE then takes part in the elongation of the autophagic membrane and its enclosure to form the autophagosome.

3.3.1 Autophagy and cardiac diseases

Under baseline conditions, autophagy represents an important homeostatic mechanism. However, excessive activation of the autophagy machinery has been suggested to be involved in the pathogenesis of various disease conditions, including cardiac diseases. LC3 activation was observed early and was well-sustained in pressure-overload cardiomyopathy mouse model (Zhu *et al.*, 2007). Autophagy activation in this model promotes cardiac remodeling. Overexpression of Beclin-1, also known as Atg6, accentuates pathological remodeling and interstitial fibrosis, whereas heterozygous knockout of Beclin-1 improves systolic function and delays cardiac remodeling. In desmin-mediated cardiomyopathy mouse model, early activation of autophagy was observed well before any measurable decline in cardiac function (Tannous *et al.*, 2008). Autophagy pathway impairment by heterozygous inactivation of Beclin-1 leads to accumulation of polyubiquitinated protein aggregates, as well as acceleration to heart failure and early mortality (Tannous *et al.*, 2008). Similarly, autophagy is activated in both ischemia and subsequent reperfusion, but via two different initiation pathways (Takagi *et al.*, 2007). The AMPK pathway drives autophagy during ischemia, while Beclin-1 initiates autophagy upon reperfusion. Autophagy during ischemia is considered a cell survival response as it helps to sustain the starved cardiomyocytes during ischemia; however, autophagy during reperfusion is viewed as a pathological response as it promotes autophagic cell death.

3.3.2 Autophagy and viral myocarditis

Autophagy also plays an important part in the host innate defense system by direct sequestration of invading pathogens (bacteria, fungi, and virus) for clearance through lysosomal degradation (Jackson *et al.*, 2005). In addition, autophagy helps antigen presentation to class II MHC in order to mount an adaptive immune response (Dengjel *et al.*, 2005). However, this innate defense machinery is subverted by certain viruses to facilitate their replication (Jackson *et al.*, 2005; Wong *et al.*, 2008). It was shown that LC3-PE expression, a hallmark of autophagosome formation, is increased after CVB3 infection with dramatic reorganization of intracellular membranes (Wong *et al.*, 2008) (Fig. 2B). Inhibition of autophagy by 3-methyladenine which targets the upstream signaling class III PI3-kinase, and by siRNA knockdown of Atg7 expression effectively block viral replication (Wong *et al.*, 2008). Recent work in mouse models also suggests that autophagy is activated *in vivo* after CVB3 infection (unpublished data). LC3-PE expression is elevated in CVB3-infected organs such as the heart, liver, and pancreas. Kemball *et al.* also reported the induction of autophagosome formation in pancreatic acinar cells in CVB3-infected mice (Kemball *et al.*, 2010). This theme of virus-induced autophagy activation is further extended to coxsackievirus B4-infected rat primary neurons (Yoon *et al.*, 2008). Nonetheless, virus-induced autophagy only serves to help viral replication without increasing protein degradation as suggested by the unchanged expression level of p62, a selective autophagy substrate, after virus infection (Wong *et al.*, 2008).

Subversion of the autophagy machinery by enteroviruses may contribute to the pathogenesis of viral myocarditis beyond impacting cardiomyocyte viability. Recent research demonstrates that cellular autophagy plays a role in nucleic acid-sensing toll-like receptor 3 (TLR3) signaling, which is necessary for the antiviral interferon pathway (Gorbea *et al.*, 2010). TLR3-deficient mice show vulnerability to CVB3 infection and develop acute myocarditis (Negishi *et al.*, 2008). Dysregulation of the autophagy pathway in CVB3-infected cardiomyocytes may interfere with TLR3-mediated antiviral response, resulting in compromised viral clearance and increased myocardial damage during viremia. In addition, autophagy is known to be a pro-survival response against apoptosis. The dysregulation of autophagy may decrease the viability of virus-infected cardiomyocytes because it cannot protect the host from virus-induced apoptosis. Furthermore, angiotensin II receptors type I & II (AT1 & AT2) regulate cardiomyocyte autophagy activity (Porrello *et al.*, 2009). AT1 expression triggers autophagy in neonatal cardiomyocytes as well as subsequent autophagic cell death, while AT2 expression counteracts AT1-induced autophagic activity. Further modulation by angiotensins may have an adverse effect on virus-infected cardiomyocytes as it may further activate autophagy, thus triggering autophagic cell death.

4. Potential therapeutics targeting viral proteases, UPS, and autophagy

The current knowledge of the roles of viral proteases and the host protein degradation systems in viral myocarditis may lead to new diagnostic and therapeutic approaches for the disease. Virus-induced SRF cleavage fragments may be utilized as a biomarker to detect acute phase myocarditis. Early diagnosis of viral myocarditis opens up the optimal timeframe for treatment. Successful medical interventions during acute infection can limit viral replication and its associated damage, limit viral spreading, as well as minimize the damage caused by immune activation. Since the viral proteases and the protein degradation systems all play important roles in viral propagation, a combinatorial therapy of highly specific viral protease inhibitors, proteasome inhibitors, and autophagy inhibitors during viremia would limit viral infection effectively. Furthermore, application of proteasome inhibitors and autophagy inhibitors provides additional benefits in immunomodulation to control the inflammatory response. On the other hand, viral myocarditis patients in the chronic phases may be managed differently. Since DCM patients have depressed proteasomal function, proteasome inhibitor treatment may further exacerbate myocardial damage. Moreover, long-term application of inhibitors against UPS will have adverse effects as demonstrated in the increased incidence of heart failure in cancer patients undergoing proteasome inhibitor treatment (Enrico *et al.*, 2007; Hacihanefioglu *et al.*, 2008).

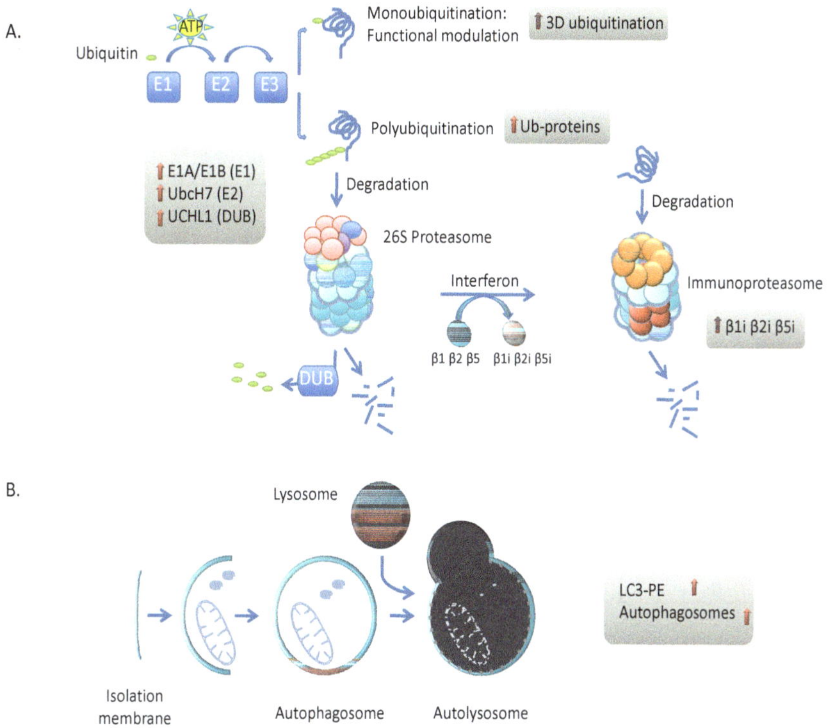

Fig. 2. Dysregulation of the host protein degradation systems in viral cardiomyopathy. The ubiquitin/proteasome system (UPS) and autophagy are the two major protein degradation mechanisms in eukaryotic cells. A. The UPS function by a cascade of enzymatic reactions (El - ubiquitin activating enzyme, E2 - ubiquitin conjugating enzyme, E3 - ubiquitin ligase) that conjugate ubiquitin, a small protein modifier, onto the target proteins. The type of ubiquitin conjugation linkage determines the target protein's fate: functional modulation or degradation. Polyubiquitinated target proteins are recognized by the 26S proteasome for degradation, whereas monoubiquitination serves to help endocytosis, endosomal sorting, DNA repair, histone regulation, and nuclear export. Ubiquitins are recycled by the deubiquitinating enzymes (DUBs). CVB3 infection causes the dysregulation of the UPS. An increased expression of ubiquitin-protein conjugates, E1A/E1B (El), UbcH7 (E2), UCH-L1 (DUB) was observed in CVB3-infected mouse hearts. Proteasome inhibitor application attenuates viral replication *in vitro* and reduces myocardial lesion and fibrosis *in vivo*. B. Autophagy begins with the enwrapping of organelles and cytoplasmic proteins by the isolation membrane which elongates and encloses to form a double-membraned vesicle called the autophagosome. The autophagosome fuses with lysosomes to degrade the sequestrated materials. Autophagy plays an important role in host defense by trapping and degrading invading pathogens. However, certain viruses including CVB3 evolve strategies to subvert autophagic mechanism to facilitate their own replication. Autophagosome formation is upregulated during CVB3 infection. Inhibition of the autophagy pathway has been shown to block viral replication *in vitro*.

5. Conclusion

Viral-induced protein cleavage and host protein degradation dysregulation play important roles in the pathogenesis of viral myocarditis and its subsequent progression to DCM. Identification of viral-induced protein cleavage fragments may allow early diagnosis of viral myocarditis, which opens up the optimal treatment window. A combination of antiviral therapies including specific viral protease inhibitors, proteasome inhibitors, and autophagy inhibitors presents new strategies for effective early viral clearance and minimization of viral-induced, inflammation-associated damage. Further studies employing system-like approaches, such as ubiquitomics, degradomics, and RNAi screens, are required to decipher the complex interactions between host and virus during different stages of viral myocarditis. Efforts in clarifying the precise functions and regulatory mechanisms of the host protein degradation systems in the disease progression of viral myocarditis will lead to novel therapeutic targets to improve treatment in different disease stages.

6. References

Abelmann WH. (1971). Virus and the heart. *Circulation* 44, 950-956.

Badorff C & Knowlton KU. (2004). Dystrophin disruption in enterovirus-induced myocarditis and dilated cardiomyopathy: from bench to bedside. *Med Microbiol Immunol* 193, 121-126.

Badorff C, Lee GH, Lamphear BJ, Martone ME, Campbell KP, Rhoads RE & Knowlton KU. (1999). Enteroviral protease 2A cleaves dystrophin: evidence of cytoskeletal disruption in an acquired cardiomyopathy. *Nat Med* 5, 320-326.

Baughman KL. (2006). Diagnosis of myocarditis: death of Dallas criteria. *Circulation* 113, 593-595.

Calabrese F, Carturan E & Thiene G. (2010). Cardiac infections: focus on molecular diagnosis. *Cardiovasc Pathol* 19, 171-182.

Chang J, Wei L, Otani T, Youker KA, Entman ML & Schwartz RJ. (2003). Inhibitory cardiac transcription factor, SRF-N, is generated by caspase 3 cleavage in human heart failure and attenuated by ventricular unloading. *Circulation* 108, 407-413.

Chau DH, Yuan J, Zhang H, Cheung P, Lim T, Liu Z, Sall A & Yang D. (2007). Coxsackievirus B3 proteases 2A and 3C induce apoptotic cell death through mitochondrial injury and cleavage of eIF4GI but not DAP5/p97/NAT1. *Apoptosis* 12, 513-524.

Cooper LT, Jr. (2009). Myocarditis. *N Engl J Med* 360, 1526-1538.

Davis FJ, Gupta M, Pogwizd SM, Bacha E, Jeevanandam V & Gupta MP. (2002). Increased expression of alternatively spliced dominant-negative isoform of SRF in human failing hearts. *Am J Physiol Heart Circ Physiol* 282, H1521-1533.

de Breyne S, Bonderoff JM, Chumakov KM, Lloyd RE & Hellen CU. (2008). Cleavage of eukaryotic initiation factor eIF5B by enterovirus 3C proteases. *Virology* 378, 118-122.

Deconinck AE, Rafael JA, Skinner JA, Brown SC, Potter AC, Metzinger L, Watt DJ, Dickson JG, Tinsley JM & Davies KE. (1997). Utrophin-dystrophin-deficient mice as a model for Duchenne muscular dystrophy. *Cell* 90, 717-727.

Dengjel J, Schoor O, Fischer R, Reich M, Kraus M, Muller M, Kreymborg K, Altenberend F, Brandenburg J, Kalbacher H, Brock R, Driessen C, Rammensee HG & Stevanovic S.

(2005). Autophagy promotes MHC class II presentation of peptides from intracellular source proteins. *Proc Natl Acad Sci U S A* 102, 7922-7927.

Depre C, Wang Q, Yan L, Hedhli N, Peter P, Chen L, Hong C, Hittinger L, Ghaleh B, Sadoshima J, Vatner DE, Vatner SF & Madura K. (2006). Activation of the cardiac proteasome during pressure overload promotes ventricular hypertrophy. *Circulation* 114, 1821-1828.

Drory Y, Turetz Y, Hiss Y, Lev B, Fisman EZ, Pines A & Kramer MR. (1991). Sudden unexpected death in persons less than 40 years of age. *Am J Cardiol* 68, 1388-1392.

Enrico O, Gabriele B, Nadia C, Sara G, Daniele V, Giulia C, Antonio S & Mario P. (2007). Unexpected cardiotoxicity in haematological bortezomib treated patients. *Br J Haematol* 138, 396-397.

Esfandiarei M & McManus BM. (2008). Molecular biology and pathogenesis of viral myocarditis. *Annu Rev Pathol* 3, 127-155.

Ferlini A, Sewry C, Melis MA, Mateddu A & Muntoni F. (1999). X-linked dilated cardiomyopathy and the dystrophin gene. *Neuromuscul Disord* 9, 339-346.

Froeschle JE, Feorino PM & Gelfand HM. (1966). A continuing surveillance of enterovirus infection in healthy children in six United States cities. II. Surveillance enterovirus isolates 1960-1963 and comparison with enterovirus isolates from cases of acute central nervous system disease. *Am J Epidemiol* 83, 455-469.

Gao G, Wong J, Zhang J, Mao I, Shravah J, Wu Y, Xiao A, Li X & Luo H. (2010). Proteasome activator REGgamma enhances coxsackieviral infection by facilitating p53 degradation. *J Virol* 84, 11056-11066.

Gao G, Zhang J, Si X, Wong J, Cheung C, McManus B & Luo H. (2008). Proteasome inhibition attenuates coxsackievirus-induced myocardial damage in mice. *Am J Physiol Heart Circ Physiol* 295, H401-408.

Gorbea C, Makar KA, Pauschinger M, Pratt G, Bersola JL, Varela J, David RM, Banks L, Huang CH, Li H, Schultheiss HP, Towbin JA, Vallejo JG & Bowles NE. (2010). A role for Toll-like receptor 3 variants in host susceptibility to enteroviral myocarditis and dilated cardiomyopathy. *J Biol Chem* 285, 23208-23223.

Grady RM, Teng H, Nichol MC, Cunningham JC, Wilkinson RS & Sanes JR. (1997). Skeletal and cardiac myopathies in mice lacking utrophin and dystrophin: a model for Duchenne muscular dystrophy. *Cell* 90, 729-738.

Griffin TA, Nandi D, Cruz M, Fehling HJ, Kaer LV, Monaco JJ & Colbert RA. (1998). Immunoproteasome assembly: cooperative incorporation of interferon gamma (IFN-gamma)-inducible subunits. *J Exp Med* 187, 97-104.

Grist NR & Reid D. (1997). Organisms in myocarditis/endocarditis viruses. *J Infect* 34, 155.

Hacihanefioglu A, Tarkun P & Gonullu E. (2008). Acute severe cardiac failure in a myeloma patient due to proteasome inhibitor bortezomib. *Int J Hematol* 88, 219-222.

Hershko A & Ciechanover A. (1998). The ubiquitin system. *Annu Rev Biochem* 67, 425-479.

Huber M, Watson KA, Selinka HC, Carthy CM, Klingel K, McManus BM & Kandolf R. (1999). Cleavage of RasGAP and phosphorylation of mitogen-activated protein kinase in the course of coxsackievirus B3 replication. *J Virol* 73, 3587-3594.

Hwang JJ, Allen PD, Tseng GC, Lam CW, Fananapazir L, Dzau VJ & Liew CC. (2002). Microarray gene expression profiles in dilated and hypertrophic cardiomyopathic end-stage heart failure. *Physiol Genomics* 10, 31-44.

Jackson WT, Giddings TH, Jr., Taylor MP, Mulinyawe S, Rabinovitch M, Kopito RR & Kirkegaard K. (2005). Subversion of cellular autophagosomal machinery by RNA viruses. *PLoS Biol* 3, e156.

Jakel S, Kuckelkorn U, Szalay G, Plotz M, Textoris-Taube K, Opitz E, Klingel K, Stevanovic S, Kandolf R, Kotsch K, Stangl K, Kloetzel PM & Voigt A. (2009). Differential interferon responses enhance viral epitope generation by myocardial immunoproteasomes in murine enterovirus myocarditis. *Am J Pathol* 175, 510-518.

Kaab S, Barth AS, Margerie D, Dugas M, Gebauer M, Zwermann L, Merk S, Pfeufer A, Steinmeyer K, Bleich M, Kreuzer E, Steinbeck G & Nabauer M. (2004). Global gene expression in human myocardium-oligonucleotide microarray analysis of regional diversity and transcriptional regulation in heart failure. *J Mol Med* 82, 308-316.

Kemball CC, Alirezaei M, Flynn CT, Wood MR, Harkins S, Kiosses WB & Whitton JL. (2010). Coxsackievirus infection induces autophagy-like vesicles and megaphagosomes in pancreatic acinar cells in vivo. *J Virol* 84, 12110-12124.

Levine B & Kroemer G. (2008). Autophagy in the pathogenesis of disease. *Cell* 132, 27-42.

Luo H, Wong J & Wong B. (2010). Protein degradation systems in viral myocarditis leading to dilated cardiomyopathy. *Cardiovasc Res* 85, 347-356.

Luo H, Zhang J, Cheung C, Suarez A, McManus BM & Yang D. (2003). Proteasome inhibition reduces coxsackievirus B3 replication in murine cardiomyocytes. *Am J Pathol* 163, 381-385.

Mao I, Liu J, Li X & Luo H. (2008). REGgamma, a proteasome activator and beyond? *Cell Mol Life Sci* 65, 3971-3980.

Mason JW. (2003). Myocarditis and dilated cardiomyopathy: an inflammatory link. *Cardiovasc Res* 60, 5-10.

McManus BM, Chow LH, Wilson JE, Anderson DR, Gulizia JM, Gauntt CJ, Klingel KE, Beisel KW & Kandolf R. (1993). Direct myocardial injury by enterovirus: a central role in the evolution of murine myocarditis. *Clin Immunol Immunopathol* 68, 159-169.

McManus BM, Gauntt CJ & Cassling RS. (1988). Immunopathologic basis of myocardial injury. *Cardiovasc Clin* 18, 163-184.

Meiners S, Dreger H, Fechner M, Bieler S, Rother W, Gunther C, Baumann G, Stangl V & Stangl K. (2008). Suppression of cardiomyocyte hypertrophy by inhibition of the ubiquitin-proteasome system. *Hypertension* 51, 302-308.

Miano JM. (2003). Serum response factor: toggling between disparate programs of gene expression. *J Mol Cell Cardiol* 35, 577-593.

Murray BW, Sultmann H & Klein J. (2000). Identification and linkage of the proteasome activator complex PA28 subunit genes in zebrafish. *Scand J Immunol* 51, 571-576.

Narula J, Chandrasekhar Y & Dec GW. (1998). Apoptosis in heart failure: a tale of heightened expectations, unfulfilled promises and broken hearts em leader. *Apoptosis* 3, 309-315.

Negishi H, Osawa T, Ogami K, Ouyang X, Sakaguchi S, Koshiba R, Yanai H, Seko Y, Shitara H, Bishop K, Yonekawa H, Tamura T, Kaisho T, Taya C, Taniguchi T & Honda K. (2008). A critical link between Toll-like receptor 3 and type II interferon signaling pathways in antiviral innate immunity. *Proc Natl Acad Sci U S A* 105, 20446-20451.

Nigro G, Comi LI, Politano L & Bain RJ. (1990). The incidence and evolution of cardiomyopathy in Duchenne muscular dystrophy. *Int J Cardiol* 26, 271-277.

Niu Z, Li A, Zhang SX & Schwartz RJ. (2007). Serum response factor micromanaging cardiogenesis. *Curr Opin Cell Biol* 19, 618-627.

Oka T, Xu J & Molkentin JD. (2007). Re-employment of developmental transcription factors in adult heart disease. *Semin Cell Dev Biol* 18, 117-131.

Okuni M, Yamada T, Mochizuki S & Sakurai I. (1975). Studies on myocarditis in childhood, with special reference to the possible role of immunological process and the thymus in the chronicity of the disease. *Jpn Circ J* 39, 463-470.

Parlakian A, Charvet C, Escoubet B, Mericskay M, Molkentin JD, Gary-Bobo G, De Windt LJ, Ludosky MA, Paulin D, Daegelen D, Tuil D & Li Z. (2005). Temporally controlled onset of dilated cardiomyopathy through disruption of the SRF gene in adult heart. *Circulation* 112, 2930-2939.

Parlakian A, Tuil D, Hamard G, Tavernier G, Hentzen D, Concordet JP, Paulin D, Li Z & Daegelen D. (2004). Targeted inactivation of serum response factor in the developing heart results in myocardial defects and embryonic lethality. *Mol Cell Biol* 24, 5281-5289.

Porrello ER, D'Amore A, Curl CL, Allen AM, Harrap SB, Thomas WG & Delbridge LM. (2009). Angiotensin II type 2 receptor antagonizes angiotensin II type 1 receptor-mediated cardiomyocyte autophagy. *Hypertension* 53, 1032-1040.

Powell SR, Samuel SM, Wang P, Divald A, Thirunavukkarasu M, Koneru S, Wang X & Maulik N. (2008). Upregulation of myocardial 11S-activated proteasome in experimental hyperglycemia. *J Mol Cell Cardiol* 44, 618-621.

Predmore JM, Wang P, Davis F, Bartolone S, Westfall MV, Dyke DB, Pagani F, Powell SR & Day SM. (2010). Ubiquitin proteasome dysfunction in human hypertrophic and dilated cardiomyopathies. *Circulation* 121, 997-1004.

Ravikumar B, Sarkar S, Davies JE, Futter M, Garcia-Arencibia M, Green-Thompson ZW, Jimenez-Sanchez M, Korolchuk VI, Lichtenberg M, Luo S, Massey DC, Menzies FM, Moreau K, Narayanan U, Renna M, Siddiqi FH, Underwood BR, Winslow AR & Rubinsztein DC. (2010). Regulation of mammalian autophagy in physiology and pathophysiology. *Physiol Rev* 90, 1383-1435.

Razeghi P, Baskin KK, Sharma S, Young ME, Stepkowski S, Essop MF & Taegtmeyer H. (2006). Atrophy, hypertrophy, and hypoxemia induce transcriptional regulators of the ubiquitin proteasome system in the rat heart. *Biochem Biophys Res Commun* 342, 361-364.

Reyes MP & Lerner AM. (1985). Coxsackievirus myocarditis--with special reference to acute and chronic effects. *Prog Cardiovasc Dis* 27, 373-394.

Rivett AJ & Hearn AR. (2004). Proteasome function in antigen presentation: immunoproteasome complexes, Peptide production, and interactions with viral proteins. *Curr Protein Pept Sci* 5, 153-161.

Seipelt J, Liebig HD, Sommergruber W, Gerner C & Kuechler E. (2000). 2A proteinase of human rhinovirus cleaves cytokeratin 8 in infected HeLa cells. *J Biol Chem* 275, 20084-20089.

Si X, Gao G, Wong J, Wang Y, Zhang J & Luo H. (2008). Ubiquitination is required for effective replication of coxsackievirus B3. *PLoS One* 3, e2585.

Si X, McManus BM, Zhang J, Yuan J, Cheung C, Esfandiarei M, Suarez A, Morgan A & Luo H. (2005). Pyrrolidine dithiocarbamate reduces coxsackievirus B3 replication through inhibition of the ubiquitin-proteasome pathway. *J Virol* 79, 8014-8023.

Si X, Wang Y, Wong J, Zhang J, McManus BM & Luo H. (2007). Dysregulation of the ubiquitin-proteasome system by curcumin suppresses coxsackievirus B3 replication. *J Virol* 81, 3142-3150.

Stansfield WE, Tang RH, Moss NC, Baldwin AS, Willis MS & Selzman CH. (2008). Proteasome inhibition promotes regression of left ventricular hypertrophy. *Am J Physiol Heart Circ Physiol* 294, H645-650.

Sun Q, Chen G, Streb JW, Long X, Yang Y, Stoeckert CJ, Jr. & Miano JM. (2006). Defining the mammalian CArGome. *Genome Res* 16, 197-207.

Szalay G, Meiners S, Voigt A, Lauber J, Spieth C, Speer N, Sauter M, Kuckelkorn U, Zell A, Klingel K, Stangl K & Kandolf R. (2006). Ongoing coxsackievirus myocarditis is associated with increased formation and activity of myocardial immunoproteasomes. *Am J Pathol* 168, 1542-1552.

Takagi H, Matsui Y, Hirotani S, Sakoda H, Asano T & Sadoshima J. (2007). AMPK mediates autophagy during myocardial ischemia in vivo. *Autophagy* 3, 405-407.

Tannous P, Zhu H, Johnstone JL, Shelton JM, Rajasekaran NS, Benjamin IJ, Nguyen L, Gerard RD, Levine B, Rothermel BA & Hill JA. (2008). Autophagy is an adaptive response in desmin-related cardiomyopathy. *Proc Natl Acad Sci U S A* 105, 9745-9750.

Wessely R, Klingel K, Santana LF, Dalton N, Hongo M, Jonathan Lederer W, Kandolf R & Knowlton KU. (1998). Transgenic expression of replication-restricted enteroviral genomes in heart muscle induces defective excitation-contraction coupling and dilated cardiomyopathy. *J Clin Invest* 102, 1444-1453.

Why HJ, Meany BT, Richardson PJ, Olsen EG, Bowles NE, Cunningham L, Freeke CA & Archard LC. (1994). Clinical and prognostic significance of detection of enteroviral RNA in the myocardium of patients with myocarditis or dilated cardiomyopathy. *Circulation* 89, 2582-2589.

Wong J, Zhang J, Si X, Gao G, Mao I, McManus BM & Luo H. (2008). Autophagosome supports coxsackievirus B3 replication in host cells. *J Virol* 82, 9143-9153.

Xiong D, Lee GH, Badorff C, Dorner A, Lee S, Wolf P & Knowlton KU. (2002). Dystrophin deficiency markedly increases enterovirus-induced cardiomyopathy: a genetic predisposition to viral heart disease. *Nat Med* 8, 872-877.

Xiong D, Yajima T, Lim BK, Stenbit A, Dublin A, Dalton ND, Summers-Torres D, Molkentin JD, Duplain H, Wessely R, Chen J & Knowlton KU. (2007). Inducible cardiac-restricted expression of enteroviral protease 2A is sufficient to induce dilated cardiomyopathy. *Circulation* 115, 94-102.

Yalamanchili P, Datta U & Dasgupta A. (1997). Inhibition of host cell transcription by poliovirus: cleavage of transcription factor CREB by poliovirus-encoded protease 3Cpro. *J Virol* 71, 1220-1226.

Yoon SY, Ha YE, Choi JE, Ahn J, Lee H, Kweon HS, Lee JY & Kim DH. (2008). Coxsackievirus B4 uses autophagy for replication after calpain activation in rat primary neurons. *J Virol* 82, 11976-11978.

Zhang X, Azhar G, Chai J, Sheridan P, Nagano K, Brown T, Yang J, Khrapko K, Borras AM, Lawitts J, Misra RP & Wei JY. (2001). Cardiomyopathy in transgenic mice with cardiac-specific overexpression of serum response factor. *Am J Physiol Heart Circ Physiol* 280, H1782-1792.

Zheng Q & Wang X. (2010). Autophagy and the ubiquitin-proteasome system in cardiac dysfunction. *Panminerva Med* 52, 9-25.

Zhu H, Tannous P, Johnstone JL, Kong Y, Shelton JM, Richardson JA, Le V, Levine B, Rothermel BA & Hill JA. (2007). Cardiac autophagy is a maladaptive response to hemodynamic stress. *J Clin Invest* 117, 1782-1793.

Part 3

Recent Advances in Myocarditis

16

Myocarditis Presenting with Ventricular Arrhythmias: Role of Electroanatomical Mapping-Guided Endomyocardial Biopsy in Differential Diagnosis

Maurizio Pieroni, Costantino Smaldone and Fulvio Bellocci
Cardiology Department, Catholic University of the Sacred Heart, Rome, Italy

1. Introduction

Myocarditis is defined as a disease characterized by myocardial inflammation associated with myocyte necrosis. It can be caused by infections, autoimmune response primarily affecting the myocardium or by systemic autoimmune or inflammatory disorders (Aretz et al., 1986). Viral infections are the most frequent cause and account for the vast majority of cases in North America and Europe (Cooper, 2009).

Cardiac symptoms that develop during myocarditis may follow after a delay of days to weeks from the beginning of the pathological process; they are quite unspecific and include fatigue, dyspnoea, palpitations, malaise and atypical chest discomfort. Even the clinical cardiac signs may be vague in many patients and generally include cardiac murmurs, gallop rhythms and other signs of heart failure and sometimes pericardial rubs when the pericardium is also involved in the inflammatory process. Myocarditis is often associated with various types of ECG abnormalities (including bundle branch blocks, Q waves resembling those related to myocardial infarction, repolarization abnormalities and QRS prolongation) and rhythm disturbance such as atrio-ventricular blocks, supraventricular tachycardias and ventricular ectopies and tachycardias. Echocardiography may reveal overt systolic dysfunction or a reduction of peak systolic velocities at TDI; moreover, regional wall motion abnormalities and diastolic dysfunction may be found (Cooper, 2009; Feldman et al. 2000). Therefore, this disease should always be considered in patients who present with rapidly progressive cardiomyopathy, chest pain with ECG anomalies that mimic an acute coronary syndrome but with normal coronary arteries or idiopathic ventricular arrhythmias. Furthermore, in young people myocarditis may be frequently responsible for sudden cardiac death, particularly after strenuous physical exertion (Doolan et al., 2004; Corrado D et al. 2001). With this regard it should be highlighted that the recognition of myocarditis in patients presenting with aborted sudden death or major ventricular arrhythmias is actually challenging in everyday clinical practice, as the diagnosis may be difficult and may require the use of invasive procedures. Nevertheless, the detection of myocarditis in patients presenting with ventricular arrhythmias may have a pivotal importance, because the identification of myocarditis as the substrate of arrhythmias is actually important for targeting therapies.

In the last decades the development of new diagnostic techniques, in particular cardiac magnetic resonance, has led to an increased recognition of myocarditis as a cause of ventricular arrhythmias. However endomyocardial biopsy still represents the gold standard for the diagnosis of myocarditis. The main criticism against a wider use of endomyocardial biopsy in the diagnostic approach to patients with ventricular arrhythmias is represented by the possible sampling error in the presence of a focal myocarditis. We recently demonstrated that three dimensional electroanatomical mapping (3D-EAM) may guide endomyocardial biopsy identifying the segments of ventricular wall presenting an abnormal voltage, thus reducing sampling error and increasing sensitivity of biopsy. The systematic association of endomyocardial biopsy with electroanatomical mapping represents a significant improvement of the diagnostic tools available to identify the substrate of ventricular arrhythmias.

In this chapter we describe the role of electroanatomical mapping-guided endomyocardial biopsy in the differential diagnosis of myocardial pathological substrates in patients with ventricular arrhythmias. We report the results of our group and other groups adopting this technique in different categories of patients, including subjects with a clinical diagnosis of arrhythmogenic right ventricular cardiomyopathy (ARVC), competitive athletes and patients with electrocardiographic diagnosis of Brugada syndrome.

2. Myocarditis and ventricular arrhythmias

Endomyocardial biopsy and autopsy findings have clearly demonstrated that myocarditis represents a frequent cause of life-threatening ventricular arrhythmias and sudden death. Post-mortem studies suggest that myocarditis is a major cause of sudden, unexpected death in adults less than 40 years of age (accounting for approximately 20% of cases - Fabre & Sheppard, 2006; Doolan et al., 2004). Indeed myocarditis may frequently cause ventricular arrhythmias associated with systolic dysfunction of left or right ventricle or both. In both its acute and chronic phase myocarditis may be associated with severe arrhythmias that can significantly affect the natural course of the disease, as they can further contribute to the deterioration of cardiac systolic and diastolic function and can be the ultimate cause of death in these patients (Magnani et al. 2006; Zeppenfeld et al. 2007; Graner et al, 2007). Mechanisms of arrhythmogenesis in the context of myocarditis include myocyte necrosis, replacement fibrosis (favoring re-entry mechanism), proarrhythmic effects of cytokines and inflammatory mediators possibly through a modulation of ion channel function.

In patients with chronic active myocarditis, the perpetuation of inflammation is often related to viral persistence or to autoimmune self-maintaining mechanisms, and replacement fibrosis seems to represent a major arrhythmogenic substrate in this case, together with the permanence of an inflammatory milieu surrounding myocardiocytes. Moreover it has been demonstrated that enteroviral persistence perpetrates myocardial damage even in the absence of overt myocardial inflammation, through the release of proteases capable of cleaving dystrophin (Andreoletti et al., 2007). This in turns causes cytoskeleletal anomalies that can affect myocyte mechanical and even electric properties and finally lead to myocyte death, possibly contributing to arrhythmogenesis.

Myocarditis may be the cause of ventricular arrhythmias even in subjects with no previous symptoms or presenting with an apparently normal heart or minimal electrocardiographic and cardiac structural abnormalities (Theleman et al., 2001; Friedman et al., 1994). Subtle abnormalities not detectable by first-line examinations such as echocardiography may be present in patients with myocarditis presenting with ventricular arrhythmias. Other imaging modalities such as cardiac magnetic resonance (CMR) and even ventricular angiography are generally needed to detect these abnormalities. In a study published in 2001 we found small aneurysms at ventricular angiography in patients with apparently idiopathic major ventricular arrhythmias; it should be underlined that all the patients enrolled in this study were also submitted to CMR that failed to detect microaneurysms in most patients (It is possible that currently used cine-sequences for functional analysis of both ventricles may enhance the diagnostic performance of CMR even in this setting). Histological examination of myocardial samples drawn from areas surrounding the aneurysms revealed the presence of active lymphocytic myocarditis with intense myocytolisis. Notably, no patient suffered from cardiac sudden death or malignant ventricular arrhythmias during a 1-year follow-up and sequential Holter recording showed progressive reduction of the arrhythmic burden. Furthermore neither heart failure episodes nor decrease of LV function were reported in the study population (Chimenti et al., 2001). Under this respect it should be noticed that inflammatory microaneurysms were also found in experimental animal models of myocarditis, namely in hamster and mice which survived to acute viral myocarditis, and they seem to cause electroanatomical abnormalities that are associated with development of severe ventricular arrhythmias; interestingly, in the inoculated animals the prognosis associated with the development of microaneurysms in the setting of experimental viral myocarditis was good with a survival similar to normal animals who had no aneurysms (Hoschino et al., 1984; Matsumori et al 1983).

Myocarditis may selectively affect the right ventricle causing structural abnormalities, including microaneurysms, and arrhythmic manifestations typical of arrhythmogenic right ventricular cardiomyopathy. In fact myocardial inflammatory infiltrates associated with myocyte necrosis and replacement fibrosis, may lead to functional and structural changes of right ventricular myocardium resembling those produced by fibrofatty replacement, and representing the substrate of abnormal voltage map and ventricular arrhythmias (Hoffmann et al, 1993; Pieroni et al., 2009). Namely, our group demonstrated that biopsy-proven myocarditis is present in up to 50% of patients fulfilling current diagnostic criteria of arrhythmogenic right ventricular cardiomyopathy at non-invasive evaluation (including cardiac magnetic resonance), moreover myocarditis was associated to the presence of low-voltage areas, as detected by 3D electro-anatomic mapping (Pieroni et al., 2009). Consistently it has been recently reported that also right ventricular sarcoidosis may mimic electroanatomic mapping features and arrhythmic presentation of arrhythmogenic right ventricular cardiomyopathy (Ott et al., 2003; Koplan et al. 2006; Vaisawala et al., 2009).

Myocarditis represents a frequent cause of ventricular arrhythmias also in competitive athletes and its recognition and differential diagnosis with other cardiomyopathies with different prognosis may have important implications for sport eligibility (Basso C et al., 2007). In fact, a recent study by our group demonstrated the presence of myocarditis, diagnosed by endomyocardial biopsy, in most elite athletes presenting with major arrhythmias and apparently normal heart. Moreover it should be emphasized that according to current diagnostic recommendations (the 2nd consensus document on Brugada Syndrome underlined the need to exclude other pathological conditions), the presence of a myocarditis should be always excluded in patients with electrocardiographic features leading to the diagnosis of Brugada syndrome. Among the pathologic conditions that can lead to a

Brugada-like phenotype, myocarditis of the right ventricle is one of the most frequently found when patients with Brugada syndrome are submitted to an extensive invasive and non-invasive evaluation (Frustaci et al., 2005; Okubo et al., 2010). In facts, a study on 18 patients with Brugada Syndrome (diagnosed according to the consensus criteria) presenting with sustained ventricular arrhythmias or syncope, revealed the presence of biopsy-proven myocarditis in most patients (Frustaci el al., 2005). The complex links between myocarditis and genetically determined arrhythmic disorders is further discussed below in this chapter.
Various studies on experimental animal models contributed to demonstrate that both autoimmune and viral myocarditis may cause major ventricular arrhythmia. Studies on murine models of myocarditis demonstrated that persistence of inflammation after the acute phase is associated with electrical abnormalities associated with ventricular arrhythmias; interestingly, a close correlation between the location of inflammatory burden (associated with myocyte necrosis), the reported electric abnormalities and the site of origin of arrhythmias was found (Kishimoto et al., 1983; Hoshino et al., 1982;). The major mechanisms involved in the genesis of arrhythmias seems to be the formation of micro-reentry circuits, favored by myocyte injury and replacement fibrosis, and triggered activity mainly due to the pro-arrhythmic effects of cytokines. Moreover it was reported that the environment surrounding myocytes could influence the electrophysiological properties of the myocardium, this phenomenon is known as electrical remodeling. As previously pointed out the inflammatory process of the myocardium may itself be arrhythmogenic, nonetheless the change in the electrophysiological properties of the myocardiocytes seems also play a role in causing the arrhythmias. Changes in expression of surface ion channels, as assessed by quantitative determination of mRNA expression, have been demonstrated in animal experimental models of both viral and autoimmune myocarditis; these changes, affecting mainly potassium and calcium channels, causes modification of the ventricular effective refractory period, which appear to be longer in myocarditis, an increase in monofasic action potential duration of the ventricular myocardium and an augment of ventricular vulnerability that ultimately favors the genesis of ventricular arrhythmias (Saito et al., 2006). Interestingly, some data suggests that these changes may be transient and can reverse after the healing of the inflammatory process. Altogether, these data further support the hypothesis that active inflammation represents a major substrate of ventricular arrhythmias and suggests that pro-arrhythmic changes of myocardial electrical properties caused by the inflammation might be, completely or partially, reversed after the healing of the inflammatory process.

2.1 Myocarditis and sudden arrhythmic death

In the last decades myocarditis has emerged as an important cause of sudden arrhythmic death also in patients with a structurally and functionally normal heart. The most striking evidence that myocarditis may be the substrate of sudden arrhythmic death is represented by a study on Air Force recruits victims of cardiac sudden death in which myocarditis was recognized as the cause of death in 40% of cases (Phillips et al., 1986)
Although no data on cardiac function before death were available in the study, the percentage of cases in which myocarditis was observed at necropsy studies indicates the high arrhythmic risk related to myocarditis. In more recent studies the percentage of myocarditis detected at necropsy in subjects with sudden arrhythmic death and an apparently normal heart ranged from 5 to 12% (Doolan et al., 2004; Thelemann et al., 2001).

In a study performed in our Institution in 1994 seventeen young patients (10 males and 7 females, aged 14 to 38 years, mean 26.4) without overt organic heart disease, who had been resuscitated from sudden cardiac arrest were submitted to noninvasive (electrocardiography, 2D-echocardiography, and magnetic resonance imaging) and invasive (coronary angiography with ergonovine testing, electrophysiologic study and biventricular angiography and endomyocardial biopsy) cardiac studies. Six to 8 biopsy fragments per patient were processed for histology and electron microscopy and read by a pathologist blinded to clinical data. Two groups of patients were distinguished by invasive and noninvasive examinations: Group 1 consisted of 9 patients with entirely normal parameters; Group 2 consisted of 8 patients with structural, nonspecific cardiac abnormalities. In this latter group, mild to moderate dilatation and hypokinesia of the left ventricle were documented in 4 patients, concentric left ventricular hypertrophy was seen in three patients, and RV dysfunction was noted in 1 patient. Histologic examination was abnormal in all patients and revealed specific lesions in 65% of them; in particular an active myocarditis was diagnosed in 6 out of 9 patients in the Group 1. In these 6 patients immunosuppressive therapy (steroids plus azathioprine) administered on top of conventional antiarrhthmic treatment led to dispappearance of ventricular arrhythmias and healing of myocardial inflammation at follow-up endomyocardial biopsies (Frustaci et al., 1994) Similarly in a study from the Padua group in a series of 273 sudden cardiac deaths victims, 76 cases (28%) presented a macroscopically normal heart: of these 60 (79%) had abnormal histology with a 36% of cases of active myocarditis (Corrado et al., 2001). These data suggest that myocarditis represents an important, frequently unrecognized and underestimated, cause of sudden arrhythmic death. Moreover these studies dramatically demonstrate that sudden arrhythmic death may represent the very first clinical manifestation of myocarditis. Accordingly the consensus document based on the two main registries on sudden arrhythmic death (the UCARE, Unexplained Cardiac Arrest Registry of Europe and the IVF-US, Idiopathic Ventricular Fibrillation Registry of United States) includes myocarditis among the subclinical disorders that may cause sudden death (UCARE, 1997).

It should be also emphasized that myocarditis is a cause of sudden arrhythmic death even in competitive athletes, more frequently exposed to viral infections of upper airways. With this regard it has been claimed but never conclusively demonstrated that exercise in the context of an active myocarditis may represent a further arrhythmic trigger.

2.1.1 Myocarditis and genetically determined arrhythmic syndromes

In the last decades several studies suggested a role for myocardial inflammation in the pathogenesis of different genetically determined arrhythmic syndromes and cardiomyopathies. In the presence of gene mutations leading to abnormal structure and/or function of structural and functional proteins, myocardial inflammation may act as a mechanism of myocardial damage, amplificating the dysfunction related to the genetic abnormalities, or rather as trigger of specific clinical manifestations, such as arrhythmias, occurring later in the natural history of the disease. Myocardial inflammation has been observed in necropsy and endomyocardial biopsy studies in genetically determined myocardial disorders, including ARVC, Brugada syndrome and hypertrophic cardiomyopathy.

In ARVC myocardial inflammation may be seen in up to 75% of hearts at autopsy, and probably it plays a role in triggering ventricular tachyarrhythmias (Thiene et al., 2001). Nobody knows whether inflammation is a reactive phenomenon to cell death, or whether it is the consequence of an infection or immune mechanism. Viruses have been detected in the myocardium of some ARVC patients and have been claimed to support an infective etiology of the disease (Bowles et al., 2002). Others say that the viruses are innocent bystanders or that spontaneous cell degeneration may serve as a milieu favoring viral settlement in the myocardium (Calabrese et al., 2006). In addition we and others demonstrated that myocarditis may present with clinical and arrhythmic features and structural right ventricular abnormalities resemblig those observed in ARVC. (Chimenti et al., 2004; Pieroni et al., 2009).

With regard to Brugada syndrome we studied 18 consecutive patients with clinical phenotype of Brugada syndrome and normal cardiac structure and function on noninvasive examinations. Clinical presentation was ventricular fibrillation in 7 patients, sustained polymorphic ventricular tachycardia in 7, and syncope in 4. All patients underwent cardiac catheterization, coronary and ventricular angiography, biventricular endomyocardial biopsy, and DNA screening of the *SCN5A* gene. Biopsy samples were processed for histology, electron microscopy, and molecular screening for viral genomes. In 14 patients histology showed a prevalent or localized right ventricular myocarditis, arrhythmogenic right ventricular cardiomyopathy in 1 patient and cardiomyopathic changes in 3. In the latter 4 patients genetic studies identified *SCN5A* gene mutations causing in vitro abnormal function of mutant proteins. In these patients, myocyte cytoplasm degeneration and a significant increase of apoptotic myocytes in right and left ventricle versus normal controls were observed (Frustaci et al., 2005). This study highlighted the complexities between the clinical manifestations of Brugada syndrome, the presence of *SCN5A* mutations, and the presence of structural heart disease and provided striking new evidence implicating myocarditis in the transient development of Brugada-like ECG abnormalities and arrhythmias.

However it still remains unclear whether myocardial inflammation may be part of the structural changes following an abnormal ion channel function, or rather right ventricular myocarditis may mimic ECG and arrhythmic features of Brugada syndrome. Further studies combining genetic analysis and accurate pathology studies are needed to clarify the complex menage a trois between abnormal gene function (whether affecting desmosomal or ion channel proteins), myocardial inflammation and inherited arrhythmic syndromes.

Myocarditis has been also observed in patients with hypertrophic cardiomyopathy and severe arrhythimic manifestations, suggesting that inflammation may act as a trigger for life-threatening ventricular arrhythmias when affecting a myocardium already prone to electrical instability (Frustaci et al., 2007). Even in this context it is not clear whether myocardial inflammation was the result of a reactive process related to ischemic myocyte necrosis or rather a superimposed autoimmune or viral process.

3. The diagnosis of myocarditis in patients with ventricular arrhythmias

Myocardial inflammation represents a potent pro-arrhythmic substrate, myocarditis should always be taken into account when facing with ventricular arrhythmias. Furthermore the detection of myocarditis as the pathological substrate underlying ventricular arrhythmias may be crucial as the identification of myocarditis as the etiology of the arrhythmias is actually important for targeting therapies and may have implications even for patients' relatives as discussed below in the chapter. In the last decades the development of new imaging techniques, in particular CMR, led to an increased recognition of myocarditis as a cause of ventricular arrhythmias.

3.1 Cardiac magnetic resonance

Cardiac Magnetic resonance offers a combination of clarity of anatomical visualization, interobserver consistency and quantitative accuracy, even when evaluating the right ventricle, which enables to overcome the major pitfalls of echocardiography. Furthermore it is characterized by the unique feature of providing some degree of tissue characterization, thus allowing to obtain non-invasively information about the presence of necrosis, fibrosis and edema. Nonetheless CMR has some limitations due to the technical difficulty in obtaining good images in patients with arrhythmias that cause high variability of cardiac cycle length and also due to safety issues related to the presence of cardiac rhythm devices. Recently a panel of international experts on CMR has published a white paper in which imaging protocols and diagnostic criteria are defined that should be used in the setting of myocarditis. According to this consensus (Friedrich et al., 2009), a diagnosis of myocarditis can be set when at least two of the following features are present: one area of non-ischemic (i.e. sparing of sub-endocardial layers of the myocardium and/or distribution of areas not consistent with coronary perfusion territories) late gadolinium enhancement (consistent with myocyte injury and scarring), global or regional signal increase in T2-weighted images (indicative of tissue oedema) and global early gadolinium enhancement (consistent with hyperemia) (Figure 1).

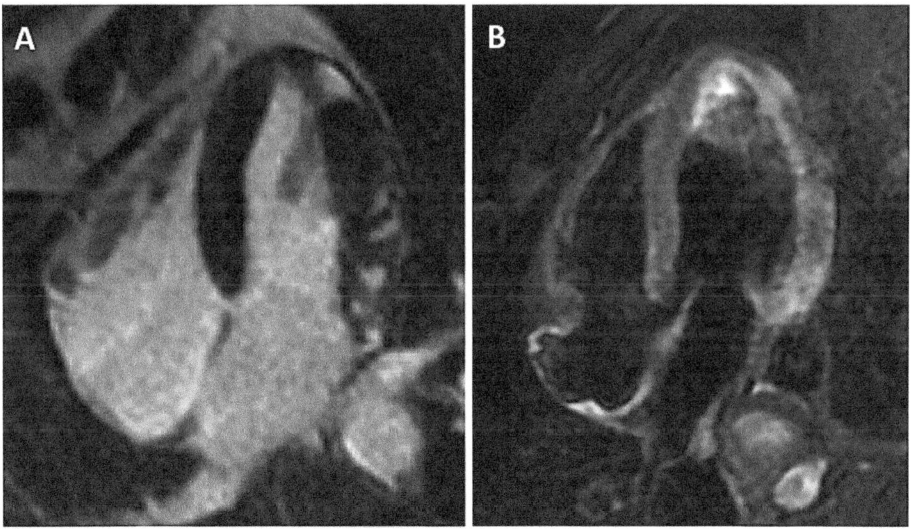

Fig. 1. Diagnosis of myocarditis through CMR in a patient with sustained ventricular arrhythmias. Evidence of spotty areas of sub-epicardial and midwall late enhancement (non-ischemic pattern) in the lateral wall (A), associated with areas of edema (high signal intensity on T2-weighted images) in the same location (B). The presence of both late enhancement and edema fulfils the criteria proposed by the consensus document.

In many studies CMR has demonstrated to be useful for the assessment of the presence of pathological substrates underlying ventricular arrhythmias. Its use allowed to detect the presence of structural cardiomyopathies including myocarditis (Ordovas et al. 2008) in up to 30% of patients. Clinical studies specifically addressing the diagnostic yield of CMR in the setting of myocarditis presenting with either arrhythmia or heart failure reported a sensitivity and specificity of more then up to 90% (Mahrholdt et al., 2004). Moreover, CMR was able to differentiate active from healing inflammation in patients presenting with chronic myocarditis.

In particular, De Cobelli and colleagues studied patients presenting with chronic myocarditis assessed with EMB and CMR; they found areas of high signal intensity in T2-weighted images in 36% of patients with histological evidence of active myocarditis, but not in patients with borderline myocarditis. They also found areas of late gadolinium enhancement in 84% and 44% of patients with active and borderline myocarditis, respectively. A midwall pattern of late enhancement was a frequent finding in patients with both active myocarditis and borderline myocarditis, whereas a subepicardial pattern was only observed in patients with histological evidence of active myocarditis (De Cobelli et al., 2004). Taken together, these data support the need to include sequences for the detection of myocardial inflammation when CMR is performed in the non-invasive diagnostic work-up of patients presenting with ventricular arrhythmias (Figure 2). In addition CMR represents an important noninvasive tool in the follow-up of patients with a diagnosis of myocarditis.

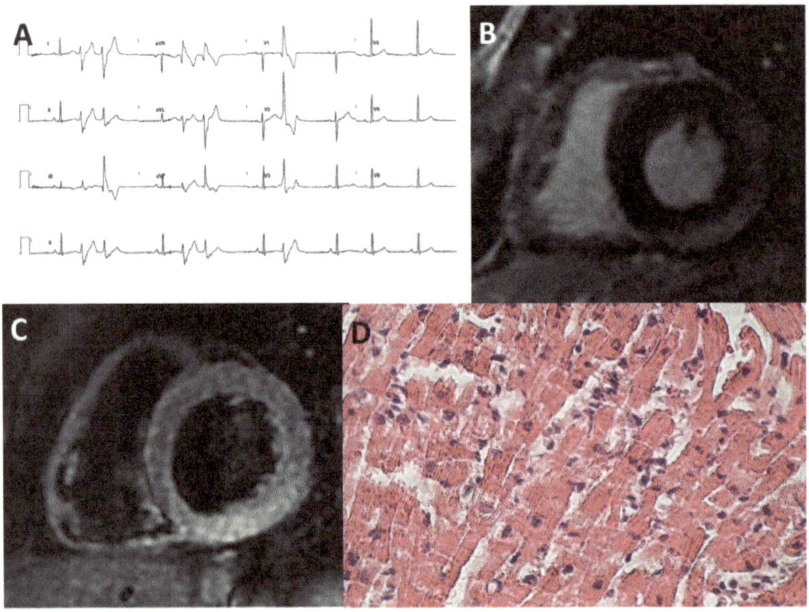

Fig. 2. CMR findings in a patient with chronic myocarditis presenting with ventricular arrhythmias. ECG shows repetitive polymorphic ventricular ectopic beats (A). CMR shows sub-epicardial late enhancement in the posterior and postero-lateral walls (B) and transmural edema in the same location (C). Histology shows the presence of active myocarditis (D).

3.2 Endomyocardial biopsy

Despite the improvement of imaging techniques, endomyocardial biopsy still represents the gold standard for the diagnosis of myocarditis as allow the recognition and the characterization of the myocardial inflammatory process, the assessment of myocyte necrosis and fibrosis as well as the possible detection of viral genomes.

A recent statement from AHA/ACC/ESC (Cooper et al., 2007) aimed to define the role of endomyocardial biopsy in the management of cardiovascular disease, identified 14 clinical scenarios in which the incremental diagnostic, prognostic and therapeutic value of endomyocardial biopsy could be estimated and compared with the procedural risks. According to this statement, in the absence of randomized clinical trials or multicenter studies, endomyocardial biopsy may be considered in the setting of unexplained ventricular arrhythmias (Clinical scenario 13) only in exceptional cases in which the perceived likelihood of meaningful prognostic and therapeutic benefit outweighs the procedural risks (Class of recommendation IIb, Level of evidence C).

Nevertheless there is growing evidence that endomyocardial biopsy may be crucial to clarify the pathological substrate and therefore the cause of otherwise unexplained ventricular arrhythmias, with a possible impact on both treatment and prognosis as detailed further in this chapter.

Accordingly a recent document from the Italian federation of Cardiology (Leone et al., 2009) suggested indications to endomyocardial biopsy different from the above-mentioned statement, in particular with regard to patients with ventricular arrhythmias. The authors graded clinical indications according to the following scheme:

- Grade 1: there are no alternative tools to obtain a definite diagnosis and the clinical implications of diagnosis are certain.
- Grade 2A: there are no alternative tools to obtain a definite diagnosis and the clinical implications of diagnosis are uncertain.
- Grade 2B: there are no alternative tools to obtain a definite diagnosis but the diagnosis has scientific but no clinical implications.
- Grade 3: there are alternative tools to obtain a definite diagnosis.

According to this grading, taking into account the potential diagnostic usefulness of endomyocardial biopsy in different myocardial disorders, the authors identified several clinical scenarios. In the presence of sustained and/or life-threatening ventricular arrhythmias, when a myocarditis is suspected or is a possible diagnosis, the grade of recommendation to perform endomyocardial biopsy is 1. Similarly in the presence of AV blocks associated with a clinical context consistent with a diagnosis of myocarditis, recommendations are Grade 2A and 2B in the presence or in the absence of left ventricular dysfunction respectively. Therefore the Italian Federation of Cardiology document seems to more adequately address the diagnostic and therapeutic issues that are frequently faced by cardiologists in everyday clinical practice when dealing with patients with severe ventricular arrhythmias or atrioventricular conduction disturbances and no evidence of ischemic heart disease or overt valvular or myocardial disease.

Both documents do also indicate how many samples are needed in different clinical conditions, how to handle and process myocardial samples, and which studies are necessary to obtain the desired diagnostic information. In the case of clinically suspected myocarditis 5 to 10 samples must be obtained to perform histology and immunohistochemistry studies and molecular bioloy studies to detect the presence of viral genomes. Samples for molecular biology must be flash-frozen in liquid nitrogen and stored at -80°C. Endomyocardial biopsy should better not be performed in patients with clinically suspected myocarditis, if immunohistochemistry and virology studies are not available.

The main criticism against a wider use of endomyocardial biopsy in the diagnostic approach to patients with ventricular arrhythmias is represented by the possible sampling error in the presence of a focal myocarditis. In fact, as previously mentioned, the myocardial inflammation in patients presenting with arrhythmias may present a patchy distribution and therefore myocardial samples drawn from a same conventional site (the right side of interventriculrar septum or the left ventricular apex) may not include myocardial tissue involved by the inflammatory process. Increasing the number of samples obtained or arbitrarily changing the site of biopsy can in part minimize sampling error, but these tricks may increase the risks of the procedure. To overcome the sampling error and increase the diagnostic sensistivity of endomyocardial biopsy, we recently demonstrated that in patients presenting with ventricular arrhythmias, electroanatomical mapping may guide the execution endomyocardial biopsy identifying the segments of ventricular wall presenting an abnormal voltage, suggesting an abnormal histological substrate (Pieroni et al, 2009; Casella & Dello Russo, 2009). This technique represents an important innovation in the field of endomyocardial biopsy as reduces sampling error and increases the sensitivity of biopsy, thus possibly reducing the number of samples needed for a complete study of myocardial tissue and therefore reducing the risks of the procedure.

3.3 Electroanatomic mapping

Electroanatomic mapping allows operators to record intracardiac electrical activation in relation to anatomic location in a cardiac chamber of interest, even during arrhythmia mapping. Several 3D-EAM systems are currently available that accomplish these tasks. When applied properly, such technology allows one to accurately determine the location of arrhythmia origin, define cardiac chamber geometry in three dimensions, delineate areas of anatomic interest, and allow catheter manipulation and positioning without fluoroscopic guidance. These systems often simplify mapping efforts and can enhance procedural success, particularly in cases in which complex arrhythmias and unusual cardiac anatomy are encountered.

The CARTO mapping system (Biosense, Diamond Bar, CA, USA) is a three-dimensional nonfluoroscopic mapping system that utilizes a low-level magnetic field (5×10^{-6} to 5×10^{-5} Tesla) delivered from three separate coils in a locator pad beneath the patient. The magnetic field strength from each coil is detected by a location sensor embedded proximal to the tip of a specialized mapping catheter. The strength of each coil's magnetic field measured by the location sensor is inversely proportional to the distance between the sensor and coil. Hence, by integrating each coil's field strength and converting this measurement into a distance, the location sensor (and therefore, catheter tip location) can be triangulated in space. The mapping catheter has proximal and distal electrode pairs, and a tip electrode capable of radiofrequency energy delivery. This catheter can be moved along a chamber's surface to record local endocardial activation times for arrhythmia mapping, while simultaneously recording location points to generate 3D chamber geometry. Validation studies have shown CARTO to have substantial accuracy in navigating to single points, in returning to prior ablation sites, and in creating a desired length of ablation line. Electrograms recorded from the specialized mapping (NaviSTAR) catheter showed excellent correlation with recordings from standard EP catheters. Moreover human validation studies have shown a good level of spatial precision and accuracy, and realistic reconstruction of chamber geometry and electroanatomic activation during arrhythmia mapping. Nevertheless in our experience, the comparison between biplane right ventricular angiography and the 3D reconstruction obtained by CARTO showed that small structures such as microaneurysms, can be missed by the mapping catheter and therefore are not properly visualized. These limitations would be partially overcome by importing CT and CMR images and merging them with 3D maps so that during mapping the catheter can be visualized inside the anatomical images.

Similar to CARTO the NavX system is a mapping and 3D nonfluoroscopic intracardiac browsing system that can reconstruct in real time geometry as well as the electric activation of the heart chamber. NavX technology makes use of six surface patch electrodes that generate, once correctly positioned, an electric filed. Within this electric field it is possible to locate in real time the position of every electrophysiology catheter employed during the procedure, including the cardiac bioptome when electically connected to the mapping system. We tested both systems in guiding endomyocardial biopsy execution. Although a comparison between the systems exceeds the scopes of this chapter, CARTO system probably offers a more detailed reconstruction of the ventricular chambers, while NavX system has the advantage of direct real time visulization of the bioptome in the 3D map. In this chapter we will refer to the CARTO system as it was more frequently used in our and other studies.

High-density mapping must be obtained in sinus rhythm (reference channel: QRS complex) by sampling at least 100 points in each chamber, uniformly distributed. The voltage maps are then edited setting the point density (fill threshold) at 15 mm and manually eliminating intracavitary points. According to current literature "electroanatomic scar" is defined as an area including at least 3 adjacent points with bipolar signal amplitude <0.5 mV; the reference value for normal endocardium is usually set at 1,5 mV. In the CARTO system the color display to identify normal and abnormal voltage myocardium ranges from red (electroanatomic scar tissue; amplitude <0.5 mV), to purple (electroanatomic normal tissue; amplitude ≥1.5 mV). Intermediate colors represent the electroanatomic border zone (amplitude >0.5 and <1.5 mV) (Figure 3).

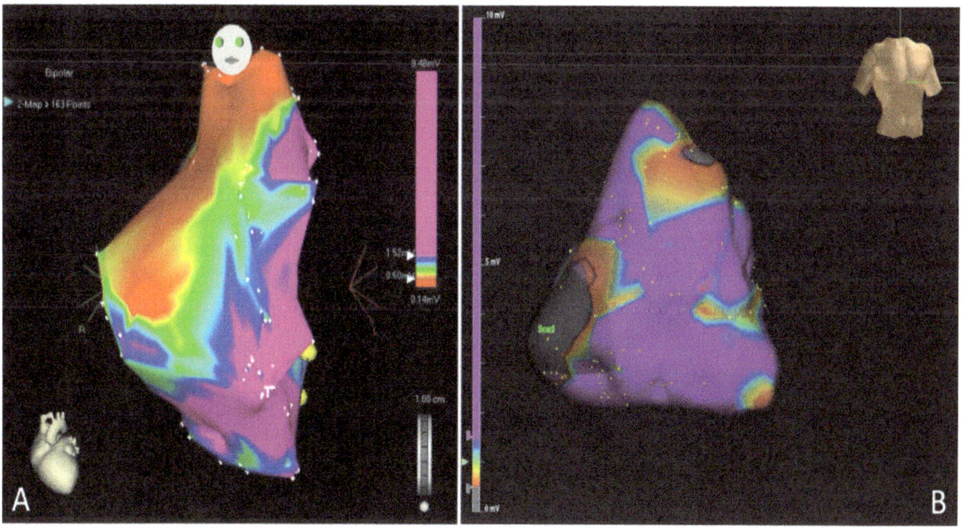

Fig. 3. Example of electroanatomic maps obtained with CARTO (A) and NavX (B) systems. For colours interpretation see text.

Adequate catheter contact should be confirmed by concordant catheter tip motion with the cardiac silhouettes on fluoroscopy and by adherence of voltage map to angiographic right ventricular shape. To avoid low voltage recordings due to poor contact, the following tools can be used: 1) the signal has to satisfy 3 stability criteria automatically detected by CARTO system in terms of cycle length, local activation time and beat-to-beat difference of the location of the catheter (<2%, <3 ms, and <4 mm, respectively); 2) both bipolar and unipolar signals are simultaneously acquired to confirm true catheter contact through the analysis of local electrogram (in particular the shape of the unipolar electrogram); 3) in the presence of a low voltage area, at least 3 additional points should be acquired in the same site to confirm the reproducibility of the voltage measurement. The anatomical distribution of the pathological areas is evaluated dividing the right ventricular voltage map into five segments: outflow tract, free (anterolateral) wall, inferior and posterior basal segments, apex, and interventricular septum.

3.4 Electroanatomic mapping-guided endomyocardial biopsy

The main limitation of endomyocardial biopsy to provide a specific diagnosis in patients with ventricular arrhythmias caused by focal myocardial diseases, (i.e. myocarditis or initial forms of arrhythmogenic right ventricular cardiomyopathy), is represented by the sampling error due to the lack of an effective guide in selecting ventricular areas where to perform biopsies. In the last years, after the development of 3D-EAM systems, we introduced a new technique for the execution of endomyocardial biopsies in patients with ventricular arrhythmias (Pieroni et al., 2009).

3.4.1 Technique

The new approach is aimed to perform endomyocardial biopsies in the ventricular segments presenting electrical abnormalities at electroanatomical mapping. When using the CARTO system, once the electroanatomical map is completed, the mapping catheter is placed in a region of interest of the ventricular wall and the preformed sheath is positioned closed to the catheter tip (Figure 4). Endomyocardial biopsy is then performed in the area with abnormal electrical properties as showed by the map. As previously mentioned, another approach we tested requires the electrical connection of the bioptome to the mapping system: the presence of the metallic jaws makes the bioptome similar to a mapping catheter and it is therefore visualized in the 3D electroanatomical map of the ventricle. In this case, the site of biopsy can be chosen "live", directly mapping the ventricular wall with the bioptome (Figure 4). The latter technique can be adopted when using the NavX mapping system. With both systems we usually performed ventricular angiography before the execution of ventricular mapping, in order to improve the anatomical accuracy of the map, as angiography still represents the gold standard to detect wall motion abnormalities and small aneurysms of the right venticle.

Although no data on specificity and sensitivity of 3D-EAM-guided vs. conventional technique are currently available in literature, it is reasonable that obtaining myocardial samples from areas of the ventricular wall presenting electrical abnormalities will probably reduce the sampling error and the need for multiple biopsies from the same patient (See below). Moreover the combination of 3D-EAM with other imaging tools such as cardiac MRI would further improve our ability to obtain samples from selected regions that present structural, functional and electrical abnormalities.

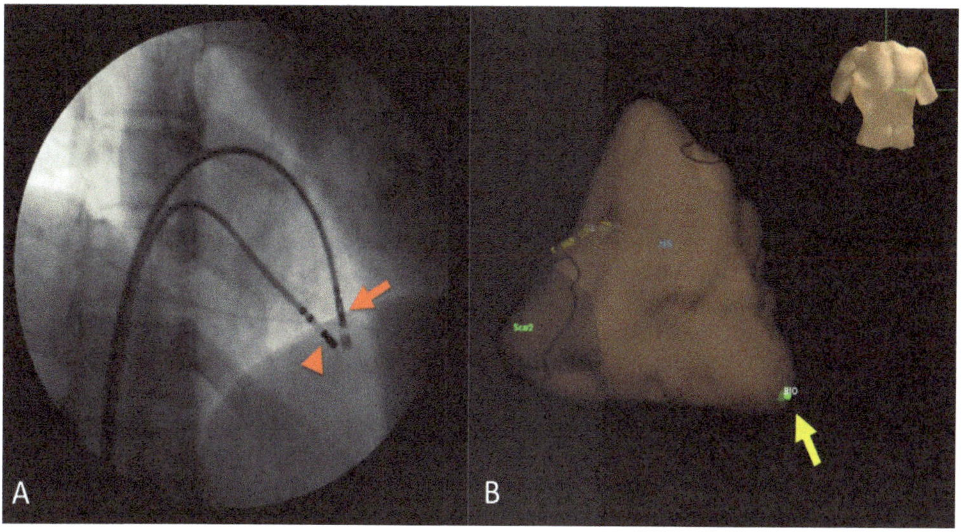

Fig. 4. 3D-EAM-guided EMB. With the CARTO system (A) the long sheath with the bioptome inside (arrow) is positioned near to the mapping catheter (arrowhead). With the NavX system (B) the bioptome tip (green point and arrow) can be directly visualized in the 3D ventricular map.

3.4.2 Safety

The execution of endomyocardial biopsies drawing myocardial samples from non conventional sites, including the right ventricular free-wall and outflow tract do not increase the risks of the procedure. Since 2006 we perfomed 3D-EAM-guided endomyocardial biopsy in more than sixty patients with about 400 samples obtained. In order to evaluate the safety of this new approach we prospectively analysed the rate of major and minor complications through continuous ECG monitoring during the procedure, ECG and 2D-echocardiography at the end the procedure and after 3 and 6 hours. Major complications included pericardial tamponade with need for pericardiocentesis, hemo- and pneumopericardium, permanent atrioventricular block requiring permanent pacemaker implantation, myocardial infarction, transient cerebral ischemic attack and stroke, severe valvular damage, and death, whereas minor complications included transient chest pain, transient ECG abnormalities, transient arrhythmias, transient hypotension, and small pericardial effusions. The major complication rate was 0% and the minor complication rate was 4.5%: minor complications were represented by small pericardial effusions in 2 patients and chest pain in 1. These rates are in line with those observed in a recent large two-centers study including 755 procedures (right, left and biventricular endomyocardial biopsy) and reporting a major and minor complication rate of 0.82% and 5.1% respectively for right ventricular endomyocardial biopsy (Yilmaz et al., 2010). In literature another study in which 3D-EAM-guided endomyocardial biopsy was performed in 22 patients, reported a higher rate of major complications (1.1%) and minor complications (5.7%), thus suggesting that the expertise of the operators besides the clinical condition and the underlying disorder may influence the safety of the procedure (Avella et al., 2008).

4. Electroanatomic mapping-guided endomyocardial biopsy in patients with ventricular arrhythmias

There is growing evidence that 3D-EAM-guided endomyocardial biopsy represent a new important tool to improve the diagnosis and the treatment of patients with arrhythmias, as well as the knowledge of the pathological substrates and mechanisms ubderlying arrhythmic syndromes. Since 2006 we performed 66 3D-EAM-guided endomyocardial biopsy procedures. In all cases the biopsies where drawn from the right ventricle, with biventricular mapping and 3D-EAM-guided biopsy being performed in 10 patients. Although data on a direct comparison between 3D-EAM-guide and conventional technique are not yet available, the 3D-EAM-guided approach seems to significantly improve the diagnostic sensitivity and specificity of endomyocardial biopsy. In fact, when applying immunohistochemistry and molecular biology techniques, a definite histologic diagnosis was obtained in all cases. The new technique was firstly adopted in a series of 30 patients with a noninvasive diagnosis of ARVC according to current diagnostic criteria (Pieroni et al., 2009). Twenty-nine (97%) of 30 patients presented an abnormal voltage map. Histology and immunohistochemistry confirmed the diagnosis of ARVC in 15 patients, while showed an active myocarditis in the remaining 15 patients (Figure 5). Patients with ARVC were not distinguishable on the basis of clinical features, presence and severity of structural and functional right ventricular abnormalities and three-dimensional 3D-EAM findings.

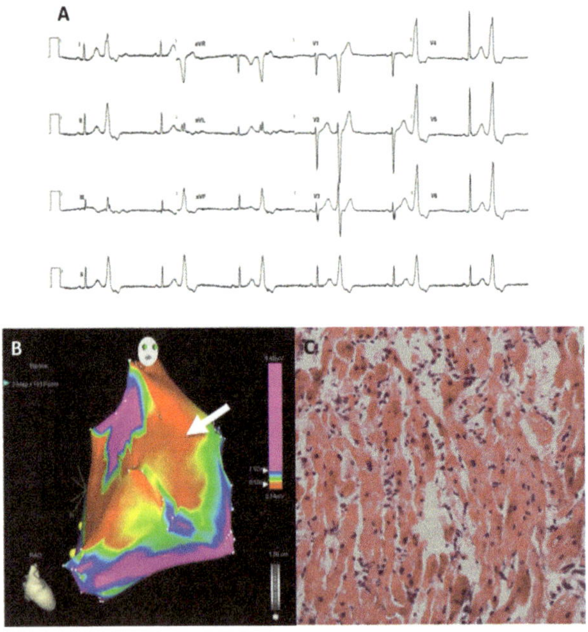

Fig. 5. 3D-EAM-guided EMB, in a patient with bigeminism due to ventricular ectopic beats with LBBB morphology and inferior axis (A). 3D-EAM shows low voltages in the outflow tract and free wall (B). Endomyocardial biopsies drawn from free wall (arrow) shows active myocarditis (C).

On the basis of clinical and histological features, a cardioverter defibrillator was implanted in 13 patients with biopsy-proven ARVC and in 1 patient only with myocarditis. At a mean follow-up of 21±8 months, 7 (47%) patients with ARVC experienced recurrence of symptomatic sustained ventricular arrhythmias with appropriate defibrillator intervention in all cases. All patients with myocarditis remained asymptomatic and free from arrhythmic events. Our study was the first to demonstrate that 3D-EAM-guided EMB may allow obtaining a differential diagnosis in patients with otherwise undistiguishable clinical, arrhythmic and imaging features. In addition our study clearly showed that patients with similar arrhythmic presentation may have a dramatically different prognosis in terms of arrhythmias' recurrence according to the underlying disorders, as only 53% of biopsy-proven ARVC patients remained free from arrhythmias at a mean follow-up of 21±8 months years, while no patients with biopsy-proven myocarditis experienced major arrhythmic events during the same time (Figure 6).

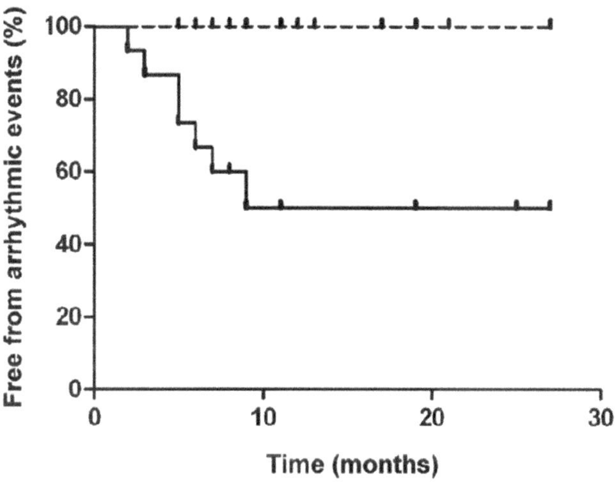

Fig. 6. Kaplan-Meier analysis of arrhythmic event-free survival depending on the histological findings (Modified from Pieroni et al. 2009).

In a more recent study (Pieroni et al unpublished data) we performed 3D-EAM-guided EMB in a series of elite competitive athletes presenting with sustained ventricular arrhythmias. We studied 13 consecutive competitive athletes with evidence of sustained ventricular arrhythmias within the previous six months on 12-lead ECG, 24-hour Holter ECG or ECG exercise testing and who were judged as having a structurally normal heart after a thorough non-invasive evaluation, including signal-averaged electrocardiogram, transthoracic echocardiogram and CMR. Depending on the presumed site of arrhythmias origin according to 12-lead ECG criteria, patients underwent right or left ventricular 3D-EAM and 3D-EAM-guided endomyocardial biopsy. Twelve (92%) patients presented at least 1 low-voltage region at 3D-EAM, while the histologic diagnosis was active myocarditis in 7 patients, and of arrhythmogenic RV cardiomyopathy in 5. In one patient the histological evidence of contraction-band necrosis allowed to unmask caffeine and ephedrine abuse.

The identification of the underlying histological substrate in patients with ventricular arrhythmias may be relevant also when radiofrequency catheter ablation (RFCA) is considered as a possible therapeutic strategy. In fact there is growing evidence that in patients with ARVC, RFCA is effective in abolishing ventricular tachycardias, but the rate or recurrence of arrhthmias with the same or a different morphology may be very high even when an epicardial approach is adopted (Dalal et al., 2007). On the contrary several reports have demonstrated that RFCA may be effective in eliminating ventricular arrhythmias in myocardial inflammatory disorders, including Chagas cardiomyopathy and sarcoidosis (Sosa et al., 1999; Sarabanda et al., 2005; Jefic et al., 2009; Henz et al., 2009). Recent reports and also our experience suggest that endocardial ablation cannot be sufficient in some patients and a combined endo-epicardial approach is required for definitive results. (See below, Clinical implications of myocarditis diagnosis)

5. Clinical implications of myocarditis diagnosis in patients with ventricular arrhythmias

Despite the improvement of diagnostic techniques in defining the characteristics and the etiology of the inflammatory process and the more specific comprehension of the mechanisms leading to myocardial damage, a specific standardized treatment of myocarditis is not yet available. However in the last decades several studies and trials have clearly demonstrated that an etiologic definition of myocarditis based on the immunohistological evaluation of inflammation and proof of viral infection by PCR on biopsies is essential for targeting appropriate treatment strategies indicating that myocarditis patients may benefit from immunosuppression, provided that viral persistence is excluded, while patients with viral persistence fail to respond favourably or deteriorate by immunosuppression.

Several studies have demonstrated the negative prognostic role of viral persistence. In a recent study Kuhl and colleagues analyzed 172 patients with dilated cardiomyopathy and biopsy-proven viral infection in endomyocardial biopsies. The authors reported a high prevalence of enteroviral and parvovirus B19 infection (32.6% and 36.6%, respectively) and found that viral persistence was associated with a progressive impairment of left ventricular ejection fraction, whereas spontaneous viral elimination was associated with a significant improvement in left ventricular function (Kuhl et al., 2005).

Autoimmunity, on the other hand, may play an outstanding role in the progression of myocardial damage and persistence of symptoms, including ventricular arrhythmias. Notably, both acute viral infection and chronic viral persistence can induce autoimmunity by mechanisms not fully elucidated. Molecular mimicry has been suggested as one mechanism to explain chronic myocarditis (Caforio et al., 2002; Rose et al., 2006) and several cellular antigens have been identified to cross-react with viral antigens, thus providing possible targets in virus-induced myocarditis. Autoantibody production also may be caused by the initial myocyte damage by viral infection, releasing increased amounts of self-antigens into the circulation. Autoantibodies against adrenergic and acetylcholine receptors contractile structures, extracellular matrix proteins, proteins involved in energy metabolism, calcium receptors and homeostasis and antistress proteins have all been detected in patients with myocarditis (Neumann et al., 1994; Pankuweit et al., 1997). Furthermore, autoimmunity is considered the main pathogenetic mechanism underlying eosinophilic, giant-cell and granulomatous myocarditis (Cihakova et al., 2008), as well as myocarditis associated with connective tissue diseases, peripartum cardiomyopathy (Ansari et al., 2002) or heart transplant, in which immunosuppression has been proven effective.

Immunosuppression is clearly recommended essentially for the treatment of eosinophilic, granulomatous, giant-cell myocarditis and lymphocytic myocarditis associated with connective tissue diseases or with the rejection of a transplanted heart. With regard to idiopathic lymphocytic myocarditis, beyond acute phase where a spontaneous resolution has been reported in up to 40% of the cases, many patients with idiopathic myocarditis and chronic heart failure are likely to benefit from immunosuppression. An up-regulation of HLA antigens in the myocardial tissue of patients with lymphocytic myocarditis has been proposed as a marker of susceptibility to beneficial effects of immunosuppression (Wojnicz et al., 2001). Recently the data from a randomized double-blind, placebo-controlled study designed to evaluate the efficacy of immunosuppression in virus-negative inflammatory cardiomyopathy have been reported (Frustaci et al., 2009). Eighty-five patients with myocarditis and chronic (>6 months) heart failure unresponsive to conventional therapy and no evidence of myocardial viral genomes were randomized to receive either prednisone and azathioprine (43 patients, Group 1) or placebo (42 patients, Group 2) in addition to conventional therapy for heart failure. Primary outcome was the 6 months improvement in left-ventricular function. Group 1 showed a significant improvement of left-ventricular ejection fraction and a significant decrease in left-ventricular dimensions and volumes compared with baseline. None of Group 2 patients showed improvement of ejection fraction, that significantly worsened compared with baseline. No major adverse reaction was registered as a result of immunosuppression. These data confirmed the efficacy of immunosuppression in virus-negative inflammatory cardiomyopathy. Lack of response in 12% of cases suggested the presence of not screened viruses or mechanisms of damage and inflammation not susceptible to immunosuppression. Antiviral therapy is a logical strategy advocated for the treatment of myocarditis in patients with evidence of viral presence in myocardial tissue. In a small phase II study 22 patients with myocarditis and biopsy-proven viral persistence (15 enteroviral and 7 adenoviral) were treated with interferon-beta $18x10^6$ IU/week for 24 weeks. Interferon-b treatment resulted in complete elimination of both enteroviral and adenoviral genomes and hemodynamic improvement, as shown by improvement of EF and amelioration of heart failure symptoms. Importantly, treatment with interferon-beta was safe and well-tolerated, with no adverse cardiac effects, and flu-like side effects could be efficiently eliminated by non-steroidal anti-inflammatory drugs (Kuhl et al., 2003). After these encouraging results, a prospective placebo-controlled randomized multicenter study, the Betaferon® in Chronic Viral Cardiomyopathy (BICC) trial, was initiated in 2002 and presented at the 2008 American Heart Association scientific sessions. The primary endpoint was virus elimination or reduction of virus load. At 24-week follow-up, compared to placebo, virus elimination and/or viral load reduction were significantly higher in the interferon group. Moreover, interferon-beta showed a good safety profile and was associated with beneficial effects on clinical secondary endpoints, such as NYHA functional class and quality of life, as assessed by Minnesota questionnaire, although echocardiographic and hemodynamic parameters were not statistically significantly different. This interesting phase II study showed proof of concept for targeted therapy based on molecular diagnosis in inflammatory cardiomyopathy. Future directions in the field of antiviral therapy include preventing direct viral damage and inhibition of viral proliferation by preventing the interaction of viruses with their cellular receptor and their consequent signalling amplification systems, such as the tyrosine kinase p56lck, phosphatase CD45 and downstream ERK1/2 (Liu et al., 2000). Therefore, additional research is required to further understand the mechanisms of viral heart disease and consequently identify new potential targets for therapy.

No specific trial or data from single-center studies on the treatment of myocarditis presenting with ventricular arrhythmias are currently available in literature. In patients with acute myocarditis, therapy for arrhythmias is essentially supportive, since arrhythmias usually resolve after the acute phase of the disease, which can last several weeks, together with the resoluton of the inflammatory process. Even in chronic myocarditis, management of ventricular arrhythmias is currently confined to antiarrhythmic drug therapy, with limited efficacy, and to implantable cardioverter-defibrillator for higher-risk patients, including those with hemodynamically unstable ventricular tachycardias (Zipes et al., 2006) and those with aborted sudden death. Radiofrequency catheter ablation has been demonstrated to be effective in reducing ventricular tachycardia occurrence in patients with Chagas cardiomyopathy and sarcoidosis. Regarding ventricular arrhythmias in patients with lymphocytic myocarditis, isolated reports suggest that RFCA may be effective, (Chauhan et al., 2008; Hama et al. 2009; Kettering et al., 2009; Zeppenfeld et al., 2007) but its safety and long-term efficacy in this setting is unclear. In our Institution we documented the safety and efficacy of RFCA in a series of consecutive patients with chronic active myocarditis presenting with drug-refractory ventricular tachycardias. We enrolled 20 pts with biopsy-proven myocarditis and drug-refractory ventricular tachycardia including 5 pts presenting with electrical storm. All patients underwent endocardial RFCA with an irrigation catheter, using contact electroanatomical mapping. Recurrence of sustained ventricular tachycardia after endocardial RFCA was treated with additional epicardial RFCA. Endocardial RFCA was acutely successful in 14 pts (70%), while in the remaining 6 pts (30%) clinical ventricular tachycardia was successfully ablated by epicardial RFCA thus demonstrating that in patients with myocarditis, RFCA of drug-refractory ventricular tachycardia is feasible, safe and effective and that epicardial RFCA should be considered as an important therapeutic option to increase success rate (Pieroni and colleagues in press).

6. Conclusion

Myocarditis represents a frequent but often underestimated cause of life-threatening ventricular arrhyhmias and sudden arrhythmic death and therefore should be always suspected in these clinical settings. The recognition of myocarditis as the cuase of ventricular arrhythmias may have dramatic implications on treatment and prognosis. Imaging techniques such as CMR have improved our ability to recognize myocardial inflammatory damage, and increased the awareness of the disease among physicians. Nevertheless EMB still represents the gold standard for the diagnosis of myocarditis as offers a immunohistological and virological characterization of thr inflammatoty process that may influence the treatment. Electroanatomic mapping-guided EMB represents a new important technique that allows increasing diagnostic sensitivity and minimizing the sampling error in patients with myocarditis presenting with arrhythmias. In the next future 3D-EAM-guide EMB will also represent an important research tool in the study of channellopathies and other genetically determined arrhythmic syndromes.

7. References

Andréoletti L, Ventéo L, Douche-Aourik F, et al. Active Coxsackieviral B infection is associated with disruption of dystrophin in endomyocardial tissue of patients who died suddenly of acute myocardial infarction. J Am Coll Cardiol 2007;50:2207-14.

Ansari AA, Fett JD, Carraway RE, et al. Autoimmune mechanisms as the basis for human peripartum cardiomyopathy. Clin Rev Allergy Immunol 2002; 23: 301-324.

Aretz HT, Billingham ME, Edwards WD, et al. Myocarditis. A histopathologic definition and classification. Am J Cardiovasc Pathol 1987;1:3-14.

Avella A, d'Amati G, Pappalardo A, et al. Diagnostic value of endomyocardial biopsy guided by electroanatomic voltage mapping in arrhythmogenic right ventricular cardiomyopathy/dysplasia. J Cardiovasc Electrophysiol. 2008;19:1127-34.

Basso C, Carturan E, Corrado D, Thiene G. Myocarditis and dilated cardiomyopathy in athletes: diagnosis, management, and recommendations for sport activity. Cardiol Clin. 2007;25:423-9.

Bowles NE, Ni J, Marcus F, Towbin JA. The detection of cardiotropic viruses in the myocardium of patients with arrhythmogenic right ventricular dysplasia/cardiomyopathy. J Am Coll Cardiol. 2002;39:892–895.

Caforio AL, Mahon NJ, Tona F,McKenna WJ. Circulating cardiac autoantibodies in dilated cardiomyopathy and myocarditis: pathogenetic and clinical significance. Eur J Heart Fail 2002; 4: 411-417.

Calabrese F, Basso C, Carturan E, Valente M, Thiene G. Arrhythmogenic right ventricular cardiomyopathy/dysplasia: is there a role for viruses? Cardiovasc Pathol. 2006;15:11–17.

Casella M, Dello Russo A. (2008). *An atlas of radioscopic catheter placement for the electrophysiologist.* Springer-Verlag. ISBN:978-1-84800-226-5, London.

Chauhan VS, Hameedullah I, Nanthakumar K, Downar E. Epicardial catheter ablation of incessant ventricular tachycardia in giant cell myocarditis. J Cardiovasc Electrophysiol 2008;19:1219.

Chimenti C, Calabrese F, Thiene G, Pieroni M, Maseri A, Frustaci A. Inflammatory left ventricular microaneurysms as a cause of apparently idiopathic ventricular tachyarrhythmias. Circulation 2001;104:168-73.

Chimenti C, Pieroni M, Maseri A, Frustaci A. Histologic findings in patients with clinical and instrumental diagnosis of sporadic arrhythmogenic right ventricular dysplasia. J Am Coll Cardiol 2004; 43: 2305 - 2313.

Cihakova D; Rose NR. Pathogenesis of myocarditis and dilated cardiomyopathy. Adv Immunol 2008; 99: 95-114.

Cooper LT, Baughman KL, Feldman AM et al. American Heart Association; American College of Cardiology; European Society of Cardiology. The role of endomyocardial biopsy in the management of cardiovascular disease: a scientific statement from the American Heart Association, the American College of Cardiology, and the European Society of Cardiology. Circulation 2007;116:2216-33.

Cooper LT. Myocarditis. N Engl J Med. 2009;360:1526–38.

Corrado D, Basso C, Thiene G. Sudden cardiac death in young people with apparently normal heart. Cardiovasc Res 2001;50:399-408.

Dalal D, Jain R, Tandri H, Dong J, Eid SM, Prakasa K, et al. Long-term efficacy of catheter ablation of ventricular tachycardia in patients with arrhythmogenic right ventricular dysplasia/cardiomyopathy. J Am Coll Cardiol 2007;50:432-40.

De Cobelli F, Pieroni M, Esposito A, et al. Delayed gadolinium-enhanced cardiac magnetic resonance in patients with chronic myocarditis presenting with heart failure or recurrent arrhythmias. J Am Coll Cardiol 2006;47:1649-54.

Doolan A, Langlois N, Semsarian C. Causes of sudden cardiac death in young Australians. Med J Aust 2004;180:110-112.

Fabre A, Sheppard MN. Sudden adult death syndrome and other non-ischaemic causes of sudden cardiac death. Heart. 2006 Mar;92(3):316-20.

Fabre A, Sheppard MN. Sudden adult death syndrome and other non-ischaemic causes of sudden cardiac death. Heart. 2006;92:316-20.

Feldman AM, McNamara D. Myocarditis. N Engl J Med. 2000;343:1388–98.

Friedman RA, Kearney DL, Moak JP, Fenrich AL, Perry JC. Persistence of ventricular arrhythmia after resolution of occult myocarditis in children and young adults. J Am Coll Cardiol 1994;24:780-3.

Friedrich MG, Sechtem U, Schulz-Menger J, Holmvang G, Alakija P, Cooper LT, White JA, Abdel-Aty H, Gutberlet M, Prasad S, Aletras A, Laissy JP, Paterson I, Filipchuk NG, Kumar A, Pauschinger M, Liu P; International Consensus Group on Cardiovascular Magnetic Resonance in Myocarditis. Cardiovascular magnetic resonance in myocarditis: A JACC White Paper. J Am Coll Cardiol. 2009;53:1475-87.

Frustaci A, Bellocci F, Olsen EG. Results of biventricular endomyocardial biopsy in survivors of cardiac arrest with apparently normal hearts. Am J Cardiol 1994;74:890-5.

Frustaci A, Priori SG, Pieroni M, et al. Cardiac histological substrate in patients with clinical phenotype of Brugada syndrome. Circulation 2005;112:3680 –7.

Frustaci A, Russo MA, Chimenti C. Randomized study on the efficacy of immunosuppressive therapy in patients with virus-negative inflammatory cardiomyopathy: the TIMIC study. Eur Heart J. 2009;30:1995-2002.

Frustaci A, Verardo R, Caldarulo M, Acconcia MC, Russo MA, Chimenti C. Myocarditis in hypertrophic cardiomyopathy patients presenting acute clinical deterioration. Eur Heart J. 2007;28:733-40.

Granér M, Lommi J, Kupari M, Raisanen-Sokolowski A, Toivonen L. Multiple forms of sustained monomorphic ventricular tachycardia as common presentation in giant-cell myocarditis. Heart 2007;93:119-21.

Hama Y, Funabashi N, Ueda M, et al. Right-sided heart wall thickening and delayed enhancement caused by chronic active myocarditis complicated by sustained monomorphic ventricular tachycardia. Circulation 2009;119:e200-3.

Henz BD, do Nascimento TA, Dietrich Cde O, et al. Simultaneous epicardial and endocardial substrate mapping and radiofrequency catheter ablation as first-line treatment for ventricular tachycardia and frequent ICD shocks in chronic chagasic cardiomyopathy. J Interv Card Electrophysiol 2009;26:195-205.

Hofmann R, Trappe HJ, Klein H, Kemnitz J. Chronic (or healed) myocarditis mimicking arrhythmogenic right ventricular dysplasia. Eur Heart J 1993;14:717–20.

Hoshino T, Matsumori A, Kawai C, Imai J. Electrocardiographic abnormalities in Syrian golden hamsters with coxsackievirus B1 myocarditis. Jpn Circ J 1982;46:1305-12.

Hoshino T, Matsumori A, Kawai C, Imai J. Ventricular aneurysms and ventricular arrhythmias complicating Coxsackie virus B1 myocarditis of Syrian golden hamsters. Cardiovasc Res. 1984;18:24-9.

Jefic D, Joel B, Good E, Morady F, Rosman H, Knight B, Bogun F. Role of radiofrequency catheter ablation of ventricular tachycardia in cardiac sarcoidosis: report from a multicenter registry. Heart Rhythm. 2009;6:189-95.

Kettering K, Kampmann C, Mollnau H, Kreitner KF, Munzel T, Weiss C. Catheter ablation of an incessant ventricular tachycardia originating from the left aortic sinus cusp in an adolescent with subacute myocarditis. Clin Res Cardiol 2009;98:66-70.

Kishimoto C, Matsumori A, Kawai C. Electrocardiographic findings in experimental murine myocarditis--arrhythmias in the chronic stage. Jpn Circ J. 1983;47:1317-21.

Koplan BA, Soejima K, Baughman K, et al. Refractory ventricular tachycardia secondary to cardiac sarcoid: electrophysiologic characteristics, mapping, and ablation. Heart Rhythm 2006;3:924 -9.

Kuhl U, Pauschinger M, Schwimmbeck PL, et al. Interferon-beta treatment eliminates cardiotropic viruses and improves left ventricular function in patients with myocardial persistence of viral genomes and left ventricular dysfunction. Circulation 2003; 107: 2793-2798.

Kuhl U, Pauschinger M, Seeberg B, et al. Viral persistence in the myocardium is associated with progressive cardiac dysfunction. Circulation 2005; 112: 1965-1970.

Leone O, Rapezzi C, Sinagra G, Angelini A, Arbustini E, Bartoloni G, Basso C, Caforio AL, Calabrese F, Coccolo F, d'Amati G, Mariesi E, Milanesi O, Nodari S, Oliva F, Perkan A, Prandstraller D, Pucci A, Ramondo A, Silvestri F, Valente M, Thiene G; Federazione Italiana di Cardiologia; Associazione per la Patologia Cardiovascolare Italiana. Consensus document on endomyocardial biopsy of the Associazione per la Patologia Cardiovascolare Italiana. G Ital Cardiol. 2009;10:3S-50S

Liu, P, Aitken, K, Kong, YY, *et al.* The tyrosine kinase p56lck is essential in coxsackievirus B3-mediated heart disease. Nat Med 2000; 6: 429-434.

Magnani JW, Danik HJ, Dec GW, Jr., DiSalvo TG. Survival in biopsy-proven myocarditis: a long-term retrospective analysis of the histopathologic, clinical, and hemodynamic predictors. Am Heart J 2006;151:463-70.

Mahrholdt H, Goedecke H, Wagner A et al. Cardiovascular magnetic resonance assessment of human myocarditis: comparison to histology and molecular pathology. Circulation 2004;109:1250-8.

Matsumori A, Kishimoto C, Kawai C, Sawada S. Right ventricular aneurysms complicating encephalomyocarditis virus myocarditis in mice. Jpn Circ J. 1983;47:1322-4.

Muratore CA, Baranchuk A. Current and emerging therapeutic options for the treatment of chronic chagasic cardiomyopathy. Vasc Health Risk Manag 2010;6:593-601.

Neumann DA, Rose NR, Ansari AA,Herskowitz A. Induction of multiple heart autoantibodies in mice with coxsackievirus B3- and cardiac myosin-induced autoimmune myocarditis. J Immunol 1994; 152: 343-350.

Ohkubo K, Watanabe I, Okumuru Y et al. Right ventricular histological substrate and conduction delay in patients with Brugada Syndrome. Int J Cardiol 2010;51:17-23).

Ordovas KG, Reddy GP, Higgins CB. MRI in nonischemic acquired heart disease. J Magn Reson Imaging. 2008;27:1195–213.

Ott P, Marcus FI, Sobonya RE, Morady F, Knight BP, Fuenzalida CE. Cardiac sarcoidosis masquerading as right ventricular dysplasia. Pacing Clin Electrophysiol. 2003;26:1498-503.

Pankuweit S, Portig I, Lottspeich F,Maisch B. Autoantibodies in sera of patients with myocarditis: characterization of the corresponding proteins by isoelectric focusing and N-terminal sequence analysis. J Mol Cell Cardiol 1997; 29: 77-84.

Phillips MP, Robinowitz M, Higgins JR, et al. Sudden cardiac death in Air Force recruits. JAMA 1986;256:2696-2699.

Pieroni M, Dello Russo A, Marzo F, et al. High prevalence of myocarditis mimicking arrhythmogenic right ventricular cardiomyopathy differential diagnosis by electroanatomic mapping-guided endomyocardial biopsy. J Am Coll Cardiol 2009;53:681-9.

Rose NR. The significance of autoimmunity in myocarditis. Ernst Schering Res Found Workshop 2006: 141-154.

Saito J, Niwano S, Niwano H, et al. Electrical remodeling of the ventricular myocardium in myocarditis: studies of rat experimental autoimmune myocarditis. Circ J 2002;66:97-103.

Sarabanda AV, Sosa E, Simoes MV, Figueiredo GL, Pintya AO, Marin-Neto JA. Ventricular tachycardia in Chagas' disease: a comparison of clinical, angiographic, electrophysiologic and myocardial perfusion disturbances between patients presenting with either sustained or nonsustained forms. Int J Cardiol 2005;102:9-19.

Sosa E, Scanavacca M, D'Avila A, Bellotti G, Pilleggi F. Radiofrequency catheter ablation of ventricular tachycardia guided by nonsurgical epicardial mapping in chronic Chagasic heart disease. Pacing Clin Electrophysiol 1999;22:128-30.

Theleman KP, Kuiper JJ, Roberts WC Acute myocarditis (predominately lymphocytic) causing sudden death without heart failure. Am J Cardiol 2001;88:1078-83.

Thiene G, Basso C. Arrhythmogenic right ventricular cardiomyopathy: An update. Cardiovasc Pathol. 2001;10:109–117.

UCARE, IVF-US. Survivors of out-of-hospital cardiac arrest with apparently normal heart. Need for definition and standardized clinical evaluation. Consensus Statement of the Joint Steering Committees of the Unexplained Cardiac Arrest Registry of Europe and of the Idiopathic Ventricular Fibrillation Registry of the United States. Circulation 1997;95:265-72.

Vasaiwala SC, Finn C, Delpriore J, et al. Prospective Study of cardiac sarcoid mimicking arrhythmogenic right ventricular dysplasia. J Cardiovasc Electrophysiol 2008;19:2000-7.

Wojnicz, R, Nowalany-Kozielska, E, Wojciechowska, C, *et al.* Randomized, placebo-controlled study for immunosuppressive treatment of inflammatory dilated cardiomyopathy: two-year follow-up results. Circulation 2001; 104: 39-45.

Yilmaz A, Kindermann I, Kindermann M, Mahfoud F, Ukena C, Athanasiadis A, Hill S, Mahrholdt H, Voehringer M, Schieber M, Klingel K, Kandolf R, Böhm M, Sechtem U. Comparative evaluation of left and right ventricular endomyocardial biopsy: differences in complication rate and diagnostic performance. Circulation. 2010;122:900-9.

Zeppenfeld K, Blom NA, Bootsma M, Schalij MJ. Incessant ventricular tachycardia in fulminant lymphocytic myocarditis: Evidence for origin in the Purkinje system and successful treatment with ablation. Heart Rhythm 2007;4:88-91.

Zipes DP, Camm AJ, Borggrefe M, et al. ACC/AHA/ESC 2006 guidelines for management of patients with ventricular arrhythmias and the prevention of sudden cardiac death--executive summary: A report of the American College of Cardiology/American Heart Association Task Force and the European Society of Cardiology Committee for Practice Guidelines (Writing Committee to Develop Guidelines for Management of Patients with Ventricular Arrhythmias and the Prevention of Sudden Cardiac Death) Developed in collaboration with the European Heart Rhythm Association and the Heart Rhythm Society. Eur Heart J 2006;27:2099-140.

17

Biomarkers of Heart Failure in Myocarditis and Dilated Cardiomyopathy

DeLisa Fairweather, Eric D. Abston and Michael J. Coronado
Johns Hopkins University Bloomberg School of Public Health
USA

1. Introduction

There are many reviews that discuss the role of biomarkers in cardiovascular disease (CVD) and heart failure (Braunwald, 2008; Chen et al., 2010; Hochholzer et al., 2010), but little information exists regarding the presence and usefulness of biomarkers for heart failure in myocarditis and dilated cardiomyopathy (DCM) patients. Heart failure (HF) is the end consequence of many CVDs including atherosclerosis, myocardial infarction, myocarditis and DCM. CVD is the leading cause of morbidity and mortality in Western nations (Roger et al., 2011), and a growing concern worldwide (Gaddam et al., 2011). As treatments for CVD prolong survival, the prevalence of chronic HF has increased. It is now estimated that 5.8 million people in the United States live with HF and over 23 million worldwide (Bui et al., 2011). Approximately 550,000 new cases of HF are diagnosed each year, with a lifetime risk for developing disease of one in five (Chen et al., 2010; Krumholz et al., 1997). Hospitalizations for HF have also increased dramatically in the United States from 402,000 in 1979 to 2.4 million in 2007 with the cost of treating HF patients estimated at $39 billion annually (Bui et al., 2011; Chen et al., 2010; Roger et al., 2011). Biomarkers have become an increasingly important clinical tool for assessing CVD and progression to HF. Biomarkers are used in early detection of sub-clinical disease, diagnosis, risk stratification, monitoring disease state, and to determine therapies (Hochholzer et al., 2010). Many biomarkers are also risk factors directly involved in the pathogenesis of disease.

2. Heart failure

In spite of advances in diagnosis and treatment, HF remains a growing medical problem associated with major hospitalization, mortality and poor prognosis. Heart failure is characterized by significantly reduced cardiac output resulting in an inability to meet the metabolic needs of the body. Most cases of HF are caused by systolic dysfunction, or reduced myocardial contractile function, as occurs during ischemic injury, pressure or volume overload and DCM. However, HF can also occur because of an inability to relax, expand or fill the ventricle resulting in diastolic dysfunction as observed during myocardial fibrosis and constrictive pericarditis (Afanasyeva et al., 2004; Kumar et al., 2005). The prevalence of HF is higher in men than women and sex is a major risk factor along with age, hypertension, left ventricular (LV) hypertrophy, valvular heart disease, obesity and diabetes (Bui et al., 2011; Roger et al., 2011) (Table 1). The New York Heart Association (NYHA) has defined four stages of HF in patients called the NYHA classification: class I) patients who have no symptoms or limitations in ordinary activities; class II) patients who have no symptoms in rest or in mild exercise, but symptoms appear with intense activity resulting in slight or mild limitations; class III) patients who have a marked limitation of activity, but no symptoms at rest; and finally class IV) patients who have symptoms when resting and who are restricted to bed or chair. This classification is still widely used in clinical practice but is not always a reliable guide to evaluate prognosis and therapy of patients with systolic HF (Hebert et al., 2011). Echocardiography is the imaging method most commonly used for the initial clinical assessment of patients with suspected HF because it is widely available, versatile, non-invasive, and has a low cost (Blauwet & Cooper, 2010). However, causative diagnosis cannot be established in a significant number of patients with HF despite significant advancement in echocardiographic techniques. Cardiac magnetic resonance imaging (MRI) is being used with increasing frequently and often provides additional information to echocardiography in patients with suspected or known HF (Blauwet & Cooper, 2010; Karamitsos & Neubauer, 2011; Olimulder et al., 2009). Although echocardiography and MRI are good at defining changes in volume, they do not assess pressure.

Nonmodifiable risk factors	Potentially controllable risk factors
Increasing age	Infections
Male gender	Inflammation
Family history	Obesity
Genetic abnormalities	Alcohol
Left ventricular hypertrophy	Stress
Myocardial infarction	Air pollution
Valvular heart disease	Diabetes mellitus
Hypersensitivity	Hypertension
	Tobacco smoking
	Hyperlipidemia

Table 1. Risk factors for developing heart failure. (Adapted from Bui et al., 2011 and Kumar et al., 2005)

The cardiac myocyte is generally considered to be a terminally differentiated cell that has lost its ability to divide or regenerate. Increased mechanical load causes an increase in the cellular content resulting in an increase in cell size termed hypertrophy (Kumar et al., 2005). The extent of hypertrophy varies depending on the underlying causes (Figure 1). Volume overload hypertrophy is characterized by dilation and an increase in muscle mass and wall thickness. Cardiac hypertrophy is also accompanied by many transcriptional and morphologic changes including generation of myofibroblasts, collagen deposition and fibrosis (Figure 1). Sustained hypertrophy and/or dilation may evolve to HF.

2.1 Myocarditis, dilated cardiomyopathy and heart failure

Myocarditis, or inflammation of the myocardium, leads to around half of all DCM cases in the United States (Roger et al., 2011). DCM is the most common form of cardiomyopathy requiring a heart transplant (Cooper, 2009, Wexler et al., 2009). Additionally, DCM contributes to approximately one third of all congestive HF cases (Jameson et al., 2005). The

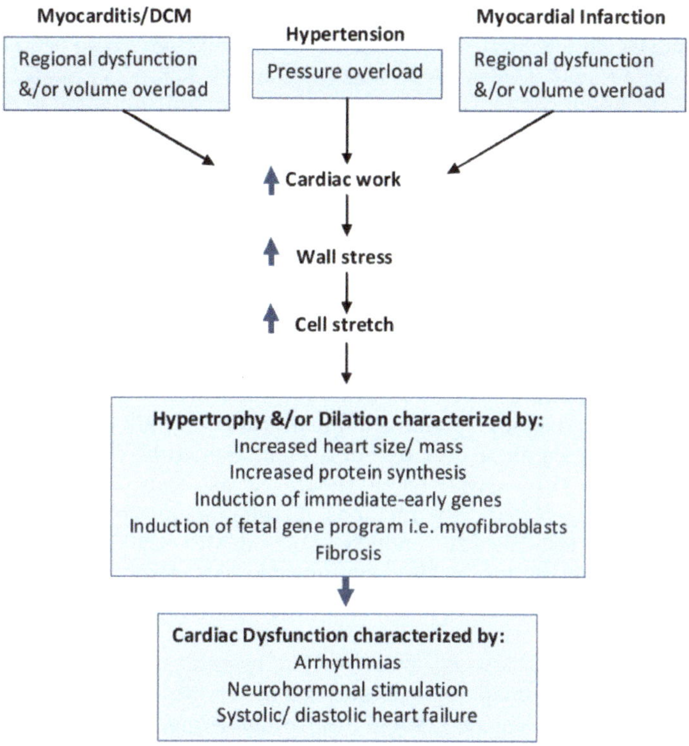

Fig. 1. Representation of the sequence of events leading to the development of heart failure. Viral infection or other causes of myocarditis lead to cardiac dysfunction resulting in increased cardiac work. Adapted from Kumar et al., 2005.

prognosis for patients with acute myocarditis varies but depends on ejection fraction (EF), clinical presentation and pulmonary artery pressure (Schultz et al., 2009). The life expectancy after diagnosis of myocarditis is 50% at 10 years and only 50% at 4 years after diagnosis of DCM (Grzybowski et al., 1996; Gupta et al., 2008). Over 20% of sudden deaths among young adults, the military, and athletes are due to myocarditis (Gupta et al., 2008). Similar to coronary artery disease and HF, myocarditis and DCM occur more frequently in men than women (Cooper, 2009; Roger et al., 2011). The clinical presentation of acute myocarditis in adults is highly variable often presenting as myocardial infarction or angina with nonspecific symptoms. Symptoms suggesting a viral infection including fever, rash, myalgias, arthralgias, fatigue, and respiratory or gastrointestinal symptoms frequently occur several days to weeks before the onset of myocarditis (Blauwet & Cooper, 2010). Electrocardiogram is widely used as a screening tool for myocarditis, but only detects about 47% of cases (Morgera et al., 1992). Echocardiography is useful for evaluating cardiac chamber size, wall thickness, systolic and diastolic function, and the presence of intramural thrombi in suspected myocarditis patients (Blauwet & Cooper, 2010). However, there is no specific echocardiographic feature for myocarditis, and patterns consistent with hypertrophy, DCM and/or ischemic heart disease can be observed in myocarditis patients. Cardiac MRI is an important noninvasive method to assess patients suspected to have acute myocarditis. Unique features of myocarditis including myocardial edema, hyperemia, increased capillary permeability due to inflammation, and fibrosis can be identified using a combination of T1 and T2-weighted images (Blauwet & Cooper, 2010; Karamitsos & Neubauer, 2011). Endomyocardial biopsy is used to verify inflammation in the heart and to assess whether certain cell populations such as eosinophils or giant cells are present in the myocardium for diagnostic purposes (i.e. eosinophilic or giant cell myocarditis). Due to the focal nature of myocarditis and the fact that foci are frequently located in the peri/myocardium, endomyocardial biopsies often miss inflammation and so often do not aid in diagnosis (Maisch, 1994; Olimulder et al., 2009). Although the complication rate is low, patients are at a risk of death from the procedure.

3. Biomarkers in heart failure

Biomarkers are frequently used in cardiovascular medicine where they provide valuable information regarding diagnosis, treatment, identification of individuals at risk for HF, and potentially the pathogenesis of disease. For a biomarker to be clinically useful it should fulfill several criteria: 1) biomarker levels should be able to be accurately assessed using widely available and cost-efficient methods, 2) biomarkers should provide additional information from the tests already conducted such as MRI, and 3) biomarker information should aid in medical decision making (Braunwald, 2008; Morrow & de Lemos, 2007). A growing list of enzymes, hormones, markers of cardiac stress or necrosis, cytokines and other biological agents have been examined as possible biomarkers for HF (Table 2). Although biomarkers are discussed in this review by category (e.g. those associated with cardiac damage or inflammation), in reality many of these biomarkers interact or are associated with one another suggesting that combinations of biomarkers are likely to provide the best assessment of HF risk. This review will focus on HF biomarkers from Table 2 that have been studied in myocarditis/ DCM patients or experimental models.

3.1 Biomarkers of cardiovascular injury or stress

Myocyte injury can occur from many causes including infections, oxidative stress, inflammation or severe ischemia (Brauanwald, 2008). Cardiac myosin is typically not used as a biomarker for HF because it is rapidly cleared from the circulation. Cardiac troponin I and T are current standard biomarkers used to diagnose acute myocardial infarction and to stratify patient risk in acute coronary syndromes (ACS) because of their long half-life in the circulation (Hochholzer et al., 2010). B-type natriuretic peptide (BNP) and N-terminal pro-brain natriuretic peptide (NT-pro-BNP) are important indicators of cardiovascular stress having the advantage of being able to distinguish acute from chronic HF. Recently ST2 has emerged as another biomarker of cardiac damage that has prognostic ability in patients suspected of HF.

3.1.1 Troponins I and T

The cardiac troponins are proteins located in myocytes that are responsible for regulating cardiac muscle contraction. Cardiac troponin is composed of three subunits that are products of different genes- troponin C, troponin I and troponin T. Compared to myosin and actin, troponins are present at low levels in the heart. However, both troponin I and T are ideally suited to detect myocardial damage because they are expressed as cardiac-specific isoforms (Agewall et al., 2011). Elevated sera troponins are associated with

Biomarker
Myocyte inury
Cardiac-specific troponins I and T
Myosin light-chain kinase I
Creatine kinase MB fraction
Myocyte stress
Brain natiuretic peptide
N-terminal pro-brain natriuretic peptide
ST2/ interleukin-33
Inflammation
C-reactive protein
Tumor necrosis factor
Fas (APO-1)
Interleukins 1, 6, 18
Galectin-3
Oxidative stress
Oxidized low-density lipoproteins
Myeloperoxidase
Urinary and plasma isoprostanes
Neurohormones
Norepinephrine
Renin
Angiotensin II
Aldosterone
Endothelin
Extracellular-matrix remodeling
Matrix metalloproteinases
Tissue inhibitors of metalloproteinases
Collagen propeptides

Table 2. Biomarkers in heart failure. (Adapted from Braunwald, 2008)

myocardial ischemia and necrosis and have been found to be excellent diagnostic and prognostic biomarkers for thrombotic ACS. But many cardiac conditions can lead to elevated troponins in addition to ACS including myocarditis, DCM and HF (Table 3). With new high-sensitivity detection methods for troponins, very minor changes in cardiac damage can be detected. Although troponins released to the circulation do not identify the type of heart damage, their levels may indicate the severity of damage (Figure 2) (Miller et al., 2007). A number of studies have been conducted examining troponin release during myocarditis, DCM or heart failure in patients (Smith et al., 1997; Brandt et al., 2001; Imazio et al., 2008; Miller et al., 2007; Peacock et al., 2008). Troponin I and T have also been found to predict the severity of myocarditis and the short-term prognosis in children with acute and fulminant myocarditis and DCM (Soongswang et al., 2002; Al-Biltagi et al., 2010). Overall, troponin levels were found to increase in relation to the severity of myocardial inflammation or ventricular wall stress caused by remodeling (Agewall et al., 2011; Miller et al., 2007). DCM patients with elevated serum troponin I levels were more dilated and had a worse outcome that troponin I-negative patients (Miettinen et al., 2008). Additionally, acute decompensated heart failure patients who were positive for troponin had a lower EF and higher in-hospital mortality, independent from other predictive values, than those who were negative for troponin (Peacock et al., 2008). Troponin T was found to be an important independent variable that predicted increased risk of death in patients with chronic HF (Latini et al., 2007). These findings demonstrate that troponin measurement is an important tool in early risk assessment of myocarditis/ DCM patients.

Condition
Acute coronary syndrome
Myocarditis
Pericarditis
Endocarditis
Dilated cardiomyopathy
Acute heart failure
Pulmonary embolism
Stroke
Sepsis
Acute aortic dissection
Tachyarrhythmias
Cardiac contusion
Tako-tsubo cardiomyopathy
Strenuous exercise e.g. marathon runners
Sympathomimetic drugs
Chemotherapy

Table 3. Cardiac conditions that can result in acutely elevated troponins. (Adapted from Agewall et al., 2011)

Interestingly, autoantibodies against circulating troponin I have been found in patients with ACS and acute myocardial infarction (Eriksson et al., 2005; Leuschner et al., 2008; Shmilovich et al., 2007). These autoantibodies were discovered because they interfered with troponin detection assays (Eriksson et al., 2005). This discovery led to the realization that autoantibodies against troponin I were also present in the sera of patients with DCM and heart failure (Miettinen et al., 2008; Shmilovich et al., 2007). One study of DCM patients found that troponin I, but not troponin I autoantibodies, were associated with dilation and poor outcome (Miettinen et al., 2008). In another study a significant number of DCM patients had autoantibodies against troponin I, but the autoantibodies were not found to bind to cardiac myocytes or activate Ca^{2+} currents (Shmilovich et al., 2007). Myocardial infarction patients with elevated troponin I autoantibodies had poor recovery of LV EF suggesting that troponin autoantibodies affect heart function (Leuschner et al., 2008). Further evidence that troponin autoantibodies may directly affect heart function comes from animal studies. PD-1 receptor deficient mice were found to develop severe DCM with high levels of autoantibodies against tropoinin I (Kaya et al., 2010; Nishimura et al., 2001). These troponin I autoantibodies were found to bind to heart tissue and to induce Ca^{2+} influx in cardiac myocytes. Inoculation of mice with recombinant troponin I with complete Freund's adjuvant was found to induce severe myocarditis and increased proinflammatory cytokines that progressed to fibrosis, DCM and heart failure (Goser et al., 2006; Kaya et al., 2008; 2010). However, this inflammatory response was only observed for troponin I but not troponin T inoculation. More research is needed to better understand the relationship of circulating troponin I and its autoantibodies in the progression of myocarditis to DCM and heart failure.

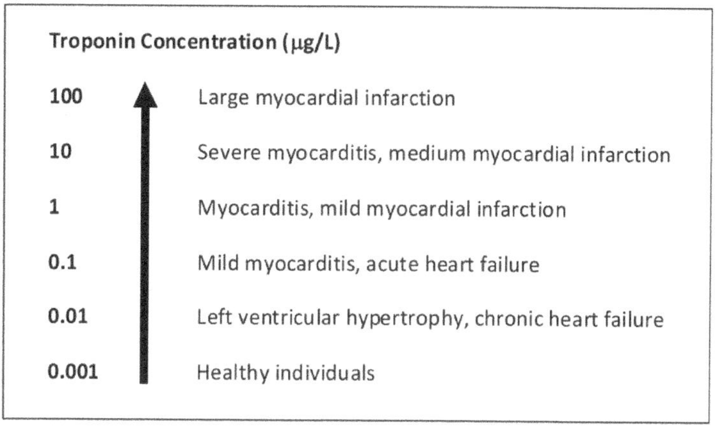

Fig. 2. Relationship between serum troponin levels and the severity of cardiac damage caused by myocarditis, heart failure or myocardial infarction. Adapted from Agewall et al., 2011.

3.1.2 BNP and NT-pro-BNP

In contrast to cardiac myosin or troponins that are released due to cell wall compromise, BNP is synthesized in healthy cardiac myocytes from its precursor NT-pro-BNP (Braunwald, 2008; Chen et al., 2010). The prohormone BNP is only released to the circulation when the ventricles become dilated, hypertrophic or during other conditions that induce wall distension and stretching, and by neurohormonal activation (Table 4). Prohormone BNP is cleaved by an endoprotease, corin, in the circulation into two polypeptides: the inactive NT-pro-BNP and the bioactive BNP. BNP causes arterial vasodilation, natriuresis and diureses while reducing the renin angiotensin system and adrenergic response (Braunwald, 2008; Palazzuoli et al., 2011). Elevated plasma BNP levels occur during hypertrophic cardiomyopathy, diastolic dysfunction and LV hypertrophy, and have been shown to be directly proportional to NYHA class and inversely related to cardiac output (Silver et al., 2004). Although few studies specifically address the topic, BNP has been found to be elevated in the serum of patients with myocarditis or DCM and in animal models of myocarditis (Grabowski et al., 2004; Miller et al., 2007; Ogawa et al., 2008; Talvani et al., 2004; Tanaka et al., 2011). Plasma BNP levels are also elevated in patients with acute myocardial infarction and this relationship persists into the late phases of cardiac remodeling (Hirayama et al., 2005). Many studies have linked higher levels of circulating BNP with heart failure diagnosis and worse outcome (Miller et al., 2007; Palazzuoli et al., 2011). BNP levels are a better predictor of death than norepinephrine or endothelin-1 (Braunwald, 2008). Several studies have found that NT-pro-BNP was better than BNP for predicting death or re-hospitalization for heart failure, probably due to the longer half-life of NT-pro-BNP in sera (Masson et al., 2006; Omland et al., 2007). However, BNP is a better predictor than NT-pro-BNP of worse outcome in ACS (Palazzuoli et al., 2011). Natriuretic peptides were also found to be useful in screening asymptomatic subjects at risk of developing HF such as those with hypertension, diabetes and coronary artery disease (Braunwald, 2008). Noncardiac conditions that increase plasma BNP levels such as age, race, obesity and renal dysfunction should be taken into consideration when using this biomarker (Table 4). Overall, BNP and NT-pro-BNP are biomarkers with a high sensitivity and specificity in predicting HF in a number of conditions including myocarditis and DCM.

Cardiac condition	Noncardiac condition
Systolic dysfunction	Acute pulmonary embolism
Diastolic dysfunction	Pulmonary hypertension
Myocarditis	Anemia
Pericarditis	Septic shock
Myocardial fibrosis	Hyperthyroidism
Dilated cardiomyopathy	*Cor pulmonale*
Heart failure	Renal failure
Valvular heart disease	
Coronary artery disease	
Hypertension	
Atrial fibrillation	

Table 4. Conditions that increase plasma natriuretic peptide levels. (Adapted from Braunwald, 2008 and Palazzuoli et al., 2011)

3.1.3 Soluble ST2

Soluble ST2 (sST2), an interleukin (IL)-1 receptor (R) (IL-1R) family member, is basally expressed by cardiomyocytes and upregulated in the heart by mechanical strain and IL-1β (Weinberg et al., 2002). The ST2 gene is known to encode at least 3 isoforms of ST2 by alternative splicing: ST2L, a transmembrane receptor; sST2, a secreted soluble form of ST2 that can serve as a decoy receptor for the ST2 ligand, IL-33; and ST2V, a variant of ST2 found in the gut of humans (Miller & Liew, 2011). ST2L is a member of the Toll-like receptor (TLR)/IL-1R superfamily that share a common structure with an extracellular domain of three linked immunglobulin-like motifs, a transmembrane segment and a cytoplasmic Toll-interleukin-1 receptor (TIR) domain. ST2L forms a complex with IL-1R accessory protein (IL-1RAcP) that is required for IL-33 signaling (Ali et al., 2007). IL-33 signaling recruits the adaptor protein MyD88 to the TIR domain leading to activation of the transcription factors NF-κB and AP-1 and production of inflammatory mediators including proinflammatory tumor necrosis factor (TNF), IL-1β, IL-6, and the T helper (Th)2-associated cytokines IL-5, IL-13 and IL-10 (Liew et al., 2010; Miller & Liew, 2011). Both ST2L and sST2 are induced in cardiomyocytes by biomechanical strain (Weinberg et al., 2002). Elevated levels of sST2 in the sera are associated with poor prognosis in patients with acute myocardial infarction or chronic heart failure where sST2 levels correlate positively with creatine kinase and negatively with EF (Weinberg et al., 2002; 2003). In patients with severe chronic NYHA class III or IV heart failure, the change in sST2 levels was an independent predictor of subsequent mortality or transplantation (Weinberg et al., 2003). IL-33 is expressed largely within fibroblasts in the heart and is thought to be released from necrotic cells due to tissue damage caused by direct damage or infection (Liew et al., 2010). IL-33 has been shown to be cardioprotective using animal models where recombinant (r)IL-33 treatment reduced hypertrophy and fibrosis following pressure overload induced by transverse aortic constriction (TAC) (Sanada et al., 2007). This effect was reversed by treating mice with sST2 prior to TAC, providing evidence that sST2 functions as a decoy receptor for IL-33. Additionally, rIL-33 treatment was found to decrease atherosclerosis in ApoE deficient mice fed a high fat diet by skewing the immune response from a Th1 to a Th2 response (Miller et al., 2008).

Currently there are no reports on the role of sST2 or IL-33 in the development of myocarditis or DCM even though sST2 is known to be a good biomarker predicting heart failure. Our laboratory is investigating the role of sST2/IL-33 signaling in an autoimmune model of coxsackievirus B3 (CVB3) myocarditis and DCM in mice. We found that IL-33 mRNA was upregulated in the heart during acute CVB3 myocarditis and chronic DCM (Figure 3A,B). Additionally, sST2 levels were elevated in the sera during acute CVB3 myocarditis in mice (Figure 3C) and correlated with poor heart function as assessed by echocardiography (not shown) or pressure-volume relationships (Figure 4). Serum sST2 is a good marker of disease because it could not be detected in the sera of undiseased mice (Figure 3C). Our findings of elevated sST2 levels in the sera of mice with CVB3 myocarditis and its relation to poor heart function suggest that sST2 may serve as a useful biomarker to predict progression to HF in myocarditis and DCM patients.

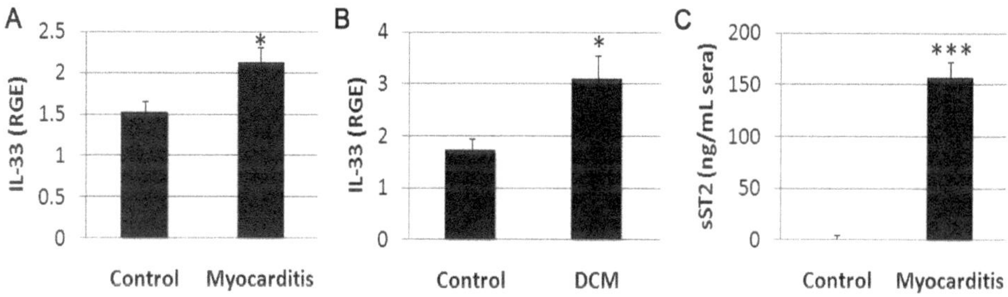

Fig. 3. IL-33 and sST2 are increased during autoimmune CVB3 myocarditis in mice. Male BALB/c mice were infected intraperitoneally with heart-passaged coxsackievirus B3 (CVB3) containing infectious CVB3 (10^3 plaque forming units) and heart proteins on day 0 and myocarditis examined at day 10 post infection (pi) and dilated cardiomyopathy (DCM) at day 90 pi. Saline inoculated age-matched mice were used as controls. Interleukin (IL)-33 mRNA was assessed by quantitative RT-PCR in the heart at day 10 (**A**) and 90 (**B**) pi and normalized to hypoxanthine phosphoribosyltransferase (HPRT) levels. sST2 levels were assessed in the sera of mice during acute myocarditis at day 10 pi by ELISA (**C**). Data are expressed as mean relative gene expression (RGE) ±standard error of the mean (SEM) in 7 to 10 mice per group. $^*P < 0.05$; $^{***}P < 0.001$.

3.2 Biomarkers of inflammation

Inflammation is important in the pathogenesis of many of the conditions that lead to HF. Traditionally, inflammatory biomarkers have been considered to be risk markers rather than risk factors because their role in disease pathogenesis is not always clear (Rao et al., 2006). Many inflammatory biomarkers found in the circulation, such as C-reactive protein (CRP),

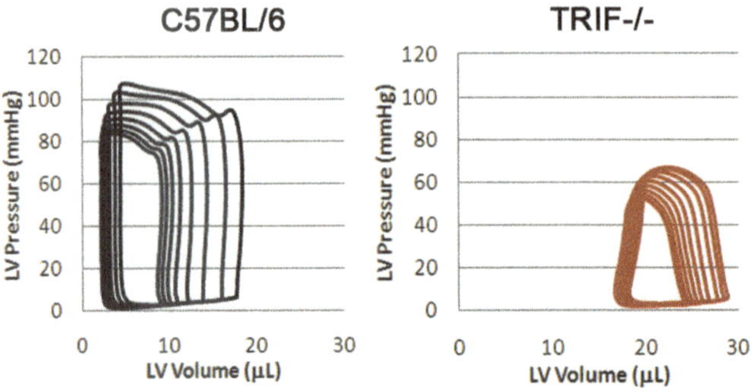

Fig. 4. Poor heart function in TRIF deficient mice is associated with elevated sST2 during acute CVB3 myocarditis. Male C57BL/6 (BL/6) or TRIF deficient (TRIF-/-) mice were infected intraperitoneally with heart-passaged coxsackievirus B3 (CVB3) containing infectious CVB3 (10^3 plaque forming units) and heart proteins on day 0 and myocarditis examined at day 10 post infection (pi) using end systolic pressure-volume relationships (ESPVR). Ees, a measure of LV end systolic stiffness/elastance, was 7.1 in BL/6 and 5.1 in TRIF-/- mice ($P = 0.04$) while V_0, the X-intercept of the ESPVR, was -5.4 in BL/6 and 26.8 in TRIF-/- mice ($P = 0.0001$). End diastolic volume (EDV) was 24±1.2 in BL/6 and 33±3.3 in TRIF-/- mice ($P < 0.01$). Thus, elevated sST2 in the sera of TRIF-/- mice (not shown) was associated with dilation and heart failure in TRIF deficient mice in an autoimmune model of CVB3 myocarditis.

IL-6 and serum amyloid A protein (SAA), are part of the acute phase response arising in the liver and although they are strongly associated with disease they may simply infer the presence of an inflammatory state. In clinical studies inflammatory mediators have been found to predict progression to HF similar to injury biomarkers and/or neurohormones (Table 2) (Mann, 2005). Inflammatory biomarkers have been shown in animal studies and the clinical setting to increase LV dysfunction, increase edema, and induce endothelial dysfunction and cardiomyocyte apoptosis, as well as other deleterious effects (Table 5).
A recent long-term study of myocarditis patients revealed that inflammation was the best predictor for the progression to HF following acute myocarditis (Kindermann et al., 2008). Viruses like CVB3, adenovirus, parvovirus B19 and hepatitis C virus are often detected in patient myocardial biopsies (Cooper, 2009; Gupta et al., 2008). Antiviral treatments such as interferon-β reduce inflammation and HF in animal models and patients, implying that viral infections are an important cause of myocarditis cases that lead to HF (Kuhl et al., 2003; Wang et al., 2007). Inflammation appears to be etiologically linked with the development of HF, not only because heart failure is a consequence of inflammatory CVDs but because patients with chronic HF that have elevated levels of inflammatory mediators have a worse prognosis (Robinson et al., 2011). Evidence exists that both cellular and auto/antibody-mediated damage contribute to the progression to DCM and HF following myocarditis (Cooper, 2009; Fairweather et al., 2008; Kallwellis-Opara et al., 2007). Similar to atherosclerosis, acute myocardial inflammation is associated with an elevated Th1 response in males (Daniels et al., 2008; Frisancho-Kiss et al., 2007; Huber and Pfaeffle, 1994; Nishikubo et al., 2007). A Th17 response has been shown to increase fibrosis leading to DCM in the experimental autoimmune myocarditis (EAM) model in mice (Baldeviano et al., 2010).

Interestingly, Th2 responses have also been implicated in the pathogenesis of myocarditis leading to HF (Afanasyeva et al., 2001; Fairweather et al., 2004a; 2004b). IFN-γ deficient mice, which have elevated IL-4 levels and a Th2 response, progress to severe DCM and HF following CVB3 myocarditis (Fairweather et al., 2004a).

Deleterious effects
Known
Left ventricular dysfunction
Pulmonary edema
Cardiomyopathy
Inflammation
Left ventricular remodeling
Endothelial dysfunction
Inducible nitric oxide synthase activation
Decreased skeletal-muscle blood flow
Anorexia and cachexia
Potential
Receptor uncoupling from adenylate cyclase
Activation of the fetal-gene program
Apoptosis of cardiac myocytes

Table 5. Deleterious effects of inflammatory biomarkers on acute and chronic heart failure. (Adapted from Anker & von Haehling, 2004; Braunwald, 2008; Mann, 2005)

3.2.1 C-reactive protein

Interest in the study of inflammatory mediators in patients with HF began in 1954 when an assay for CRP was first developed (Braunwald, 2008). CRP is an acute phase protein synthesized in the liver in response to IL-6 and released to the circulation during inflammation (Pepys & Hirschfield, 2003). Its levels are synergistically increased by IL-1β. In phagocytes CRP has been shown to bind Fcγ receptor I and II and to function in the clearance of apoptotic and necrotic cells (Devaraj et al., 2009; Rhodes et al., 2011). In 1956 a study was published showing that CRP was detectible in the sera of 30 out of 40 patients with chronic HF, and that elevated CRP levels were associated with more severe disease (Braunwald, 2008; Elster et al., 1956). Since then many studies have shown that CRP independently predicts adverse outcomes in patients with acute or chronic HF (Braunwald, 2008; Osman et al., 2006). Higher levels of CRP are associated with more severe HF and independently associated with morbidity and mortality (Anand et al., 2005). Additionally, elevated CRP levels identified asymptomatic elderly individuals who were at a high risk of developing HF in the future (Vasan et al., 2003). The main problem with CRP as a biomarker is that it lacks specificity for CVD. That is, CRP levels are elevated in the sera during most conditions that increase inflammation such as acute or chronic infection, cigarette smoking, ACS and some autoimmune diseases (Pepys & Hirschfield, 2003; Perez-De-Lis et al., 2010; Rhodes et al., 2011). There is increasing evidence that CRP may be able to exert direct proinflammatory effects on the heart by increasing matrix metalloproteinase-1 (MMP)-1 and IL-8 in endothelial cells and by increasing CD11b and CC-chemokine receptor 2 (CRR2) in monocytes, for example (Table 6) (Devaraj et al., 2009; Osman et al., 2006; Venugopal et al., 2005).

Endothelial cells	Monocyte-macrophages	Smooth muscle cells
Increased VCAM, ICAM-1, E-selectin, MCP-1 and monocyte adhesion	Increased tissue factor	Increased AT-1 and VSMC migration and proliferation
Increased PAI-1, IL-8, CD40/CD40L, MMP-1, ET-1 and M-CSF	Increased superoxide and myeloperoxidase	Increased neointimal formation *in vivo*
Decreased tPA	Increased proinflammatory cytokines (e.g. TNF) and decreased IL-10	Increased iNOS
Decreased prostacyclin	Increased CD11b and CCR2	Increased ROS
Increased superoxide and iNOS	Promoted oxLDL uptake and decreases cholesterol efflux	Increased tissue factor
Promoted endothelial dysfunction *in vivo*	Increased MMPs and HMGB1	
Impaired EPC number and function *in vitro*	Increased M-CSF and proliferation	

Table 6. Inflammatory effects of C-reactive protein. (Adapted from Devaraj et al., 2009) Abbreviations: AT, angiotensin receptor; CCR2, CC-chemokine receptor-2; CD40L, CD40 ligand; EPC, endothelial progenitor cell; ET, endothelin; HMGB1, high-mobility group protein B1; ICAM, intercellular adhesion molecule; IL, interleukin; iNOS, inducible nitric oxide synthase; MCP, monocyte chemotactic protein; M-CSF, macrophage colony-stimulating factor; MMP, matrix metalloproteinase; oxLDL, oxidative low-density lipoprotein; PAI, plasminogen activator inhibitor; ROS, reactive oxygen species; TNF, tumor necrosis factor; tPA, tissue plasminogen activator; VCAM, vascular cell adhesion molecule; VSMC, vascular smooth muscle cell.

Although many studies have examined the relationship between serum CRP levels and HF, few studies have examined CRP levels in myocarditis patients. In one study, 31 patients with clinical and histological evidence of lymphocytic myocarditis were found to have elevated plasma CRP levels that correlated positively with the NYHA functional class (Kaneko et al., 2000; Osman et al., 2006). Five of these patients who died of HF during the study had significantly higher levels of CRP, suggesting that CRP measurement may be a useful tool for determining prognosis in myocarditis patients. A separate study found that 80% of patients with clozapine-induced myocarditis (an antipsychotic drug used to treat schizophrenic symptoms) had elevated levels of CRP compared to a control group (Ronaldson et al., 2010). Several studies have examined CRP levels in idiopathic/ non-ischemic DCM patients where CRP levels have been found to independently predict disease outcome (Ishikawa et al., 2006; Kaneko et al., 1999; Senes et al., 2008). CRP levels increased with the severity of symptoms and the level of systolic impairment in DCM patients, while ongoing statin treatment was found to decrease CRP levels (De Gennaro et al., 2008). Interestingly, CRP has been found to co-express with TNF, macrophages and complement in the myocardium of DCM patients suggesting that CRP may play a role in the pathogenesis of disease (Satoh et al., 2005; Zimmermann et al., 2009). One of the obstacles to understanding the role of CRP in myocarditis and DCM is that mouse CRP appears only in trace amounts during the acute phase response (Pepys & Hirschfield, 2003). Instead of CRP mice upregulate serum amyloid P component (SAP), which is a non-acute phase protein in humans. Thus, CRP deficient or transgenic mice may provide only limited information on the role of CRP in HF promotion.

3.2.2 Cytokines: TNF, IL-1β and IL-18

The inability of hemodynamic factors to fully explain HF cases led to the hypothesis that cytokines released from cardiac tissue and/or inflammatory cells also contribute to disease progression. According to the "cytokine hypothesis", HF develops because cytokine cascades that are activated following myocardial injury or stress exert deleterious effects on heart function (Table 5) (Anker & von Haehling, 2004; Braunwald, 2008; Seta et al., 1996). Cytokines can induce hemodynamic abnormalities and/or direct toxic effects on the heart. Since the original report in 1990 by Levine et al. there have been many studies showing that an increase in circulating TNF levels directly relates to a patient's NYHA classification and predicts patient mortality (Anker & von Haehling, 2004; Mann, 2005; Seta et al., 1996; Vasan et al., 2003). Similar relationships between IL-1β, IL-6 or IL-18 and HF have been found (Anker & von Haehling, 2004; Hedayat et al., 2010; Jefferis et al., 2011; Vasan et al., 2003). Cardiac myocyte hypertrophy, contractile dysfunction, cardiac myocyte apoptosis and extracellular matrix (ECM) remodeling contribute critically to the progression from cardiac injury to HF (Hedayat et al., 2010).

More than any other category of biomarker (Table 2), the role of cytokines in the pathogenesis of myocarditis and DCM has been studied by researchers (Fairweather & Rose, 2005; Hedayat et al., 2010). TNF, IL-1β and IL-18 have all been shown to play a role in myocarditis by inducing myocyte hypertrophy, contractile dysfunction, myocyte apoptosis and contributing to ECM remodeling, a step critical in the progression from myocarditis to DCM (Cain et al., 1999; Fairweather et al., 2004a; 2004b; Hedayat et al., 2010). In one study, TNF mRNA expression was found to be elevated more often in myocarditis patients when viral genomes were also detected, and greater mRNA levels of TNF and its receptor TNFRI correlated with impaired cardiac function (Calabrese et al., 2004). In a mouse model of CVB3 myocarditis, TNF was found to increase CD1d expression on lymphocytes resulting in increased inflammation in males (Huber, 2010). However, viral replication and acute CVB3 myocarditis was not altered in TNFRI deficient mice (Fairweather et al., 2005). Out of the 13 or so TLRs that have been described so far in humans and mice, TLR4 is unique in its ability to work with the inflammasome to produce bioactive IL-1β and IL-18 in the heart (Fairweather et al., 2003; Vallejo, 2011). TLR2 and TLR4 signaling increase TNF levels, and TLR2 can act with TLR4 to increase IL-1β levels (Vallejo, 2011). TLR4 mRNA expression has been found to be higher in patients with myocarditis than controls, and to correlate with viral RNA levels in the heart (Satoh et al., 2003). Myocarditis patients with active viral replication had higher levels of TLR4 that was associated with lower systolic function. In a mouse model of CVB3 myocarditis, our laboratory found that TLR4 deficient mice develop reduced acute inflammation and lower IL-1β and IL-18 levels in the heart (Fairweather et al., 2003). The importance of TLR4 signaling in a strictly autoimmune model of myocarditis was demonstrated by Nishikubo et al. where TLR4 signaling was found to be necessary to mount a Th1-type immune response (Nishikubo et al., 2007). We have shown that TLR4 is upregulated on macrophages and mast cells during the innate immune response to CVB3 and during acute CVB3 myocarditis and this response results in increased inflammation and progression to DCM and HF in males compared to females (Frisancho-Kiss et al., 2007; 2009; Onyimba et al., 2011). A Th1 response in male mice was found to be due to TLR4-derived IL-

18, which was originally named IFN-γ-inducing factor, rather than to a classical IL-12/STAT4-induced Th1 response (Frisancho-Kiss et al., 2006). We were surprised to find that TLR4 was expressed on alternatively activated M2 macrophages (induced by Th2 cytokines) rather than classically activated M1 macrophages (induced by Th1 cytokines) within the heart during acute CVB3 myocarditis (Fairweather & Cihakova 2009; Frisancho-Kiss et al., 2009). These CD11b+GR1+F4/80+ M2 macrophages expressed TLR4 and IL-1β (Frisancho-Kiss et al., 2009). We, and others, have shown that IL-1β is particularly important in the cardiac remodeling that leads to fibrosis, DCM and HF following acute myocarditis (Blyszczuk et al., 2009; Cihakova et al., 2008 Fairweather et al., 2004a; 2006). Further work is needed to better understand the role of innate TLRs and cytokine production/regulation in the heart in order to determine whether anti-cytokine therapies will be effective once disease has progressed to the point of being clinically apparent (Mann, 2005). Another area that needs to be addressed in animal models is the relationship between sera levels of proinflammatory cytokines and the stage of disease (i.e. acute myocarditis vs. DCM) and whether increases in sera levels of cytokines predict HF.

3.3 Biomarkers of extracellular matrix remodeling

Remodeling of the ventricles plays an important role in the progression to HF (Braunwald, 2008). The extracellular matrix provides a framework for cardiac myocytes, mediates cell adhesion and cell-to-cell communication, mediates diastolic stiffness, promotes cell survival or apoptosis, and is a reservoir for growth factors and cytokines (Liu et al., 2006). Release of cytokines and growth factors at the site of tissue injury and by inflammatory cells induces fibroblast proliferation and deposition of collagen, which is the primary component of the ECM resulting in scar tissue (Figure 5). Profibrotic cytokines, such as TNF and IL-1β, and growth factors, like transforming growth factor (TGF)β1 and fibroblast growth factor (FGF), induce collagen production from fibroblasts. Normally a balance exists between matrix metalloproteinases (MMPs) that proteolytically degrade fibrillar collagen and tissue inhibitors of MMPs (TIMPs). However, during inflammatory CVDs an imbalance in MMPs and TIMPs contributes to collagen deposition, ventricular dilatation and remodeling resulting in DCM and HF. The activity of MMPs has been shown to be increased in the progression to HF (Bradham et al., 2002; Tyagi et al., 1996). Serum MMP9, for example, has been found to predict CVD mortality better than other traditional prognostic markers such as cholesterol, CRP or IL-6 (Blankenberg et al., 2003; Liu et al., 2006).

The progression from myocarditis to fibrosis, DCM and HF has been well documented in clinical studies and animal models (Fairweather et al., 2004a; Kania et al., 2009; Looi et al., 2010). Studies in our laboratory have revealed a two-stage process where increases in profibrotic mediators during acute CVB3 myocarditis, which occurs from day 8 to 12 post infection, result in a gradual remodeling that progresses to fibrosis and DCM by day 35 post infection (Figure 5) (Fairweather et al., 2004a; 2006; Fairweather & Rose, 2007). In both animal and human studies of DCM, genes associated with extracellular matrix remodeling and fibrosis are upregulated with disease (Piro et al., 2010; Yung et al., 2004). TNF, IL-1β, IL-4, IL-6, IL-17 and TGF-β have all been found to initiate remodeling (Baldeviano et al., 2010; Blyszczuk et al., 2009; Fairweather et al., 2004a; Heymans, 2006; Kania et al., 2009). There are many MMPs, but only 4 known TIMPS. MMPs are upregulated in the heart during EAM and during viral myocarditis (Marchant & McManus, 2009; Tang et al., 2007; Westermann et al., 2010). Individual MMPs and TIMPs have been found to differ in their effects on myocarditis in rodents (Liu et al., 2006; Marchant & McManus, 2009; Westermann et al., 2010). For example, MMP9 deficient mice had increased CVB3 replication and inflammation, and worse heart function than wild type controls, indicating that MMP9 protects the heart from CVB3 myocarditis (Cheung et al., 2008). In contrast, TIMP-1 deficient mice were protected from CVB3 myocarditis indicating that TIMP-1 increases disease (Crocker et al., 2007). Although a number of studies have examined the role of MMPs and TIMPs in myocarditis, the relationship between serum levels of these factors and the progression to DCM and HF is not yet clear from animal models.

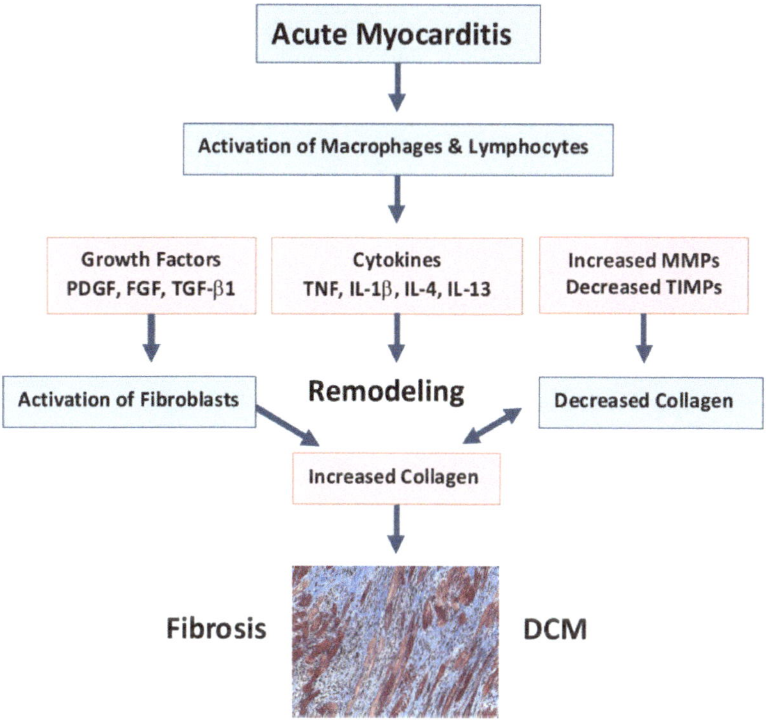

Fig. 5. Development of fibrosis and DCM following acute myocarditis. Macrophages and lymphocytes present within the myocardium during acute myocarditis release profibrotic cytokines such as tumor necrosis factor (TNF), interleukin (IL)-1β, IL-4 and IL-13 that activate fibroblasts to release collagen. Inflammation additionally stimulates the release of growth factors like platelet-derived growth factor (PDGF), fibroblast growth factor (FGF) and transforming growth factor (TGF)-β1, which act with cytokines to increase collagen production. Cytokines and growth factors released from inflammatory cells and cardiac tissues contribute to pathology. Normally a balance exists between matrix metalloproteinases (MMPs) that proteolytically degrade fibrillar collagen and tissue inhibitors of MMPs (TIMPs). However, during acute myocarditis an imbalance in MMPs and TIMPs contributes to collagen deposition, ventricular dilatation and remodeling resulting in dilated cardiomyopathy (DCM) and heart failure.

3.4 Thrombosis biomarkers

Atherosclerosis is a major initiator of thrombi formation that can restrict blood flow and lead to a heart attack (Carter, 2005). Cardiac mural thrombi can arise from a myocardial infarction, infection, inflammation (e.g. myocarditis) or rheumatic heart disease, for example. Although research has led to a clear understanding of conditions that induce thrombosis, the precise pathology leading to disease remains unclear. Thrombi can develop anywhere in the cardiovascular system like in the ventricular or atrial chambers, arteries, veins or capillaries. The size and shape of individual thrombi vary depending on the circumstances leading to their development. They often are found at sites of endothelial injury. Once thrombi have formed (acute) they may accumulate more platelets and fibrin and grow larger, or dislodge and travel to other sites, or be removed by fibrinolytic activity, and finally they can attract inflammation, undergo remodeling with deposition of collagen and be reincorporated into the vessel or myocardium (Kumar et al., 2005) (Figure 6).

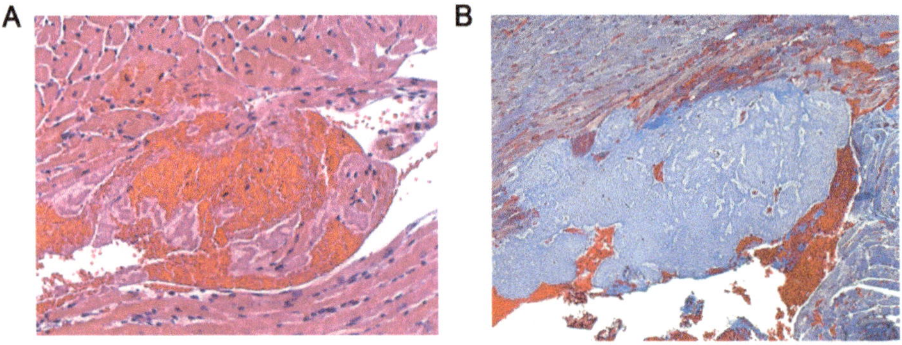

Fig. 6. Mural thrombi develop during acute CVB3 autoimmune myocarditis in mice and reincorporate into the myocardium. Male BALB/c mice were infected intraperitoneally with heart-passaged coxsackievirus B3 (CVB3) containing infectious CVB3 (10^3 plaque forming units) and heart proteins on day 0 and thrombus formation examined at day 10 post infection (pi) during acute myocarditis (**A**) or during chronic myocarditis/DCM at day 35 pi (**B**). H&E staining shows ventricular mural thrombus at day 10 pi (magnification, x100) (**A**). Masson's trichrome stains bright blue revealing collagen composition of mural integrated ventricular thrombus at day 35 pi (magnification, x100) (**B**).

Damage of cardiac tissue by viruses and inflammation is known to release tissue factor (TF), the main initiator of the coagulation cascade that results in the formation of fibrin and thrombotic clots (Mackman, 2009). Mural thrombi are known to occur in viral models of myocarditis in mice as well as in myocarditis patients (Antoniak et al., 2008; Kojima et al., 1988; Kuh & Seo, 2005). Furthermore, DCM patients demonstrate a high frequency of LV thrombi and prothrombotic characteristics like high levels of circulating fibrinogen and antithrombin III (Abdo et al., 2010). Many studies have shown that TF can increase inflammation by stimulating release of IL-6, a cytokine that along with TNF and IL-1β has been strongly associated with poor CVD outcome (Braunwald, 2008; Carter, 2005; Mackman, 2009; Rao et al., 2006). Complement components also contribute to thrombosis by depositing at sites of tissue damage and by activating platelets (Fairweather et al., 2006; Peerschke et al.,

2010). Eosinophils are potent inducers of ECM remodeling, releasing many profibrotic factors including IL-1β, IL-6, TGF-β, MMPs, and TIMPs (Shamri et al., 2011). Additionally, eosinophils release potent prothrombotic agents such as major basic protein, eosinophilic cationic protein, and eosinophil peroxidase, as well as directly and/or indirectly activating TF (Ames et al., 2010). Eosinophilia, fibrosis and thrombosis are characteristics of eosinophilic cardiovascular diseases like Churg Strauss syndrome, a form of vasculitis, hypereosinophilic syndrome, eosinophilic myocarditis and giant cell myocarditis (Ames et al., 2010; Cooper, 2000; 2009; Kleinfeldt et al., 2010; Rezaizadeh et al., 2010). Circulating biomarkers that may indicate a hypercoagulable state include complement C3, C4, IL-6, fibrinogen or antithrombin III (Abdo et al., 2010). Complement components were recently found to be elevated in the sera of mycarditis and DCM patients (Cooper et al., 2010). We have found that complement receptor 1 deficient mice, a receptor that regulates C3 levels, develop severe CVB3 myocarditis, dilation and HF with elevated levels of IL-1β in the heart and fibrosis (Fairweather et al., 2006). Overactivation of the terminal complement complex (C5b-9) has been shown to contribute to the progression of myocarditis to DCM in mice, indicating the importance of complement in regulating disease (Zwaka et al., 2002). Overall, these findings suggest that biomarkers of coagulation and/or thrombosis are likely to be important indicators of progression to DCM and HF following myocarditis.

4. Conclusions

Biomarkers are an important clinical tool for assessing progression to heart failure. DCM often leads to HF, and myocarditis is an important cause of acute (sudden death) and chronic (arising from DCM) forms of HF. Even though myocarditis is known to be an important cause of HF, few clinical studies have been conducted to determine the presence or usefulness of HF biomarkers in predicting adverse outcomes in myocarditis patients. Studies that have been conducted in myocarditis/DCM patients or animal models suggest that many of the biomarkers used to assess the likelihood of progression to heart failure in other CVDs will also provide useful information in myocarditis/DCM patients. More studies examining the ability of circulating HF biomarkers to predict poor outcome and HF in animal models of myocarditis/DCM are needed. Animal models will also provide valuable information on the potential role of HF biomarkers in the pathogenesis of disease. This knowledge is critical in determining the ability of therapies targeted to these biomarkers to prevent disease progression.

5. Acknowledgements

The authors thank Adriana Bucek for technical assistance and Norman Barker for photography. The research discussed by the authors in this review was funded by a National Institutes of Health Grant HL087033 to Dr. Fairweather.

6. References

Abdo, A.S., Kemp, R., Barham, J. & Geraci, S.A. (2010) Dilated cardiomyopathy and role of antithrombotic therapy. *American Journal of Medical Science* 339: 557-560.

Afanasyeva, M., Wang, Y., Kaya, Z., Park, S., Zilliox, M.J., Schofield, B.H., Hill, S.L. & Rose, N.R. (2001) Experimental autoimmune myocarditis in A/J mice is an interleukin-4-dependent disease with a Th2 phenotype. *American Journal of Pathology* 159: 193-203.

Afanasyeva, M., Georgakopoulos, D., Fairweather, D., Caturegli, P., Kass, D.A. & Rose, N.R. (2004) A novel model of constrictive pericarditis associated with autoimmune heart disease in interferon-γ knockout mice. *Circulation* 110: 2910-2917.

Agewall, S., Giannitsis, E., Jernbert, T. & Katus, H. (2011) Troponin elevation in coronary vs. non-coronary disease. *European Heart Journal* 32: 404-411.

Al-Biltagi, M., Issa, M., Hagar, H.A., Abdel-Hafez, M. & Aziz, N.A. (2010) Circulationg cardiac troponin levels and cardiac dysfunction in children with acute and fulminant viral myocarditis. *Acta Paediatrica* 99: 1510-1516.

Ali, S., Huber, M., Kollewe, C., Bischoff, S.C., Falk, W. & Martin, M.U. (2007) IL-1 receptor accessory protein is essential for IL-33-induced activation of T lymphocytes and mast cells. *Proceedings from the National Academy of Sciences USA* 104: 18660-18665.

Ames, P.R.J., Margaglione, M., Mackie, S. & Alves, J.D. (2010) Eosinophilia and thrombophilia in Churg Strauss syndrome: a clinical and pathogenetic overview. *Clinical Applied Thrombosis/ Hemostasisis* 16: 628-636.

Anand, I.S., Latini, R., Florea, V.G., Kuskowski, M.A., Rector, T., Masson, S., Signorini, S., Mocarelli, P., Hester, A., Glazer, R., Cohn, J.N. & Val-HeFT Investigators. (2005) C-reactive protein in heart failure: prognostic value and the effect of valsartan. *Circulation* 112: 1428-1434.

Anker, S.D. & von Haehling, S. (2004) Inflammatory mediators in chronic heart failure: an overview. *Heart* 90: 464-470.

Antoniak, S., Boltzen, U., Riad, A., Kallwellis-Opara, A., Rohde, M., Dorner, A., Tschope, C., Noutsias, M., Pauschinger, M., Schultheiss, H.-P. & Rauch, U. (2008) Viral myocarditis and coagulopathy: increased tissue factor expression and plasma thrombogenicity. *Journal of Molecular and Cellular Cardiology* 45: 118-126.

Baldeviano, G.C., Barin, J.G., Talor, M.V., Srinivasan, S., Bedja, D., Zheng, D., Gabrielson, K., Iwakura, Y., Rose, N.R. & Cihakova, D. (2010) Interleukin-17A is dispensable for myocarditis but essential for the progression to dilated cardiomyopathy. *Circulation Research* 106: 1646-1655.

Blankenberg, S. (2003) Plasma concentrations and genetic variation of matrix metalloproteinase 9 and prognosis of patients with cardiovascular disease. *Circulation* 107: 1579-1585.

Blauwet, L.A. & Cooper, L.T. (2010) Myocarditis. *Progress in Cardiovascular Diseases* 52: 274-288.

Blyszczuk, P., Kania, G., Dieterle, T., Marty, R.R., Valaperti, A., Berthonneche, C., Pedrazzini, T., Berger, C.T., Dirnhofer, S., Matter, C.M., Penninger, J.M., Luscher, T.F. & Eriksson, U. (2009) Myeloid differentiation factor-88/interleukin-1 signaling controls cardiac fibrosis and heart failure progression in inflammatory dilated cardiomyopathy. *Circulation Research* 105: 912-920.

Bradham, W.S., Moe, G., Wendt, K.A., Scott, A.A., Konig, A., Romanova, M., Naik, G. & Spinale, F.G. (2002) TNF-alpha and myocardial matrix metalloproteinases in heart failure: relationship to LV remodeling. *American Journal of Physiology and Heart Circulation Physiology* 282: H1288-H1295.

Brandt, R.R., Filzmaier, K. & Hanrath, P. (2001) Circulation cardiac troponin I in acute pericarditis. *American Journal of Cardiology* 87: 1326-1328.

Braunwald, E. (2008) Biomarkers in heart failure. *New England Journal of Medicine* 358: 2148-2159.

Bui, A.L., Horwich, T.B. & Fonarow G.C. (2011) Epidemiology and risk profile of heart failure. *Nature Reviews Cardiology* 8: 30-41.

Cain, B.S., Meldrum, D.R., Dinarello, C.A., Meng, X., Joo, K.S., Banjeree, A. & Harken, A.H. (1999) Tumor necrosis factor-alpha and interleukin-1beta synergistically depress human myocardial function. *Critical Care Medicine* 27: 1309-1318.

Calabrese, F., Carturan, E., Chimenti, C., Pieroni, M., Agostini, C., Angelini, A., Crosato, M., Valente, M., Boffa, G.M., Furstaci, A. & Thiene, G. (2004) Overexpression of tumor necrosis factor (TNF)alpha and TNFalpha receptor I in human viral myocarditis: clinicopathologic correlations. *Molecular Pathology* 17: 1108-1118.

Carter, A.M. (2005) Inflammation, thrombosis and acute coronary syndromes. *Diabetes Vascular Disease* Research 2: 113-121.

Chen, W.-C., Tran, K.D. & Maisel, A.S. (2010) Biomarkers in heart failure. *Heart* 96: 314-320.

Cheung, C., Marchant, D., Walker, E.K., Luo, Z., Zhang, J., Yanagawa, B., Rahmani, M., Cox, J., Overall, C., Senior, R.M., Luo, H. & McManus, B.M. (2008) Ablation of matrix metalloproteinase-9 increases severity of viral myocarditis in mice. *Circulation* 117: 1574-1582.

Cihakova, D., Barin, J. G., Afanasyeva, M., Kimura, M., Fairweather, D., Berg, M., Talor, M.V., Baldeviano, G.C., Frisancho-Kiss, S., Gabrielson, K., Bedja, D. & Rose, N.R. (2008) Interleukin-13 protects against experimental autoimmune myocarditis by regulating macrophage differentiation. *American Journal of Pathology* 172: 1195-1208.

Cooper, L.T. Jr. (2000) Giant cell myocarditis: diagnosis and treatment. *Herz* 3: 291-298.

Cooper, L.T. Jr. (2009) Myocarditis. *New England Journal of Medicine* 360: 1526-1538.

Cooper, L.T. Jr., Onuma, O.K., Sagar, S., Oberg, A.L., Mahoney, D.W., Asmann, Y.W. & Liu, P. (2010) Genomic and proteomic analysis of myocarditis and dilated cardiomyopathy. *Heart Failure Clinics* 6: 75-85.

Crocker, S.J., Frausto, R.F., Whitmire, J.K., Benning, N., Milner, R. & Whitton, J.L. (2007) Amelioration of coxsackievirus B3-mediated myocarditis by inhibition of tissue inhibitors of matrix metalloproteinase-1. *American Journal of Pathology* 171: 1762-1773.

Daniels, M.D., Hyland, K.V., Wang, K. & Engman, D.M. (2008) Recombinant cardiac myosin fragment induces experimental autoimmune myocarditis via activation of Th1 and Th17 immunity. *Autoimmunity* 41: 490-499.

De Gennaro, L., Brunetti, N.D., Cuculo, A., Pellegrino, P.L. & Di Biase, M. (2008) Systemic inflammation in nonischemic dilated cardiomyopathy. *Heart Vessels* 23: 445-450.

Devaraj, S., Singh, U. & Jialal, I. (2009) The evolving role of C-reactive protein in atherothrombosis. *Clinical Chemistry* 55: 229-238.

Elster, S.K., Braunwald, E. & Wood, H.F. (1956) A study of C-reactive protein in the serum of patients with congestive heart failure. *American Heart Journal* 51: 533-541.

Eriksson, S., Hellman, J. & Pettersson, K. (2005) Autoantibodies against cardiac troponins. *New England Journal of Medicine* 352: 98-100.

Fairweather, D. & Cihakova, D. (2009) Alternatively activated macrophages in infection and autoimmunity. *Journal of Autoimmunity* 33: 222-230.

Fairweather, D. & Rose, N.R. (2005) Inflammatory heart disease: a role for cytokines. *Lupus* 14: 646-651.

Fairweather, D. & Rose, N.R. (2007) Coxsackievirus-induced myocarditis in mice: a model of autoimmune disease for studying immunotoxicity. *Methods* 41: 118-122.

Fairweather, D., Yusung, S., Frisancho(-Kiss), S., Barrett, M., Gatewood, S., Steele, R. & Rose, N.R. (2003) IL-12Rβ1 and TLR4 increase IL-1β and IL-18-associated myocarditis and coxsackievirus replication. *Journal of Immunology* 170: 4731-4737.

Fairweather, D., Frisancho-Kiss, S., Yusung, S.A., Barrett, M.A., Gatewood, S.J.L., Davis, S.E., Njoku, D.B. & Rose, N.R. (2004a) IFN-γ protects against chronic viral myocarditis by reducing mast cell degranulation, fibrosis, and the profibrotic cytokines TGF-β_1, IL-1β, and IL-4 in the heart. *American Journal of Pathology* 165: 1883-1894.

Fairweather, D., Frisancho-Kiss, S., Gatewood, S., Njoku, D., Steele, R., Barrett, M. & Rose, N.R. (2004b) Mast cells and innate cytokines are associated with susceptibility to autoimmune heart disease following coxsackievirus B3 infection. *Autoimmunity* 37: 131-145.

Fairweather, D., Frisancho-Kiss, S., Yusung, S.A., Barrett, M.A., Davis, S.E., Steele, R.A., Gatewood, S.J.L. & Rose, N.R. (2005) IL-12 protects against coxsackievirus B3-induced myocarditis by increasing IFN-γ and macrophage and neutrophil populations in the heart. *Journal of Immunology* 174: 261-269.

Fairweather, D., Frisancho-Kiss, S., Njoku, D.B., Nyland, J.F., Kaya, Z., Yusung, S.A., Davis, S.E., Frisancho, J.A., Barrett, M.A. & Rose, N.R. (2006) Complement receptor 1 and 2 deficiency increases coxsackievirus B3-induced myocarditis and heart failure by increasing macrophages, IL-1β and immune complex deposition in the heart. *Journal of Immunology* 176: 3516-3524.

Fairweather, D., Frisancho-Kiss, S. & Rose, N.R. (2008) Sex differences in autoimmune disease from a pathologic perspective. *American Journal of Pathology* 173: 600-609.

Frisancho-Kiss, S., Nyland, J.F., Davis, S.E., Frisancho, J.A., Barrett, M.A., Rose, N.R. & Fairweather, D. (2006) Sex differences in coxsackievirus B3-induced myocarditis: IL-12Rβ1 signaling and IFN-γ increase inflammation in males independent from STAT4. *Brain Research* 1126: 139-147.

Frisancho-Kiss, S., Davis, S.E., Nyland, J.F., Frisancho, J.A., Cihakova, D., Rose, N.R. & Fairweather, D. (2007) Cutting Edge: Cross-regulation by TLR4 and T cell Ig mucin-3 determines sex differences in inflammatory heart disease. *Journal of Immunology* 178: 6710-6714.

Frisancho-Kiss, S., Coronado, M.J., Frisancho, J.A., Lau, V.M., Rose, N.R., Klein, S.L. & Fairweather, D. (2009) Gonadectomy of male BALB/c mice increases Tim-3^+ alternatively activated M2 macrophages, Tim-3^+ T cells, Th2 cells and Treg in the heart during acute coxsackievirus-induced myocarditis. *Brain Behavior and Immunity* 23: 649-657.

Gaddam, K.K., Ventura H.O. & Lavie C.J. (2011) Metabolic syndrome and heart failure- the risk, paradox and treatment. *Current Hypertension Research* 13: 142-148.

Goser, S., Andrassy, M., Buss, S.J., Leuschner, F., Volz, C.H., Ottl, R., Zittrich, S., Blaudeck, N., Hardt, S.E., Pfitzer, G., Rose, N.R., Katus, H.A. & Kaya, Z. (2006) Cardiac troponin I but not cardiac troponin T induces severe autoimmune inflammation in the myocardium. *Circulation* 114: 1693-1702.

Grabowski, M., Karpinski, G.J., Filipiak, K., Rdzanek, A., Pietrasik, A., Wretwoski, D., Rudowski, R. & Opolski, G. (2004) Diagnostic value of BNP in suspected perimyocarditis- a preliminary report. *Kardiology Pol.* 61: 451-458.

Grzybowski, J., Bilinska, Z.T., Ruzyllo, W., Kupsc, W., Michalak, E., Szczesniewska, D., Poplawska, W. & Rydlewska-Sadowska, W. (1996) Determinants of prognosis of nonischemic dilated cardiomopathy. *Journal of Cardiac Failure* 2: 77-85.

Gupta, S., Markham, D.W., Drazner, M.H. & Mammen, P.P.A. (2008) Fulminant myocarditis. *Nature Clinical Practice* 5: 693-706.

Hebert, K., Macedo, F.Y., Trahan, P., Tamariz, L., Dias, A., Palacio, A. & Arcement, L.M. (2011) Routine serial echocardiography in systolic heart failure: is it time for the heart failure guidelines to change? *Congestive Heart Failure* 17: 85-89.

Hedayat, M., Mahmoudi, M.J., Rose, N.R. & Rezaei, N. (2010) Proinflammatory cytokines in heart failure: double-edged swords. *Heart Failure Reviews* 15: 543-562.

Heymans, S. (2006) Inflammation and cardiac remodeling during viral myocarditis. *Ernst Schering Research Foundation Workshop* 55: 197-218.

Hirayama, A., Kusuoka, H., Yamamoto, H., Sakata, Y., Asakura, M., Higuchi, Y., Mizuno, H., Kashiwase, K., Ueda, Y., Okuyama, Y., Hori, M. & Kodama, K. (2005) Serial changes in plasma brain natriuretic peptide concentration at the infarct and non-infarct sites in patients with left ventricular remodeling after myocardial infarction. *Heart* 91: 1573-1577.

Hochholzer, W., Morrow, D.A. & Giugliano, R.P. (2010) Novel biomarkers in cardiovascular disease: update 2010. *American Heart Journal* 160: 583-594.

Huber, S.A. (2010) Tumor necrosis factor-alpha promotes myocarditis in female mice infected with coxsackievirus B3 through upregulation of CD1d on hematopoeitic cells. *Viral Immunology* 23: 79-86.

Huber, S.A. & Pfaeffle, B. (1994) Differential Th1 and Th2 cell responses in male and female BALB/c mice infected with coxsackievirus group B type 3. *Journal of Virology* 68: 5126-5132.

Imazio, M., Cecchi, E., Demichelis, B., Chinaglia, A., Lerna, S., Demarie, D., Ghisio, A., Pomari, F., Belli, R. & Trinchero, R. (2008) Myopericarditis versus viral or idiopathic acute pericarditis. *Heart* 94: 498-501.

Ishikawa, C., Tsutamoto, T., Fujii, M., Sakai, H., Tanaka, T. & Horie, M. (2006) Prediction of mortality by high-sensitivity C-reactive protein and brain natriuretic peptide in patients with dilated cardiomyopathy. *Circulation Journal* 70: 857-863.

Jameson, J.N., Kasper, D., Harrison, T.R., Braunwald, E., Fauci, A.S., Hauser, S.L. & Longo, D.L. (2005) Harrison's Principles of Internal Medicine. McGraw-Hill Medical Publishing Division, New York.

Jefferis, B.J., Papacosta, O., Owen, C.G., Wannamethee, S.G., Humphries, S.E., Woodward, M., Lennon, L.T., Thomson, A., Welsh, P., Rumley, A., Lowe, G.D. & Whincup, P.H. (2011) Interleukin 18 and coronary heart disease: prospective study and systematic review. *Atherosclerosis* April 8 [Epub ahead of print].

Kallwellis-Opara, A., Dorner, A., Poller, W.-C., Noutsias, M., Kuhl, U., Schultheiss, H.-P. & Pauschinger, M. (2007) Autoimmunological features in inflammatory cardiomyopathy. *Clinical Research Cardioliology* 96: 469-480.

Kaneko, K., Kanda, T., Yamauchi, Y., Hasegawa, A., Iwasaki, T., Arai, M., Suzuki, T., Kobayashi, I. & Nagai, R. (1999) C-reactive protein in dilated cardiomyopathy. *Cardiology* 91: 215-219.

Kaneko, K., Kanda, T., Hasegawa, A., Suzuki, T., Kobayashi, I. & Nagai, R. (2000) C-reactive protein as a prognostic marker in lymphocytic myocarditis. *Japan Heart Journal* 41: 41-47.

Kania, G., Blyszczuk, P. & Eriksson, U. (2009) Mechanisms of cardiac fibrosis in inflammatory heart disease. *Trends in Cardiovascular Medicine* 19: 247-252.

Karamitsos, T.D. & Neubauer, S. (2011) Cardiovascular magnetic resonance in heart failure. *Current Cardiology Report* doi: 10.1007/s11886-011-0177-2.

Kaya, Z., Goser, S., Buss, B.J., Leuschner, F., Ottl, R., Li, J., Volkers, M., Zittrich, S., Pfitzer, G., Rose, N.R. & Katus, H.A. (2008) Identification of cardiac troponin I sequence motifs leading to heart failure by induction of myocardial inflammation and fibrosis. *Circulation* 118: 2063-2072.

Kaya, Z., Katus, H.A. & Rose, N.R. (2010) Cardiac troponins and autoimmunity: their role in the pathogenesis of myocarditis and of heart failure. *Clinical Immunology* 134: 80-88.

Kindermann, I., Kindermann, M., Kandolf, R., Klingel, K., Bultmann, B., Muller, T., Lindinger, A. & Bohm, M. (2008) Predictors of outcome in patients with suspected myocarditis. *Circulation* 118: 639-648.

Kleinfeldt, T., Nienaber, C.A., Kische, S., Akin, I., Turan, R.G., Korber, T., Schneider, H. & Ince, H. (2010) Cardiac manifestation of the hypereosinophilic syndrome: new insights. *Clinical Research Cardioliology* 99: 419-427.

Kojima, J., Miyazaki, S., Fujiwara, H., Kumada, T. & Kawai, C. (1988) Recurrent left ventricular mural thrombi in a patient with acute myocarditis. *Heart Vessels* 4: 120-122.

Krumholz, H.M., Want, Y., Parent, E.M., Mockalis, J., Petrillo, M. & Radford, M.J. (1997) Quality of care for elderly patients hospitalized with heart failure. *Archives of Internal Medicine* 157: 2242-2247.

Kuh, J.H. & Seo, Y. (2005) Transatrial resection of a left ventricular thrombus after acute myocarditis. *Heart Vessels* 20: 230-232.

Kuhl, U., Pauschinger, M., Schwimmbeck, P.L., Seeberg, B., Lober, C., Noutsias, M., Poller, W. & Schultheiss, H.P. (2003) Interferon-beta treatment eliminates cardiotropic viruses and improves left ventricular function in patients with myocardial persistence of viral genomes and left ventricular dysfunction. *Circulation* 107: 2793-2798.

Kumar, V., Abbas, A.K. & Fausto, N. (2005) *Robbins and Cotran Pathologic Basis of Disease*, 7th edn. Elsevier Saunders, Philadelphia.

Latini, R., Masson, S., Anand, I.S., Missov, E., Carlson, M., Vago, T., Angelici, L., Barlera, S., Parrinello, G., Maggioni, A.P., Tognoni, G., Cohn, J.N. & Val-HeFT Investigators. (2007) Prognostic value of very low plasma concentrations of troponin T in patients with stable chronic heart failure. *Circulation* 116: 1242-1249.

Leuschner, F., Li, J., Goser, S., Reinhardt, L., Ottl, R., Bride, P., Zehelein, J., Pfitzer, G., Remppis, A., Giannitsis, E., Katus, H.A. & Kaya, Z. (2008) Absence of autoantibodies against cardiac troponin I predicts improvement of left ventricular function after acute myocardial infarction. *European Heart Journal* 29: 1949-1955.

Levine, B., Kalman, J., Mayer, L., Fillit, H.M. & Packer, M. (1990) Elevated circulating levels of tumor necrosis factor in severe chronic heart failure. *New England Journal of Medicine* 323: 236-241.

Liew, F.Y., Pitman, N.I. & McInnes, I.B. (2010) Disease-associated funcitons of IL-33: the new kid in the IL-1 family. *Nature Reviews Immunology* 10: 103-110.

Liu, P., Sun, M. & Sader, S. (2006) Matrix metalloproteinases in cardiovascular diseae. *Canadian Journal of Cardiology* 22(Suppl. B): 25B-30B.

Looi, J.L., Edwards, C., Armstrong, G.P., Scott, A., Patel, H., Hart, H. & Christiansen, J.P. (2010) Characteristics and prognostic importance of myocardial fibrosis in patients with dilated cardiomyopathy assessed by contrast-enhanced cardiac magnetic resonance imaging. *Clinical Medicine Insights in Cardiology* 4: 129-134.

Mackman, N. (2009) The many faces of tissue factor. *Journal of Thombosis and* Haemostasis 7: 136-139.

Maisch, B. (1994) Pericardial diseases, with a focus on etiology, pathogenesis, pathophysiology, new diagnostic imaging methods, and treatment. *Current Opinion in Cardiology* 9: 379-388.

Mann, D.L. (2005) Targeted anticytokine therapy and the failing heart. *American Journal of Cardiology* 95(Suppl): 9C-16C.

Marchant, D. & McManus, B.M. (2009) Matrix metalloproteinases in the pathogenesis of viral heart disease. *Trends in Cardiovascular Medicine* 19: 21-26.

Masson, S., Latini, R., Anand, I.S., Vago, T., Angelici, L., Barlera, S., Missov, E.D., Clerico, A., Tognoni, G., Cohn, J.N. & Val-HeFT Investigators. (2006) Direct comparison of B-type natriuretic peptide (BNP) and amino-terminal proBNP in a large population of patients with chronic and symptomatic heart failure: the Valsartan Heart Fialure (Val-HeFT) data. *Clinical Chemistry* 52: 1528-1538.

Miettinen, K.H., Eriksson, S., Magga, J., Tuomainen, P., Kuusisto, J., Vanninen, E.J., Turpeinen, A., Punnonen, K.R., Pettersson, K. & Peuhkurinen, K.J. (2008) Clinical significance of troponin I efflux and troponin autoantibodies in patients with dilated cardiomyopathy. *Journal of Cardiac Failure* 14: 481-488.

Miller, A.M. & Liew, F.Y. (2011) The IL-33/ST2 pathway- a new therapeutic target for cardiovascular disease. *Pharmacology and Therapeutics* Feb 26 [Epub ahead of print].

Miller, W.L., Hartman, K.A., Burritt, M.F., Burnett, J.C. & Jaffe, A.S. (2007) Troponin, B-type natriuretic peptides and outcomes in severe heart failure: differences between ischemic and dilated cardiomyopathies. *Clinical Cardiology* 30: 245-250.

Miller, A.M., Xu, D., Asquith, D.L., Denby, L., Li, Y., Sattar, N., Baker, A.H., McInnes, I.B. & Liew, F.Y. (2008) IL-33 reduces the development of atherosclerosis. *Journal of Experimental Medicine* 205: 339-346.

Morgera, T., Di Lenarda, A., Dreas, L., Pinamonti, B., Humar, F., Bussani, R., Silvestri, F., Chersevani, D. & Camerini, F. (1992) Electrocardiography of myocardtiis revisited: clinical and prognostic significance of electrocardiographic changes. *American Heart Journal* 124: 455-467.

Morrow, D.A. & de Lemos, J.A. (2007) Benchmarks for the assessment of novel cardiovascular biomarkers. *Circulation* 115: 949-952.

Nishikubo, K., Imanaka-Yoshida, K., Tamaki, S., Hiroe, M., Yoshida, T., Adachi, Y. & Yasutomi, Y. (2007) Th1-type immune responses by Toll-like receptor 4 signaling are required for the development of myocarditis in mice with BCG-induced myocarditis. *Journal of Autoimmunity* 29: 146-153.

Nishimura, H., Okazaki, T., Tanaka, Y., Nakatani, K., Hara, M., Matsumori, A., Sasayama, S., Mizoguchi, A., Hiai, H., Minato, N. & Honjo, T. (2001) Autoimmune dilated cardiomyopathy in PD-1 receptor deficient mice. *Science* 291: 319-322.

Ogawa, T., Veinot, J.P., Kuroski de Bold, M.L., Georgalis, T. & de Bold, A.J. (2008) Angiotensin II receptor antagonism reverts the selective cardiac BNP upregulation and secretion observed in myocarditis. *American Journal of Physiology and Heart Circulation Physiology* 294: H2596-H2603.

Olimulder, M.A., van Es, J. & Galjee, M.A. (2009) The importance of cardiac MRI as a diagnostic took in viral myocarditis-induced cardiomyopathy. *Netherlands Heart Journal* 17: 481-486.

Omland, T., Sabatine, M.S., Jablonski, K.A., Rice, M.M., Hsia, J., Wergeland, R., Landaas, S., Rouleau, J.L., Domanski, M.J., Hall, C., Pfeffer, M.A., Braunwald, E. & PEACE Investigators. (2007) Prognostic value of B-type natriuretic peptides in patients with stable coronary artery disease: the PEACE Trial. *Journal of American College of Cardiology* 50: 205-214.

Onyimba, J.A., Coronado, M.J., Garton, A.E., Kim, J.B., Bucek, A., Bedja, D., Gabrielson, K.L., Guilarte, T.R. & Fairweather, D. (2011) The innate immune response to coxsackievirus B3 predicts progression to cardiovascular disease and heart failure in male mice. *Biology of Sex Differences* 2: 2.

Osman, R., L'Allier, P.L., Elgharib, N. & Tardif, J.-C. (2006) Critical appraisal of C-reactive protein throughout the spectrum of cardiovascular disease. *Vascular Health and Risk Management* 2: 221-237.

Palazzuoli, A., Antonelli, G., Quantrini, I. & Nuti, R. (2011) Natriuretic peptides in heart failure: where we are, where we are going. *Internal Emergency Medicine* 6: 63-68.

Peacock, W.F. 4th, DeMarco, T., Fonarow, G.C., Diercks, D., Wynne, J., Apple, F.S., Wu, A.H. & ADHERE Investigators. (2008) Cardiac troponin and outcome in acute heart failure. *New England Journal of Medicine* 15: 2117-2126.

Peerschke, E.I., Yin, W. & Ghebrehiwet, B. (2010) Complement activation on platelets: implications for vascular inflammation and thrombosis. *Molecular Immunolunology* 47: 2170-2175.

Pepys, M.B. & Hirschfield, G.M. (2003) C-reactive protein: a critical update. *The Journal of Clinical Investigation* 111: 1805-1812.

Perez-De-Lis, M., Akasbi, M., Siso, A., Diez-Cascon, P., Brito-Zeron, P., Diaz-Lagares, C., Ortiz, J., Perez-Alvarez, R., Ramos-Casals, M. & Coca, A. (2010) Cardiovascular risk factors in primary Sjogren's syndrome: a case-control study in 624 patients. *Lupus* 19: 941-948.

Piro, M., Bona, R.D., Abbate, A., Biasucci, L.M. & Crea, F. (2010) Sex-related differences in myocardial remodeling. *Journal of the American College of Cardiology* 55: 1057-1065.

Rao, M., Jaber, B.L. & Balakrishnan, V.S. (2006) Inflammatory biomarkers and cardiovascular risk: association or cause and effect? *Seminars in Dialysis* 19: 129-135.

Rezaizadeh, H., Sanchez-Ross, M., Kaluski, E., Klapholz, M., Haider, B. & Gerula, C. (2010) Acute eosinophilic myocarditis: diagnosis and treatment. *Acute Cardiac Care* 12: 31-36.

Rhodes, B., Furnrohr, B.G. & Vyse, T.J. (2011) C-reactive protein in rheumatology: biology and genetics. *Nature Reviews Rheumatology* April 5 [Epub ahead of print].

Robinson, T., Smith, A. & Channer, K.S. (2011) Reversible heart failure: the role of inflammatory activation. *Postgraduate Medical Journal* 87: 110-115.

Roger, V.L., Go, A.S., Lloyd-Jones, D.M., Adams, R.J., Berry, J.D., Brown, T.M., Carnethon, M.R., Dai, S., de Simone, G., Ford, E.S., Fox, C.S., Fullerton, H.J., Gillespie, C., Greenlund, K.J., Hailpern, S.M., Heit, J.A., Ho, P.M., Howard, V.J., Kissela, B.M., Kittner, S.J., Lackland, D.T., Lichtman, J.H., Lisabeth, L.D., Makuc, D.M., Marcus, G.M., Marelli, A., Matchar, D.B., McDermott, M.M., Meigs, J.B., Moy, C.S., Mozaffarian, D., Mussolino, M.E., Nichol, G., Paynter, N.P., Rosamond, W.D., Sorlie, P.D., Stafford, R.S., Turan, T.N., Turner, M.B., Wong, N.D., Wylie-Rosett, J., American Heart Association Statistics Committee and Stroke Statistics Subcommittee. (2011) Heart disease and stroke statistics- 2011 update. *Circulation* 123: e18-e209.

Ronaldson, K.J., Taylor, A.J., Fitzgerald, P.B., Topliss, D.J., Elsik, M. & McNeil, J.J. (2010) Diagnostic characteristics of clozapine-induced myocarditis identified by an analysis of 38 cases and 47 controls. *Journal of Clinical Psychiatry* 71: 976-981.

Sanada, S., Hakuno, D., Higgins, L.J., Schreiter, E.R., McKenzie, A.N.J. & Lee R.T. (2007) IL-33 and ST2 comprise a critical biomechanically induced and cardioprotective signaling system. *The Journal of Clinical Investigation* 117: 1538-1549.

Satoh, M., Nakamura, M., Akatsu, T., Iwasaka, J., Shimoda, Y., Segawa, I. & Hiramori, K. (2003) Expression of Toll-like receptor 4 is associated with enteroviral replication in human myocarditis. *Clinical Science (London)* 104: 577-584.

Satoh, M., Nakamura, M., Akatsu, T., Shimoda, Y., Segawa, I. & Hiramori, K. (2005) C-reactive protein co-expresses with tumor necrosis factor-alpha in the myocardium in human dilated cardiomyopathy. *European Journal Heart* 7: 748-754.

Schultz, J.C., Hilliard, A.A., Cooper, L.T. & Rihal, C.S. (2009) Diagnosis and treatment of viral myocarditis. *Mayo Clinical Proceedings* 84: 1001-1009.

Senes, M., Erbay, A.R., Yilmaz, F.M., Topkaya, B.C., Zengi, O., Dogan, M. & Yucel, D. (2008) Coenzyme Q10 and high-sensitivity C-reactive protein in ischemic and idiopathic dilated cardiomyopathy. *Clinical Chemistry Laboratory Medicine* 46: 382-386.

Seta, Y., Shan, K., Bozkurt, B., Oral, H. & Mann, D.L. (1996) Basic mechanisms in heart failure: the cytokine hypothesis. *Journal of Cardiac Failure* 2: 243-249.

Shamri, R., Xenakis. J.J. & Spencer, L.A. (2011) Eosinophils in innate immunity: an evolving story. *Cell Tissue Research* 343: 57-83.

Shmilovich, H., Danon, A., Binah, O., Roth, A., Chen, G., Wexler, D., Keren, G. & George, J. (2007) Autoantibodies to cardiac troponin I in patients with idiopathic dilated and ischemic cardiomyopathy. *International Journal of Cardiology* 117: 198-203.

Silver, M.A., Maisel, A., Yancy, C.W., McCullough, P.A., Burnett, J.C. Jr., Francis, G.S., Mehra, M.R., Peacock, W.F. 4th, Fonarow, G., Gibler, W.B., Morrow, D.A., Hollander, J. & BNP Consensus Panel. (2004) NBP Consensus Panel 2004: A clinical approach for the diagnostic, prognostic, screening, treatment monitoring, and therapeutic roles of natriuretic peptides in cardiovascular diseases. *Congestive Heart Failure* 10(Suppl. 3): 1-30.

Smith, S.C., Ladenson, J.H., Mason, J.W., & Jaffe, A.S. (1997) Elevations of cardiac troponin I associated with myocarditis. Experimental and clinical correlates. *Circulation* 95: 163-168.

Soongswang, J., Durongpisitkul, K., Ratanarapee, S., Leowattana, W., Nana, A., Laohaprasitiporn, D., Akaniroj, S., Limpimwong, N. & Kangkagate, C. (2002) Cardiac troponin T: its role in the diagnosis of clinically suspected acute myocarditis and chronic dilated cardiomyopathy in children. *Pediatric Cardiology* 23: 531 535.

Talvani, A., Rocha, M.O., Barcelos, L.S., Gomes, Y.M., Ribeiro, A.L. & Teixeira, M.M. (2004) Elevated concentrations of CCL2 and tumor necrosis factor-alpha in chagasic cardiomyopathy. *Clinical Infectious Disease* 38: 943-950.

Tanaka, K., Ito, M., Kodama, M., Tomita, M., Kimura, S., Hoyano, M., Mitsuma, W., Hirono, S., Hanawa, H. & Aizawa, Y. (2011) Sulfated polysaccharide fucoidan ameliorates experimental autoimmune myocarditis in rats. *Journal of Cardiovascular Pharmacology and Therapy* 16: 79-86.

Tang, Q., Huang, J., Qian, H., Xiong, R., Shen, D., Wu, H., Bian, Z. & Wei, X. (2007) Microarray analysis reveals the role of matrix metalloproteinases in mouse experimental autoimmune myocarditis induced by cardiac myosin peptides. *Cell Molecular Biology Letters* 12: 176-191.

Tyagi, S.C., Campbell, S.E., Reddy, H.K., Tjahja, E. & Voelker, D.J. (1996) Matrix metalloproteinase activity expression in infracted, noninfarcted and dilated cardiomyopathic human hearts. *Molecular Cell Biochemistry* 155: 13-21.

Vallejo, J.G. (2011) Roleof Toll-like receptors in cardiovascular diseases. *Clinical Science* 121: 1-10.

Vasan, R.S., Sullivan, L.M., Roubenoff, R., Dinarello, C.A., Harris, T., Benjamin, E.J., Sawyer, D.B., Levy, D., Wilson, P.W., D'Agostino, R.B. & Framingham Heart Study. (2003) Inflammatory markers and risk of heart failure in elderly subjects without prior myocardial infarction: the Framingham Heart Study. *Circulation* 107: 1486-1491.

Venugopal, S.K., Devaraj, S. & Jialal, I. (2005) Effect of C-reactive protein on vascular cells: evidence for a proinflammatory, proatherogenic role. *Current Opinion in Nephrology and Hypertension* 14: 33-37.

Wang, Y.-X., da Cunha, V., Vincelette, J., White, K., Velichko, S., Xu, Y., Gross, C., Fitch, R.M., Halks-Miller, M., Larsen, B.R., Yajima, T., Knowlton, K.U., Vergona, R., Sullivan, M.E. & Croze, E. (2007) Antiviral and myocyte protective effects of murine interferon-β and -α2 in coxsackievirus B3-induced myocarditis and epicarditis in BALB/c mice. *American Journal of Physiology and Heart Circulation Physiology* 293: H69-H76.

Weinberg, E.O., Shimpo, M., De Keulenaer, G.W., MacGillivray, C., Tominaga, S., Solomon, S.D., Rouleau, J.L. & Lee, R.T. (2002) Expression and regulation of ST2, an interleukin-1 receptor family member, in cardiomyocytes and myocardial infarction. *Circulation* 106: 2961-2966.

Weinberg, E.O., Shimpo, M., Hurwitz, S., Tominaga, S., Rouleau, J.L. & Lee, R.T. (2003) Identification of serum soluble ST2 receptor as a novel heart failure biomarker. *Circulation* 107: 721-726.

Westermann, D., Savvatis, K., Schultheiss, H.P. & Tschope, C. (2010) Immunomodulation and matrix metalloproteinases in viral myocarditis. *Journal of Molecular and Cellular Cardiology* 48: 468-473.

Wexler, R.K., Elton, T., Pleister, A. & Feldman, D. (2009) Cardiomyopathy: an overview. *American Family Physician* 79: 778-784.

Yung, C.K., Helperin, V.L., Tomaselli, G.F. & Winslow, R.L. (2004) Gene expression profiles in end-stage human idiopathic dilated cardiomyopathy: altered expression of apoptotic and cytoskeletal genes. *Genomics* 83: 281-297.

Zimmermann, O., Bienek-Ziolkowski, M., Wolf, B., Vetter, M., Baur, R., Mailander, V., Hombach, V. & Torzewski, J. (2009) Myocardial inflammation and non-ischaemic heart failure: is there a role for C-reactive protein? *Basic Research in Cardiology* 104: 591-599.

Zwaka, T.P., Manolov, D., Ozdemir, C., Marx, N., Kaya, Z., Kochs, M., Hoher, M., Hombach, V & Torzewski, J. (2002) Complement and dilated cardiomyopathy: a role of sublytic terminal complement complex-induced tumor necrosis factor-alpha synthesis in cardiac myocytes. *American Journal of Pathology* 161: 449-457.

18

A Proteomic Approach to Investigate Myocarditis

Andrea Carpentieri*, Chiara Giangrande*, Piero Pucci and Angela Amoresano
Department of Organic Chemistry and Biochemistry, Facoltà di Scienze Biotecnologiche, Federico II University of Naples, Naples, Italy

1. Introduction

Myocarditis is an inflammatory disease of the cardiac muscle which might be related to viral (mainly parvovirus B19 and many others), protozoan (*Borrellia burgdoferi, Trypanosoma cruzi, Toxoplasma gondi*), bacterial (*Brucella, Corynebacterium diphtheriae, Gonococcus, Haemophilus influenzae, Actinomyces, Tropheryma whipplei, Vibrio cholerae, Borrelia burgdorferi, Leptospira, Rickettsia*), fungal (*Aspergillus*) and other non viral pathogens (Rezkalla SH et al., 2010, Blauwet LA et al., 2010, Cihakova D et al., 2010) infections; It has been reported, however, that this kind of inflammation might be caused by an hypersensitivity response to drugs (Kühl U et al., 2009). The final effect in each case is represented by myocardial infiltration of immunocompetent cells following any kind of cardiac injury.

Myocarditis presents with many symptoms, from chest pain that spontaneously resolves without treatment to cardiogenic shock and sudden death (Kühl U et al., 2010, Taylor CL et al 2010). The major long-term consequence is dilated cardiomyopathy with chronic heart failure(Lv H et al. 2011, Stensaeth KH et al 2011).

Nowadays, diagnostic tools available for this disease are mainly related to general investigations (such as electrocardiography) and analysis of the most abundant serum proteins, whose alteration is related to cardiac pathology, even if it's not specifically connected to myocarditis itself. Here we propose preliminary speculations on the serum proteins profiling (both in the expression level and in the characterization of post translational modifications) and on free peptides identification in myocardytis affected patients (compared to healthy individual), that could be helpful in finding specific markers for this pathology.

As many other inflammatory events this disease involves in fact different kinds of biological macromolecules, here we focus in particular on proteins. More than 50% of total protein content in a cell is post translationally modified. The pattern of Post Translational Modifications (PTMs) on proteins constitute a molecular code that dictates protein conformation, cellular location, macromolecular interactions and activities, depending on cell type, tissue and environmental conditions (Diernfellner AC et al., 2011, Savidge TC,

* Equally contributed to the work.

2011, Hao P et al.,2011). It is very well known that biological function of many proteins is strictly related to the presence of the appropriate set of PTMs. Most importantly, PTMs deregulation might be involved in the development of diseases , in fact, as a consequence of many pathologies, PTMs set might be altered (Dell A et al., 2001, Kim YJ. Et al 1997, Dube DH. Et al., 2005, Granovsky M. Et al 2000).

Proteomics investigations offer all useful tools to deeply investigate this kind of alterations. Two dimensional electrophoresis coupled with software mediated image analysis, affinity chromatographies and especially Mass Spectrometry (MS) present high levels of sensitivity, accuracy and reproducibility and these are all fundamental requirements that this kind of study needs.

As previously described by our group (Carpentieri A, Giangrande C, et al., 2010), serum glycoproteome characterization might be crucial in clinical investigation. In fact we showed that the *N*-glycan profiling of serum glycoproteins extracted from myocarditis affected donors compared to the ones of healthy people shows many peculiarities. We demonstrated that many of the extracted oligosaccharides are in fact incomplete or truncated structures whilst others show a high level of fucosylation, all these results fully matched previously published data about the glycosylation in proteins during chronic inflammation events (Dell A et al., 2001, Kim YJ. Et al 1997, Dube DH. Et al., 2005, Granovsky M. Et al 2000, Carpentieri A, Giangrande C, et al., 2010).

Thanks to the high sensitivity of the most modern analytical techniques, several research groups focus the research at level of peptides rather than at protein level (Taylor-Papadimitriou J. et al., 1994 Amado F et al., 2010, Menschaert G et al. 2010). In fact, these endogenous peptides are referred to as the peptidome. Initially, peptidomic analyses were conducted as a method to study neuropeptides and peptide hormones; these are signaling molecules that function in a variety of physiological processes (Ludwig M. 2011, Colgrave ML et al., 2011). Recent studies have found large numbers of cellular peptides with half-lives of several seconds, raising the possibility that they may be involved in biological functions (Gorman PM et al 2003).

Here we propose preliminary data to show molecular basis of myocarditis using a proteomic approach. The analyses were focused on the serum proteins profiling, namely the study of the expression level and the characterization of glycoproteins involved in the pathology. A classical two-dimensional gel electrophoresis procedure to obtain protein maps and a "gel-free" comparison of the glycoproteomes in healthy and myocarditis human sera by using advanced mass spectrometry were reported. Free peptides identification in myocardytis affected patients (compared to healthy individual), was achieved in order to provide possible specific markers for this pathology.

2. Materials and methods

2.1 Materials

Human serum samples from 8 healthy donors (all Caucasian 4 males and 4 females aged between 60 and 80 years, all other clinical informations were covered by laws on privacy) and from 5 myocarditis affected patients (all Caucasian 3 males and 2 females aged between 60 and 85 years, all other clinical informations were covered by laws on privacy), respectively, have been obtained from the "Servizio Analisi" Policlinico, Napoli. Aliquots of serum samples from different donors were pooled in order to obtain an average overview of glycoforms distribution.

Guanidine, dithiothreitol (DTT), trypsin, α-cyano-4-hydroxycinnamic acid were purchased from Sigma. Iodoacetamide (IAM), tris(hydroxymethyl)aminomethane, calcium chloride and ammonium bicarbonate (AMBIC) were purchased from Fluka as well as the MALDI matrix 2,5-, α-cyano-4-hydroxycinnamic. Methanol, trifluoroacetic acid (TFA) and acetonitrile (ACN) are HPLC grade type from Carlo Erba, whereas the other solvents are from Baker. Gel filtration columns PD-10 are from Pharmacia, the HPLC ones from Phenomenex, whereas the pre-packed columns Sep-pak C-18 are from Waters.
Comassie Brilliant Blue was from Bio-Rad. PNGase F were purchased from Boheringer. Ion exchange resins Dowex H+ (50W-X8 50-100 mesh) was provided by BDH. Concanavalin A sepharose resin was purchased from Amersham Biosciences.

2.2 Protein concentration determination

Sera protein concentration was determined by Bradford assay method, using bovine serum albumin (BSA) as standard. Known amounts of BSA were diluted in 800 µL of H2O and then mixed to 200 µL of Comassie Brilliant Blue. 5 different BSA concentrations were determined by measuring absorbance at 595 nm and used to obtain a linear calibration curve. Three different sera dilutions were measured at 595 nm. Absorbance data were interpoled on the calibration curve, allowing the determination of protein concentration in the different samples.

2.3 Serum depletion

The depletion of the most abundant proteins from each serum sample was performed using Multiple Affinity Removal Spin Cartridges from Agilent. The procedure was performed at room temperature according to manufacturer's instructions and then immediately frozen to -20°C.

2.4 Free peptides analysis

300 µL acetonitrile was added to 100 µL of serum, incubated at room temperature for 30 minutes and then centrifuged at 13000 rpm. Supernatants were collected and concentrated by vacuum centrifugation (SAVANT) and resuspended in 20 µL formic acid 0.1%. Samples were desalted by C18 Zip Tip (Millipore) and diluted 100 times prior mass spectrometry analyses.

LC/MS-MS HPLC-Chip/Q-TOF 6520

Peptides were analyzed by a HPLC-Chip/Q-TOF 6520 (Agilent Technologies). The capillary column works at a flow of 4 µL/min, concentrating and washing the sample in a 40 nL enrichment column. The sample was then fractionated on a C18 reverse-phase capillary column (75 µm~43 mm in the Agilent Technologies chip) at flow rate of 400 nl/min, with a linear gradient of eluent B (0.2% formic acid in 95% acetonitrile) in A (0.2% formic acid in 2% acetonitrile) from 7% to 60% in 50 min.
Data were acquired through MassHunter software (Agilent Technologies). Proteins identification was achieved by using Mascot software (Matrix science), with a tolerance of 10 ppm on peptide mass, 0.6 Da on MS/MS, and choosing methionine oxidation and glutamine conversion in pyro-glutamic acid as variable modifications.

MALDI-TOF/TOF

Peptides were also analyzed by MALDI-TOF/TOF using a 4800 Plus MALDI-TOF/TOF (Applied Biosystems). Samples were mixed on MALDI plate to the matrix consisting of a solution of 10 mg/mL α-cyano-4-hydroxycinnamic, whose preparation consisted in the resuspension of α-cyano-4-hydroxycinnamic in water and acetonitrile 10:1 (v/v). The instrument was calibrated using a mixture of standard peptides (Applied Biosystems). Spectra were register even in reflector positive. MS/MS spectra were performed with CID using air as collision gas. Spectra were manually interpreted.

2.5 2D-gel electrophoresis

IEF (first dimension) was carried out on non-linear wide-range immobilized pH gradients (pH 4-7; 7 cm long IPG strips; GE Healthcare, Uppsala, Sweden) and achieved using the EttanTM IPGphorTM system (GE Healthcare, Uppsala, Sweden). Analytical-run IPG-strips were rehydrated with 125µg□ of total proteins in 125µl of rehydratation buffer (urea 8 M, CHAPS 2%, 0,5% (v/v) IPG Buffer, bromophenol blue 0,002%) for 12 h at 20°C. The strips were then focused according to the following electrical conditions at 20°C: 500 V for 30 min, from 1000 V for 30 min, 5000 V until a total of 15000 Vt was reached. After focusing IPG strips were equilibrated for 15 min in 6 M urea, 30% (vol/vol) glycerol, 2% (wt/vol) SDS, 0.05 M Tris-HCl, pH 6.8, 2% (wt/vol) DTT, and subsequently for 15 min in the same urea/SDS/Tris buffer solution but substituting the 2% (wt/vol) DTT with 2.5% (wt/vol) iodoacetamide. The second dimension was carried out on 12% polyacrylamide gels at 25 mA/gel constant current until the dye front reached the bottom of the gel. MS gel was stained with colloidal comassie.

2.6 Image analysis

Gels images were acquired with an Epson expression 1680 PRO scanner. Computer-aided 2-D image analysis was carried out using the ImageMasterTM 2D Platinum software (GE Healthcare, Uppsala, Sweden). Differentially expressed spots were selected for MS analysis.

In order to find differentially expressed proteins, comassie stained gel image of serum proteins from healthy individual was matched with the one of myocarditis affected patient. The apparent isoelectric points and molecular masses of the proteins were calculated with ImageMaster 2D Platinum 6.0 using identified proteins with known parameters as references.

Relative spot volumes (%V) (V=integration of OD over the spot area; %V = V single spot/V total spot) were used for quantitative analysis in order to decrease experimental errors. The normalized intensity of spots on three replicate 2-D gels was averaged and standard deviation was calculated for each condition.

2.7 Protein identification by mass spectrometry

In situ digestion

Protein spots were excised from the gel and destained by repetitive washes with 0.1 M NH_4HCO_3 pH 7.5 and acetonitrile. Enzymatic digestion was carried out with trypsin (12.5 ng/µl) in 10 mM ammonium bicarbonate buffer pH 7.8. Gel pieces were incubated at 4 °C for 2 h. Trypsin solution was then removed and a new aliquot of the same solution was added; samples were incubated for 18 h at 37 °C. A minimum reaction volume was used as to obtain the complete rehydratation of the gel. Peptides were then extracted by washing the gel particles with 10mM ammonium bicarbonate and 1% formic acid in 50% acetonitrile at room temperature.

Mass spectrometry and protein identification

LC-MS/MS analyses were performed as previously described for free peptides.
Mass spectrometric obtained data were used for protein identification using the software MASCOT that compare peptide masses obtained by MS and MS/MS data of each tryptic digestion with the theoretical peptide masses from all the proteins accessible in the databases (Peptide Mass Fingerprinting, PMF). Database searches were performed in NBCI databank (National Center for Biotechnology Information), restricting the analysis to the pertinent taxonomies. The parameters used for the identification were: tolerance of 10 ppm on peptide mass, 0.6 Da on MS/MS, and cysteine carbamidomethylation as fixed modification. Variable modifications were methionine oxidation, glutamine conversion in pyro-glutamic acid, and asparagine deamidation.

2.8 Boronate affinity chromatography

Glycoproteins were purified using PBA-bound agarose (Sigma-Aldrich, Munich, Germany). 500 μl of sample previously diluted (1 : 1) with equilibration buffer (50 mM taurine/NaOH, pH 8.7, containing 3–10 mM $MgCl_2$) was incubated with 200 μl of pre-washed immobilized ligand resin for 1 h on ice and with gentle shaking. After transfer of the resin into 1,5 ml eppendhorf tubes, the non-binding fraction was collected by low speed centrifugation (10 s, 500 × g). The resin was then thoroughly rinsed with equilibration buffer (six washes of 150 μl each) and 1 N NaCl (three washes of 150 μl each). For final elution of the bound fraction, a total of six washes (150 μl each) with taurine buffer containing 50 mM sorbitol were used. Three successive fractions (150 μl each) were pooled before further analysis.

2.9 Deglycosylation

Glycopeptides were lyophilized, resuspended in 10 mM AMBIC and incubated with PNGase F (5 U), for 12-16 h at 37°C. Deglycosylation was carried out also on unbound peptides, in order to release the glycans not recognized by Boronate affinity chromatography.

3. Results and discussion

3.1 Free peptides analysis

The analyses to investigate the "peptidomic" both in healthy and in pathological samples were accomplished by using a gel-free approach. The peptide component of the eluted fraction was analyzed by tandem mass spectrometry. The stringency of scoring parameters of the MASCOT algorithm minimized the number of false positive identifications. Most MS/MS spectra giving positive hits were derived from doubly and triply charged precursor ions that resulted predominantly in y-ion series.
Triplicate LC-MS/MS analysis of supernatants after ACN precipitation of serum proteins, showed the occurrence of many free peptides in both analyzed sera. As reported in Table 1, the total number of detected and identified peptides was 41. Among these, 9 peptides were unique in the pathologic sample. It should be noted that some peptides were identified in both samples.

m/z	RT	Sequence	Peptide	Protein	H/M ratio
567.95	17.09	QAGAAGSRMNFRPGVLS	(650-666)	**Q14624** Inter-alpha-trypsin inhibitor heavy chain H4	H:not detected
513.78	17.70	YYLQGAKIPKPEASFSPR	(627-644)	**Q14624** Inter-alpha-trypsin inhibitor heavy chain H4	H:not detected
823.17	22.11	MNFRPGVLSSRQLGLPGPPDVPDH AAYHPF	(658-687)	**Q14624** Inter-alpha-trypsin inhibitor heavy chain H4	H:not detected
1005.98	22.78	QLGLPGPPDVPDHAAYHPF	(669-687)	**Q14624** Inter-alpha-trypsin inhibitor heavy chain H4	0.68±0.18
757.71	19.96	SRQLGLPGPPDVPDHAAYHPF	(667-687)	**Q14624** Inter-alpha-trypsin inhibitor heavy chain H4	0.27±0.09
681.85	22.07	PGVLSSRQLGLPGPPDVPDHAAYHP F	(662-687)	**Q14624** Inter-alpha-trypsin inhibitor heavy chain H4	0.18±0.03
576.90	20.69	PGVLSSRQLGLPGPPDVPDHAAYHP FR	(662-688)	**Q14624** Inter-alpha-trypsin inhibitor heavy chain H4	H:not detected
379.71	0.55	LAEGGGVR	(28-35)	**P02671** Fibrinogen alpha chain	25±3.11
453.24	3.65	FLAEGGGVR	(27-35)	**P02671** Fibrinogen alpha chain	2.48±0.57
510.76	11.29	DFLAEGGGVR	(26-35)	**P02671** Fibrinogen alpha chain	1.33±0.76
539.27	11.70	GDFLAEGGGVR	(25-35)	**P02671** Fibrinogen alpha chain	3.15±1.02
597.77	15.59	SGEGDFLAEGGGV	(22-34)	**P02671** Fibrinogen alpha chain	0.85±0.23
603.79	12.57	EGDFLAEGGGVR	(24-35)	**P02671** Fibrinogen alpha chain	2.42±0.63
632.30	13.50	GEGDFLAEGGGVR	(23-35)	**P02671** Fibrinogen alpha chain	2.72±0.71
655.28	16.03	DSGEGDFLAEGGGV	(21-34)	**P02671** Fibrinogen alpha chain	1.23±0.36
675.81	13.67	SGEGDFLAEGGGVR	(22-35)	**P02671** Fibrinogen alpha chain	2.32±0.58
690.80	16.13	ADSGEGDFLAEGGGV	(20-34)	**P02671** Fibrinogen alpha chain	3.25±0.82
733.33	14.04	DSGEGDFLAEGGGVR	(21-35)	**P02671** Fibrinogen alpha chain	1.59±0.12
768.85	14.08	ADSGEGDFLAEGGGVR	(20-35)	**P02671** Fibrinogen alpha chain	6.16±1.01
851.71	13.58	SSSYSKQFTSSTSYNRGDSTFES	(576-598)	**P02671** Fibrinogen alpha chain	0.65±0.17

m/z	RT	Sequence	Peptide	Protein	H/M ratio
693.06	13.06	SSSYSKQFTSSTSYNRGDSTFESKS	(576-600)	**P02671** Fibrinogen alpha chain	M: not detected
733.83	14.48	SSSYSKQFTSSTSYNRGDSTFESKSY	(576-601)	**P02671** Fibrinogen alpha chain	M: not detected
619.75	17.89	QGVNDNEEGFF	(31-41)	**P02675** Fibrinogen beta chain	3.25±0.89
663.26	16.54	QGVNDNEEGFFS	(31-42)	**P02675** Fibrinogen beta chain	1.97±0.41
696.28	17.64	QGVNDNEEGFFSA	(31-43)	**P02675** Fibrinogen beta chain	2.31±0.53
404.55	18.90	RIHWESASLL	(1310-1319)	**P01024** Complement C3	H: not detected
402.22	14.29	THRIHWESASLLR	(1308-1320)	**P01024** Complement C3	H: not detected
445.25	16.98	SKITHRIHWESASLL	(1305-1319)	**P01024** Complement C3	H: not detected
415.20	7.60	HWESASL	(1312-1318)	**P01024** Complement C3	H: not detected
471.74	16.21	HWESASLL	(1312-1319)	**P01024** Complement C3	H: not detected
851.07	22.22	TLEIPGNSDPNMIPDGDFNSYVR	(957-979)	**P0C0L4** Complement C4-A	H: not detected
1054.53	25.86	DDPDAPLQPVTPLQLFEGR	(1429-1447)	**P0C0L4** Complement C4-A	H: not detected
489.96	20.26	RHPDYSVVLLLR	(169-180)	**P02768** Serum Albumin	0.43±0.17
417.91	16.67	KFQNALLVRY	(426-435)	**P02768** Serum Albumin	H: not detected
547.31	16.25	KVPQVSTPTLVEVSR	(438-452)	**P02768** Serum Albumin	H: not detected
868.11	21.57	AVPPNNSNAAEDDLPTVELQGVVPR	(14-38)	**P00488** Coagulation factor XIII A	2.40±0.84
920.14	21.09	RAVPPNNSNAAEDDLPTVELQGVVPR	(13-38)	**P00488** Coagulation factor XIII A	23.60±3.61
837.93	21.39	TAFGGRRAVPPNNSNAAEDDLPTVELQGVVPR	(7-38)	**P00488** Coagulation factor XIII A	91.32±7.39
781.37	17.84	TATSEYQTFFNPR	(315-327)	**P00734** Prothrombin	H: not detected
868.46	25.47	TGIFTDQVLSVLKGEE	(86-101)	**P02655**Apolipoprotein C-II	H: not detected
572.95	12.91	DALSSVQESQVAQQAR	(45-60)	**P02656**Apolipoprotein C-III	H: not detected
803.76	21.14	AATVGSLAGQPLQERAQAWGERL	(210-232)	**P02649**Apolipoprotein E	0.02

Table 1. List of free peptides identified by LC-MS/MS. Averaged area of chromatographic peaks from healthy(H) and myocarditis (M) ratio, indicates that some of them were differently represented. Peptide sequences were validated by MALDI-TOF/TOF analyses too.

As a whole, the LC-MS/MS proved to be a very sensitive and reproducible analysis which led to the identification of very weakly present peptides, these data were confirmed by another fragmentation technique, MALDI-TOF/TOF. As Fig. 1 shows, the fragmentation pattern of the peptide -ADSGEGDFLAEGGGVR- (from alpha fibrinogen protein) confirm what we found using LC-MS/MS analysis. Some of these peptides are related to different proteolytic activities on proteins involved in acute phase or inflammatory events, such as myocarditis itself. Among identified peptides, the molecular species , namely, peptide 662-668 from inter-alpha-trypsin inhibitor heavy chain H4 and peptide 1305-1319 from complement C3 correspond to free bioactive peptides, whose activity might be related again to inflammatory events (van den Broek I et al, 2010, ter Weeme M, et al, 2009). Preliminary qualitative and quantitative differences were detected in the analysis of the peptidomas from healthy and pathological samples. In fact, as reported in the Table 1 , averaged area of each peak of all detected peptides resulted to be different, showing that some of them were differently represented in each sample. The above mentioned peptides from complement C3 and inter-alpha trypsin inhibitor were poorly represented in the healthy serum samples, whereas fibrinogen alpha chain peptides were strongly represented in these sera, as well as coagulation factor XIII A peptides.

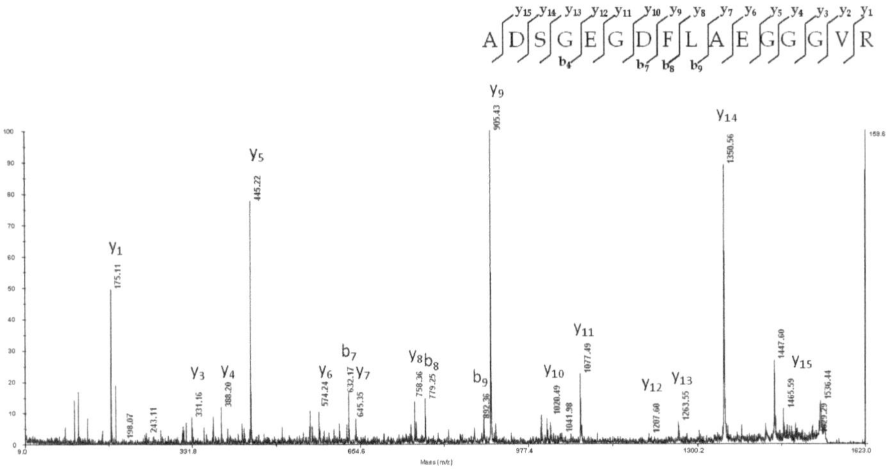

Fig. 1. Positive ion mode MALDI-TOF/TOF fragmentation spectrum of m/z 1536.44 corresponding to peptide 20-35 from fibrinogen alpha chain protein from healthy serum.

3.2 The proteins profile from 2D-electrophoresis is different

After depletion of the most abundant proteins, a two dimensional electrophoretic separation of the two sera samples was performed, thus leading to the construction of 2D protein maps of healthy and myocarditis samples. Each gel was blue comassie stained. Image analysis was performed on the two sets of 2D maps (from healthy control and pathologic sera) clearly showing that the protein profile is quite different, as reported in figure 2. The protein spots which resulted to be differentially expressed in the two samples were then submitted to mass spectral identification. Fig 2 shows all the spots we chose.

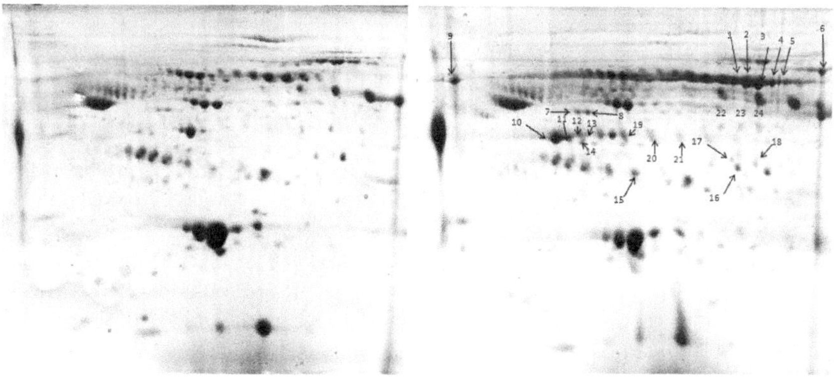

(a) (b)

Fig. 2. Two-dimensional electrophoresis gels of healthy (A) and myocarditis affected (B) sera proteins. Arrows and numbers in (B) correspond to numbers of identified spots in Table 2.

It should be underlined that all the spots we further analysed were taken from the pathologic serum and results are summarized in Table 2.

Spot	Accession number	Protein
1	P02790	Hemopexin
2	P02790	Hemopexin
3	P02790	Hemopexin
4	P02790	Hemopexin
5	P02790	Hemopexin
6	P02787	Serotransferrin
7	P01008	Antithrombin III
8	P01008	Antithrombin III
9	P01011	Alpha-1 antichymotrypsin
10	P01024	Complement C3
11	P04196	Histidine rich glycoprotein
12	P01024	Complement C3
13	P00738	Haptoglobin
14	P04196	Histidine rich glycoprotein
15	Q14624	Inter-alpha-trypsin inhibitor heavy chain H4
16	P08603	Complement factor H
17	P08603	Complement factor H
18	P03952	Plasma kallikrein
19	P06727	Apolipoprotein A-IV
20	P00738	Haptoglobin
21	P00738	Haptoglobin
22	P36955	Pigment epithelium-derived factor
23	P36955	Pigment epithelium-derived factor
24	P36955	Pigment epithelium-derived factor

Table 2. List of proteins identified by LC-MS/MS of spots excised from two-dimensional gels of sera taken from myocarditis affected patients.

Proteins excised from the gel were reduced alkylated and, in situ, digested with trypsin. The resulting peptide mixtures were directly analysed by LC-MS/MS according to the peptide mass fingerprinting procedure. MS and MS-MS obtained data were used to search for a non-redundant sequence using the in-house MASCOT software, taking advantage of the specificity of trypsin and of the taxonomic category of the samples. The number of measured masses that matched within the given mass accuracy of 20 ppm was recorded and the proteins that had the highest number of peptide matches were examined.

Thanks to this approach, we could identify many proteins differently expressed in the two sera. Among identified proteins, hemopexin (Dooley H et al., 2010) , complement C3 (Adamsson Eryd S et al., 2011, Onat A et al., 2011), plasma kallikrein (Kolte D et al.,2011) are undoubtedly related to inflammatory events and most interestingly they resulted clearly over expressed in the pathologic sample.

A preliminary speculation on identified proteins might involve the function of hempopexin. As shown by literature data (Dooley H et al., 2010, : Mauk MR et al., 2011, Larsen R et al.,2010), hemopexin is a serum protein with the very well known function of scavenging the heme released or lost by the turnover of heme proteins such as haemoglobin or by haemolysis caused by parasitic infection, and thus protects the body from the oxidative damage that free heme can cause (Larsen R et al.,2010). Myocarditis itself it's not related to haemolysis phenomena, but some viral infections may cause it, therefore, finding a very high level of hempoxin in a myocarditis affected patient might be a putative marker of the inflammation itself (quite common are in fact viral myocarditis).

Moreover we found some connections between differently expressed proteins in pathologic serum and identified free peptides; in particular we could detect some free peptides some peptides from proteins Complement C3, Inter-alpha-trypsin inhibitor heavy chain H4, Antithrombin III which results over expressed in pathologic serum, (see Tab 1).

3.3 Boronate affinity chromatography

The third part of this work focus on the investigation of one of the most important post-translational modification, the glycosylation. The importance of investigation of post-translational modifications (PTM) is notably increased in the proteomic era, as they play a critical role in cellular functioning and they vary in response to environmental stimuli, signalling modulators or development of diseases (Laurell E et al., 2011). PTMs can affect biological functions thus playing a critical role in cellular functioning. Moreover, they can vary in response to environmental stimuli, thus finely tuning cellular mechanisms and their deregulation might be involved in the development of diseases. A huge number of different types of PTMs have been identified but only a few are reversible and important for regulation of biological processes (Wu C et al. 2011). The pattern of PTMs on proteins constitute a molecular code that dictates protein conformation, cellular location, macromolecular interactions and activities, depending on cell type, tissue and environmental conditions. Understanding this code is the major challenge of proteomics in post-genomic era. Existing methodologies for PTMs identification essentially rely on specific enrichment procedures able to selectively increase the amount of modified peptides. These procedures have to be integrated with sophisticated mass spectrometric experiments to address the identifications of PTMs. The development of a variety of new technologies for exploring the structures of the sugar chains has opened up a new frontier in the glycomics field. Moreover recent progress in mass spectrometry led to new challenges in glycomics, including the development of rapid glycan enrichment. Recently our group introduced an easy to handle strategy to give preliminary insights for the comparison of glycoproteomes in healthy and pathological human sera, by using a single Con A affinity chromatography step coupled with mass spectrometry techniques. The strategy led both to the identification of 69 different glycosylation sites within 49 different proteins and to the definition of the glycosylation patterns. Moreover, glycoform distribution in myocarditis and hepatic carcinoma has been reported. The analysis of glycan profiling, once extracted from serum glycopeptides, is essential for comparative studies on different sera samples thus providing a useful tool for the development of screening procedures (Carpentieri A, Giangrande C, et al., 2010).

In this paper, a different simple and rapid procedure to obtain an overview of the glycosylation sites profiling in the two samples was accomplished. This was achieved by enriching for the N-linked glycopeptides resulting from trypsin digestion of sera samples in order to enhance the identification of N-glycosylation sites using LC-MS/MS. The analyses have been carried out by using healthy sera as control.

To reduce the complexity of the whole sample, Boronate affinity purification was rapidly performed in batch after tryptic digestion. Thanks to the vicinal diols binding capacity no discrimination on the basis of the glycan type was performed thus, in a proof of principle, all glycopeptides could be selected. The recovered glycopeptides were then deglycosylated by PNGase F treatment and the peptide mixtures directly analysed by LC-MS/MS.

The analyses were performed on intact serum samples without any pre-purification step or removal of most abundant proteins. The peptide component of the eluted fraction was analysed by tandem mass spectrometry. Similar analyses were carried out on the unbound Boronate fractions, mainly containing non-glycosylated peptides.

The data were then pooled and summarised in Table 3. The results presented here demonstrated that Boronate affinity chromatography on serum tryptic digests is a useful tool to enhance the detection by LC-MS/MS of glycopeptide. Another advantage of the strategy relies on the fact that it was performed on glycopeptides instead of glycoproteins, therefore there were no SDS-PAGE step, no isolation of the individual glycoproteins and no *in situ* digestion. This allowed the detection of less abundant glycopeptides together with the most represented ones, such as those deriving from albumins or immunoglobulins.

As shown in Table 3, all the selected peptides still contained the conserved N-glycosylation motif (Asn-X-Ser/Thr), thus indicating that N-glycosylation peptides were isolated with high selectivity. This analysis led both to the localization of the modification sites and identification of glycoproteins.

The presence of a putative N-glycosylation site was confirmed by the fact that peptides mass was increase of 1 Da, due to the conversion of Asn into Asp after PNGase F incubation. However, some non-specific peptides, namely non-glycosylated peptides, were detected in the eluted Boronate fraction, and identified as belonging to most abundant proteins like albumin.

Spontaneous deamidation seems rather unlikely for generating the results presented, although it cannot be excluded completely. Most MS/MS spectra giving positive hits were derived from doubly charged precursor ions that resulted predominantly in y-ion series.

As a whole, using Boronate affinity approach we could confirm the previously identified glycosylation sites based on ConcanavalinA enrichment and 5 more glycosylation sites were identified thus refining previous data (Carpentieri A, Giangrande C, et al., 2010) on myocarditis glycoproteome.

	Protein	Sequence	Peptide
P01011	Alpha-1-antichymotrypsin	YTGN*ASALFILPDQDKH,M	268-283
P02763	Alpha-1-acid glycoprotein	SVQEIQATFFYFTPN*KTEDTIFLR[H,M] QDQCIYN*TTYLNVQR[H,M]	58-81 87-101
P01009	Alpha-1-antitrypsin	YLGN*ATAIFFLPDEGKH,M QLAHQSN*STNIFFSPVSIATAFAMLSL GTKH ADTHDEILEGLNFN*LTEIPEAQIHEGF QELLRH,M	268-283 64-93 94-125
P01023	Alpha-2-macroglobulin	SLGNVN*FTVSAEALESQELCGTEVPS VPEHGRKH	864-886
P43652	Afamin	DIENFN*STQKH,M YAEDKFN*ETTEKH	28-37 396-407
P01008	Antithrombin III	LGACN*DTLQQLMEVFKH,M SLTFN*ETYQDISELVYGAKH,M	124-139 183-201
P04114	Apolipoprotein B-100	FN*SSYLQGTNQITGRH,M FVEGSHN*STVSLTTKH AEEEMLEN*VSLVCPKM YDFN*SSMLYSTAKM	1522-1536 3405-3419 27-41 3462-3474
P05090	Apolipoprotein D	ADGTVNQIEGEATPVN*LTEPAKM	83-104
P02749	Apolipoprotein H	VYKPSAGN*NSLYRH LGN*WSAMPSCKM	155-167 251-261
O75882	Attractin	IDSTGN*VTNELRH,M GPVKMPSQAPTGNFYPQPLLN*SSMC LEDSRH	411-422 1023-1052
P00450	Ceruloplasmin	EHEGAIYPDN*TTDFQRH,M EN*LTAPGSDSAVFFEQGTTRH,M	129-144 396-414
P08603	Complement factor H	ISEEN*ETTCYMGKH MDGASN*VTCINSRH,M IPCSQPPQIEHGTIN*SSRM SPDVIN*GSPISQKH	907-919 1024-1036 868-885 212-224
P10909	Clusterin	LAN*LTQGEDQYYLRH,M	372-385
Q8IWV2	Contactin-4	LN*GTDVDTGMDFRM	64-76
P05156	Complement factor 1	FLNN*GTCTAEGKH,M	100-111
P01024	Complement C3	TVLTPATNHMGN*VTFTIPANRH	74-94
P0C0L4	Complement C4-A	GLN*VTLSSTGRH,M	1326-1336
P02748	Complement component C9	AVN*ITSENLIDDVVSLIRH,M	413-430
Q14517	Protocadherin-fat 1	QVYN*LTVRAKDKM FSMDYKTGALTVQN*TTQLRSRM	994-1005 1930-1950
P02765	Alpha-2-HS-glycoprotein	VCQDCPLLAPLN*DTRH,M AALAAFNAQNN*GSNFQLEEISRH	145-159 166-187
Q03591	Complement factor H related protein 1	LQNNENN*ISCVERH	120-132

	Protein	Sequence	Peptide
Q13439	Golgin subfamily A member 4	HN*STLKQLMREFNTQLAQKH	1990-2008
P02790	Hemopexin	SWPAVGN*CSSALRH,M ALPQPQN*VTSLLGCTHH,M	181-193 447-462
P00738	Haptoglobin	VVLHPN*YSQVDIGLIKH,M MVSHHN*LTTGATLINEQWLLTTAKH,M NLFLN*HSEN*ATAKH,M	236-251 179-202 203-215
P04196	Histidine rich glycoprotein	VEN*TTVYYLVLDVQESDCSVLSRH VIDFN*CTTSSVSSALANTKH,M	61-83 121-139
P05155	Plasma protease C1 inhibitor	VGQLQLSHN*LSLVILVPQNLKH,M	344-364
P01857	Ig alpha-1 chain C region	LSLHRPALEDLLLGSEAN*LTCTLTGLRH	127-153
P01859	Ig gamma-2 chain C region	TKPREEQFN*STFRH TPLTAN*ITKH	168-180 200-208
P01860	Ig gamma-1 chain C region	EEQYN*STYRH,M	136-144
P01591	Immunoglobulin J chain	EN*ISDPTSPLRH,M	48-58
P40189	Interleukin-6 receptor beta	QQYFKQN*CSQHESSPDISHFERM	812-833
P56199	Integrin alpha-1	SYFSSLN*LTIRM	1096-1106
P29622	Kallistatin	DFYVDEN*TTVRH	232-242
P01042	Kininogen-1	LNAENN*ATFYFKH,M	389-400
P11279	Lysosome-associated membrane glycoprotein 1	DPAFKAAN*GSLRM	314-325
P01871	Ig mu chain C region	YKN*NSDISSTRH GLTFQQN*ASSMCVPDQDTAIRM	44-54 204-223
Q9HC10	Otoferlin	NEMLEIQVFN*YSKVFSNKH,M	59-76
Q5VU65	Nuclear pore membrane glycoprotein 210-like	EVVVN*ASSRH	1551-1559
Q9Y5E7	Protocadherin beta 2	ETRSEYN*ITITVTDFGTPRM	414-432
P36955	Pigment epithelium derived factor	VTQN*LTLIEESLTSEFIHDIDRH	282-303
P27169	Serum paraoxanase/arylesterase1	HAN*WTLTPLKH	250-259
P49908	Selenoprotein P	EGYSN*ISYIVVNHQGISSRH	79-97
Q9Y275	Tumor necrosis factor ligand superfamily member 13B	CIQNMPETLPN*NSCYSAGIAKM	232-252

	Protein	Sequence	Peptide
P40225	Thrombopoietin	IHELLN*GTRGLFPGPSRRM	250-267
P02787	Serotransferrin	QQQHLFGSN*VTDCSGNFCLFRH,M CGLVPVLAENYN*KSDNCEDTPEAGY FAVAVVKM	622-642 421-452
P07996	Thrombospondin 1	VVN*STTGPGEHLRH,M	1065-1077
P04004	Vitronectin	NN*ATVHEQVGGPSLTSDLQAQSKM	85-107
P25311	Zinc-alpha-2-glycoprotein	DIVEYYN*DSN*GSHVLQGRH,M	100-117
P02766	Transthyretin	ALGISPFHEHAEVVFTA**N***DSGPR[H]	101-123

Table 3. LC/MSMS analysis for the identification of glycosylation sites, H indicates peptides deriving from healthy serum and M indicates the ones from myocarditis serum.

4. Conclusions

In biomedical applications, a comparative approach is usually employed to identify proteins that are up and down regulated in a disease specific manner for use as diagnostic markers or therapeutic targets. This report represents an overview of the investigation at molecular level of myocarditis by using a proteomic approach .

Serum proteins (including the N-glycosylation sites profiling) and glycoproteins and free peptides occurring in human sera from healthy donors were compared to the ones from myocarditis patients. This procedure, allowed the identification of several N-glycosylation sites by a single-step proteomic approach, contemporarily probing an entire complex sample by LC-MS/MS. Thanks to the depletion of the serum most abundant proteins, we could detect some of the very weakly represented free peptides, whose presence is connected to the pathology itself. The high resolution, the sensitivity and the reproducibility of the used techniques led to the identification of some up regulated proteins in the serum from a myocarditis affected patient, all these proteins are connected to inflammatory events and one in particular (hemopexin) opens the way to new speculations in serum proteins as a specific marker for pathologic state.

Finally, this proteomic approach represents a new opportunity for therapeutics and early diagnostics, for the screening of proteic biomarkers in pathological status. Finding a biomarker molecule that precisely indicates certain kind of pathology, is something quite difficult to achieve since it requires a huge background in many different fields of clinical investigation. Here we contribute with putative diagnostic species that could really be helpful for an early diagnosis myocarditis event.

5. Acknowledgments

This work was supported by grants from the INBB, Ministero dell'Universita` e della Ricerca Scientifica (Progetti di Rilevante Interesse Nazionale 2002, 2003, 2005, 2006; FIRB 2001). Support from the National Center of Excellence in Molecular Medicine (MIUR - Rome) and from the Regional Center of Competence (CRdC ATIBB, Regione Campania – Naples) is gratefully acknowledged. The authors declare that this paper is novel and does not overlap with any already published articles.

6. References

Adamsson Eryd S, Smith JG, Melander O, Hedblad B, Engström G.Inflammation-sensitive proteins and risk of atrial fibrillation: a population-based cohort study. Eur J Epidemiol. 2011 Mar 19 18;144(4):539-50.

Amado F, Lobo MJ, Domingues P, Duarte JA, Vitorino R. Salivary peptidomics.Expert Rev Proteomics. 2010 Oct;7(5):709-21.

Blauwet LA, Cooper LT. Myocarditis. Prog Cardiovasc Dis. 2010 Jan-Feb;52(4):274-88.

Carpentieri A, Giangrande C, Pucci P, Amoresano A. Glycoproteome study in myocardial lesions serum by integrated mass spectrometry approach: preliminary insights. Eur J Mass Spectrom (Chichester, Eng). 2010;16(1):123-49.

Cihakova D, Rose NR. Pathogenesis of myocarditis and dilated cardiomyopathy. Adv Immunol. 8;99:95-114.

Colgrave ML, Xi L, Lehnert SA, Flatscher-Bader T, Wadensten H, Nilsson A, Andren PE, Wijffels G. Neuropeptide profiling of the bovine hypothalamus: Thermal stabilization is an effective tool in inhibiting post-mortem degradation. Proteomics. 2011 Apr;11(7):1264-76.

Dell A, Morris HR. Glycoprotein structure determination by mass spectrometry. Science. 291,2351-2356 (2001).

Diernfellner AC, Schafmeier T. Phosphorylations: making the Neurosporacrassa circadian clock tick. FEBS Lett. 2011 Mar 28 [Epub ahead of print] .

Dooley H, Buckingham EB, Criscitiello MF, Flajnik MF. Emergence of the acute-phase protein hemopexin in jawed vertebrates. Mol Immunol. 2010 Nov-Dec;48(1-3):147-52.

Dube DH. Bertozzi CR. Glycans in cancer and inflammation--potential for therapeutics and diagnostics. Nat Rev Drug Discov. 4, 477-88 (2005).

Gorman PM, Yip CM, Fraser PE, Chakrabartty A. Alternate aggregation pathways of the Alzheimer beta-amyloid peptide: Abeta association kinetics at endosomal pH. J Mol Biol. 2003 Jan 24;325(4):743-57.

Granovsky M. Fata J. Pawling J. Muller WJ. Khokha R. Dennis JW. Suppression of tumor growth and metastasis in Mgat5-deficient mice. Nat Med. 6, 306-12 (2000).

Hao P, Guo T, Sze SK. Simultaneous analysis of proteome, phospho- and glycoproteome of rat kidney tissue with electrostatic repulsion hydrophilic interaction chromatography. PLoS One. 2011 Feb 23;6(2)

Herrero M, Ibañez E, Cifuentes A. Capillary electrophoresis-electrospray-mass spectrometry in peptide analysis and peptidomics. Electrophoresis. 2008 May;29(10):2148-60

Kim YJ. Varki A. Perspectives on the significance of altered glycosylation of glycoproteins in cancer. Glycoconj J. 14, 569-76 (1997).

Kolte D, Bryant J, Holsworth D, Wang J, Akbari P, Gibson G, Shariat-Madar Z. Biochemical characterization of a novel high-affinity and specific plasma kallikrein inhibitor. Br J Pharmacol. 2011 Apr;162(7):1639-49.

Kühl U, Schultheiss HP. Myocarditis in children. Heart Fail Clin. 2010 Oct;6(4):483-96,.

Kühl U, Schultheiss HP. Viral myocarditis: diagnosis, aetiology andmanagement. Drugs. 2009 Jul 9;69(10):1287-302.

Larsen R, Gozzelino R, Jeney V, Tokaji L, Bozza FA, Japiassú AM, Bonaparte D, Cavalcante MM, Chora A, Ferreira A, Marguti I, Cardoso S, Sepúlveda N, Smith A, Soares MP.

A central role for free heme in the pathogenesis of severe sepsis. Sci Transl Med. 2010 Sep 29;2(51):51.

Laurell E, Beck K, Krupina K, Theerthagiri G, Bodenmiller B, Horvath P, Aebersold R, Antonin W, Kutay U. Phosphorylation of Nup98 by multiple kinases is crucial for NPC disassembly during mitotic entry. Cell. 2011 Feb. [Epub ahead of print]

Ludwig M. Are neuropeptides brain hormones? J Neuroendocrinol. 2011 Apr;23(4):381-2.

Lv H, Havari E, Pinto S, Gottumukkala RV, Cornivelli L, Raddassi K, Matsui T, Rosenzweig A, Bronson RT, Smith R, Fletcher AL, Turley SJ, Wucherpfennig K, Kyewski B, Lipes MA. Impaired thymic tolerance to α-myosin directs autoimmunityto the heart in mice and humans. J Clin Invest. 2011 Mar 23. [Epub ahead of print]

Mauk MR, Smith A, Grant Mauk A. An alternative view of the proposed alternative activities of hemopexin. Protein Sci. 2011 Mar 14. [Epub ahead of print]

Menschaert G, Vandekerckhove TT, Baggerman G, Schoofs L, Luyten W, VanCriekinge W. Peptidomics coming of age: a review of contributions from abioinformatics angle. J Proteome Res. 2010 May 7;9(5):2051-61.

Onat A, Can G, Rezvani R, Cianflone K. Complement C3 and cleavage products in cardiometabolic risk. Clin Chim Acta. 2011 Mar 23. [Epub ahead of print]

Rezkalla SH, Kloner RA. Influenza-related viral myocarditis. WMJ. 2010 Aug;109(4):209-13.

Stensaeth KH, Hoffmann P, Fossum E, Mangschau A, Sandvik L, Klow NE. Cardiac magnetic resonance visualizes acute and chronic myocardial injuries in myocarditis. Int J Cardiovasc Imaging. 2011 Feb 24.

Taylor CL, Eckart RE. Chest pain, ST elevation, and positive cardiac enzymes in an austere environment: Differentiating smallpox vaccination-mediated myocarditis and acute coronary syndrome in operation Iraqi freedom. J Emerg Med. 30

Taylor-Papadimitriou J. Epenetos AA. Exploiting altered glycosylation patterns in cancer: progress and challenges in diagnosis and therapy. Trends Biotechnol. 12, 227-33 (1994).

ter Weeme M, Vonk AB, Kupreishvili K, van Ham M, Zeerleder S, Wouters D, Stooker W, Eijsman L, Van Hinsbergh VW, Krijnen PA, Niessen HW. Activated complement is more extensively present in diseased aortic valves than naturally occurring complement inhibitors: a sign of ongoing inflammation. Eur J Clin Invest. 2010 Jan;40(1):4-10. Epub 2009 Oct 15.

van den Broek I, Sparidans RW, Schellens JH, Beijnen JH. Sensitive liquid chromatography/tandem mass spectrometry assay for absolute quantification of ITIH4-derived putative biomarker peptides in clinical serum samples. Rapid Commun Mass Spectrom. 2010 Jul 15;24(13):1842-50.

Wu C, Parrott AM, Fu C, Liu T, Marino SM, Gladyshev VN, Jain MR, Baykal AT, Li Q, Oka S, Sadoshima J, Beuve A, Simmons WJ, Li H. Thioredoxin 1-Mediated Post-Translational Modifications: Reduction, Transnitrosylation, Denitrosylation and Related Proteomics Methodologies. Antioxid Redox Signal. 2011 Apr 1.

Acute Myocarditis – A Trigger of Cardiac Autoimmunity? Expected Insights from the Etiology, Titre-Course, and Effect on Survival of Cardiac Autoantibodies (ETiCS) Study

Roland Jahns et al.*

University Hospital of Würzburg, Department of Internal Medicine I, Cardiology, Comprehensive Heart Failure Centre CHFC/IFB, Würzburg, Germany

1. Introduction

Progressive cardiac dilatation and pump failure of unknown aetiology - termed "idiopathic" dilated cardiomyopathy (DCM) (Richardson et al., 1996; Maron et al., 2006) - represents one of the main causes of severe heart failure in Western populations with an annual incidence of about 100 and a prevalence of 300-400 patients per year (American Heart Association, 2009). The large majority of cases are thought to arise from an initial (mostly viral) infection leading to acute myocardial inflammation. Acute myocarditis may either heal (about one third of the cases) or progress to a chronic inflammatory process with continued fibrotic repair, subsequent dilatation of the left and/or right ventricle and -finally- severe congestive heart failure (about another third of the patients). Progression to DCM appears to occur particularly, when associated (a) with chronic inflammation of the myocardium due to viral persistence (Kühl et al., 2005) and/or (b) with the development of autoantibodies directed against distinct sarcoplasmatic or myocyte membrane proteins that are essential for cardiac function (Freedman & Lefkowitz, 2004; Jahns et al., 2006). The latter findings are further strengthened by the fact that patients with DCM often have alterations in both, their innate and their adaptive immune system (Limas, 1997; Luppi et al., 1998; Jahns et al., 2006; Mahrholdt et al., 2006). Thus, under certain conditions an initial acute inflammatory reaction may proceed into a kind of low-grade inflammation (MacLellan & Lusis, 2003) facilitating the development of abnormal or misled immune responses to the primary (infectious)

*Nikolas Deubner[1], Valérie Biovin[2], Alida L.P. Caforio[3], Stephan B. Felix[4], Michael Fu[5], Martin J. Lohse[2], and Georg Ertl[1]

1 *University Hospital of Würzburg, Department of Internal Medicine I,Cardiology, Comprehensive Heart Failure Centre CHFC/IFB, Würzburg, Germany;*

2 *University of Würzburg, Institute for Pharmacology and Toxicology, Würzburg, Germany;*

3 *University of Padua, Division of Cardiology, Dpt. of Cardiologic, Thoracic and Vascular Sciences, Padua, Italy;*

4 *University of Greifswald, Department of Internal Medicine B – Cardiology, Greifswald,Germany;*

5 *University of Gothenburg, Department of Molecular and Clinical Medicine, Gothenburg, Sweden.*

trigger (MacLellan & Lusis, 2003; Freedman & Lefkowitz, 2004; Kühl et al., 2005; Smulski et al., 2006; Maekawa et al., 2007). More recently, a detailed molecular analysis of T cell infiltrates in human endomyocardial biopsies (EMBs) from both, patients with acute myocarditis and patients with (post-)inflammatory DCM revealed an increased expression of CD3d, CD3z, and T cell receptor beta constant region (TRBC) in both disease entities. However, differential expression of functional T cell markers was found in DCM EMBs only (dominance of Th1 markers, regulatory [FoxP3] T cells, and cytotoxic T cells (CTLs)) and not in acute myocarditis. Additionally, in DCM EMBs some Th2 marker genes were increased, indicating that a Th2 response (required for T/B cell interactions) also participates in the T cell infiltrates in DCM (Noutsias et al., 2011). This might explain, why a substantial number of DCM patients have been found to develop cross-reacting antibodies and/or autoantibodies to different cardiac self-antigens, including mitochondrial proteins (e.g., adenine nucleotide translocator, lipoamide and pyruvate dehydrogenase (Schultheiss & Bolte, 1985; Schultheiss et al., 1988; Pohlner et al., 1997; Schulze et al., 1999)), sarcoplasmatic proteins (e.g., actin, laminin, myosin, troponin (Neumann et al., 1990; Caforio et al., 2002; Okazaki et al., 2003; Göser et al., 2006; Li et al., 2006)), and membrane proteins (e.g., cell surface adrenergic or muscarinergic receptors (Fu, L.X.M. et al., 1993; Magnusson et al., 1994; Jahns et al., 1999; Christ et al., 2006)).

Irrespective of whether development of DCM is primarily due to chronic myocardial infection (Kühl et al., 1996) or to abnormalities in the adaptive or innate immune system (Luppi et al., 1998; Eriksson et al., 2003), in both cases cardiac tissue injury is believed to be mediated mainly by cytokines and/or heart-specific autoantibodies (Caforio et al., 1995; Limas, 1997; Eriksson et al., 2003). However, the pathophysiological relevance of each of the aforementioned cardiac autoantibodies (aabs) is far from clear. Low titers of autoantibodies to various house-keeping antigens can also be detected in healthy subjects as a part of the natural immunological repertoire (Rose, 2001).

In addition, under physiological conditions at least the intracellularly localized cardiac antigens are not easily accessible for the immune system. Thus, the mechanisms by which autoimmune-mediated myocardial injury is initiated are mostly based on indirect or circumstantial evidence (Limas, 1997). The potential pathophysiological - and thus clinical - relevance of a heart-specific autoantibody depends on its disease-inducing or -aggravating potential, which in turn is supposed to be associated with both the *accessibility* and the *functional relevance* of its target. Therefore, autoantibodies directed against cell surface key constituents, and in particular aabs that have the potential to affect myocardial contraction and relaxation (e.g. , by interaction with the cardiac beta1-adrenoceptor (beta1-AR)) and/or the M2-muscarinic acetylcholine receptor (M2-AchR)) represent key candidates involved in the initiation and/or progression of DCM (Fu et al. 1993, 2008; Magnusson et al., 1996; Limas, 1997; Engelhardt et al., 2004; Jahns et al., 2004; Freedman & Lefkowitz, 2004). Whereas anti-muscarinic antibodies (exhibiting an agonist-like effect on cardiac M2-AchR) have been associated with negative chronotropic effects at the sinuatrial level (e.g., sinus node dysfunction, atrial fibrillation (Wang et al., 1996; Baba et al., 2004)), functionally activating anti-beta1-AR antibodies have been associated with both the occurrence of severe arrhythmias at the ventricular level, and the development of (maladaptive) left ventricular hypertrophy, finally switching to left ventricular enlargement and progressive heart failure (Jahns et al., 1999, 2006; Iwata et al., 2001; Engelhardt et al., 2004; Störk et al., 2006). In addition, both autoantibodies seem to target the (easily accessible) second extracellular loop of the respective receptors.

To generate an autoimmune response, myocyte membrane proteins (including receptors) must be degraded to small oligopeptides able to form a complex with a major histocompatibility (MHC) class II or human leukocyte antigen (HLA) molecule of the host (Hoebeke et al., 1996). In previous clinical studies autoimmunity has been found to be associated with certain HLA- and MHC class II-phenotypes (Limas, 1996), and also with the expression and/or activity of the T-lymphocyte antigen 4 (CTLA-4) - known as a potent (indirect) suppressor of the immune system (Golden et al., 2005). Therefore, another important point to consider in the development of (human) post-inflammatory and/or post-ischemic cardiomyopathy is the patients' genetic pre-disposition, which will determine both, the susceptibility to self-directed immune reactions and the phenotypic expression of the myocardial disease (MacLellan & Lusis, 2003; Limas et al., 2004).
On this background the following book-chapter will review current knowledge and recent experimental and clinical evidence for the potential role of cardiac autoantibodies in the pathogenesis of DCM focussing on the rationale and expected insights from the prospective diagnostic multicentre **E**tiology, **Ti**tre-**C**ourse, and (effect on) **S**urvival of cardiac autoantibodies (**ETiCS**) study.

2. Rationale and scope of the ETiCS study

Evidence for a pathophysiologic role of autoimmunity in human heart disease has substantially increased during the past two decades, but the true prevalence and clinical impact of cardiac autoantibodies (aabs) in human heart disease are still unclear, as are the events leading to their formation, their frequency of appearance, and their kinetics (that is, their patterns of clearance and/or persistence).
In this regard, the investigator-initiated diagnostic multicentre ETiCS study will prospectively address the hypothesis that a first inflammatory (i.e., acute myocarditis (AMitis)) or ischemic injury of the myocardium (i.e., first acute myocardial infarction (FAMI)) may trigger the development of heart-directed autoimmune reactions (**Fig. 1**).

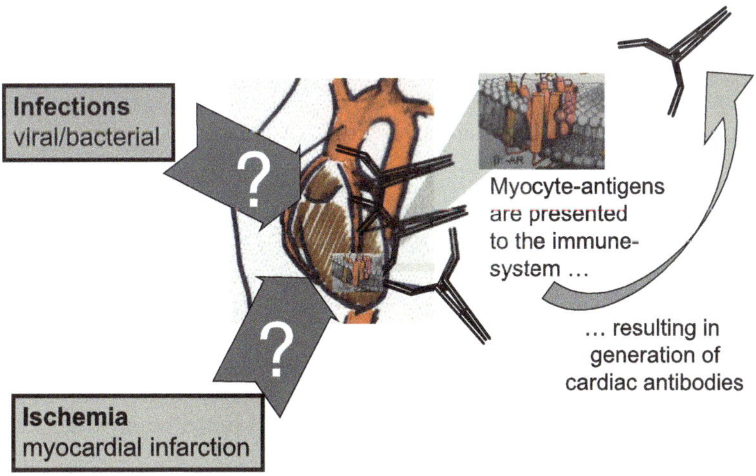

Fig. 1. Formation of autoantibodies against myocardial self-antigens.

Immunogenicity is defined as the property of a molecule to induce an immune response (Hoebeke, 1996). To serve as a potential antigen, myocyte constituents (e.g., cardiac membrane receptors) must be degraded by proteolysis into small fragments (oligopeptides), and one or several of the generated fragments must be able to form a complex with one of the major histocompatibility complexes (class II-MHCs) or human leukocyte antigen (HLA) molecules of the host. When presented to T cells (Harding et al., 1990; Mobini et al., 1999) antigenic parts of such myocyte-derived (self) peptides may engender an immunological response. Acute inflammatory processes are supposed to enhance the occurence of self-directed immune responses (e.g., acute viral or bacterial myocarditis and/or acute ischemic events (Borda et al., 1984; Latif et al., 1993; Kühl et al., 1996; Limas, 1997; Noutsias et al., 1999; Liu & Mason, 2001; Rose, 2001; Caforio et al., 2002)).

Therefore, we assume that a first substantial inflammatory or ischemic myocyte damage - through liberation of a "critical amount" of cardiac self-antigens previously hidden to the immune system - might induce and perpetuate a disease-causing and/or -modulating autoimmune reaction that deteriorates cardiac function and ultimately results in progressive heart failure.

As a consequence, the ETiCS study has been designed to provide a maximum of sequential clinical and serological data from patients after a first inflammatory or ischemic cardiac event. The development/prevalence and titre-course (clearance/persistence) of distinct cardiac aabs after 0, 3, 6, and 12 months of either event will be prospectively assessed and correlated with the corresponding cardiac functional parameters, cardiac imaging (echocardiography, cardiac magnetic resonance imaging), and clinical outcome. A limited number of ETiCS sub-studies will focus on components of the patients' immune system potentially involved in the generation of cardiac receptor-aabs - including a search for pre-disposing genotypes (Limas et al., 2004; Caforio & Iliceto, 2008) - and on the possible impact of conformational adrenoceptor-aabs on renal function (Boivin et al., 2001).

Expanding the scope of ETiCS beyond adrenoceptor-directed autoimmunity other known cardiac aabs will be investigated by the respective expert core centres, including aabs against the muscarinic acetylcholine receptor 2 (Fu, L.X.M. et al., 1993), against troponin I (Göser et al., 2006), organ-specific and skeletal muscle cross-reactive anti-heart-aabs (Caforio et al., 2007), and cardio-depressant aabs (Felix et al., 2002). This joint venture will enable a comprehensive characterisation of heart-directed autoimmunity after inflammatory or ischemic disruption of myocardial integrity, and allow for cross-correlations of the titre-course and prognostic impact of all cardiac aabs prospectively analyzed.

3. Design of the ETiCS study

The prospective ETiCS study complies with the standards of Good Clinical Practice (GCP) and has been approved by the Ethics committees of all participating institutions. Within a two years-period ETiCS will include 400 patients with a first cardiac event, 200 of them with acute myocarditis (AMitis), and 200 patients with a first myocardial infarction (FAMI; acute ST-elevation MI only, without any history or signs of previous myocardial infarction). After inclusion and baseline assessment, the patients will undergo three follow-up visits after 3, 6, and 12 months (Fig. 2). Diagnosis of acute myocarditis is based on at least one major and two minor clinical criteria and/or symptoms (see table 1) and must be confirmed by endomyocardial biopsy (EMB) using either the WHO/ISFC (Richardson et al., 1996; Elliott et al., 2008) or the Dallas criteria (Aretz et al., 1987). This proceeding is in full accordance with the actual AHA/ACC/ESC scientific statement on the role of EMB in the management of cardiovascular disease (Cooper et al., 2007), which strongly recommends EMB in acute myocarditis because of its potential relevance for outcome and therapeutic decisions (Kindermann et al., 2008; Frustaci et al., 2009). In addition, immunohistology and molecular analysis of the EMBs may also significantly contribute to further elucidate the clinical impact of heart-directed autoimmune reactions.

Suspicion of acute myocarditis (One major and two minor criteria fulfilled)	
Major criteria	**ST/T wave changes in the electrocardiograms (ECG) Ventricular arrhythmia (ECG) Pericardial effusion on echocardiography Impairment of LVEF on echocardiography with CAD excluded by coronary angiography (no stenosis >50%)**
Minor criteria	**Dyspnea, new onset within the past 30 days Chest pain, new onset within the past 30 days Palpitations, new onset within the past 30 days History of infection within the past 30 days Fever >38.0° C within the past 30 days**

Table 1. Diagnostic criteria for suspicion of acute myocarditis.

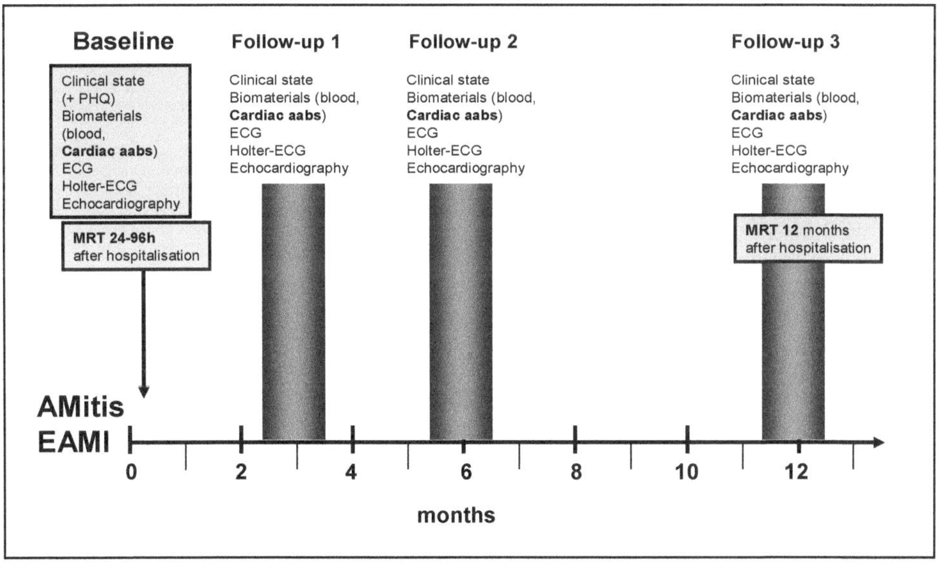

Fig. 2. Time schedule of the follow-up examinations in the ETiCS study.

Echocardiography and cardiac magnetic resonance imaging (cMRI) will be carried out in all patients within 24 to 96 hours of hospitalisation and one year after the respective cardiac event. Follow-up visits at 3, 6, and 12 months comprise a detailed patient history including medication, physical examination, a standardized health questionnaire, echocardiography, ECG, Holter-ECG, and blood sampling (**Fig. 2**). The sequentially obtained blood samples will serve to determine the time course of formation and the titre-course (clearance/persistence) of distinct cardiac aabs at 0, 3, 6, and 12 months after inflammatory or ischemic cardiac injury (AMitis, FAMI). Three-hundred healthy subjects with normal blood pressure, ECG, and exercise-stress test will serve as a control collective (male to female ratio 1:1, n=50 per five-years age range, no history of myocardial infarction, diabetes, or peripheral vascular disease). The primary endpoint of the planned cross-sectional analyses is the association of a specific cardiac aab status at diagnosis (aab-positive/aab-negative) with (a) the change in cardiac function as derived from sequential echocardiograms and cMRI (baseline *versus* 12 months), and (b) the severity and clinical course of the index disease. Longitudinal primary endpoints are titre-changes of a given cardiac aab over time, conversion rates (persistence/clearance), and the "time to first cardiovascular event" (see table 2 for definition of composite endpoints). Pre-specified secondary endpoints for each of the different cardiac aabs at diagnosis are time to cardiovascular death and time to all-cause death (table 2).

Primary endpoint: prospective ETiCS study
Titre course of conformational cardiac aabs
Secondary endpoints: prospective ETiCS study
Change in left ventricular enddiastolic diameter
Change in left ventricular ejection fraction
Occurrence of ventricular arrhythmias
Change of clinical NYHA classification
Severity of inflammation as assessed by EMB/cMRI
Time to cardiovascular death/all-cause death
Composite endpoints
Cardiovascular Death
Myocardial infarction
Resuscitation (successful or not successful)
ICD discharge, if appropriate
Cardiac transplantation
Sudden cardiac death
Death due to progressive heart failure
Death due to myocardial infarction

Table 2. Pre-defined endpoints of the ETiCS study.

4. ETiCS substudies

4.1 Immunobiology of heart-directed autoreactivity

This substudy attempts to unravel the step-by-step changes occurring in a patients' immune system whilst autoantibody-mediated immune cardiomyopathy develops after inflammatory or ischemic myocardial injury, including the time course and cell types (T and B cell subpopulations) involved in the generation of cardiac aabs. The reactivity and prevalence of receptor (auto)antigen-specific T and B cell populations will be assessed by antigenic recall assays as well as FACS and Elispot analyses. In addition, the respectively activated immunologic paths will be derived from the Th1/Th2/Th17 cytokine profiles determined in the sera from cardiac autoantibody-positive patients with acute myocarditis (including an analysis of the corresponding EMBs (Noutsias et al, 2011)) or acute transmural myocardial infarction. Since the cytotoxic T-lymphocyte antigen 4 (CTLA-4) is a potent (indirect) suppressor of the immune system, its mutation or hampered expression might promote hyperreactivity to autoantigens (Golden et al., 2005). Thus, in all ETiCS patients CTLA-4 expression and CTLA-4 alleles will be determined by FACS and by PCR, respectively. In addition, in all patients the HLA-DR/DQ and MHC class II haplotypes (Limas et al., 2004; Caforio & Iliceto, 2008) will be determined and correlated with the formation and titre-course of distinct cardiac aabs in order to unravel the individual genetic susceptibility for heart-directed autoimmune reactions.

4.2 Adrenoceptor-autoantibodies and their impact on kidney function

The possible clinical implications of adrenoceptor-directed autoimmunity have gained increasing interest in human heart disease. By contrast, the renal effects of functionally active adrenoceptor-aabs have been almost neglected. Previous immuno-histologic studies on the rat kidney strongly suggest that functionally stimulating adrenoceptor aabs are capable of modulating the secretion of renin from the juxtaglomerular cells *via* renal beta1-AR and, also, to increase the sodium-reabsorption in the distal tubulus (Boivin et al., 2001). Thus, through renal beta1-AR-mediated activation of the renin-angiotensin-aldosterone-system (RAAS) and/or augmentation of the circulating blood volume such aabs might contribute to further worsening of the prognosis of antibody-positive heart failure patients.
To assess the impact of adrenoceptor-aabs on kidney function (and clinical outcome), a number of pre-specified renal functional parameters will be sequentially determined in all ETiCS patients (e.g. serum *versus* urine creatinine/sodium/pH; glomerular filtration rate (GFR), urinary protein excretion). Primary endpoints are the relationship between antibody-titres and renal function at baseline and the "time to first cardiovascular event", adjusted for renal function. Secondary endpoints include the change in renal function dependent on the formation and conversion rates (clearance/persistence) of adrenoceptor-aabs.
These data might furnish a rationale for the development of novel therapeutic strategies to protect the kidney(s) from functional adrenoceptor-aabs in aab-positive heart failure patients.

5. Conclusion and expected insights from the ETiCS study

In the last two decades, much knowledge has accumulated with respect to the possible pathophysiologic and clinical implications of heart-directed aabs (Jahns et al., 2006; Fu, M., 2008).
Homologies between cardiomyocyte surface molecules (in particular membrane receptors) and viral or bacterial proteins have been proposed as a mechanism for the elaboration of endogenous cardiac autoantibodies by antigen mimicry (Elies et al., 1996; Hoebeke et al., 1996). Chagas' heart disease, a slowly evolving inflammatory cardiomyopathy, is one of the best investigated examples to highlight this mechanism. The disease is induced by the protozoon *Trypanosoma cruzi*. About 30% of the Chagas' patients develop antibodies that cross-react between the ribosomal P2beta-protein of *T. cruzi* and some specific amino acids present in the second extracellular loop of the human beta1-adrenoceptor (Elies et al., 1996).

Because the large majority of functionally active beta1-aabs detected in DCM patients seem to be directed against the same receptor loop, it was speculated that these antibodies might also originate from molecular mimicry between the beta1-adrenoceptor and hitherto non-identified viral pathogen (Hoebeke, 1996). Another example is Chlamydia-associated heart disease, which in BALBc mice appears to be induced by antigen mimicry between Chlamydia antigens and the alpha-myosin heavy chain molecule, resulting in activation of autoreactive T- and B-cells (Bachmaier et al., 1999).

However, irrespective of (potentially occurring) immunologic cross-reactions, to date no prospective clinical study has ever addressed the key question, whether structural damage to the heart muscle (e.g., necrosis or apoptosis) is a mandatory pre-requisite for the formation of heart-directed aabs.

In general, the immune system will not attack cardiac self-proteins. On a susceptible genetic background, however, this self-inhibition of immune effector cells after cardiac injury may be hampered. It is presently unclear, whether this autoreactivity depends on the kind and extent of injury, the kind and amount (or "dose") of self-antigens presented, or the kind and quality of the subsequently engaged immunologic paths. Regarding the latter aspect, a recent analysis of the expression of functional T cell markers in EMBs from patients with acute myocarditis and patients with chronic (post-inflammatory) DCM found an increased expression of CD3d, CD3z, and TRBC in both disease entities, whereas Th1 (more than) Th2 marker-genes as well as regulatory and cytotoxic T cells were differentially up-regulated in DCM EMBs only (Noutsias et al., 2011). Interestingly, in human DCM biopsies any clues for a Th17 response were lacking, which is in sharp contrast to findings in murine models of (experimental) autoimmune myocarditis (Valaperti et al., 2008). Nevertheless, from these recent molecular data it seems clear now that in human DCM a Th2 response also participates in the myocardial T cell infiltrates and serves as a pre-requisite for the stimulation (that is, maturation) of autoreactive B cells that, e.g., produce cardiac autoantibodies.

In acute myocarditis diffuse and/or focal inflammation causes structural damage to the heart. If myocardial inflammation persists, in a majority of cases cardiac function does not recover and finally may result in severe DCM. Acute ischemia also causes structural damage to the heart and to date represents the most common aetiology of heart failure. Thus, a structured follow up of patients with either disease is both pathophysiologically and clinically relevant.

The ETiCS study will follow such patients 3, 6, and 12 months after their index events, because the formation of autoreactive immunoglobulin G (IgG) is supposed to take place within the first 6 weeks (up to three months) after the index event.

A variety of autoreactive IgG have been identified, but only few of them have been investigated more in detail. Because myocyte surface receptors are easily accessible to circulating autoantibodies, the cardiac beta1-adrenergic receptor (which is the predominant adrenocepter subtype in the heart) and the M2-muscarinic acetylcholine receptor represent key targets for autoreactive antibodies that might affect heart function to some extent.

To generate an autoimmune response, membrane receptors must be degraded to small oligopeptides able to form a complex with a MHC class II or HLA molecule of the host (Hoebeke, 1996). In case of the human beta1-adrenoceptor, a computer-based search for potential immunogenic amino-acid streches within this (seven) transmembrane spanning protein revealed, that the only portion of the molecule containing B- and T-cell epitopes (and accessible to antibodies) was in fact the predicted second extracellular receptor loop (beta1-ECII). This might explain the successful use of ECII-mimicking peptides for the induction of specific anti-beta1-ECII antibodies in different animal-models (Magnusson et al., 1996; Jahns et al., 2004, 2006). Finally, by isogenic transfer of anti-beta1-ECII antibodies in a human-analogous rat model the (autoimmune-)attack against the hearts of healthy recipients by activating anti-beta1-antibodies has been identified as a possible cause of heart failure (Jahns et al., 2004).

In the last decade several research groups have independently shown that anti-beta1-ECII-antibodies preferentially recognize native membrane beta1-receptors in various immunological assays (cell-ELISA, immunoprecipitation, immunofluorescence), indicating that such antibodies or autoantibodies are conformational (Jahns et al., 1999, 2006; Fu 2008). In addition, functional tests revealed that such anti-beta1-ECII may also act as allosteric regulators of beta1-adrenoceptor activity through modulation of cellular cAMP-production and/or cAMP-dependent protein kinase (PKA) activity (Wallukat et al., 1991; Limas et al., 1992; Jahns et al., 1999; Nikolaev et al., 2007). The use of different screening-techniques renders direct comparisons of the available data difficult, however. Hence, so far reported prevalences should be always interpreted in the context of the detection method utilised. Nevertheless, taken all these reports together, there is wide consent that a substantial fraction of patients with DCM and ICM, but only very few healthy subjects have ciculating functionally active adrenoceptor-aabs (Wallukat et al., 1991; Magnusson et al., 1994; Jahns et al., 1999). An association of such aabs with impaired cardiac function (Jahns et al., 1999), a higher incidence of ventricular arrhythmias (Iwata et al., 2001; Störk et al., 2006), and a higher incidence of sudden cardiac death (Iwata et al., 2001) have been demonstrated. In addition, a previous clinical follow-up study also implies an increased risk for (cardiovascular) mortality in adrenoceptor aab-positive DCM patients (Störk et al., 2006).

To further analyse the time-course and sequentially engaged immunologic processes in autoimmune-mediated heart disease, the ETiCS study will prospectively follow the evolution of cardiac morphology and function after a first inflammatory or ischemic myocyte damage. In total 400 patients will benefit from a structured follow-up and best standard available medical care. The central hypothesis of ETiCS is that both inflammatory and ischemic myocardial injury may trigger a sequence of immunologic reactions which result in the formation of functionally active cardiac receptor-aabs (Jahns et al., 2006). Thus, the pre-specified primary endpoint is the titre of receptor-aabs at diagnosis compared to 3, 6, and 12 months after the index event. Since these aabs are thought to confer additional risk, pre-specified secondary endpoints of the ETiCS study comprise occurrence of life-threatening arrhythmias, changes in cardiac diameters and function, changes in clinical status, time to cardiovascular death, and time to all-cause death.

Endomyocardial biopsies will allow for a correlation of cardiac aab-titres with the severity of myocardial inflammation (Aretz et al., 1987; Elliott et al., 2008; Kindermann et al., 2008) , with the kind of T cells engaged (Th1 vs. Th2-response, Treg, CTLs (Noutias et al. 2011)), and with the presence and/or activity of infective agents detected (that is, the type and load of pre-specified viral/microbial pathogens, as determined by PCR (Kühl et al., 2005)).

Once available, the results of the ETiCS study will significantly contribute to a number of important diagnostic, pathophysiologic and prognostic issues in autoantibody-mediated heart disease (Fu, M., 2008). We expect insights on the role of inflammatory (and ischemic) cardiac damage in triggering autoimmune processes (including the involved immunologic paths), and on the relevance of heart-directed autoimmune reactions for the initiation or progression of heart failure (Jahns et al., 2006). In particular, we might learn and better understand whether -and if so, then to which extent- the specific target of a heart-directed autoantibody, but also its respective titre and biological activity and -last not least- its respective kinetics (that is, antibody-persistence or -clearance over time) relate to the complex process of cardiac wounding and healing. Different cardiac aabs might have distinct propensities to induce a certain cardiac phenotype, and the ETiCS study will allow for a differentiation of such features in a prospective manner. Thereby, additional prognostic markers for patients with an unfavourable course of autoimmune heart failure might be recognised and, as a consequence, conventional treatment modalities could be optimized earlier and/or novel -more specific- treatment strategies could be developed.

6. Future perspectives and therapeutic implications

Despite available treatment guidelines, the recent progress in conventional pharmacotherapy, and promising novel device-based therapeutic approaches, the outcome of patients suffering from heart failure remains unsatisfactory. This has stimulated the search for causal treatment strategies aiming to block or neutralize factors thought to play a role in heart failure progression.

In a large number of neurologic, rheumatologic, and endocrine disorders autoimmune phenomena have been recognised as main disease-causing factors. Their relevance in human heart disease and failure, however, still need to be substantiated (Jahns et al., 2006; Fu, M., 2008) although preliminary clinical data suggest that the presence of certain cardiac aabs clearly worsens the prognosis of patients with idiopathic DCM (Störk et al., 2006). Therapeutic strategies known from other autoimmune disorders, such as application of peptide-ligands (for multiple sclerosis (Warren et al., 2006)) or immunoadsorption of disease-causing aabs (for myasthenia gravis (Tzartos et al., 2008)) might thus also offer treatment options for a variety of human cardiac disorders.

In this regard, recent *in vitro* experiments with functionally active receptor-aabs isolated from a smaller number of DCM-patients indicate, that aab-induced adrenoceptor activation might be abrogated by incubation with epitope-mimicking peptides (Nikolaev et al., 2007; Jahns et al. 2010). Although clinical *in vivo* data with epitope-derived antibody-scavengers are still lacking, the latter *in vitro* findings together with the results from the ETiCS study should stimulate further research in the field of specifically antibody-directed therapeutic strategies.

In addition to established anti-adrenergic drugs like cardioselective beta-blockers such strategies might comprise (a) the aforementioned epitope-derived peptides as antibody-scavengers (Jahns et al., 2010), (b) an elimination of functionally active cardiac aabs by selective or non-selective immunoadsorption (studies currently under way (Felix & Staudt, 2008; Müller et al., 2008)), or (c) the direct targeting/suppression of autoantibody-producing B cells and/or plasma-cells themselves (Neubert et al., 2008).

At least in animal models of antibody-induced immune-cardiomyopathy and -nephropathy some of these novel therapeutic approaches have already been successfully applied (Jahns et al., 2005; Matsui et al., 2006; Neubert et al., 2008; Jahns et al., 2010). Hence, the results from the clinical (diagnostic) ETiCS study might also furnish a basis for and accelerate further pre-clinical development of such novel therapeutic approaches and agents targeting at cardio-noxious aabs, and -hopefully- for a faster transfer into clinical practice. Moreover, by initiating a joint venture of the leading European research institutes in the field of cardiac autoimmunity, ETiCS could equally serve as a starting point for future common efforts to further understand and therapeutically modulate the immune system with respect to immune-mediated (post-inflammatory) human cardiac disorders.

7. Acknowledgements

The investigator-initiated ETiCS study receives public funding from the German Ministry for Education and Research (Bundesministerium für Bildung und Forschung, BMBF Project number 01ES0816). The ETiCS study has been acknowledged by the German Competence Network Heart Failure (CNHF, subproject 6b), and has equally been associated to the BMBF-funded Comprehensive Heart Failure Centre, University Hospital of Würzburg (CHFC, associated project C4). All authors had full access to the data and have read and approved the final article and have declared no conflicts of interest.

8. References

American Heart Association, Dallas (2009). Heart disease and stroke statistics - 2009 update. A report from the American Heart Association Statistics Committee and Stroke Statistics Subcommittee. *Circulation* 119: 480-486.

Aretz, H.T., Billingham, M.E., Edwards, W.D., Factor, S., Fallon, J.T., Fenoglio, J.J., Jr., Olsen, E. & Schoen, F.J. (1987). Myocarditis. A histopathologic definition and classification. *Am. J. Cardiovasc. Pathol.* 1,1: 3-14.

Baba, A., Yoshikawa, T., Fukuda, Y., Sugiyama, T., Shimada, M., Akaishi, M., Tsuchimoto, K., Ogawa, S. & Fu M (2004). Autoantibodies against M2-muscarinic acetylcholine receptors: new upstream targets in atrial fibrillation in patients with dilated cardiomyopathy. *Eur. Heart J.* 25: 1108-1115.

Bachmaier, K., Neu, N., de la Maza, L.M., Pal, S., Hessel, A., Penninger, J.M. (1999). Chlamydia infections and heart disease linked through antigenic mimicry. *Science* 283: 1335-1339.

Boivin, V., Jahns, R., Gambaryan, S., Ness, W. & Lohse, M. (2001). Immunofluorescent imaging of beta1- and 2-adrenergic receptors in rat kidney. *Kidney Int.* 59: 515-531.

Borda, E., Pascual, J., Cossio, P., Vega, M., Araña, R. & Sterin-Borda, L. (1984). A circulating IgG in Chagas disease which binds to β-adrenoceptor of myocardium and modulates its activity. *Clin. Exp. Immunol.* 57: 679-685.

Caforio, A.L., Goldman, J.H., Baig, M., Keeling, P.J., Bottazzo, G.F. & McKenna, W.J. (1995). Organ-specific cardiac autoantibodies in dilated cardiomyopathy - an update. *Eur. Heart J.* 16, Suppl.O: 68-70.

Caforio, A.L. & Iliceto, S. (2008). Genetically determined myocarditis: clinical presentation and immunological characteristics. *Curr. Opin. Cardiol.* 23,3: 219-226.

Caforio, A.L., Mahon, N.G., Baig, M., Tona, F., Murphy, R.T., Elliott, P.M.& McKenna, W.J. (2007). Prospective familial assessment in dilated cardiomyopathy: cardiac autoantibodies predict disease development in asymptomatic relatives. *Circulation* 115,1: 76-83.

Caforio, A.L., Mahon, N.J., Tona, F. & McKenna, W.J. (2002). Circulating cardiac autoantibodies in dilated cardiomyopathy and myocarditis: pathogenetic and clinical significance. *Eur. J. Heart Fail.* 4: 411-417.

Christ, T., Schindelhauer, S., Wettwer, E., Wallukat, G. & Ravens, U. (2006). Interaction between autoantibodies against the beta1-adrenoceptor and isoprenaline in enhancing L-type Ca^{2+} current in rat ventricular myocytes. *J. Mol. Cell Cardiol.* 41: 716-723.

Cooper, L.T., Baughman, K.L., Feldman, A.M., Frustaci, A., Jessup, M., Kuhl, U., Levine, G.N., Narula, J., Starling, R.C., Towbin, J. & Virmani, R. (2007). The role of endomyocardial biopsy in the management of cardiovascular disease: a scientific statement from the American Heart Association, the American College of Cardiology, and the European Society of Cardiology. Endorsed by the Heart Failure Society of America and the Heart Failure Association of the European Society of Cardiology. *J. Am. Coll. Cardiol.* 50,19: 1914-1931.

Elies R., Ferrari I, Wallukat G, Lebesgue D, Chiale P, Elizari M, Rosenbaum M, Hoebeke J, Levin MJ (1996) Structural and functional analysis of the B cell epitopes recognized by anti-receptor autoantibodies in patients with Chagas' disease. J. Immunol. 157: 4203-4211

Elliott, P., Andersson, B., Arbustini, E., Bilinska, Z., Cecchi, F., Charron, P., Dubourg, O., Kuhl, U., Maisch, B., McKenna, W.J., Monserrat, L., Pankuweit, S., Rapezzi, C., Seferovic, P., Tavazzi, L. & Keren, A. (2008). Classification of the cardiomyopathies: a position statement from the European Society Of Cardiology Working Group on Myocardial and Pericardial Diseases. *Eur. Heart J.* 29,2: 270-276.

Engelhardt, S., Hein, L., Dyachenkow, V., Kranias, E.G., Isenberg, G. & Lohse, M.J. (2004). Altered calcium handling is critically involved in the cardiotoxic effects of chronic beta-adrenergic stimulation. *Circulation* 109: 1154-1160.

Eriksson, U., Ricci, R., Hunziker, L., Kurrer, M.O., Oudit, G.Y., Watts, T.H., Sonderegger, I., Bachmaier, K., Kopf, M. & Penninger, J.M. (2003). Dendritic cell-induced autoimmune heart failure requires cooperation between adaptive and innate immunity. *Nat. Med.* 9,12: 1484-1490.

Felix, S.B. & Staudt, A. (2008). Immunoadsorption as a teatment option in dilated cardiomyopathy. *Autoimmunity* 41,6: 484-489.

Felix, S.B., Staudt, A., Landsberger, M., Grosse, Y., Stangl, V., Spielhagen, T., Wallukat, G., Wernecke, K.D., Baumann, G. & Stangl, K. (2002). Removal of cardiodepressant antibodies in dilated cardiomyopathy by immunoadsorption. *J. Am. Coll. Cardiol.* 39,4: 646-652.

Freedman, N.J. & Lefkowitz, R.J. (2004). Anti-beta1-adrenergic receptor antibodies and heart failure: causation, not just correlation. *J. Clin. Invest.* 113: 1379-1382.

Frustaci, A., Russo, M.A. & Chimenti, C. (2009). Randomized study on the efficacy of immunosuppressive therapy in patients with virus-negative inflammatory cardiomyopathy: the TIMIC study. *Eur. Heart J.* 30,16: 1995-2002.

Fu, L.X.M., Magnusson, Y., Bergh, C.H., Waagstein, F., Hjalmarson, Å. & Hoebeke, J. (1993). Localization of a functional autoimmune epitope on the second extracellular loop of the human muscarinic acetylcholine receptor 2 in patients with idiopathic dilated cardiomyopathy. *J. Clin. Invest.* 91: 1964-1968.

Fu, M. (2008). Autoimmunity and idiopathic dilated cardiomyopathy: where we stand? *Autoimmunity* 41,6: 415-418.

Golden, B., Levin, L., Ban, Y., Concepcion, E., Greenberg, D.A. & Tomer, Y. (2005). Genetic analysis of families with autoimmune diabetes and thyroiditis: evidence for common and unique genes. *J. Clin. Endocrinol. Metab.* 90,8: 4904-4911.

Göser, S., Andrassy, M., Buss, S.J., Leuschner, F., Volz, C.H., Öttl, R., Zittrich, S., Blaudeck, N., Hardt, S.E., Pfitzer, G., Rose, N.R., Katus, H.A. & Kaya, Z. (2006). Cardiac troponin I but not cardiac troponin T induces severe autoimmune inflammation in the myocardium. *Circulation* 114: 1693-1702.

Harding, C.V., Unanue, E.R. & Slot, J.M. (1990). Functional and ultrastructural evidence for intracellular formation of major histocompatibility complex class II-peptide complexes during antigen processing. *Proc. Natl. Acad. Sci. USA* 87: 5553-5557.

Hoebeke, J. (1996). Structural basis of autoimmunity against G protein-coupled membrane receptors. *Int. J. Cardiol.* 54: 103-111.

Iwata, M., Yoshikawa, T., Baba, A., Anzai, T., Mitamura, H. & Ogawa, S. (2001). Autoantibodies against the second extracellular loop of beta1-adrenergic receptors predict ventricular tachycardia and sudden death in patients with idiopathic dilated cardiomyopathy. *J. Am. Coll. Cardiol.* 37: 418-424.

Jahns, R., Boivin, V., Hein, L., Palm, D., Nikolaev, V.O., Müller, J., Angermann, C.E., Ertl, G. & Lohse, M.J. (2005). A new cyclic receptor-peptide prevents development of heart dilatation and failure induced by antibodies activating cardiac beta1-adrenergic receptors. *Circulation* 112, suppl.II: 5 (120).

Jahns, R, Boivin, V., Hein, L., Triebel, S., Angermann, C.E., Ertl, G & Lohse M.J. (2004). Direct evidence for a beta1-adrenergic receptor directed autoimmune attack as a cause of idiopathic dilated cardiomyopathy. *J. Clin. Invest.* 113:1419-1429.

Jahns, R., Boivin, V. & Lohse, M.J. (2006). Beta1-adrenergic receptor function, autoimmunity, and pathogenesis of dilated cardiomyopathy. *Trends Cardiovasc. Med.* 16: 20-24.

Jahns, R., Boivin, V., Inselmann, G., Lohse, M. & Boege, F. (1999). Autoantibodies activating human beta1-adrenergic receptors are associated with reduced cardiac function in chronic heart failure. *Circulation* 99: 649-654.

Jahns, R., Schlipp, A., Boivin, V. & Lohse, M.J. (2010). Targeting receptor-antibodies in immune-cardiomyopathy. *Semin. Thromb. Hemost.* 36: 212-218.

Kindermann, I., Kindermann, M., Kandolf, R., Klingel, K., Bultmann, B., Müller, T., Lindinger, A. & Böhm, M. (2008). Predictors of outcome in patients with suspected myocarditis. *Circulation* 118,6: 639-648.

Kühl, U., Noutsias, M., Seeberg, B. & Schultheiss, H.P. (1996). Immunohistological evidence for a chronic intramyocardial inflammatory process in dilated cardiomyopathy. *Heart* 75,3: 295-300.

Kühl, U., Pauschinger, M., Noutsias, M., Seeberg, B., Bock, T., Lassner, D., Poller, W., Kandolf, R. & Schultheiss, H.P. (2005). High prevalence of viral genomes and multiple viral infections in the myocardium of adults with idiopathic left ventricular dysfunction. *Circulation* 111: 887-893.

Kühl, U., Pauschinger, M., Seeberg, B., Lassner, D., Noutsias, M., Poller, W. & Schultheiss, H.P. (2005). Viral persistence in the myocardium is associated with progressive cardiac dysfunction. *Circulation* 112: 1965-1970.

Latif, N., Baker, C.S., Dunn, M.J., Keeling, P.J. & Botazzo, G.F. (1993). Frequency and specificity of antiheart antibodies in patients with dilated cardiomyopathy detected using SDS-page and Western blotting. *J. Am. Coll. Cardiol.* 22: 1378-1384.

Li, Y., Heuser, J.S., Cunningham, L.C., Kosanke, S.D. & Cunningham, M.W. (2006). Mimicry and antibody-mediated cell signaling in autoimmune myocarditis. *J. Immunol.* 177: 8234-8240.

Limas, C.J. (1996). Autoimmunity in DCM and the major histocompatibility complex. *Int. J. Cardiol.* 54: 113-116.

Limas, C.J. (1997). Cardiac autoantibodies in dilated cardiomyopathy. *Circulation* 95: 1979-1980.

Limas, C.J., Goldenberg, I.F. & Limas, C. (1992). Assessment of immune modulation of beta-adrenergic pathways in human dilated cardiomyopathy: influence of methodologic factors. *Am. Heart J.* 123: 967-970.

Limas, C.J., Iakovis, P., Anyfantakis, A., Kroupis, C. & Cokkinos, D.V. (2004). Familial clustering of autoimmune diseases in patients with dilated cardiomyopathy. *Am. J. Cardiol.* 93: 1189-1191.

Liu, P. & Mason, J. (2001). Advances in the understanding of myocarditis. *Circulation* 104: 1076-1082.

Luppi, P., Rudert, W.A., Zanone, M.M., Stassi, G., Trucco, G., Finegold, D., Boyle, G.J., Del Nido, P., McGowan, F.X. & Trucco, M. (1998). Idiopathic dilated cardiomyopathy. A superantigen-driven autoimmune disease. *Circulation* 98: 777-785.

MacLellan, W.R. & Lusis, A.J. (2003). Dilated cardiomyopathy: learning to live with yourself. *Nat. Med.* 9: 1455-1456.

Maekawa, Y., Ouzounian, M., Opavsky, M.A. & Liu, P.P. (2007). Connecting the missing link between dilated cardiomyopathy and viral myocarditis. *Circulation* 115: 5-8.

Magnusson, Y., Hjalmarson, Å. & Hoebeke, J. (1996). Beta1-adrenoceptor autoimmunity in cardiomyopathy. *Int. J. Cardiol.* 54: 137-141.

Magnusson, Y., Wallukat, G., Waagstein, F., Hjalmarson, Å. & Hoebeke, J. (1994). Autoimmunity in idiopathic DCM. Characterization of antibodies against the beta1-adrenoceptor with positive chronotropic effect. *Circulation* 89,6: 2760-2767.

Mahrholdt, H., Wagner, A., Deluggi, C.C., Kispert, E., Hager, S., Meinhardt, G., Vogelsberg, H., Fritz, P., Dippon, J., Bock, C.-T., Klingel, K., Kandolf, R. & Sechtem, U. (2006). Presentation, patterns of myocardial damage, and clinical course of viral myocarditis. *Circulation* 114: 1581-1590.

Maron, B.J., Towbin, J.A., Thiene, G., Antzelevitch, C., Corrado, D., Arnett, D., Moss, A.J., Seidman, C.E. & Young, J.B. (2006). Contemporary definitions and classification of the cardiomyopathies: an American Heart Association Scientific Statement from the Council on Clinical Cardiology, Heart Failure and Transplantation Committee; Quality of Care and Outcomes Research and Functional Genomics and Translational Biology Interdisciplinary Working Groups; and Council on Epidemiology and Prevention. *Circulation* 113: 1807-1816.

Matsui, S., Fu, M., Hayase, M., Katsuda, S., Yamaguchi, N., Teraoka, K., Kurihara, T.W., Murano, H. & Takekoshi, N. (2006). Transfer of immune components from rabbit autoimmune cardiomyopathy into severe combined immunodeficiency (SCID) mice induces cardiomyopathic changes. *Autoimmunity* 39,2: 121-128.

Mobini, R., Magnusson, Y., Wallukat, G., Viguier, M., Hjalmarson, Å. & Hoebeke, J. (1999). Probing the immunological properties of the extracellular domains of the human beta1-adrenoceptor. *J. Autoimmun.* 13,2: 179-186.

Müller, I.I., Klingel, K., Nikolaev, V.O., Jahns, R., Gawatz, M.P. & Weig, H.J. (2008). Immunoadsorption in a 40 year old man with dilated cardiomyopathy and underlying active myocarditis. *Clin. Res. Cardiol.* 22: 138-140.

Neubert, K., Meister, S., Moser, K., Weisel, F., Maseda, D., Amann, K., Wiethe, C., Winkler, T.H., Kalden, J.R., Manz, R.A. & Voll, R.E. (2008). The proteasome inhibitor bortezemib depletes plasma cells and protects mice with lupus-like disease from nephritis. *Nat. Med.* 14: 748-755.

Neumann, D.A., Burek, C.L., Baughman, K.L., Rose, N.R. & Herskowitz, A. (1990). Circulating heart-reactive antibodies in patients with myocarditis or cardiomyopathy. *J. Am. Coll. Cardiol.* 16: 839-846.

Nikolaev, V.O., Boivin, V., Störk, S., Angermann, C.E., Ertl, G., Lohse, M.J.& Jahns, R. (2007). A novel fluorescent method for the rapid detection of functional beta1-adrenergic receptor autoantibodies in heart failure. *J. Am. Coll. Cardiol.* 50: 423-431.

Noutsias, M., Seeberg, B., Schultheiss, H.P. & Kühl, U. (1999). Expression of cell adhesion molecules in dilated cardiomyopathy: evidence for endothelial activation in inflammatory cardiomyopathy. *Circulation* 99,16: 2124-2131.

Noutias, M., Rohde, M., Göldner, K., Block, A., Blunert K., Hemaidan, L., Hummel M., Blohm, J.H., Lassner, D., Kühl, U. , Schultheiss, H.P., Volk, H.D. & Kotsch, K. (2011). Expression of functional T cell markers and T cell receptor Vbeta repertoire in endomyocardial biopsies from patients presenting with acute myocarditis and dilated cardiomyopathy. *Eur. J. Heart Fail.* 13,6: 611-618.

Okazaki, T., Tanaka, Y., Nishio, R., Mitsuiye, T., Mizoguchi, A., Wang, J., Ishida, M., Hiai, H., Matsumori, A., Minato, N. & Honjo, T. (2003). Autoantibodies against cardiac troponin I are responsible for dilated cardiomyopathy in PD-1-deficient mice. *Nat. Med.* 9,12: 1477-1483.

Pohlner, K., Portig, I., Pankuweit, S., Lottspeich, F. & Maisch, B. (1997). Identification of mitochondrial antigens recognized by the antibody in sera of patients with dilated cardiomyopathy by two-dimensional gel electrophoresis and protein sequencing. *Am. J. Cardiol.* 80: 1040-1045.

Richardson, P., McKenna, W., Bristow, M., Maisch, B., Mautner, B., O'Connell, J., Olsen, E., Thiene, G., Goodwin, J., Gyarfas, I., Martin, I.& Nordet, P. (1996). Report of the 1995 World Health Organization/International Society and Federation of Cardiology Task Force on the Definition and Classification of cardiomyopathies. *Circulation* 93,5: 841-842.

Rose, N.R. (2001). Infection, mimics, and autoimmune disease. *J. Clin. Invest.* 107: 943-944.

Schultheiss, H.P. & Bolte, H.D. (1985). Immunological analysis of autoantibodies against the adenine nucleotide translocator in dilated cardiomyopathy. *J. Mol. Cell Cardiol.* 17: 603-617.

Schultheiss, H.P., Kühl, U., Janda, I., Melzner, B., Ulrich, G. & Morad, M. (1988). Antibody-mediated enhancement of calcium permeability in cardiac myocytes. *J. Exp. Med.* 168: 2102-2109.

Schulze, K., Witzenbichler, B., Christmann, C. & Schultheiss, H.P. (1999). Disturbance of myocardial energy metabolism in experimental virus myocarditis by antibodies against the adenine nucleotid translocator. *Cardiovasc. Res.* 44: 91-100.

Smulski, C., Labovsky, V., Levy, G., Hontebeyrie, M., Hoebeke, J. & Levin, M.J. (2006). Structural basis of the cross-reaction between an antibody to the trypanosoma cruzi ribosomal P2beta protein and the human beta1-adrenergic receptor. *FASEB J.* 20: 1396-1406.

Störk, S., Boivin, V., Horf, R., Hein, L., Lohse, M.J., Angermann, C.E. & Jahns, R. (2006). Stimulating autoantibodies directed against the cardiac beta1-adrenergic receptor predict increased mortality in idiopathic cardiomyopathy. *Am. Heart J.* 152: 697-704.

Tzartos, S.J., Bitzopoulou, K., Gavra, I.M., Kordas, G.H., Jacobson, L., Kostelidou, K.M., Lagoumintzis, G., Lazos, O., Poulas, K., Sideris, S., Sotiriadis, A., Trakas, N. & Zisimopoulou, P. (2008). Antigen-specific apheresis of pathogenic autoantibodies from myasthenia gravis sera. *Ann. N. Y. Acad. Sci.* 1132: 291-299.

Valaperti, A., Marty, R.R., Kania, G., Germano, D., Mauermann, N., Dirnhofer, S., Leimenstoll, B., Blyszczuk, P., Dong, C., Müller, C., Hunziker, L. & Eriksson, U. (2008): CD11b+ monocytes abrogate Th17 CD4+ T cell-mediated experimental autoimmune myocarditis. *J. Immunol.* 180: 2686-2695.

Wallukat, G., Morwinski, M., Kowal, K., Förster, A., Boewer, V. & Wollenberger, A. (1991). Autoantibodies against the beta-adrenergic receptor in human myocarditis and dilated cardiomyopathy: beta-adrenergic agonism without desensitization. *Eur. Heart J.* 12,1: 178-181.

Wang, W.Z., Zhao, R.R., Wu, B.W., Jin, X.H., Zuh, L., Hjalmarson, Ǻ. & Fu, M. (1996). Effects of anti-peptide antibodies against human M2 muscarinic receptors on cardiac function of rats in vivo. *Blood Pressure* 3: 25-27

Warren, K.G., Catz, I., Ferenczi, L.Z. & Krantz, M.J. (2006). Intravenous synthetic peptide MBP8298 delayed disease progression in an HLA Class II-defined cohort of patients with progressive multiple sclerosis: results of a 24-moth double-blind placebo-con-trolled clinical trial and 5 years of follow-up treatment. *Eur. J. Neurol.* 13: 887-895.

20

Nucleic Acid-Based Strategies for the Treatment of Coxsackievirus-Induced Myocarditis

Decheng Yang
Department of Pathology and Laboratory Medicine, University of British Columbia, The Institute for Heart and Lung Health, St. Paul's Hospital, Vancouver, B. C., Canada

1. Introduction

Viral myocarditis is the most common heart disease in infants, children, young adults and pregnant women. Although a number of viruses from different genera, such as adenovirus, hepatitis C virus (HCV), parvoviruses and cytomegalovirus have been reported to cause myocarditis (Bowles et al., 2003; Kindermann et al., 2008; Kuhl et al., 2005a; Kuhl et al., 2005b; Kyto et al., 2005; Mahrholdt et al., 2006; Matsumori, 2005; Matsumori et al., 2006), coxsackievirus, particularly coxsackievirus B3 (CVB3), is generally considered the primary etiological agent of myocarditis (Blauwet, 2010; Kuhl et al., 2005a; Mahrholdt et al., 2006). CVB3 infection of the heart is often persistent and enters the chronic phase, leading to dilated cardiomyopathy (DCM)(Andreoletti et al., 2009; L. T. Cooper, Jr., 2009; Kuhl et al., 2005b; Yajima& Knowlton, 2009), a squelae of viral myocarditis characterized by ventricular chamber dilation, increased wall thickness, weaker beating and abnormal heart function. Patients with DCM eventually develop into congestive heart failure.

To date, there is no clinically proven specific treatment available for viral myocarditis and DCM. Patients with DCM eventually need heart transplantation as the final treatment (Schultz et al., 2009). The managements for viral myocarditis are usually supportive therapies, such as improvements in cardiophysiology with medicine used to treat other kinds of heart diseases, and application of non-specific antiviral agents to decrease the viral load. The former measurements include administration of angiotensin-converting enzyme inhibitor or angiotensin receptor blockade, beta-adrenergic blockade, diuretics, etc (Dennert et al., 2008; Rose, 2009; Schultz et al., 2009); the later measurements include application of type I interferons or nucleotide analogs such as ribavirin, which is reviewed elsewhere (Blauwet, 2010; Dennert& Crijns& Heymans, 2008; Schultz et al., 2009). If myocarditis was caused by an autoimmune disorder, it would be appropriately treated by immunosuppression (Rose, 2009; Schultz et al., 2009). However, the effectiveness of treatment with immunosuppressive therapies has not reached a consensus amongst different studies. This can probably be attributed to the difficulty of confirmation and diagnosis of the etiology and pathogenesis of myocarditis. Thus it is very important to distinguish infectious and autoimmune disease since the same methods of treatment will not be optimal for both forms of heart muscle diseases. The diagnostic gold standard is endomyocardial biopsies with the histological Dallas criteria, in association with new immunohistochemical and viral PCR analyses of cardiac tissues (L. T. Cooper et al., 2007). In case of confirmed autoimmune-related disease and lack of detectable viral infection, an immunosuppressive treatment combining corticoids and azathioprine may be beneficial to the patients (Frustaci et al., 2003). However, if the disease is primarily caused by viral infections, more specific antiviral agents would be the ideal drugs of choice. In recent years, the search for such antiviral drugs has become a new trend in drug development for treatment of viral myocarditis. The strategies for developing such antivirals include i) screening chemical compounds, such as Pleconaril, capable of interacting with picornavirus (particularly human rhinovirus) antireceptor to block viral entry of the host cells (Groarke& Pevear, 1999; Kaiser et al., 2000; Reisdorph et al., 2003), ii) application of herb medicine to reduce viral load or boost immune responses to limit viral replication (Si et al., 2007; Y. F. Wang et al., 2009), iii) development of small peptide inhibitors of viral proteases to block CVB3 replication cycle (Maghsoudi et al., 2010) and iv) production of recombinant soluble protein of coxsackievirus-adenovirus receptor (CAR) fused to a human immunoglobulin (sCAR-Fc) to block coxsackievirus B3 entry (Pinkert et al., 2009; Werk et al., 2009; Yanagawa et al., 2003; Yanagawa et al., 2004). Another very attractive and promising trend in drug development is the nucleic acid (NA)-based approach to target viral genome or cellular genes to block viral translation and transcription. These strategies include design and synthesis of antisense oligonucleotide (ASON), ribozyme, short interfering RNA (siRNA) and artificial microRNA (miRNA). In this chapter we will focus our discussion on the recent state of this group of antiviral agents for the treatment of myocarditis caused by CVB3 and other viruses that have been recently reported as causal agents of myocarditis.

2. CVB3 genome organization and its receptor

CVB3, a member of enterovirus in the *Picornaviridae* family, is a positive single-stranded, non-enveloped RNA virus. Its genome is ~7.4 kb long containing a single long open reading frame (encoding 11 proteins) flanking by the 5′ and 3′untranslated regions (UTRs) (Klump et al., 1990). The 5′UTR is unusually long (741 nucleotides (nt)) and harbors a number of *cis*-acting translational elements, such as internal ribosomal entry site (IRES) and cloverleaf sequence (Cheung et al., 2007; Z. Liu et al., 1999; Verma et al., 2010; Yang et al., 1997), which are crucial structures for viral translation and transcription. The 3′UTR is a 99-nt long segment attached with a poly-A tail. The 3′UTR folds to form kissing-loop tertiary structures, which are believed to play a role in facilitating viral transcription of the negative strand of CVB3 replication intermediate (Melchers et al., 1997; J. Wang et al., 1999). The viral genomic RNA can directly serve as a mRNA template for translation of a single long polyprotein, which is processed by viral proteases to produce eleven individual proteins, among which four are structural proteins, VP1-VP4, and seven are non-structural proteins including proteases, 2A and 3C, as well as a RNA-dependent RNA polymerase 3D. These three enzymatic proteins play important roles in viral life cycle and pathogenesis (Knowlton, 2008).

CVB3 is a cardiotropic virus. It infects cardiomyocytes by endocytosis through viral receptor CAR (coxsackie and adenovirus receptor) colocalized with tight junction protein (e.g., occludin) (Raschperger et al., 2006). Structural analysis of CAR D1 domain supports the proposed function of CAR as a mediator of cell adhesion (Honda et al., 2000) in the junction complexes of epithelial cells in many tissues (Cohen et al., 2001). It is also known that CAR binding site (anti-receptor) on CVB3 particle lies in the canyon on the capsid surface. Upon attachment of CVB3 particles to CAR, the receptor changes conformation to form the viral A-particle, a product of the interactions between CVB3 and CAR, which then allows for the release of viral RNA into host cells and begins viral translation and transcription. The observation that soluble CAR can function as a virus trap leading to inactive A-particles has been suggested as a strategy for CVB3 therapy (Pinkert et al., 2009; Werk et al., 2009; Yanagawa et al., 2004). Depending on the different combination of viral strains and mouse models in study of CVB3 infection, a CVB3 co-receptor called decay accelerating factor (DAF, CD55) is sometimes also necessary for CVB3 entry of the host cells (Freimuth et al., 2008; Shafren et al., 1997). Thus, genes encoding CAR and DAF are important candidates for study of viral tropism and rationale targets for antiviral drug design.

3. NA-based antiviral strategies

3.1 Antisense oligonucleotide (ASON)

ASON is probably the earliest NA-based antiviral agent developed. They are designed to bind a complementary sequence in the target mRNA to form RNA-DNA heteroduplexes. These double-stranded hybrid sequences are recognized by RNase H, which digests the RNA strand in the duplex, releasing the ASON to bind another target and so on, effectively silencing the encoded gene (Walder & Walder, 1988). Certain ASONs are not capable of activation of RNase H; instead they inhibit gene translation by steric competition with the translational machinery. In addition, ASONs, if bound to pre-mRNA at intron-exon junctions, can disrupt mRNA splicing (Munroe, 1988). Furthermore, ASONs can also disrupt RNA trafficking by occupying protein-RNA interaction sequences necessary for correct intracellular localization. For example, hnRNP A2 response element (A2RE) is identified as a key sequence required for the trafficking of myelin basic protein (Shan et al., 2000).

Due to major problems including instability, non-specific delivery and unwanted side effects of the ASONs, the structure of this molecule has been modified extensively at different components (i.e., the bases, sugar or phosphate backbone) and has entered its third generation (Fig. 1). The first generation of chemical modification was designed to enhance nuclease resistance of ASON in serum (Stein et al., 1997). The representative of such is the phosphorothioate (PS) oligonucleotide (ON), in which one of the non-bridging oxygen atoms in the phosphodiester bond is replaced by sulfur, intended to prevent cleavage by nucleases. Early antiviral PS-modified ASONs exhibited the antisense properties of phosphodiester ASONs, such as the ability to induce RNase H activation, while showing enhanced stability *in vitro* for up to 48 hours (Hoke et al., 1991); reviewed in (Kurreck, 2003). One notable property of PS-ASON is their tendency to form aptamers, i.e., nonspecific interactions with proteins due to its negative charge. This is disadvantageous intracellularly because aptamer interactions can impede ASON interaction with its intended target, and hence its function. Conversely, the tendency for PS-ASONs to bind serum proteins albumin and alpha-2 macroglobulin in circulation actually improves their bio-distribution throughout the body *in vivo* and prevents them from being cleared for excretion (Crooke et al., 1996).

Another strategy to increase the stability of ASONs is the addition of alkyl groups at the 2′ position of the ribose. 2′-*O*-methyl (OMe) and 2′-*O*-methoxy-ethyl (MOE) substitutions sterically shield the backbone from nuclease access, and also increase affinity to the target, shown by increased T_m, thus stabilizing the duplex (Cotten et al., 1991). 2′-*O*-alkyl ASONs

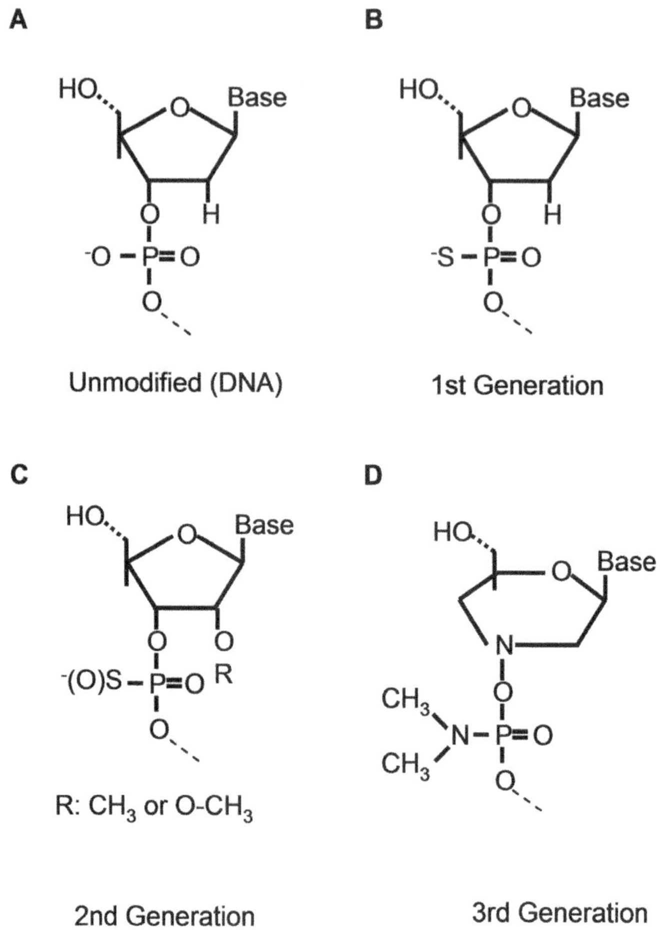

Fig. 1. Structures of certain nucleic acid analogs used to synthesize different generation ASONs. (A) unmodified deoxyribonucleotide. (B) Phosphorothioate modification of the phosphodiester backbone replaces the non-bridging oxygen with a sulfur atom. (C) Second generation ASONs with a 2′-akyl or 2′-methoxy ethyl groups further stabilize the molecule. (D) Phosphorodiamidate morpholino oligos have a modified backbone and modified sugar ring and are electrically neutral.

are also less toxic than PS-ASONs (Cotten et al., 1991); however, the 2′-*O*-alkyl group simultaneously shields heteroduplexed ASON-RNA from RNase H and therefore cannot induce direct cleavage of the target RNA. These modified ASONs function mainly by blocking translation via steric hindrance of elongating ribosome. In order to retain the advantage of the RNAse H mechanism while still conferring some benefits of 2′-O-alkyl protection, chimeric oligos containing both 2′ unmodified and 2′-modified DNAs, called gapmers, were conceived. Gapmers are typically end-modified, allowing a normal DNA-RNA heteroduplex to form mid-strand, although they may also consist of centre-modified

ASON flanked by normal DNA, or more commonly, phosphorothioate-linked DNA so as to capitalize on the advantages of both types of modifications (Turner et al., 2006). Both designs also reduce the polyanionic side effects of the phosphorothioate modification (Monia et al., 1993). 2′-O-alkyl modified ASONs and mixed backbone gapmer ASONs represent a second generation of ASON.

Third generation ASONs are phosphorodiamidate morpholino oligonucleotides (PMOs). PMOs are nonionic DNA analogues originally proven in loss of function knockdown studies in developmental systems such as zebrafish. The success and limitations of their usage have been recently reviewed comprehensively (Amantana& Iversen, 2005; Heasman, 2002). PMOs have an altered structure in which the ribose is replaced by a morpholine moiety and phosphorodiamidate (O-PONH$_2$-O) linkers are used instead of phosphodiester bonds. Thus PMOs are resistant to digestion by nucleases and are electrically neutral, a property that reduces nonspecific interactions with intracellular proteins. Morpholinos form base pairs with target sequences, but the binding ability is no greater than binding of analogous DNA and RNA oligomers, necessitating the use of relatively long 25-base oligomers for antisense inhibition. In addition, PMO-RNA hybrids do not activate RNase H. Therefore, the mechanism by which the PMOs inhibit protein synthesis is via binding the critical mRNA elements, such as the mRNA 5′UTR or the start codon region, to prevent ribosomes from binding or scanning. Alternatively, PMOs may occupy the mRNA splice recognition site to block the normal posttranscriptional processing required for synthesis of the functional protein. A good example is the report on therapeutic application of PMOs to correct aberrant splicing of mutated β-globin precursor mRNA (Lacerra et al., 2000).

The limitations of PMOs are their low cellular uptake levels as compared to unmodified ASONs. To address this shortcoming, PMOs can be conjugated to certain positive peptide carriers such as arginine-rich HIV-TAT and *drosophila* antennapedia sequences (Cardarelli et al., 2007). Because PMOs have a standard phosphodiester linkage and are uncharged, the addition of a positive peptide conjugate does not cause the same aptamer interaction as that caused by PS-ASON, which contains negative oxygen atoms.

3.2 Ribozymes

Ribozymes are catalytically active small RNA (~30-100 nts) molecules that act as enzymes to specifically cleave single strand RNA without the need of proteins. A major therapeutic advantage of ribozymes is the ability to make them *trans-acting* and to confer specificity to virtually cleave any target sequence (Peracchi, 2004). This can be achieved by fusing the ribozyme core sequence at the 5′ and 3′ ends with the sequences that are complementary to the target sequence. Of the nine groups of ribozymes, the hammerhead and hairpin ribozymes have received a great deal of attention (Scherer& Rossi, 2003). Hammerhead ribozymes, originally identified from plant viroid and viroid RNA, are composed of about 30 nts and have minimal requirements for the cleavage site, in which virtually any motif with the dinucleotide sequence UU, UC or UA can be targeted (Haseloff& Gerlach, 1992). For this reason, hammerhead ribozyme is very popular for the design of therapeutic ribozymes. On the other hand, the hairpin ribozyme has a more complex structure and requirements for target sequences, with a preference for GUC and cleavage occurring directly upstream of the G residue (Kore et al., 1998).

An advantage of ribozyme over ASON is its catalytic mode of action, which should in principle require a much lower concentration of ribozymes as compared to non-catalytic

ASONs. In addition, chemical modifications of ribozyme can increase its stability and improve therapeutic potential (Gonzalez-Carmona et al., 2006; Jakobsen et al., 2007). Antiviral ribozymes have been extensively tested in different gene therapy settings (Haasnoot et al., 2007). On the other hand, ribozyme also has its limitation, which is that target site selections are limited due to sequence requirements at the cleavage site and to structural constrains that interfere with ribozyme function to a higher extent (Frese, 2006). Therefore, the selection of appropriate target sites is of utmost importance which can not be predicted but must rather be determined empirically and which depends on the particular ribozyme used.

3.3 RNAi-based strategies

The term of RNA interference (RNAi) refers to a cellular process by which a double-strand RNA (dsRNA) sequence specifically inhibits the expression of a gene. This very efficient process of posttranscriptional gene silencing (PTGS) was discovered first in plant (Napoli et al., 1990) and served as a protection against viruses and genetic instability arising from transposons (Bartel, 2004). Accumulated evidence suggests that RNAi also plays a role in the antiviral defense mechanism in mammalian cells (Bennasser et al., 2005; Berkhout& Jeang, 2007; Cullen, 2006; Lecellier et al., 2005). These findings fuel the interests of the researchers to use RNAi not only for study of gene regulation but also for antiviral drug development (Lecellier et al., 2005; Otsuka et al., 2007).

The specificity of RNA silencing is mediated by small RNAs called short interfering RNAs (siRNA) and microRNA (miRNA). Both types of RNAs are generated by members of the Dicer family. This group of class III endoribonucleases cleaves double stranded non-coding RNA into fragments with a length of 21-25 nts. For siRNA, the long dsRNA or transgene-expressed short hairpin RNA (shRNA) is cleaved by Dicer. These RNAs are assembled into a multi-component complex, known as the RNA-induced silencing complex (RISC), which incorporates a single strand (antisense strand) of the siRNA serving as a guide sequence to silence the target gene (Hannon, 2002; Tomari& Zamore, 2005) (Fig. 2). For miRNA, this endogenous gene regulator is processed from primary RNA (priRNA) transcripts of non-coding regions or introns of protein-coding polymerase II transcripts. They are processed by RNase III Drosha to approximately 70-nt long pre-miRNAs, which are transported into cytoplasm by exportin-5 and are cleaved by Dicer to become the functional miRNA. Similar to siRNA, they also form a RISC with Argonaut proteins (having RNse H activity) and bind to their target mRNAs. The modes of actions of siRNA and miRNA depend on the degree of complementation between the siRNA or miRNA and their target sequences. siRNAs usually target coding regions by complementary base-paring and induce sequence-specific cleavage of mRNA substrate (Caudy et al., 2003); however, miRNA preferentially recognize target sequences in the 3′UTR of mRNAs and this target site is often in multi-copy (Brennecke et al., 2005; Grimson et al., 2007; Krek et al., 2005; Lewis et al., 2003). The binding of the miRNA often takes place with an incomplete homology, although a perfect base-pairing in the seed region (positions nt 2-8 from 5′ end of the antisense strand) of miRNA forms the core of interaction. Depending on the complete or partial homology between the miRNA and mRNA, the result can be cleavage of the target mRNA or repression of translation (Fig. 2) (Doench et al., 2003; Parker et al., 2005).

The precise mechanisms of RNAi-mediated suppression of gene expression have been studied extensively and made significant progress. The proposed mechanisms include the translation suppression by blocking the binding and scanning of ribosome and other

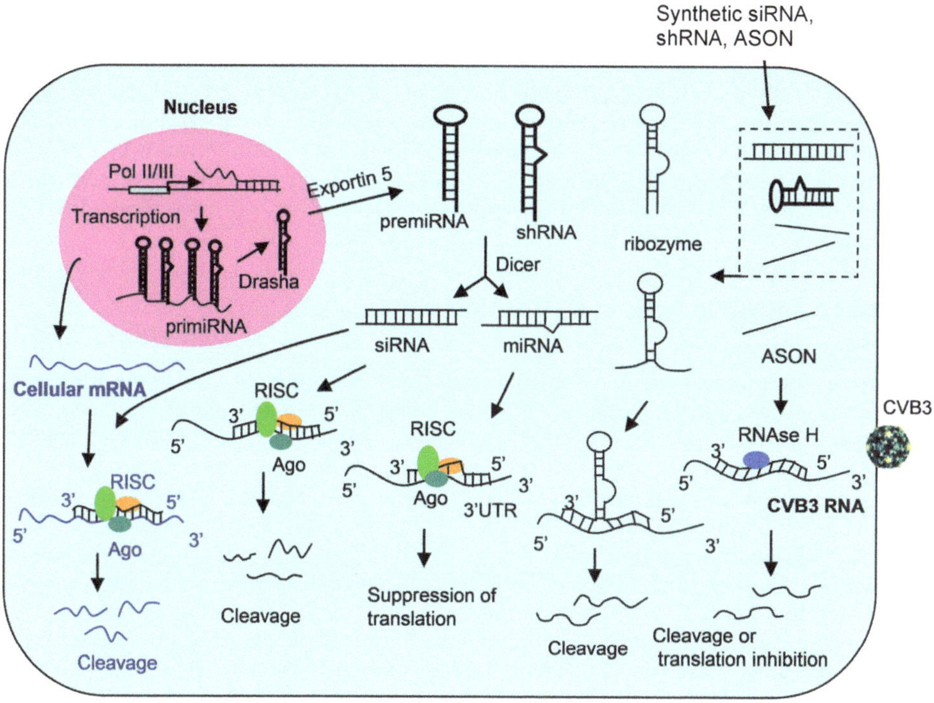

Fig. 2. NA-based antiviral strategies for pathogens of viral myocarditis. Antiviral nucleic acids can either be transfected into cells or expressed intracellularly. ASONs hybridize to viral mRNA to induce RNase H-mediated cleavage of RNA strand of the DNA-RNA duplexes. Some modified ASONs cannot induce RNase H but they have a high affinity for the target and inhibit translation by steric hindrance of ribosome or splicing. Binding of ribozymes to the target sequence can trigger cleavage of the viral RNA. siRNAs incorporated in the RISC target the viral RNA by perfect sequence complementation and induce cleavage of the target sequence by RNAse H activity of Ago protein. miRNAs (or AmiRNAs) target viral RNA by imperfect sequence complementation and induce gene silencing by destabilizing mRNAs (e.g., 3′ deadenylation or 5′ de-capping) and suppression of translation initiation and elongation. In addition, siRNAs can also target cellular genes (e.g., CAR and signal molecules) involved in viral entry and replication.

initiation factors on the mRNA or by disassociation of the premature translation initiation complexes. According to an alternative model, the mRNA destabilization is via miRNA-induced 3′ end de-adenylation or 5′ end de-capping, which results in degradation of mRNA after cleavage. Recently, some other mechanisms have been suggested. As review of the detailed mechanisms of RNAi action is beyond the scope of this article, the readers can refer to the recent reviews (Bartel, 2009; Carthew& Sontheimer, 2009; Q. Liu, Paroo, Z., 2010; Moazed, 2009). It should be pointed out that RNAi strategies for antiviral design have some advantages over the ASONs. Although they all cleave target mRNAs by RNase H, the modified ASON DNA induces activation of RNase H and cleavage of target sequence in nucleus, while the dsRNA functions primarily in cytoplasm. Ago2, the most important component of the RISC, is located in the p-bodies (Sen & Blau, 2005). Its cytoplasm localization is critically important for anti-coxsackievirus action as this virus is replicated only in cytoplasm. In addition, in the case of RNAi, an endogenous cellular pathway is followed, which could explain the high efficiency with which siRNAs are able to reach 1000 times higher than the ASON in cleavage of the same target molecule (Bertrand et al., 2002; Grunweller et al., 2003). However, the limitations for RNAi are present (Hemida et al., 2010); similar to the ribozymes, the selection of the suitable target for binding is restricted, particularly for miRNA, as the search for effective targeting sites are often limited in the 3′UTR of mRNA.

4. NA-based antivirals against CVB3 infection

4.1 Anti-CVB3 ASONs

CVB3, one of the most frequently used model systems for study of viral replication and pathogenesis, is also widely employed for evaluation of NA-based antiviral agents. The early investigations mainly focused on the application of the second and third generations of the ASONs. McManus and coworkers are one of the pioneer groups to study the potential possibility to inhibit CVB3 replication using ASONs. Their earliest work using regular ASONs to target the different sites of 5′UTR of CVB3 genome successfully mapped the IRES by *in vitro* translation inhibition assay (Yang et al., 1997). This study provided useful information for the design of ASON for inhibiting CVB3 replication *in vitro* and in mouse models. Later, they used PS-ASONs targeting the 5′ and 3′UTRs as well as the start codon region and found that the oligomers targeting the 5′ and 3′ proximate ends of the CVB3 genome are the most effective candidates to inhibit viral replication in HeLa cells. Each of these two ASONs resulted in ~80% reduction of viral particle production, which is followed by the candidates targeting the IRES and the initiation codon region (A. Wang et al., 2001). The importance of these sites for ASON binding was further confirmed by *in vivo* evaluation using a murine myocarditis model, although the antiviral efficiency is not as high as that obtained from *in vitro* evaluation (Yuan et al., 2004).

To improve the stability of the oligomers, our group designed eight phosphorodiamidate morpholino oligomers (PMO) targeting both the sense and antisense strands of the CVB3 replication intermediate. To increase the efficiency of drug internalization, the PMO were conjugated to a cell-penetrating arginine-rich peptide. These modified ASONs were evaluated in HeLa cells and HL-1 cardiomyocytes in culture and in a murine myocarditis model (Yuan et al., 2006). One of the oligomers, designed to target a sequence in the 3′ portion of the CVB3 IRES, was found to be especially potent against CVB3. Treatment of cells with this oligomer prior to CVB3 infection produced an approximately 3-$\log_{10}$ decrease in viral titer and largely protected cells from a virus-induced cytopathic effect. A similar antiviral effect was observed when this oligomer treatment began shortly after the virus infection period. A/J mice receiving intravenous administration of this oligomer once prior to and once after CVB3 infection showed an ~2-$\log_{10}$-decreased viral titer in the myocardium at 7 days post infection and a significantly decreased level of cardiac tissue damage, compared to the controls (Yuan et al., 2006).

In addition to the many ASON reports, another strategy using CpG containing oligodeoxynucleotide to activate antiviral immunity has been reported (Cong et al., 2007). The mechanism is that the C-type of CpG oligomer can induce anti-CVB3 activity in human peripheral blood mononuclear cells (PBMCs) through the induction of synthesis of natural mixed interferons.

4.2 Antiviral ribozymes

Ribozyme as an antiviral agent has been tested for many virus infections; however, report on anti-CVB3 has not been documented. Here, we will take HCV as an example to briefly discuss the potential application of ribozyme for the treatment of HCV infection, as many recent reports found that HCV is a new causal agent of myocarditis (Matsumori, 2005; Matsumori et al., 2006). To investigate the potential application of synthetic, stabilized ribozymes for the treatment of chronic HCV infection, Macejak *et al.* designed and synthesized hammerhead ribozymes targeting 15 conserved sites in the 5′UTR of HCV RNA including the IRES (Macejak et al., 2000). It was shown that the inhibitory activity of ribozyme targeting site at nucleotide 195 of HCV RNA exhibited a sequence-specific dose response, required an active catalytic ribozyme core, and was dependent on the presence of the HCV 5′UTR. In an investigation of new genetic approaches on the management of this infection, six hammerhead ribozymes directed against a conserved region of the plus strand and minus strand of the HCV genome were isolated from a ribozyme library that was expressed using recombinant adenovirus vectors (Macejak et al., 2001). Treatment with synthetic stabilized anti-HCV ribozymes and vector-expressed HCV ribozymes has the potential to aid in treatment of patients who are infected with HCV by reducing the viral burden through specific targeting and cleavage of the viral genome. Gonzalez-Carmona and colleagues used RNA transcripts from a construct encoding a HCV-5'-NCR-luciferase fusion protein to test four chemically modified HCV specific ribozymes in a cell-free system and in HepG2 or CCL13 cell lines. They found that ribozyme (Rz1293) showed an inhibitory activity of translation of more than 70% thus verifying that the GCA 348 cleavage site in the HCV loop IV is an accessible target site in cell culture and may be suitable for the development of novel optimized hammerhead structures (Gonzalez-Carmona et al., 2006).

4.3 Anti-CVB3 siRNAs

RNAi-mediated antiviral strategies can achieve much higher efficiency than ASONs. Thus, recent studies have focused on the design and evaluation of anti-CVB3 siRNAs. This group of small double-stranded RNAs, as a silencer of target gene expression, can virtually inhibit any genes of virus and cell if the site of targeting within the gene is unique. Thus, the target search for anti-CVB3 siRNAs is not only concentrating on CVB3 genome but also extending to the host cellular genes required for viral infection or replication.

4.3.1 Targeting the CVB3 genome

CVB3 genome harbors many *cis*-acting sequence elements for viral transcription and translation, such as the 5′ and 3′ UTRs, the IRES and other segments for binding of transcription and translation initiation factors. In addition, the viral genome also encodes many essential enzymes for CVB3 multiplication, such as proteases 2A and 3C as well as the RNA-dependent RNA polymerase 3D. These structures are rationale targets for design of anti-CVB3 siRNAs. This hypothesis has been tested by a number of groups. The earlier selection of the siRNA targets was focused on CVB3 protease 2A. Almost at the same time, two groups independently found that inhibition of 2A protease by specific siRNAs significantly reduced CVB3 replication. The first group by Yuan et al., evaluated five siRNAs targeting the 5′UTR, AUG start codon, VP1, 2A and 3D, respectively and found that siRNA targeting 2A (nts 3543-3561) showed strongest anti-CVB3 activity in HeLa cells, resulting in 92% reduction of viral replication and siRNAs targeting VP1, 3D and the 5′UTR showed modest antiviral effects, respectively. By mutational analysis of the mechanism of siRNA action, they found that siRNA functions by targeting the positive strand of the virus and requires a perfect sequence match in the central region of the target, but mismatches were more tolerated near the 3′ end than the 5′end of the antisense strand (Yuan et al., 2005). This finding on the targeting of siRNA to positive strand of CVB3 was further supported by a later study using siRNA targeting the CVB3 3D gene (Schubert et al., 2007). The second group that studied siRNA targeting CVB3 2A by Merl and co-workers evaluated antiviral activity of siRNA-2A (nts 3637-3657) *in vitro* and in highly susceptible type I interferon receptor-knockout mice. They found that siRNA-2A led to significant reduction of viral tissue titers, attenuated tissue damage and prolonged survival of mice (Merl et al., 2005). It is very interesting to point out that although the two groups used different targeting sequences within the 2A RNA, they all achieved high efficiency of antiviral effects. However, the later work by Racchi et al., which used these two siRNAs together to transfect HeLa cells and then infect with CVB3 did not potentiate the anti-CVB3 effect compared with an equimolar concentration of either siRNA (Racchi et al., 2009).

CVB3 RNA polymerase 3D is probably the most frequently used target for design of anti-CVB3 siRNAs as it is the only viral enzyme involved in CVB3 RNA replication. To date, at least a half dozen of studies on 3D have been reported. The earlier *in vitro* investigations using either un-modified or LNA-modified siRNAs or plasmid vector-expressed shRNAs all achieved significant reduction of viral replication in CVB3-infected HeLa or Cos-7 cells (Ahn et al., 2005; Schubert et al., 2005; Schubert et al., 2007; Werk et al., 2005; Yuan et al., 2005). The *in vivo* evaluation using mouse models also showed very promising results. One study employing transient transfection for *in vivo* mouse models demonstrated that two of the six candidate siRNAs targeting 3D and VP1, respectively, exerted strong anti-CVB3 effects in viral replication, accompanied by attenuated pancreatic tissue damage (J. Y. Kim et al., 2007). Another *in vivo* study is the intravenous treatment of mice with an adeno-associated virus vector (AAV2.9) expressing a shRNA targeting 3D (Fechner et al., 2008). Intravenous injection of recombinant AAV2.9 significantly attenuated the cardiac dysfunction compared to vector-treated control mice on day 10 after CVB3 infection. Recently, a study by combination of soluble CAR receptor (sCAR-Fc) and siRNA targeting 3D achieved a synergistic effect in antiviral effect in human myocardial fibroblast cell culture (Werk et al., 2009).

Other less frequently used CVB3 target genes are protease 3C, structural protein VP1 and non-structural protein 2C. Like protease 2A, protease 3C also plays an important role in the viral life cycle by processing CVB3 polyproteins to generate mature individual structural and non-structural proteins after initial cleavage by 2A (Chau et al., 2007; L. E. C. Leong, Cornell, C. T., Semler, B. L., , 2002). One study designed three siRNAs targeting genes encoding 3C, 2A and 3D of CVB4. Evaluation by transfection of rhabdomyosarcoma (RD) cells demonstrated that siRNA-3C was the most potent siRNA among these three in inhibition of CVB4 replication. This antiviral activity was followed by siRNAs targeting 3D and 2A (Tan, 2010). The difference in efficiency of these siRNAs was discussed by these authors and they proposed that this may be due to the differences in function of these viral enzymes, which are encoded by these regions: the 3C region encodes a protease 3C which is responsible for majority of the cleavage of the viral polyprotein (L. E. C. Leong, Cornell, C. T., Semler, B. L., , 2002) and 3C as well as its precursor 3CD also plays an important role at the level of viral transcription (Parsley et al., 1999). Protease 3C has been shown to be critical for interaction with the cloverleaf structures found at the 5′UTR of the viral genome to deliver the 3D to the replication complex (L. E. Leong et al., 1993). They also indicated that since the function of 3C is required prior to 3D, a down-regulation in 3C would have a detrimental effect on viral transcription as available 3D would not be able to carry out replication of CVB4 replication without the assistance of 3C. The authors' discussion seems to be reasonable; however, according to the order (timing) of action for these enzymes, 2A cleaves the polyprotein prior to 3C's cleavage. For this situation, it may be difficult to explain why the siRNAs targeting 2A did not achieve a more efficacious anti-CVB3 activity than siRNA targeting 3C. Obviously, many issues relating to the mechanisms of action need to be further studied. However, according to the present reports, one point is clear that 2A, 3C and 3D are three important targets for design anti-CVB3 siRNAs.

Viral structural protein VP1 was also a selected target for testing anti-CVB3 siRNAs; however, the data from literature often showed a lower effectiveness of the siRNA targeting this structural gene as compared to that targeting other genes (Ahn et al., 2005; J. Y. Kim et al., 2007; Yuan et al., 2005). Due to the absence of a proof-reading activity in 3D, the mutation rate for RNA viruses is as high as 10^{-3} -10^{-4} (Cann, 2005). Thus, in recent years, the discovery of the occurrence of escape mutants due to siRNA treatment of HCV, poliovirus and HIV infections (Boden et al., 2003; Gitlin et al., 2005; Wilson& Richardson, 2005) greatly encouraged researchers to search for new approaches to counteract the drug resistance. One direction is the application of multiple distinct siRNAs or a siRNA pool to target more than one target genes of the virus (Merl& Wessely, 2007; Nygardas et al., 2009). The other direction is the identification of conserved *cis*-acting replication elements (CRE) (van Ooij et al., 2006). Theoretically, the 5'- and 3'-UTRs are the ideal target regions for siRNAs as they harbor a number of conserved *cis*-acting elements. However, studies with poliovirus and CVB3 found that siRNA residing in these regions are less efficient than siRNAs targeting on other regions (e.g., the coding region and particularly the non-structural coding region) in inducing antiviral activity (Gitlin& Stone& Andino, 2005; Merl& Wessely, 2007; Saleh et al., 2004; Yuan et al., 2005). This low antiviral potency seems to be due to the highly ordered structure of the UTRs itself, as well as the formation of the protein-RNA complexes in the region, which may block the access of the RISC complexes to its target sequences. To address this issue, Lee and coworkers selected a CRE within the coding region of 2C. Evaluation in HeLa cells demonstrated the downregulation of virus replication and attenuation of cytotoxicity in various strains and clinic isolates. Cells treated with this siRNA were resistant to the emergence of viable escape mutants and showed sustained antiviral ability (Lee et al., 2007). Based on this study, a similar experiment using siRNA targeting CRE of CVA24 2C was conducted and the authors reported the similar observations (Jun et al., 2008). These findings from *in vitro* studies were further solidified by *in vivo* evaluation, in which recombinant lentivirus was employed to express shRNAs targeting the CRE of CVB3 2C. Mice injected intraperitoneally with recombinant lentiviruses had significant reductions in viral titers, viral myocarditis and proinflammatory cytokines as well as improved survival rate, after being challenged with CVB3 (Y. J. Kim et al., 2008). Recently, this CRE was further confirmed for a number of enteroviruses, by using a novel program and *in vitro* evaluation (Lee et al., 2009).

4.3.2 Targeting host cellular genes

Another approach to fight the drug resistance caused by escape mutants is the selection of therapeutic targets within the host cellular genes that are necessary for virus entry or viral replication. In this regard, the CAR receptor which is shared by CVB3 and adenovirus is an attractive candidate since both CVB3 and adenovirus are considered as the common causal agents of myocarditis. To date, two studies have been reported to silence CAR expression with specific siRNAs. One study reported that transfection of HeLa cells with siRNAs, siCAR2 or siCAR9, almost completely silenced the expression of CAR and that further analysis by viral plaque assay revealed ~60% reduction of CVB3 particle formation (Werk et al., 2005). Another study using cardiac-derived HL-1 cell line and primary neonatal cardiomyocytes (PNCMs) demonstrated that treatment with recombinant adenoviruses expressing shRNAs against CAR resulted in almost completely silencing of CAR expression in both HL-1 cells and PNCMs. CAR knockout resulted in inhibition of CVB3 infections by up to 97% in HL-1 and up to 90% in PNCMs. Adenoviruses were inhibited by only 75% in HL-1, but up to 92% in PNCMs (Fechner et al., 2007).

Another host gene, the tissue inhibitor of matrix metalloproteinase-1 (TIMP-1), has been suggested to be a potential target for siRNA to ameliorate CVB3-induced myocarditis. This suggestion is based on the investigation of Crocker and colleagues on a new role of TIMP-1 in exacerbating CVB-induced myocarditis (Crocker et al., 2007). They found that TIMP-1 expression was induced in the myocardium by CVB3 infection. Surprisingly, TIMP-1 knockout mice exhibited a profound attenuation of myocarditis, with increased survival. The amelioration of disease in TIMP-1 knockout mice was not attributable to either an altered T-cell response to the virus or to reduced viral replication. These data allowed the authors to propose and prove a novel function for TIMP-1: its highly localized up-regulation might arrest the matrix metalloproteinase (MMP)-dependent migration of inflammatory cells at the sites of infection thereby anatomically focusing the adaptive immune response. Finally, the benefits of TIMP-1 blockage in treating CVB myocarditis were confirmed by administration of siRNAs targeting TIMP-1, which diminished CVB3-induced myocarditis. However, this improvement of the disease is not due to the changes of viral titers, as demonstrated by viral plaque assay (Crocker et al., 2007).

Recently, the active investigations on CVB3-induced signal transduction pathways have provided new avenues for the search of therapeutic targets for the treatment of myocarditis. Since CVB3, like other picornaviruses, requires the activation of certain signal pathways for initiating their life cycle, inactivation of some signal molecules in the signal cascade with specific siRNAs would block CVB3 replication. Such kind of studies that have been documented thus far include i) the knockdown of ubiquitin expression by siRNAs to down-regulate the ubiquitination and subsequent alteration of protein function and/or degradation (Si et al., 2008); ii) silencing of proteosome activator REGγ to inhibit the REGγ-mediated degradation of several important intracellular proteins (Gao, 2010), such as cyclin-dependent kinase inhibitors p21, p16 and p19 and tumor suppressor p53; and iii) knockdown of genes critical important for autophagy formation, these genes include ATG7, Beeclin-1 and VPS34 (J. Wong et al., 2008). Although these target genes mentioned above have been tested *in vitro* using specific siRNAs in signal transduction studies and showed promising outcomes, their potential serving as a therapeutic target for treatment of CVB3 infection needs a further evaluation by pharmacological study in animal models.

4.4 Anti-CVB3 artificial miRNAs

miRNAs are a group of recently discovered new regulators of gene expression. These endogenous regulators control one third of human gene expression (Bartel, 2009; Q. Liu,

Paroo, Z., 2010). Thus, endogenous miRNAs are important targets for gene therapy and artificial miRNAs (AmiRNA) are useful tools for inhibiting disease-causing gene expression (Z. Liu et al., 2008; Sall et al., 2008). In this regard, although numerous studies have been documented for treatment of cancers, cardiovascular diseases, genetic diseases and other viral infections, only one study on anti-CVB3 from our group has been published so far. Here, I briefly summarize our work on design and evaluation of anti-CVB3 AmiRNAs (Ye et al., 2011). We constructed three short hairpin AmiRNAs (AmiR-1, -2 and -3) targeting the stem-loop of the 3'UTR of CVB3 with mismatches at the middle region of the target. Transfection of HeLa cells showed over-expression of these mature AmiRNAs as determined by real time quantitative RT-PCR. After these AmiRNA-expressing cells were infected with CVB3, the viral titers were reduced ~100 folds in cell cultures treated with AmiR-1 or AmiR-2 but not that treated with AmiR-3, at 24 h post infection. Mutational analysis of the targeting sites of AmiRNAs demonstrated that the central region but not the seed region of AmiRNAs is more tolerant to target mutation. In this study we also performed targeted delivery of the AmiRNAs to host cells through ligand-receptor interactions, which will be discussed in next section.

5. Drug delivery

NA-based agents are inefficiently taken up by mammalian cells and would therefore benefits from additional vehicles or modifications that facilitate drug delivery. Depending on transient delivery or long-term treatment, the delivery approaches can be divided into non-viral delivery of chemically synthesized agents and viral delivery of drug-expressing cassettes (Table 1). For the non-viral delivery measures, they can be further divided into unspecific and cell-type specific delivery. The former method has been widely used for delivery of many chemically synthesized ASONs, ribozymes and siRNAs as well as plasmids encoding shRNAs through transfection of tissue culture cells, hydrodynamic transduction/transfection of mice or intravenous (IV) injection of mice via tails using cationic lipoplexes or liposomes. The successful examples for inhibition of viral pathogens of myocarditis includes deliveries of i) ASONs targeting CVB3 IRES (Yuan et al., 2006) and both ends of the CVB3 genome (A. Wang et al., 2001), ii) siRNAs targeting CVB3 2A (Merl et al., 2005; Yuan et al., 2005) and 3D (Ahn et al., 2005; Schubert et al., 2005; Schubert et al., 2007), iii) plasmids expressing shRNAs targeting 3D and VP1 (J. Y. Kim et al., 2007) and vi) ribozymes targeting HCV RNA (Gonzalez-Carmona et al., 2006). For the cell-type specific method, proper modification and conjugation of 'naked' raw therapeutic molecules are required to achieve targeted delivery. The different chemical modifications described earlier for ASONs are applicable to all NA-based agents. The conjugation of these antivirals can be achieved by covalent linkage of a ligand to the molecules, which enables the drug internalization via specific interactions between the ligand and its receptor. The ligands can be an antibody, vitamin, short peptide, RNA aptamer, folic acid, etc. The details were reviewed elsewhere (X. Ye & Yang, 2009). By this strategy, we have specifically delivered siRNAs targeting CVB3 2A to HeLa (cancer) cells, a cell line susceptible to CVB3, through interactions between folate and its receptor highly expressed on the surface of all cancer cells but not the normal cells (Zhang et al., 2009). This study was carried out by covalent linkage of the siRNA targeting CVB3 2A to a bacterial phage-29 packaging RNA (pRNA). This small pRNA (~170 nts) can form dimer, trimer and hexamer by base pairing through its

Category	Target	Model system	Delivery route	Reference
PS-ASON	5′ & 3′UTRs, IRES, start codon,	HeLa cell, mice	Transfection	Wang 2003
PS-ASON	3′end of CVB3	HL-1 cells, mice	Transfection, IV injection	Yuan 2004
MOP-ASON	IRES, 5′ & 3′UTR, start codon, minus strand	HeLa, HL-1 cell, mice	Transfection and IV injection	Yuan 2006
CpG oligoer	no	PBMCs	Treatment	Cong 2007
siRNA	2A, VP1, 3D	HeLa cells	Transfection	Yuan 2005
siRNA	2A	HeLa cells, mice	Hydrodynamic,	Merl 2005
	2A	HeLa cells	Transfection	Racchi 2009
	2A	HeLa cells	pRNA vector	Zhang 2009
shRNA	3D	HeLa cells	Transfection of double expression plasmid	Schubert 2005
siRNA	3D, VP1	HeLa cells	Transfection	Ahn 2005
LNA-siRNA	3D	Cos-7 cells	Transfection	Schubert 2007
siRNA	siRNA pool	LLC-MK2 cells	Transfection	Nygardas 2009
shRNA	VP1, 3D, 5′ & 3′UTR	Cos-7 cells, mice	hydrodynamic, transfectin of plasmid	Kim J-Y 2007
siRNA & sCAR-Fc	3D	HMF	Transfection	Werk D 2009
shRNA	3D	HeLa, PNCMs, Mice	Transduction, IV, AAV vector	Fechner 2008
siRNA (CVB4)	3D, 3C, 2A	RD cells	Transfection	Tan , 2010
shRNA	2C	Mice	IP injection, lentivirus vecotr	Lee 2007
shRNA (CVA24)	2C	HeLa, HCC	Transfection, plasmid	Jun 2008
siRNA (enteroviruses)	2C	HeLa, Vero cells	Transfection	Lee 2009
shRNA	CAR	HL-1, PNCMs	Adenovirus vector	Fecherner 2007
siRNA	TIMP-1	Mice	IV injection	Crocker 2007
siRNA	CAR, 3D	HeLa,Cos-7 cells	Transfection	Werk 2005
siRNA	Ubiquitin	HeLa cells	Transfection	Si 2008
siRNA	ATG7, Beclin-,VPS34	HeLa cells	Transfection	Wong 2008
siRNA	Proteasome activator REGγ	HeLa cells	Transfection	Gao G 2010

Abbreviations: LNA: locked nucleic acid; RD: rhabdomyosarcoma; PBMC: peripheral blood mononuclear cell; HMF: human myocardial fibroblast; HCC: human conjunctive cell.

Table 1. NA-based agents for the treatment of CVB3 infection.

left- and right-hand loops (P. Guo, 2002) (Fig. 3). Thus, this pRNA multimer can carry multiple siRNAs and has the potential to overcome issues associated with drug resistance of viruses (P. Guo, 2005). In addition, this small pRNA vector has lower immunogenicity than big DNA vectors. Thus it is a safe vehicle for transportation of antiviral drugs (S. Guo et al., 2006). We labeled, by *in vitro* transcription, the 5′end of the pRNA with AMP-folic acid,

which guided the targeted delivery of siRNAs via ligand-receptor interactions and achieved strong inhibition of CVB3 replication (Zhang et al., 2009). The effectiveness of this strategy on targeted delivery of NA-based drugs was further solidified in targeted delivery of AmiRNAs to inhibit CVB3 replication (X. Ye, Liu, Z., Hemida, G. M., and Yang, D. C., 2011).
Viral vector-mediated delivery of NA-based agents is another promising approach for treatment of persistent infection such as CVB3, HCV and many other viruses. This is because that the vector-encoded shRNA can produce relative long-term and continuous silencing. Most viral vectors are modified viruses, which can be applied to deliver a cargo sequence to cells. Currently the most commonly used viral vectors for the delivery of NA-based drugs are derived from the adenovirus, adeno-associated viruses (AAV) and lentiviruses. These vectors have been widely used and have achieved exciting promise (Fechner et al., 2008; Henry et al., 2006; Kuhlmann et al., 2008). Recent trends in further improvement of these vectors focus on modifications of their structure to increase the capability for targeted delivery. The efforts of this goal can be summarized into three categories (X. Ye & Yang, 2009): i) the genetic and chemical modifications of the vector to express a unique chimeric surface protein, such as adenovirus capsid proteins: fiber knob, penton and hexon. The common strategy is the insertion of a foreign peptide into fiber knob, which enables the vector to be capable of binding the specific cellular receptor (Koizumi et al., 2003; Mizuguchi& Hayakawa, 2002); ii) incorporation of heterologous protein from another virus with a restricted range of tissue tropism to the viral envelope; this approach is also called pseudotyping. An example of this strategy is the pseudotyping of lentivirus vector with the neurotropic rabies virus glycoprotein allows retro-axonal and trans-synoptic spread, thereby enhancing the transgene expression within the brain (L. F. Wong et al., 2004); and iii) the application of a tissue-specific promoter to express the vector-carried gene in a specific organ or cell type. An impressive finding has been reported regarding the utilization of cardiac myosin light chain 2v promoter and the hypoxia-response element by AAV vector to express vascular endothelial growth factor, an angiogenic factor, specifically in myocardium, leading to cardiac functional improvement (Su et al., 2004). Here we will briefly discuss the delivery of NA-based antivirals using these viral vectors for CVB3 infection.
Adenovirus is known to share the CAR receptor with CVB3. This receptor is highly expressed on the surface of cardiomyocytes. Thus, adenovirus-derived vector is an ideal carrier for delivery of NA-based antivirals to the heart. This vector has successfully delivered shRNAs targeting the CAR gene in a cardiac-derived HL-1 cell line and isolated PNCMs, resulting in the strong reduction of replication of both CVB3 and adenovirus (Fechner et al., 2007). Lentivirus vectors are derived from HIV. They have the ability to transduce quiescent as well as proliferating cells, thus increasing their therapeutic ranges. Particularly, after pseudotyping with G glycoprotein of vesicular stomatitis virus, they can transduce almost any cell type (Kurreck, 2009). Kim Y-J et al. constructed recombinant lentiviruses that express shRNAs targeting the CRE within CVB3 2C. Intraperitoneal injection of mice with these viruses clearly showed a protective effect against viral myocarditis by elimination of CVB3 infection and reducing pro-inflammatory cytokines, such as IL6 and INF-α. (Y. J. Kim et al., 2008). AAVs are attractive vectors for gene transfer since they efficiently transduce target cells and are nonpathogenic for humans. Fechner H et al. have employed a pseudotyped AAV2.9 vector, carrying the most cardiotropic AAV capsid currently known to successfully transduce PNCMs. This vector expressed siRNAs targeting CVB3 3D and reduced CVB3 replication by >3 $\log_{10}$ steps. Further evaluation by

intravenous injection of mice demonstrated significant reduction of virus titers and improvement of heart function compared to the control. This study showed for the first time that intravenously injected AAV2.9 has the potential to target RNAi to the heart and suggests AVV2.9-shRNA vectors as a novel therapeutic approach for cardiac disorders (Fechner et al., 2008).

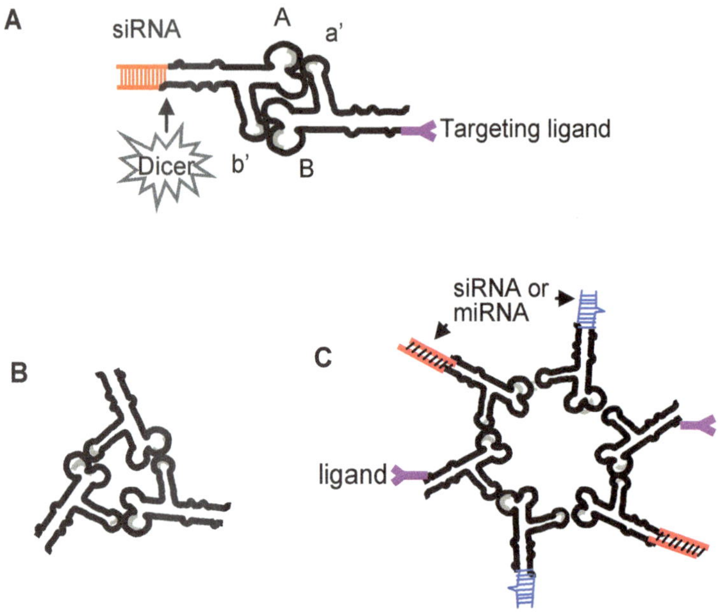

Fig. 3. Structural schematic of packaging RNA (pRNA) multimers as a drug targeted delivery vehicle. (A) pRNA dimer forms through the base-paring between the loops of an A'b-pRNA-siRNA and a B'a-pRNA-ligand. The shaded areas on the loops indicate the base-pair interactions between the monomers. siRNA is released when intracellular Dicer cleaves the dsRNA, which is indicated by an arrow. (B) pRNA trimers can be stoichiometrically formed by hand-in-hand loop interactions, which contains 1:1:1 of their linked conjugates. (C) hexamers allow for a customizable, combined therapy where multiple drugs may be added to the same complex.

6. Concluding remarks

NA-based gene silencing techniques have been successfully used in drug development. The major progress on ASON research is the chemical modifications and ligand conjugation to enhance drug stability and efficacy of delivery. The emergence of RNAi-mediated gene silencing techniques further provided new hope for this regard. Basically, siRNA silencing techniques can be used against any viral infection. Two major obstacles must, however, be overcome before it can become a broadly applicable standard therapy: the question of their specificity and efficient delivery to target cells. As siRNA can potentially cause off-site targeting and activate the immune system, minimizing the undesired effects must be considered in the drug design. Immense efforts have been undertaken to develop carrier system with which siRNAs can be delivered to their target cells. Despite great advances in the last years, further developments are still required to get systematically applied siRNAs to their required sites of action. Here, viral vectors systems for shRNA expression cassettes offer additional options for efficient and organ-specific delivery. However, this approach must be first overcome the reservations based on the negative experience with gene therapy. As discussed earlier, pRNA is a promising vehicle for targeted delivery of NA-based therapeutic molecules. For treatment of myocarditis, a myocardium-specific ligand such as peptides from the CVB3 antireceptor protein or RNA apatamers of cardiomyocytes should be identified, which will be used to replace folic acid on the pRNA vector.

Very recent advances in the understanding of miRNA biology and particularly their association with the molecular pathogenesis of a variety of diseases have served as a theoretical basis for drug development. On the one hand, miRNA, as one of the key factors for regulation of viral replication, tissue tropism and latency, are the ideal targets for inhibition. In this regard, construction of mRNAs that contain multiple tandem binding sites of a given miRNA may be useful to produce decoys or "miRNA sponges" to inhibit the function of a specific miRNA. In addition, chemically synthesized antisense RNA oligomers ('antagomirs') targeting a miRNA of interest could be also a promising approach to inhibit miRNA activity (Ebert et al., 2007; Krutzfeldt et al., 2005). Other strategies include i) overexpression of specific miRNAs using an expression vector to achieve a long-term effect of reversing the imbalance of miRNA expression caused by infections, and ii) introduction of pre-miRNA mimetics for transient replacement of a down-regulated miRNA. On the other hand, miRNA can serve as a useful tool for therapy. Since miRNA is tolerable to target mutation at its center region, application of multiple artificial miRNAs to target the 3'UTR and/or other regions of CVB3 RNA may improve the drug resistance. Given the immense interest in NA-based drug research and the rapid progress made in this field and other areas such as nano-biotechnology for drug delivery, the coming years are likely to see an increasing range of clinical applications, particularly for the RNAi-based drug candidates. The realization of the potential of NA-based therapies to address human viral pathogens suggests that this field has a very promising future.

7. Acknowledgements

My special thanks go to my students, Postdoctoral Fellows and Research Associates, whose tireless efforts contributed to the advances of my research group. I also thank Paul Hanson for his critical reading of this manuscript and Xin Ye for his help on preparing the manuscript. The work was supported by grants from the Canada Institute of Health Research and the Heart and Stroke Foundation of British Columbia & Yukon.

8. References

Ahn, J., Jun, E. S., Lee, H. S., Yoon, S. Y., Kim, D., Joo, C. H., Kim, Y. K.& Lee, H. (2005). A small interfering RNA targeting coxsackievirus B3 protects permissive HeLa cells from viral challenge. *The Journal of Virology*, 79(13), 8620-8624.

Amantana, A.& Iversen, P. L. (2005). Pharmacokinetics and biodistribution of phosphorodiamidate morpholino antisense oligomers. *Current Opinion in Pharmacology*, 5(5), 550-555.

Andreoletti, L., Leveque, N., Boulagnon, C., Brasselet, C.& Fornes, P. (2009). Viral causes of human myocarditis. *Archives Of Cardiovascular Diseases*, 102(6-7), 559-568.

Bartel, D. P. (2004). MicroRNAs: genomics, biogenesis, mechanism, and function. *Cell*, 116(2), 281-297.

Bartel, D. P. (2009). MicroRNAs: target recognition and regulatory functions. *Cell*, 136(2), 215-233.

Bennasser, Y., Le, S. Y., Benkirane, M.& Jeang, K. T. (2005). Evidence that HIV-1 encodes an siRNA and a suppressor of RNA silencing. *Immunity*, 22(5), 607-619.

Berkhout, B.& Jeang, K. T. (2007). RISCy business: MicroRNAs, pathogenesis, and viruses. *The Journal of Biological Chemistry*, 282(37), 26641-26645.

Bertrand, J. R., Pottier, M., Vekris, A., Opolon, P., Maksimenko, A.& Malvy, C. (2002). Comparison of antisense oligonucleotides and siRNAs in cell culture and in vivo. *Biochemical and Biophysical Research Communications*, 296(4), 1000-1004.

Blauwet, L. A., Cooper, L. T. (2010). Myocarditis. *Progress in Cardiovascular Diseases*, 52, 274-288.

Boden, D., Pusch, O., Lee, F., Tucker, L.& Ramratnam, B. (2003). Human immunodeficiency virus type 1 escape from RNA interference. *The Journal of Virology*, 77(21), 11531-11535.

Bowles, N. E., Ni, J., Kearney, D. L., Pauschinger, M., Schultheiss, H. P., McCarthy, R., Hare, J., Bricker, J. T., Bowles, K. R.& Towbin, J. A. (2003). Detection of viruses in myocardial tissues by polymerase chain reaction. evidence of adenovirus as a common cause of myocarditis in children and adults. *Journal of the American College of Cardiology*, 42(3), 466-472.

Brennecke, J., Stark, A., Russell, R. B.& Cohen, S. M. (2005). Principles of microRNA-target recognition. *PLoS Biology*, 3(3), e85.

Cann, A. (2005). Genome. 4th ed. *In* "Principles of Molecular Virology", pp. 78-79. Elsevier Academic Press, 9780120887897, San Diego, CA.

Cardarelli, F., Serresi, M., Bizzarri, R., Giacca, M.& Beltram, F. (2007). In vivo study of HIV-1 Tat arginine-rich motif unveils its transport properties. *Molecular Therapy*, 15(7), 1313-1322.

Carthew, R. W.& Sontheimer, E. J. (2009). Origins and Mechanisms of miRNAs and siRNAs. *Cell*, 136(4), 642-655.

Caudy, A. A., Ketting, R. F., Hammond, S. M., Denli, A. M., Bathoorn, A. M., Tops, B. B., Silva, J. M., Myers, M. M., Hannon, G. J.& Plasterk, R. H. (2003). A micrococcal nuclease homologue in RNAi effector complexes. *Nature*, 425(6956), 411-414.

Chau, D. H., Yuan, J., Zhang, H., Cheung, P., Lim, T., Liu, Z., Sall, A.& Yang, D. (2007). Coxsackievirus B3 proteases 2A and 3C induce apoptotic cell death through mitochondrial injury and cleavage of eIF4GI but not DAP5/p97/NAT1. *Apoptosis*, 12(3), 513-524.

Cheung, P., Lim, T., Yuan, J., Zhang, M., Chau, D., McManus, B.& Yang, D. (2007). Specific interaction of HeLa cell proteins with coxsackievirus B3 3'UTR: La autoantigen binds the 3' and 5'UTR independently of the poly(A) tail. *Cellular Microbiology*, 9(7), 1705-1715.

Cohen, C. J., Shieh, J. T., Pickles, R. J., Okegawa, T., Hsieh, J. T.& Bergelson, J. M. (2001). The coxsackievirus and adenovirus receptor is a transmembrane component of the tight junction. *Proceedings of the National Academy of Sciences U S A*, 98(26), 15191-15196.

Cong, Z., Wan, M., Wu, X., Wang, L., Hu, X., Yang, F., Bao, M., Zhang, X., Chen, J.& Yu, Y. (2007). A CpG oligodeoxynucleotide inducing anti-coxsackie B3 virus activity in human peripheral blood mononuclear cells. *FEMS Immunology and Medical Microbiology*, 51(1), 26-34.

Cooper, L. T., Baughman, K. L., Feldman, A. M., Frustaci, A., Jessup, M., Kuhl, U., Levine, G. N., Narula, J., Starling, R. C., Towbin, J.& Virmani, R. (2007). The role of endomyocardial biopsy in the management of cardiovascular disease: a scientific statement from the American Heart Association, the American College of Cardiology, and the European Society of Cardiology. Endorsed by the Heart Failure Society of America and the Heart Failure Association of the European Society of Cardiology. *Journal of the American College of Cardiology*, 50(19), 1914-1931.

Cooper, L. T., Jr. (2009). Myocarditis. *The New England Journal of Medicine*, 360(15), 1526-1538.

Cotten, M., Oberhauser, B., Brunar, H., Holzner, A., Issakides, G., Noe, C. R., Schaffner, G., Wagner, E.& Birnstiel, M. L. (1991). 2'-O-methyl, 2'-O-ethyl oligoribonucleotides and phosphorothioate oligodeoxyribonucleotides as inhibitors of the in vitro U7 snRNP-dependent mRNA processing event. *Nucleic Acids Research*, 19(10), 2629-2635.

Crocker, S. J., Frausto, R. F., Whitmire, J. K., Benning, N., Milner, R.& Whitton, J. L. (2007). Amelioration of coxsackievirus B3-mediated myocarditis by inhibition of tissue inhibitors of matrix metalloproteinase-1. *The American Journal of Pathology*, 171(6), 1762-1773.

Crooke, S. T., Graham, M. J., Zuckerman, J. E., Brooks, D., Conklin, B. S., Cummins, L. L., Greig, M. J., Guinosso, C. J., Kornbrust, D., Manoharan, M., Sasmor, H. M., Schleich, T., Tivel, K. L.& Griffey, R. H. (1996). Pharmacokinetic properties of several novel oligonucleotide analogs in mice. *Journal of Pharmacology and Experimental Therapeutics*, 277(2), 923-937.

Cullen, B. R. (2006). Is RNA interference involved in intrinsic antiviral immunity in mammals? *Nature Immunology*, 7(6), 563-567.

Dennert, R., Crijns, H. J.& Heymans, S. (2008). Acute viral myocarditis. *European Heart Journal*, 29(17), 2073-2082.

Doench, J. G., Petersen, C. P.& Sharp, P. A. (2003). siRNAs can function as miRNAs. *Genes & Development*, 17(4), 438-442.

Ebert, M. S., Neilson, J. R.& Sharp, P. A. (2007). MicroRNA sponges: competitive inhibitors of small RNAs in mammalian cells. *Nature Methods*, 4(9), 721-726.

Fechner, H., Pinkert, S., Wang, X., Sipo, I., Suckau, L., Kurreck, J., Dorner, A., Sollerbrant, K., Zeichhardt, H., Grunert, H. P., Vetter, R., Schultheiss, H. P.& Poller, W. (2007). Coxsackievirus B3 and adenovirus infections of cardiac cells are efficiently inhibited by vector-mediated RNA interference targeting their common receptor. *Gene Therapy*, 14(12), 960-971.

Fechner, H., Sipo, I., Westermann, D., Pinkert, S., Wang, X., Suckau, L., Kurreck, J., Zeichhardt, H., Muller, O., Vetter, R., Erdmann, V., Tschope, C.& Poller, W. (2008). Cardiac-targeted RNA interference mediated by an AAV9 vector improves cardiac function in coxsackievirus B3 cardiomyopathy. *Journal of Molecular Medicine*, 86(9), 987-997.

Freimuth, P., Philipson, L.& Carson, S. D. (2008). The coxsackievirus and adenovirus receptor. *Current Topics in Microbiology and Immunology*, 323, 67-87.

Frese, M., Bartenschlager, R. (2006). Inhibition of hepatitis C virus by nucleic acid-based antiviral approaches. *In* "New Concept of Antiviral Therapy" (E. a. H. Bogner, A., Ed.), pp. 47-86. Springer, 0387310460.

Frustaci, A., Chimenti, C., Calabrese, F., Pieroni, M., Thiene, G.& Maseri, A. (2003). Immunosuppressive therapy for active lymphocytic myocarditis: virological and immunologic profile of responders versus nonresponders. *Circulation*, 107(6), 857-863.

Gao, G., Wong, J., Zhang, J., Mao, I., Shravah, J, Wu, Y., Xiao, A., Li, X., Luo, H. (2010). Proteasome activator REGgamma enhances coxsackieviral infection by faciliating p53 degradation. *The Journal of Virology*, 84(21), 11056-11066.

Gitlin, L., Stone, J. K.& Andino, R. (2005). Poliovirus escape from RNA interference: short interfering RNA-target recognition and implications for therapeutic approaches. *J Virol*, 79(2), 1027-1035.

Gonzalez-Carmona, M. A., Schussler, S., Serwe, M., Alt, M., Ludwig, J., Sproat, B. S., Steigerwald, R., Hoffmann, P., Quasdorff, M., Schildgen, O.& Caselmann, W. H. (2006). Hammerhead ribozymes with cleavage site specificity for NUH and NCH display significant anti-hepatitis C viral effect in vitro and in recombinant HepG2 and CCL13 cells. *Journal of Hepatology*, 44(6), 1017-1025.

Grimson, A., Farh, K. K., Johnston, W. K., Garrett-Engele, P., Lim, L. P.& Bartel, D. P. (2007). MicroRNA targeting specificity in mammals: determinants beyond seed pairing. *Molecular Cell*, 27(1), 91-105.

Groarke, J. M.& Pevear, D. C. (1999). Attenuated virulence of pleconaril-resistant coxsackievirus B3 variants. *Journal of Infectious Diseases*, 179(6), 1538-1541.

Grunweller, A., Wyszko, E., Bieber, B., Jahnel, R., Erdmann, V. A.& Kurreck, J. (2003). Comparison of different antisense strategies in mammalian cells using locked nucleic acids, 2'-O-methyl RNA, phosphorothioates and small interfering RNA. *Nucleic Acids Research*, 31(12), 3185-3193.

Guo, P. (2002). Structure and function of phi29 hexameric RNA that drives the viral DNA packaging motor: review. *Progress in Nucleic Acid Research and Molecular Biology*, 72, 415-472.

Guo, P. (2005). Bacterial virus phi29 DNA-packaging motor and its potential applications in gene therapy and nanotechnology. *Methods in Molecular Biology*, 300, 285-324.

Guo, S., Huang, F.& Guo, P. (2006). Construction of folate-conjugated pRNA of bacteriophage phi29 DNA packaging motor for delivery of chimeric siRNA to nasopharyngeal carcinoma cells. *Gene Therapy*, 13(10), 814-820.

Haasnoot, J., Westerhout, E. M.& Berkhout, B. (2007). RNA interference against viruses: strike and counterstrike. *Nature Biotechnology*, 25(12), 1435-1443.

Hannon, G. J. (2002). RNA interference. *Nature*, 418(6894), 244-251.

Haseloff, J.& Gerlach, W. L. (1992). Simple RNA enzymes with new and highly specific endoribonuclease activities. 1988. *Biotechnology*, 24, 264-269.

Heasman, J. (2002). Morpholino oligos: making sense of antisense? *Developmental Biology*, 243(2), 209-214.

Hemida, M. G., Ye, X., Thair, S.& Yang, D. (2010). Exploiting the therapeutic potential of microRNAs in viral diseases: expectations and limitations. *Molecular Diagnosis & Therapy*, 14(5), 271-282.

Henry, S. D., van der Wegen, P., Metselaar, H. J., Tilanus, H. W., Scholte, B. J.& van der Laan, L. J. (2006). Simultaneous targeting of HCV replication and viral binding with a single lentiviral vector containing multiple RNA interference expression cassettes. *Molecular Therapy*, 14(4), 485-493.

Hoke, G. D., Draper, K., Freier, S. M., Gonzalez, C., Driver, V. B., Zounes, M. C.& Ecker, D. J. (1991). Effects of phosphorothioate capping on antisense oligonucleotide stability, hybridization and antiviral efficacy versus herpes simplex virus infection. *Nucleic Acids Research*, 19(20), 5743-5748.

Honda, T., Saitoh, H., Masuko, M., Katagiri-Abe, T., Tominaga, K., Kozakai, I., Kobayashi, K., Kumanishi, T., Watanabe, Y. G., Odani, S.& Kuwano, R. (2000). The coxsackievirus-adenovirus receptor protein as a cell adhesion molecule in the developing mouse brain. *Brain Research. Molecular Brain Research*, 77(1), 19-28.

Jakobsen, M. R., Haasnoot, J., Wengel, J., Berkhout, B.& Kjems, J. (2007). Efficient inhibition of HIV-1 expression by LNA modified antisense oligonucleotides and DNAzymes targeted to functionally selected binding sites. *Retrovirology*, 4, 29.

Jun, E. J., Nam, Y. R., Ahn, J., Tchah, H., Joo, C. H., Jee, Y., Kim, Y. K.& Lee, H. (2008). Antiviral potency of a siRNA targeting a conserved region of coxsackievirus A24. *Biochemical and Biophysical Research Communications*, 376(2), 389-394.

Kaiser, L., Crump, C. E.& Hayden, F. G. (2000). In vitro activity of pleconaril and AG7088 against selected serotypes and clinical isolates of human rhinoviruses. *Antiviral Research*, 47(3), 215-220.

Kim, J. Y., Chung, S. K., Hwang, H. Y., Kim, H., Kim, J. H., Nam, J. H.& Park, S. I. (2007). Expression of short hairpin RNAs against the coxsackievirus B3 exerts potential antiviral effects in Cos-7 cells and in mice. *Virus Research*, 125(1), 9-13.

Kim, Y. J., Ahn, J., Jeung, S. Y., Kim, D. S., Na, H. N., Cho, Y. J., Yun, S. H., Jee, Y., Jeon, E. S., Lee, H.& Nam, J. H. (2008). Recombinant lentivirus-delivered short hairpin RNAs targeted to conserved coxsackievirus sequences protect against viral myocarditis and improve survival rate in an animal model. *Virus Genes*, 36(1), 141-146.

Kindermann, I., Kindermann, M., Kandolf, R., Klingel, K., Bultmann, B., Muller, T., Lindinger, A.& Bohm, M. (2008). Predictors of outcome in patients with suspected myocarditis. *Circulation*, 118(6), 639-648.

Klump, W. M., Bergmann, I., Muller, B. C., Ameis, D.& Kandolf, R. (1990). Complete nucleotide sequence of infectious Coxsackievirus B3 cDNA: two initial 5' uridine residues are regained during plus-strand RNA synthesis. *The Journal of Virology*, 64(4), 1573-1583.

Knowlton, K. U. (2008). CVB infection and mechanisms of viral cardiomyopathy. *Current Topics in Microbiology and Immunology*, 323, 315-335.

Koizumi, N., Mizuguchi, H., Utoguchi, N., Watanabe, Y.& Hayakawa, T. (2003). Generation of fiber-modified adenovirus vectors containing heterologous peptides in both the HI loop and C terminus of the fiber knob. *The Journal of Gene Medicine*, 5(4), 267-276.

Kore, A. R., Vaish, N. K., Kutzke, U.& Eckstein, F. (1998). Sequence specificity of the hammerhead ribozyme revisited; the NHH rule. *Nucleic Acids Research*, 26(18), 4116-4120.

Krek, A., Grun, D., Poy, M. N., Wolf, R., Rosenberg, L., Epstein, E. J., MacMenamin, P., da Piedade, I., Gunsalus, K. C., Stoffel, M.& Rajewsky, N. (2005). Combinatorial microRNA target predictions. *Nature Genetics*, 37(5), 495-500.

Krutzfeldt, J., Rajewsky, N., Braich, R., Rajeev, K. G., Tuschl, T., Manoharan, M.& Stoffel, M. (2005). Silencing of microRNAs in vivo with 'antagomirs'. *Nature*, 438(7068), 685-689.

Kuhl, U., Pauschinger, M., Noutsias, M., Seeberg, B., Bock, T., Lassner, D., Poller, W., Kandolf, R.& Schultheiss, H. P. (2005a). High prevalence of viral genomes and multiple viral infections in the myocardium of adults with "idiopathic" left ventricular dysfunction. *Circulation*, 111(7), 887-893.

Kuhl, U., Pauschinger, M., Seeberg, B., Lassner, D., Noutsias, M., Poller, W.& Schultheiss, H. P. (2005b). Viral persistence in the myocardium is associated with progressive cardiac dysfunction. *Circulation*, 112(13), 1965-1970.

Kuhlmann, K. F., Gouma, D. J.& Wesseling, J. G. (2008). Adenoviral gene therapy for pancreatic cancer: where do we stand? *Digestive Surgery*, 25(4), 278-292.

Kurreck, J. (2003). Antisense technologies. Improvement through novel chemical modifications. *Eur J Biochem*, 270(8), 1628-1644.

Kurreck, J. (2009). RNA interference: from basic research to therapeutic applications. *Angewandte Chemie International Edition*, 48(8), 1378-1398.

Kyto, V., Vuorinen, T., Saukko, P., Lautenschlager, I., Lignitz, E., Saraste, A.& Voipio-Pulkki, L. M. (2005). Cytomegalovirus infection of the heart is common in patients with fatal myocarditis. *Clinical Infectious Diseases*, 40(5), 683-688.

Lacerra, G., Sierakowska, H., Carestia, C., Fucharoen, S., Summerton, J., Weller, D.& Kole, R. (2000). Restoration of hemoglobin A synthesis in erythroid cells from peripheral blood of thalassemic patients. *Proceedings of the National Academy of Sciences U S A*, 97(17), 9591-9596.

Lecellier, C. H., Dunoyer, P., Arar, K., Lehmann-Che, J., Eyquem, S., Himber, C., Saib, A.& Voinnet, O. (2005). A cellular microRNA mediates antiviral defense in human cells. *Science*, 308(5721), 557-560.

Lee, H. S., Ahn, J., Jee, Y., Seo, I. S., Jeon, E. J., Jeon, E. S., Joo, C. H., Kim, Y. K.& Lee, H. (2007). Universal and mutation-resistant anti-enteroviral activity: potency of small interfering RNA complementary to the conserved cis-acting replication element within the enterovirus coding region. *Journal of General Virology*, 88(Pt 7), 2003-2012.

Lee, H. S., Ahn, J., Jun, E. J., Yang, S., Joo, C. H., Kim, Y. K.& Lee, H. (2009). A novel program to design siRNAs simultaneously effective to highly variable virus genomes. *Biochemical and Biophysical Research Communications*, 384(4), 431-435.

Leong, L. E., Walker, P. A.& Porter, A. G. (1993). Human rhinovirus-14 protease 3C (3Cpro) binds specifically to the 5'-noncoding region of the viral RNA. Evidence that 3Cpro has different domains for the RNA binding and proteolytic activities. *The Journal of Biological Chemistry*, 268(34), 25735-25739.

Leong, L. E. C., Cornell, C. T., Semler, B. L., (2002). Processing determinants and functions of cleavage products of picornavirus polyproteins. *In* "Molecular biology of Picornaviruses" (B. L. Semler, wimmer, E., Ed.), pp. 187-197. ASM Press, 9781555812102, Washington, DC.

Lewis, B. P., Shih, I. H., Jones-Rhoades, M. W., Bartel, D. P.& Burge, C. B. (2003). Prediction of mammalian microRNA targets. *Cell*, 115(7), 787-798.

Liu, Q., Paroo, Z. (2010). Biochemical Principles of small RNA pathway. *Annual Review of Biochemistry*, 79, 295-319.

Liu, Z., Carthy, C. M., Cheung, P., Bohunek, L., Wilson, J. E., McManus, B. M.& Yang, D. (1999). Structural and functional analysis of the 5' untranslated region of coxsackievirus B3 RNA: In vivo translational and infectivity studies of full-length mutants. *Virology*, 265(2), 206-217.

Liu, Z., Sall, A.& Yang, D. (2008). MicroRNA: An emerging therapeutic target and intervention tool. *International Journal of Molecular Sciences*, 9(6), 978-999.

Macejak, D. G., Jensen, K. L., Jamison, S. F., Domenico, K., Roberts, E. C., Chaudhary, N., von Carlowitz, I., Bellon, L., Tong, M. J., Conrad, A., Pavco, P. A.& Blatt, L. M. (2000). Inhibition of hepatitis C virus (HCV)-RNA-dependent translation and replication of a chimeric HCV poliovirus using synthetic stabilized ribozymes. *Hepatology*, 31(3), 769-776.

Macejak, D. G., Jensen, K. L., Pavco, P. A., Phipps, K. M., Heinz, B. A., Colacino, J. M.& Blatt, L. M. (2001). Enhanced antiviral effect in cell culture of type 1 interferon and ribozymes targeting HCV RNA. *Journal of Viral Hepatitis*, 8(6), 400-405.

Maghsoudi, N., Tafreshi, N., Khodagholi, F., Zakeri, Z., Esfandiarei, M., Hadi-Alijanvand, H., Sabbaghian, M., Maghsoudi, A. H., Sajadi, M., Zohri, M., Moosavi, M.& Zeinoddini, M. (2010). Targeting enteroviral 2A protease by a 16-mer synthetic peptide: inhibition of 2Apro-induced apoptosis in a stable Tet-on HeLa cell line. *Virology*, 399(1), 39-45.

Mahrholdt, H., Wagner, A., Deluigi, C. C., Kispert, E., Hager, S., Meinhardt, G., Vogelsberg, H., Fritz, P., Dippon, J., Bock, C. T., Klingel, K., Kandolf, R.& Sechtem, U. (2006). Presentation, patterns of myocardial damage, and clinical course of viral myocarditis. *Circulation*, 114(15), 1581-1590.

Matsumori, A. (2005). Hepatitis C virus infection and cardiomyopathies. *Circulation Research*, 96(2), 144-147.

Matsumori, A., Shimada, T., Chapman, N. M., Tracy, S. M.& Mason, J. W. (2006). Myocarditis and heart failure associated with hepatitis C virus infection. *Journal of Cardiac Failure*, 12(4), 293-298.

Melchers, W. J., Hoenderop, J. G., Bruins Slot, H. J., Pleij, C. W., Pilipenko, E. V., Agol, V. I.& Galama, J. M. (1997). Kissing of the two predominant hairpin loops in the coxsackie B virus 3' untranslated region is the essential structural feature of the origin of replication required for negative-strand RNA synthesis. *The Journal of Virology*, 71(1), 686-696.

Merl, S., Michaelis, C., Jaschke, B., Vorpahl, M., Seidl, S.& Wessely, R. (2005). Targeting 2A protease by RNA interference attenuates coxsackieviral cytopathogenicity and promotes survival in highly susceptible mice. *Circulation*, 111(13), 1583-1592.

Merl, S.& Wessely, R. (2007). Anti-coxsackieviral efficacy of RNA interference is highly dependent on genomic target selection and emergence of escape mutants. *Oligonucleotides*, 17(1), 44-53.

Mizuguchi, H.& Hayakawa, T. (2002). Enhanced antitumor effect and reduced vector dissemination with fiber-modified adenovirus vectors expressing herpes simplex virus thymidine kinase. *Cancer Gene Therapy*, 9(3), 236-242.

Moazed, D. (2009). Small RNAs in transcriptional gene silencing and genome defence. *Nature*, 457(7228), 413-420.

Monia, B. P., Lesnik, E. A., Gonzalez, C., Lima, W. F., McGee, D., Guinosso, C. J., Kawasaki, A. M., Cook, P. D.& Freier, S. M. (1993). Evaluation of 2'-modified oligonucleotides containing 2'-deoxy gaps as antisense inhibitors of gene expression. *The Journal of Biological Chemistry*, 268(19), 14514-14522.

Munroe, S. H. (1988). Antisense RNA inhibits splicing of pre-mRNA in vitro. *EMBO J*, 7(8), 2523-2532.

Napoli, C., Lemieux, C.& Jorgensen, R. (1990). Introduction of a Chimeric Chalcone Synthase Gene into Petunia Results in Reversible Co-Suppression of Homologous Genes in trans. *Plant Cell*, 2(4), 279-289.

Nygardas, M., Vuorinen, T., Aalto, A. P., Bamford, D. H.& Hukkanen, V. (2009). Inhibition of coxsackievirus B3 and related enteroviruses by antiviral short interfering RNA pools produced using phi6 RNA-dependent RNA polymerase. *Journal of General Virology*, 90(Pt 10), 2468-2473.

Otsuka, M., Jing, Q., Georgel, P., New, L., Chen, J., Mols, J., Kang, Y. J., Jiang, Z., Du, X., Cook, R., Das, S. C., Pattnaik, A. K., Beutler, B.& Han, J. (2007). Hypersusceptibility to vesicular stomatitis virus infection in Dicer1-deficient mice is due to impaired miR24 and miR93 expression. *Immunity*, 27(1), 123-134.

Parker, J. S., Roe, S. M.& Barford, D. (2005). Structural insights into mRNA recognition from a PIWI domain-siRNA guide complex. *Nature*, 434(7033), 663-666.

Parsley, T. B., Cornell, C. T.& Semler, B. L. (1999). Modulation of the RNA binding and protein processing activities of poliovirus polypeptide 3CD by the viral RNA polymerase domain. *The Journal of Biological Chemistry*, 274(18), 12867-12876.

Peracchi, A. (2004). Prospects for antiviral ribozymes and deoxyribozymes. *Rev Med Virol*, 14(1), 47-64.

Pinkert, S., Westermann, D., Wang, X., Klingel, K., Dorner, A., Savvatis, K., Grossl, T., Krohn, S., Tschope, C., Zeichhardt, H., Kotsch, K., Weitmann, K., Hoffmann, W., Schultheiss, H. P., Spiller, O. B., Poller, W.& Fechner, H. (2009). Prevention of cardiac dysfunction in acute coxsackievirus B3 cardiomyopathy by inducible expression of a soluble coxsackievirus-adenovirus receptor. *Circulation*, 120(23), 2358-2366.

Racchi, G., Klingel, K., Kandolf, R.& Grassi, G. (2009). Targeting of protease 2A genome by single and multiple siRNAs as a strategy to impair CVB3 life cycle in permissive HeLa cells. *Methods & Findings in Experimental & Clinical Pharmacology*, 31(2), 63-70.

Raschperger, E., Thyberg, J., Pettersson, S., Philipson, L., Fuxe, J.& Pettersson, R. F. (2006). The coxsackie- and adenovirus receptor (CAR) is an in vivo marker for epithelial tight junctions, with a potential role in regulating permeability and tissue homeostasis. *Experimental Cell Research*, 312(9), 1566-1580.

Reisdorph, N., Thomas, J. J., Katpally, U., Chase, E., Harris, K., Siuzdak, G.& Smith, T. J. (2003). Human rhinovirus capsid dynamics is controlled by canyon flexibility. *Virology*, 314(1), 34-44.

Rose, N. R. (2009). Myocarditis: infection versus autoimmunity. *Journal of Clinical Immunology*, 29(6), 730-737.

Saleh, M. C., Van Rij, R. P.& Andino, R. (2004). RNA silencing in viral infections: insights from poliovirus. *Virus Research*, 102(1), 11-17.

Sall, A., Liu, Z., Zhang, H. M., Yuan, J., Lim, T., Su, Y.& Yang, D. (2008). MicroRNAs-based therapeutic strategy for virally induced diseases. *Current Drug Discovery Technologies*, 5(1), 49-58.

Scherer, L. J.& Rossi, J. J. (2003). Approaches for the sequence-specific knockdown of mRNA. *Nat Biotechnol*, 21(12), 1457-1465.

Schubert, S., Grunert, H. P., Zeichhardt, H., Werk, D., Erdmann, V. A.& Kurreck, J. (2005). Maintaining inhibition: siRNA double expression vectors against coxsackieviral RNAs. *Journal of Molecular Biology*, 346(2), 457-465.

Schubert, S., Rothe, D., Werk, D., Grunert, H. P., Zeichhardt, H., Erdmann, V. A.& Kurreck, J. (2007). Strand-specific silencing of a picornavirus by RNA interference: evidence for the superiority of plus-strand specific siRNAs. *Antiviral Research*, 73(3), 197-205.

Schultz, J. C., Hilliard, A. A., Cooper, L. T., Jr.& Rihal, C. S. (2009). Diagnosis and treatment of viral myocarditis. *Mayo Clinic Proceedings*, 84(11), 1001-1009.

Sen, G. L.& Blau, H. M. (2005). Argonaute 2/RISC resides in sites of mammalian mRNA decay known as cytoplasmic bodies. *Nature Cell Biology*, 7(6), 633-636.

Shafren, D. R., Williams, D. T.& Barry, R. D. (1997). A decay-accelerating factor-binding strain of coxsackievirus B3 requires the coxsackievirus-adenovirus receptor protein to mediate lytic infection of rhabdomyosarcoma cells. *The Journal of Virology*, 71(12), 9844-9848.

Shan, J., Moran-Jones, K., Munro, T. P., Kidd, G. J., Winzor, D. J., Hoek, K. S.& Smith, R. (2000). Binding of an RNA trafficking response element to heterogeneous nuclear ribonucleoproteins A1 and A2. *The Journal of Biological Chemistry*, 275(49), 38286-38295.

Si, X., Gao, G., Wong, J., Wang, Y., Zhang, J.& Luo, H. (2008). Ubiquitination is required for effective replication of coxsackievirus B3. *PLoS One*, 3(7), e2585.

Si, X., Wang, Y., Wong, J., Zhang, J., McManus, B. M.& Luo, H. (2007). Dysregulation of the ubiquitin-proteasome system by curcumin suppresses coxsackievirus B3 replication. *The Journal of Virology*, 81(7), 3142-3150.

Stein, D., Foster, E., Huang, S. B., Weller, D.& Summerton, J. (1997). A specificity comparison of four antisense types: morpholino, 2'-O-methyl RNA, DNA, and phosphorothioate DNA. *Antisense and Nucleic Acid Drug Development*, 7(3), 151-157.

Su, H., Joho, S., Huang, Y., Barcena, A., Arakawa-Hoyt, J., Grossman, W.& Kan, Y. W. (2004). Adeno-associated viral vector delivers cardiac-specific and hypoxia-inducible VEGF expression in ischemic mouse hearts. *Proceedings of the National Academy of Sciences U S A*, 101(46), 16280-16285.

Tan, E. L., Wong, A. P. Y., Poh, C. L. (2010). Development of potential antiviral stratey against coxswackievirus B4. *Virus Research*, 150, 85-92.

Tomari, Y.& Zamore, P. D. (2005). Perspective: machines for RNAi. *Genes & Development*, 19(5), 517-529.

Turner, J. J., Fabani, M., Arzumanov, A. A., Ivanova, G.& Gait, M. J. (2006). Targeting the HIV-1 RNA leader sequence with synthetic oligonucleotides and siRNA: chemistry and cell delivery. *Biochimica et Biophysica Acta*, 1758(3), 290-300.

van Ooij, M. J., Vogt, D. A., Paul, A., Castro, C., Kuijpers, J., van Kuppeveld, F. J., Cameron, C. E., Wimmer, E., Andino, R.& Melchers, W. J. (2006). Structural and functional characterization of the coxsackievirus B3 CRE(2C): role of CRE(2C) in negative- and positive-strand RNA synthesis. *Journal of General Virology*, 87(Pt 1), 103-113.

Verma, B., Bhattacharyya, S.& Das, S. (2010). Polypyrimidine tract-binding protein interacts with coxsackievirus B3 RNA and influences its translation. *Journal of General Virology*, 91(Pt 5), 1245-1255.

Walder, R. Y.& Walder, J. A. (1988). Role of RNase H in hybrid-arrested translation by antisense oligonucleotides. *Proceedings of the National Academy of Sciences U S A*, 85(14), 5011-5015.

Wang, A., Cheung, P. K., Zhang, H., Carthy, C. M., Bohunek, L., Wilson, J. E., McManus, B. M.& Yang, D. (2001). Specific inhibition of coxsackievirus B3 translation and replication by phosphorothioate antisense oligodeoxynucleotides. *Antimicrobial Agents and Chemotherapy*, 45(4), 1043-1052.

Wang, J., Bakkers, J. M., Galama, J. M., Bruins Slot, H. J., Pilipenko, E. V., Agol, V. I.& Melchers, W. J. (1999). Structural requirements of the higher order RNA kissing element in the enteroviral 3'UTR. *Nucleic Acids Research*, 27(2), 485-490.

Wang, Y. F., Wang, X. Y., Ren, Z., Qian, C. W., Li, Y. C., Kaio, K., Wang, Q. D., Zhang, Y., Zheng, L. Y., Jiang, J. H., Yang, C. R., Liu, Q.& Zhang, Y. J. (2009). Phyllaemblicin B inhibits Coxsackie virus B3 induced apoptosis and myocarditis. *Antiviral Research*, 84(2), 150-158.

Werk, D., Pinkert, S., Heim, A., Zeichhardt, H., Grunert, H. P., Poller, W., Erdmann, V. A., Fechner, H.& Kurreck, J. (2009). Combination of soluble coxsackievirus-adenovirus receptor and anti-coxsackievirus siRNAs exerts synergistic antiviral activity against coxsackievirus B3. *Antiviral Res*, 83(3), 298-306.

Werk, D., Schubert, S., Lindig, V., Grunert, H. P., Zeichhardt, H., Erdmann, V. A.& Kurreck, J. (2005). Developing an effective RNA interference strategy against a plus-strand RNA virus: silencing of coxsackievirus B3 and its cognate coxsackievirus-adenovirus receptor. *Biological Chemistry*, 386(9), 857-863.

Wilson, J. A.& Richardson, C. D. (2005). Hepatitis C virus replicons escape RNA interference induced by a short interfering RNA directed against the NS5b coding region. *The Journal of Virology*, 79(11), 7050-7058.

Wong, J., Zhang, J., Si, X., Gao, G., Mao, I., McManus, B. M.& Luo, H. (2008). Autophagosome supports coxsackievirus B3 replication in host cells. *The Journal of Virology*, 82(18), 9143-9153.

Wong, L. F., Azzouz, M., Walmsley, L. E., Askham, Z., Wilkes, F. J., Mitrophanous, K. A., Kingsman, S. M.& Mazarakis, N. D. (2004). Transduction patterns of pseudotyped lentiviral vectors in the nervous system. *Molecular Therapy*, 9(1), 101-111.

Yajima, T.& Knowlton, K. U. (2009). Viral myocarditis: from the perspective of the virus. *Circulation*, 119(19), 2615-2624.

Yanagawa, B., Spiller, O. B., Choy, J., Luo, H., Cheung, P., Zhang, H. M., Goodfellow, I. G., Evans, D. J., Suarez, A., Yang, D.& McManus, B. M. (2003). Coxsackievirus B3-associated myocardial pathology and viral load reduced by recombinant soluble human decay-accelerating factor in mice. *Laboratory Investigation*, 83(1), 75-85.

Yanagawa, B., Spiller, O. B., Proctor, D. G., Choy, J., Luo, H., Zhang, H. M., Suarez, A., Yang, D.& McManus, B. M. (2004). Soluble recombinant coxsackievirus and adenovirus receptor abrogates coxsackievirus b3-mediated pancreatitis and myocarditis in mice. *Journal of Infectious Diseases*, 189(8), 1431-1439.

Yang, D., Wilson, J. E., Anderson, D. R., Bohunek, L., Cordeiro, C., Kandolf, R.& McManus, B. M. (1997). In vitro mutational and inhibitory analysis of the cis-acting translational elements within the 5' untranslated region of coxsackievirus B3: potential targets for antiviral action of antisense oligomers. *Virology*, 228(1), 63-73.

Ye, X., Liu, Z., Hemida, G. M., and Yang, D. C. (2011). Mutation tolerance and targeted delivery of anti-coxsackievirus artificial microRNAs using folate conjugated baterial phage phi29 pRNA. *PLoS One*, 6(6), e21215.

Ye, X.& Yang, D. (2009). Recent advances in biological strategies for targeted drug delivery. *Cardiovascular and Hematological Disorders - Drug Targets*, 9(3), 206-221.

Yuan, J., Cheung, P. K., Zhang, H., Chau, D., Yanagawa, B., Cheung, C., Luo, H., Wang, Y., Suarez, A., McManus, B. M.& Yang, D. (2004). A phosphorothioate antisense oligodeoxynucleotide specifically inhibits coxsackievirus B3 replication in cardiomyocytes and mouse hearts. *Laboratory Investigation*, 84(6), 703-714.

Yuan, J., Cheung, P. K., Zhang, H. M., Chau, D.& Yang, D. (2005). Inhibition of coxsackievirus B3 replication by small interfering RNAs requires perfect sequence match in the central region of the viral positive strand. *The Journal of Virology*, 79(4), 2151-2159.

Yuan, J., Stein, D. A., Lim, T., Qiu, D., Coughlin, S., Liu, Z., Wang, Y., Blouch, R., Moulton, H. M., Iversen, P. L.& Yang, D. (2006). Inhibition of coxsackievirus B3 in cell cultures and in mice by peptide-conjugated morpholino oligomers targeting the internal ribosome entry site. *The Journal of Virology*, 80(23), 11510-11519.

Zhang, H. M., Su, Y., Guo, S., Yuan, J., Lim, T., Liu, J., Guo, P.& Yang, D. (2009). Targeted delivery of anti-coxsackievirus siRNAs using ligand-conjugated packaging RNAs. *Antiviral Research*, 83(3), 307-316.

Permissions

The contributors of this book come from diverse backgrounds, making this book a truly international effort. This book will bring forth new frontiers with its revolutionizing research information and detailed analysis of the nascent developments around the world.

We would like to thank Daniela Cihakova, MD, PhD, for lending her expertise to make the book truly unique. She has played a crucial role in the development of this book. Without her invaluable contribution this book wouldn't have been possible. She has made vital efforts to compile up to date information on the varied aspects of this subject to make this book a valuable addition to the collection of many professionals and students.

This book was conceptualized with the vision of imparting up-to-date information and advanced data in this field. To ensure the same, a matchless editorial board was set up. Every individual on the board went through rigorous rounds of assessment to prove their worth. After which they invested a large part of their time researching and compiling the most relevant data for our readers. Conferences and sessions were held from time to time between the editorial board and the contributing authors to present the data in the most comprehensible form. The editorial team has worked tirelessly to provide valuable and valid information to help people across the globe.

Every chapter published in this book has been scrutinized by our experts. Their significance has been extensively debated. The topics covered herein carry significant findings which will fuel the growth of the discipline. They may even be implemented as practical applications or may be referred to as a beginning point for another development. Chapters in this book were first published by InTech; hereby published with permission under the Creative Commons Attribution License or equivalent.

The editorial board has been involved in producing this book since its inception. They have spent rigorous hours researching and exploring the diverse topics which have resulted in the successful publishing of this book. They have passed on their knowledge of decades through this book. To expedite this challenging task, the publisher supported the team at every step. A small team of assistant editors was also appointed to further simplify the editing procedure and attain best results for the readers.

Our editorial team has been hand-picked from every corner of the world. Their multi-ethnicity adds dynamic inputs to the discussions which result in innovative outcomes. These outcomes are then further discussed with the researchers and contributors who give their valuable feedback and opinion regarding the same. The feedback is then collaborated with the researches and they are edited in a comprehensive manner to aid the understanding of the subject.

Apart from the editorial board, the designing team has also invested a significant amount of their time in understanding the subject and creating the most relevant covers. They scrutinized every image to scout for the most suitable representation of the subject and create an appropriate cover for the book.

The publishing team has been involved in this book since its early stages. They were actively engaged in every process, be it collecting the data, connecting with the contributors or procuring relevant information. The team has been an ardent support to the editorial, designing and production team. Their endless efforts to recruit the best for this project, has resulted in the accomplishment of this book. They are a veteran in the field of academics and their pool of knowledge is as vast as their experience in printing. Their expertise and guidance has proved useful at every step. Their uncompromising quality standards have made this book an exceptional effort. Their encouragement from time to time has been an inspiration for everyone.

The publisher and the editorial board hope that this book will prove to be a valuable piece of knowledge for researchers, students, practitioners and scholars across the globe.

List of Contributors

Vedide Tavli and Baris Guven
Izmir Dr Behcet Uz Children's Hospital, Department of Pediatric Cardiology, Izmir

Rafid Fayadh Al-Aqeedi
Hamad Medical Corporation, Cardiology and Cardiovascular Surgery Department, Qatar

Andréoletti Laurent
Head of the clinical and molecular Virology Unit, University medical centre and EA research team at the Medicine Faculty of Reims, France

Yukihiro Ikegami and Choichiro Tase
Fukushima Medical University, Japan

Hesham R. Omar and Hany Abdelmalak
Internal Medicine Department, Mercy Hospital and Medical Center, Chicago, Illinois, USA

Engy Helal
Emergency Department, Agouza Police Hospital, Cairo, Egypt

Yara Mikhaeil
Northwestern University, Feinberg School of Medicine, USA

Ahmed Fathy
Cardiology Department, National Heart institute, Cairo, Egypt

Julián González, Roberto Guerri-Guttenberg, Daniel Grana, Francisco Azzato and José Milei
Instituto de Investigaciones Cardiológicas Prof. Dr. A. Taquini - UBA - CONICET, Argentina

Nicolas Hanabergh and James P. Morgan
Steward Carney Hospital, Dorchester, Steward St. Elizabeth's Medical Center, Boston and Tufts University School of Medicine, Boston, United States of America

Simona Claudia Cambrea
"Ovidius" University, Faculty of Medicine, Romania

Vien Khach Lai, Muhammad Zeeshan Afzal, Muhammad Ashraf and Khawaja Husnain Haider
Department of Pathology, University of Cincinnati, Cincinnati, OH, USA

Pamela J. Lincez, Marine Walic and Marc S. Horwitz
Department of Microbiology and Immunology, University of British Columbia, Canada

Volker Ruppert
Klinik für Kardiologie, Philipps-Universität Marburg, Germany

Thomas Meyer
Klinik für Psychosomatische Medizin und Psychotherapie, Georg-August-Universität Göttingen, Germany

S.A. Huber
Department of Pathology, University of Vermont, Colchester, Vermont, U.S.A.

David Marchant, Farshid S. Garmaroudi and Bruce M. McManus
UBC James Hogg Research Centre, Institute for Heart + Lung Health, St. Paul's Hospital, University of British Columbia, Canada

Kenichi Watanabe and Somasundaram Arumugam
Department of Clinical Pharmacology, Faculty of Pharmaceutical Sciences, Niigata, Japan
University of Pharmacy and Applied Life Sciences, Niigata, Japan

Rajarajan A. Thandavarayan
Department of Clinical Pharmacology, Faculty of Pharmaceutical Sciences, Niigata, Japan
University of Pharmacy and Applied Life Sciences, Niigata, Japan
Department of Functional and Analytical Food Sciences, Niigata University of Pharmacy and Applied Life Sciences, Niigata, Japan

Makoto Kodama
First Department of Medicine, Niigata University Graduate School of Medical and Dental Sciences, Niigata, Japan

Jerry Wong and Honglin Luo
James Hogg Research Center, Providence Heart and Lung Institute, St. Paul's Hospital and Department of Pathology and Laboratory Medicine, University of British Columbia, Vancouver, BC, Canada

Maurizio Pieroni, Costantino Smaldone and Fulvio Bellocci
Cardiology Department, Catholic University of the Sacred Heart, Rome, Italy

DeLisa Fairweather, Eric D. Abston and Michael J. Coronado
Johns Hopkins University Bloomberg School of Public Health, USA

Andrea Carpentieri, Chiara Giangrande, Piero Pucci and Angela Amoresano
Department of Organic Chemistry and Biochemistry, Facoltà di Scienze Biotecnologiche, Federico II University of Naples, Naples, Italy

Roland Jahns
University Hospital of Würzburg, Department of Internal Medicine I, Cardiology, Comprehensive Heart Failure Centre CHFC/IFB, Würzburg, Germany

Nikolas Deubner and Georg Ertl
University Hospital of Würzburg, Department of Internal Medicine I,Cardiology, Comprehensive Heart Failure Centre CHFC/IFB, Würzburg, Germany

Valérie Biovin and Martin J. Lohse
University of Würzburg, Institute for Pharmacology and Toxicology, Würzburg, Germany

Alida L.P. Caforio
University of Padua, Division of Cardiology, Dpt. of Cardiologic, Thoracic and Vascular Sciences, Padua, Italy

Stephan B. Felix
University of Greifswald, Department of Internal Medicine B - Cardiology, Greifswald, Germany

Michael Fu
University of Gothenburg, Department of Molecular and Clinical Medicine, Gothenburg, Sweden

Decheng Yang
Department of Pathology and Laboratory Medicine, University of British Columbia, The Institute for Heart and Lung Health, St. Paul's Hospital, Vancouver, B. C., Canada